THIRD EDITION

COMPLEMENTARY THERAPIES

IN REHABILITATION

Evidence for Efficacy in Therapy, Prevention, and Wellness

THIRD EDITION

COMPLEMENTARY THERAPIES
IN REHABILITATION

Evidence for Efficacy in Therapy, Prevention, and Wellness

Edited by:

Carol M. Davis, DPT, EdD, MS, FAPTA

Professor, Department of Physical Therapy
University of Miami, Miller School of Medicine
Miami, Florida

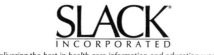

SLACK
INCORPORATED

Delivering the best in health care information and education worldwide www.slackbooks.com

ISBN: 978-1-55642-866-1

Copyright © 2009 by SLACK Incorporated

The procedures and practices described in this book should be implemented in a manner consistent with the professional standards set for the circumstances that apply in each specific situation. Every effort has been made to confirm the accuracy of the information presented and to correctly relate generally accepted practices. The authors, editor, and publisher cannot accept responsibility for errors or exclusions or for the outcome of the material presented herein. There is no expressed or implied warranty of this book or information imparted by it. Care has been taken to ensure that drug selection and dosages are in accordance with currently accepted/recommended practice. Due to continuing research, changes in government policy and regulations, and various effects of drug reactions and interactions, it is recommended that the reader carefully review all materials and literature provided for each drug, especially those that are new or not frequently used. Any review or mention of specific companies or products is not intended as an endorsement by the author or publisher.

SLACK Incorporated uses a review process to evaluate submitted material. Prior to publication, educators or clinicians provide important feedback on the content that we publish. We welcome feedback on this work.

Published by: SLACK Incorporated
                6900 Grove Road
                Thorofare, NJ 08086 USA
                Telephone: 856-848-1000
                Fax: 856-848-6091
                www.slackbooks.com

Contact SLACK Incorporated for more information about other books in this field or about the availability of our books from distributors outside the United States.

Library of Congress Cataloging-in-Publication Data

Complementary therapies in rehabilitation : evidence for efficacy in therapy, prevention, and wellness / edited by Carol M. Davis. -- 3rd ed.
      p. ; cm.
  Includes bibliographical references and index.
  ISBN 978-1-55642-866-1 (hardcover : alk. paper) 1. Alternative medicine. 2. Rehabilitation. I. Davis, Carol M.
  [DNLM: 1. Complementary Therapies--methods. 2. Rehabilitation--methods. 3. Holistic Health. WB 320 C737 2008]
  R733.C656 2008
  615.5--dc22
                                2008027062

Printed in the United States of America.

Last digit is print number: 10   9   8   7   6   5   4   3   2   1

Dedication

This book is dedicated to all those people who are willing to hold an open mind and a positive attitude about the findings of the "new science" as those findings are articulated, and particularly, this book is dedicated to those helping to move science forward for the good of improved patient care, in spite of having to bear the consequences of heightened personal ostracism and criticism.

Contents

SECTION I: INTRODUCTION

SECTION II: THE SCIENCE THAT SUPPORTS COMPLEMENTARY THERAPIES

SECTION III: BODY WORK

SECTION IV: MIND/BODY WORK

SECTION V: ENERGY WORK

Acknowledgments

In this, the third edition, once again I am grateful to so many people for their support in helping me put all this together.

To my authors who agreed to update their evidence sections: thank you so much for your diligence in searching and reporting the latest evidence from peer reviewed literature, and indicating to me the pleasure of being asked to contribute to this update.

To my DPT students in the University of Miami Miller School of Medicine, Class of 2007: thank you for sharing your peer review searches and articles with me to send to the authors to get them started on some of the new findings in the literature. **And to all my wonderful students and graduates at the University of Miami Department of Physical Therapy,** your excitement with learning about and experiencing complementary therapies, and your appreciation for being challenged to critique the literature gives me faith in the future of the use of holistic therapies in our profession and in rehabilitation.

To my boss, Sherrill H. Hayes, PhD, PT: thank you for the encouragement to continue in my research and writing in this area, in spite of uninformed attack and criticism from colleagues who seem threatened by the developments in science that they refuse to read. Your faith in me and in the knowledge that science never stands still has served as the foundation for all my scholarship. I can never thank you enough for your support and friendship.

To my mentor, dear friend and colleague, Geneva R. Johnson, PhD, PT, FAPTA: I am so grateful for you continuous support, advice and friendship, and for sharing your futuristic vision of how physical therapy can be even more responsive to patients. Your belief in me and your appreciation of my work sustains me in indescribable ways.

To my friend, colleague and teacher, John F. Barnes, PT: thank you for your support and friendship. I so admire your love of science and I appreciate your diligent sharing with me the latest scientific articles and texts. You model for all of us compassion and courage to carry on with what we who practice energy-based myofascial release have found to be so helpful for patients when other therapeutic approaches have failed. Your gifts to healing, I believe, are unparalleled in our time.

To my friends at SLACK Incorporated: John Bond, Publisher; Debra Toulson, Managing Editor; Amy McShane and Brien Cummings, Acquisitions Editors; Rob Smentek, Senior Project Editor; and Michelle Gatt and her marketing team, thank you for your detailed attention to the production of this new edition, and for your ongoing friendship. The SLACK team is an author's dream. May I never take your kind attention to my work for granted.

Finally, I acknowledge the love and support of my family and close friends who assure me that what I create is interesting to them, and important to the improvement of health care. Thank you to my twin sister, Susan and her husband, and my brother, Bill Doughty, and thank you to my friends Meryl Cohen, Jamiss Sebert, and Patricia Calhoun. I feel blessed beyond measure to have you in my life.

About the Editor

Carol M. Davis, DPT, EdD, MS, FAPTA received her undergraduate degree in biology from Lycoming College, an MS in physical therapy from Case Western Reserve University, and a Doctorate in Humanistic Studies (psychology and philosophy) in the School of Education at Boston University and a clinical doctorate in physical therapy from Mass General Institute of Health Professions.

As a faculty member at the University of Miami Miller School of Medicine, Dr. Davis has served as Clinical Assistant Professor with Family and Internal Medicine from 1983 to 1985, where she coordinated the Fellowship in Clinical Geriatrics, and from 1987 to now serves as Professor and Assistant Chair of the Department of Physical Therapy. Additionally, she has held the positions of clinical staff and clinical instructor at Massachusetts General Hospital, Assistant Professor at the University of Alabama in Birmingham, and Assistant Professor and Co-Chair ad interim of physical therapy at Sargent College of Boston University.

She is an internationally recognized speaker and consultant in teaching and developing curriculum in attitudes and values, ethics, geriatrics, and complementary therapies in rehabilitation. Dr. Davis authored the book, *Patient Practitioner Interaction: An Experiential Manual for Developing the Art of Health Care*, now in its fourth edition, and with Dr. Christine Williams, she coauthored the text *Therapeutic Interaction in Nursing*, all published by SLACK Incorporated.

Today, Dr. Davis is an active researcher, teacher, and practicing physical therapist in Miami, Florida. She conducts research in complementary therapies, clinical geriatrics, and ethics; teaches entry-level doctoral students and PhD students in physical therapy; and treats patients. She has studied Myofascial Release (Barnes Method) since 1989 and uses it regularly as a complement to her physical therapy treatments. In 2003, she was awarded the Catherine Worthingham Fellow award for a lifetime of outstanding service to the profession by the American Physical Therapy Association.

Contributing Authors

Brent Anderson PhD, PT, OCS is a licensed Physical Therapist and Orthopedic Certified Specialist for more than 13 years and is a leading authority in performing arts medicine and Pilates-evolved techniques for rehabilitation. He lectures widely at national and international symposia and consults with professional dance companies, schools, and conservatories throughout the world. In addition, he owns and operates two of the nation's most comprehensive Pilates conditioning and physical therapy centers. These highly successful studios have become the model for many other Pilates studios worldwide.

Brent received his degree in physical therapy at University of California, San Francisco in 1989 and his PhD in physical therapy at the University of Miami in 2005. He currently serves as voluntary faculty at the University of Miami, Department of Physical Therapy. His doctoral thesis explored the impact of Pilates rehabilitation on chronic low back pain using psycho-emotional wellness and quality of life measures. Brent is a 15-year member of the American Physical Therapy Association for which he formerly served as President of its Performing Arts Special Interest Group. He is also a longtime member of the International Association for Dance Medicine and Science.

Ellen Zambo Anderson, PT, MA, GCS received her bachelor's degree in physical therapy from West Virginia University and her master's degree in movement sciences from Columbia University. She is an associate professor of physical therapy in the Department of Rehabilitation and Movement Sciences at the University of Medicine and Dentistry of New Jersey. Ms. Anderson has written several book chapters about complementary therapies and has presented nationally on incorporating complementary alternative medicine into a physical therapy plan of care. She is coauthor with Judith E. Deutsch of *Complementary Therapies for Physical Therapy*.

John F. Barnes, PT graduated in physical therapy from the University of Pennsylvania in 1960. He is President and Director of the Myofascial Release Treatment Centers and National Myofascial Release Seminars located in Paoli, Pennsylvania, and Sedona, Arizona, where he and his staff treat people referred from all over the world when medicine, surgery, and traditional therapies have failed. John Barnes has educated more than 50,000 people in his workshop series over the past 30 years across the United States and Canada. He is the author of two books: *Myofascial Release* and *Healing Ancient Wounds: The Renegade's Wisdom*.

Jennifer M. Bottomley, PhD, MS, PT has a bachelor's degree in physical therapy from the University of Wisconsin, Madison and an advanced master's degree in physical therapy from the MGH Institute of Health Professionals in Boston, Massachusetts. She has a combined intercollegiate doctoral degree in gerontology and health science and service administration and a PhD from The Union Institute in Health Science in service administration, legislation, and policy management with a specialty in gerontology. She has practiced since 1974 in acute care, home care, outpatient clinics, nursing homes, and long-term care facilities. Currently, she works as an independent consultant setting up rehabilitation services in nursing homes and outpatient, assisted living, home, and community settings throughout the United States and serves on advisory boards for the Office of the Surgeon General and the Office on Women's Health in the Department of Health and Human Services. In 2007, she was appointed to a White House Interdisciplinary Medicare Reform Advisory Board. She is director of rehabilitation services for the Committee to End Elder Homelessness/HEARTH. Jennifer is the recent past President of the Section on Geriatrics of the American Physical Therapy Association and is a nationally renowned speaker and educator. She has done clinical research in the areas of nutrition and exercise, foot care in the elderly, wound care, diabetes and peripheral vascular disease interventions, balance and falls in the Alzheimer's population, T'ai Chi as an alternative exercise form, and social policy development (inclusive of the managed care perspective) for the elderly. She has coauthored a text with Carole

B. Lewis entitled *Geriatric Rehabilitation: A Clinical Approach, 3rd Edition,* and edited the *Quick Reference Dictionary for Physical Therapy, 2nd Edition* published by SLACK Incorporated in 2004.

Judith E. Deutsch, PT, PhD received her BA in Human Biology from Stanford, her MS in physical therapy from University of Southern California and her PhD in pathokinesiology from New York University. She completed a post-doctoral fellowship in rehabilitation research at University of Medicine and Dentistry of NJ. Dr. Deutsch is Professor and Director of the Research in Virtual Environments and Rehabilitation Sciences (Rivers) in the Doctoral Programs in Physical Therapy at the University of Medicine and Dentistry of New Jersey. Her current research includes the development and testing of virtual reality rehabilitation systems to improve functional mobility, use of motor imagery to improve walking for people post-stroke, and use of structural integarion (Rolfing) in rehabilitation populations. She is the Editor in Chief of the *Journal of Neurologic Physical Therapy* and a member of the Editorial Board of the *Journal of Neural Engineering Research.* She is coauthor with Ellen Zambo Anderson of *Complementary Therapies for Physical Therapy.*

Barbara Funk, MS, OTR, CHT graduated with a master's degree in occupational therapy from Boston University in 1979. She is Senior Occupational Therapist at the Rehabilitation Institute of Michigan and adjunct professor at Wayne State University and serves as a consultant to physicians and fellow therapists. She has been practicing occupational therapy for 29 years expanding her knowledge base and skills in several different areas including certification in hand therapy, training in lymphedema management (Klose and Norton Miller), John Barnes' myofascial release, craniosacral therapy, and therapeutic touch.

Mary Lou Galantino, PT, MS, PhD is Professor, Physical Therapy at Richard Stockton College of New Jersey and Adjunct Research Scholar at the University of Pennsylvania. She attained her bachelor's degree in physical therapy from the University of Pittsburgh, an advanced master's degree in physical therapy from Texas Woman's University, and her PhD from Temple University in the Psychoeducational Program where she completed her research in the use of T'ai Chi for people living with AIDS. Mary Lou edited a book in 1992, *Clinical Assessment and Treatment of HIV: Rehabilitation of a Chronic Illness,* published by SLACK Incorporated, and another text in 2002 entitled *AIDS and Complementary & Alternative Medicine.* She initiated the HIV Special Interest Group of the Oncology Section of the American Physical Therapy Association and wrote a manuscript entitled *Issues in HIV Rehabilitation.* Her research includes the use of electroacupuncture and complementary therapies, and she conducts workshops on the management of chronic diseases. She has done outreach work with the Lakota Indians in South Dakota and continues to explore the medicinal aspects of Native American cultures.

Mary Lou was the guest editor for the September 2000 issue of *Orthopaedic Physical Therapy Clinics of North America,* a special issue dedicated to complementary and alternative medicine. Her publications and clinical work have culminated in an National Institutes of Health postdoctoral award in complementary medicine at the University of Pennsylvania from 2002 to 2005, where she completed research on the psychological and physiological correlates of the impact of meditation on the stress of health care professionals.

Deborah A. Giaquinto-Wahl, MSPT, ATC received her bachelor's degree in physiology at the University of California, Davis in 1986. She then went on to become a certified athletic trainer and the assistant trainer at the Sacramento City College. Returning to graduate school she received her master's degree in physical therapy at the University of Miami in 1990. Debbie directed her post-graduate studies in manual therapy and happened upon craniosacral therapy 10 years ago and has utilized it ever since. Debbie serves as a teaching assistant for craniosacral courses through the Upledger Institute in Palm Beach Gardens, Florida, and utilizes these techniques daily in her practice near Annapolis, Maryland.

Janet Kahn, PhD, MT is a research Assistant Professor in Psychiatry at the University of Vermont, is a massage therapist who specializes in treating people with chronic pain. She is a longtime advocate of research on massage, having served as President of the American Massage Therapy Association Foundation (now the Massage Therapy Foundation) from 1996-2000 and currently as Director of Research for the Massage Therapy Research Consortium, a collaborative of 11 massage schools across North America. Dr. Kahn also serves as Executive Director of the Integrative Healthcare Policy Consortium, which initiates public policy to secure Americans' access to high quality integrated health care services and directs the public health care agenda to health promotion and illness prevention. Dr. Kahn lives in Burlington Vermont, where she breathes clean air and sails the waters of Lake Champlain.

Patrick J. LaRiccia, MD, MSCE is Attending Physician in the Department of Medicine at Penn-Presbyterian Medical Center and the Department of Rehabilitation Medicine at the Hospital of the University of Pennsylvania in Philadelphia. He also serves as Clinical Associate in Rehabilitation Medicine at the University of Pennsylvania School of Medicine, Philadelphia, Pennsylvania.

Teresa M. Miller, PT, PhD, GCFP, is currently a Clinical Assistant Professor in the Physical Therapy Program at the State University of New York, Downstate Medical Center in Brooklyn, NY. Dr. Miller was initially exposed to the Feldenkrais Method® while a BS student in Downstate's physical therapy program from 1979 to 1981. She was exposed to the method again in 1986 by a fellow PT while working in a large teaching hospital. She joined a study group with two PTs who were trained in the Feldenkrais Method—Harold Rosenthal and Steven Frieder—and began applying the concepts they taught her to patient care. After completing her MS in school psychology at St. John's University in 1993, she joined the faculty of Downstate's PT Program. In 1996, she enrolled in the East Coast Feldenkrais Training and received her certification in the Feldenkrais Method® in 1999. She completed her PhD in physical therapy from Temple University in 2007 and is currently involved in several research projects related to the Feldenkrais Method®.

Susan Morrill Ramsey, PT, MA has been practicing holistic physical therapy for more than 20 years. She received her bachelor's degree in physical therapy from Ithaca College in New York, and received her master's degree in applied psychology from the University of Santa Monica in California. She has been a professor of physical therapy, teaching both traditional and holistic physical therapy for more than 15 years. At Harcum College in Bryn Mawr, Pennsylvania, she designed and was primary professor in the Holistic Studies Certificate Program for Health Care Professionals. Susan is a nationally known expert in the area of complementary therapies. She regularly contributes a column on complementary therapies to the magazine *Advance for Physical Therapists*. She has maintained her own practice, Holistic Physical Therapy Services, for more than 15 years. Newly relocated to Portland, Maine, Susan provides highly individualized physical therapy treatment that focuses on the specific needs of the client. Susan also offers sessions in Therapeutic Touch, aromatherapy, holistic stress management counseling, and holistic health consultation.

G. Kesava Reddy, PhD obtained his doctorate in biochemistry from the University of Madras, India in 1990. Following his postdoctoral research training in the Department of Biochemistry and Molecular Biology at the University of Kansas Medical Center, he joined as a senior research associate in the Department of Physical Therapy and Rehabilitation Sciences at the University of Kansas Medical Center and became a faculty member in that department in 1996. Globally, Dr. Reddy is recognized as one of the leading scientists in the connective tissue research. His primary research involved gaining a better understanding of the role of the connective tissue in health and disease and its response to various physical modality interventions during tissue repair and wound healing. He has published a number of research papers in several peer-reviewed journals and presented his research work at the national as well as international conferences.

Sangeeta Singg, PhD received her MA in sociology from Mississippi State University and MS and PhD in psychology from Texas A & M University—Commerce. She is a professor of psychology and Director of the Graduate Counseling Psychology Program at the Angelo State University, San Angelo, Texas. She is also a licensed psychologist in the State of Texas and has practiced and taught psychology for over 25 years. Her research interests and publications are in the areas of counseling training, student personal responsibility, childhood sexual abuse, self-esteem, post-traumatic stress disorder, depression, color preference and color therapy, memory, alternative methods of healing, grief, and suicide.

Neil I. Spielholz, PT, PhD, FAPTA is Professor Emeritus at the University of Miami School of Medicine, Division of Physical Therapy and Adjunct Associate Professor of Rehabilitation at the New York University Medical Center where he completed his PhD in neurophysiology in 1972. Dr. Spielholz has a long history as a physical therapist clinician, educator and researcher and has authored two well-known texts on electrodiagnosis and nerve conduction. He is the author of 13 book chapters and over 40 peer-reviewed research publications. He serves on the editorial boards of eight different scientific journals and was awarded the Hislop award for outstanding contributions to the professional literature from the American Physical Therapy Association. In 2001, he was named a Catherine Worthingham Fellow of the American Physical Therapy Association. Dr. Spielholz keeps an open mind with regard to the clinical efficacy of complementary and alternative therapies. He was successful in challenging the federal government on behalf of the APTA when they refused to honor the research findings substantiating the use of electrical stimulation to facilitate wound healing. He has long been interested in the quality of the research and substantiation of the assertions about the efficacy of magnets and did an extensive search into the historical and contemporary literature on the clinical effectiveness of the use of magnets for this edition.

Kerri Sowers, DPT was a graduate student in physical therapy at Richard Stockton College of New Jersey when she contributed to the chapter on acupuncture.

James Stephens, PT, PhD, GCFP was originally trained as a biologist. While earning his PhD in neuroscience, he participated in a workshop with Moshe Feldenkrais that galvanized his interest in pursuing study of this method. With no Feldenkrais training on the horizon, he studied physical therapy at Hahnemann University where he earned a degree in 1983. He earned his Feldenkrais certification in the Toronto (1987) training. Jim worked for 10 years in physical therapy practices at Temple University Hospital and Moss Rehab Hospital in Philadelphia where he integrated Feldenkrais Method into physical therapy treatment of his patients. He has also maintained a private Feldenkrais practice through to the present time. In 1994, Jim began his academic career teaching in physical therapy programs first at Widener University then at Temple University. During this time, he began a research program investigating outcomes of Feldenkrais interventions with different groups of people. This has so far resulted in more than 50 peer-reviewed papers, journal articles, abstracts, and presentations. Jim is a member of the APTA neurology section where he has served as a reviewer and is chair of the Research Committee of the Feldenkrais Guild of North America whose mission is to promote research involving the Feldenkrais Method. He is currently teaching on-line courses at Temple and Drexel Universities while in transition to a new position.

Matthew J. Taylor, PT, PhD, RYT is the founder of Dynamic Systems Rehabilitation, PLLC of Scottsdale, Arizona. The clinic is based on a fusion of classical yoga therapeutic principles and his doctoral work in modern transformation learning theory. He is a US Army/Baylor University graduate with 8 years of active duty acute orthopedic care experience. He then returned to the Midwest where he established a private practice with an integrated health club that grew from a staff of two to 17 over 15 years in a town of 3500 people. His doctoral work investigated a yoga-based back school. He is currently serving on the board of directors of the International Association of Yoga Therapists and is their representative on the board of the Academic Consortium for Complementary and Alternative Health Care. In addition to a busy clinical practice, he leads continuing education workshops for health care and yoga professionals. Widely published on integrative rehabilitation from a clinical perspective, his practice has also been featured numerous times for its integrative organizational model. He has been both a principal organizer and presenter of the first two Symposiums on Yoga Therapy and Research.

Diane Zuck, MA, PT received her certificate in physical therapy at the University of Pennsylvania and her master's degree in movement sciences from Columbia University. After 35 years of practice and teaching, she retired in 2005. She was a physical therapist in the deaf-blind program at the Perkins School for the Blind in Watertown, Massachusetts, and designed and implemented classes for students with dual sensory deficits, such at those who are deaf and blind. She facilitated activities that feature a human and animal connection and maintained a small Alexander private practice.

Foreword

This book is the most thorough and up-to-date compendium on the complementary therapies available today. The first two editions of *Complementary Therapies in Rehabilitation* contributed enormously to a long-awaited shift in our health care systems. The reason: physicians, patients, therapists and health care administrators needed this vital information to help them understand and explain what complementary therapies are all about and to see how these approaches can fit into the health care system. Every facility that has begun to include these approaches has seen immediate benefits in terms of both patient satisfaction and reduction of costs.

It is remarkable that such an important book could be made even better, but that is what has happened with this new and expanded edition. It is a work that should bring satisfaction to the editor and contributors and publisher because of the beneficial influence it will have on patient outcomes. Stated differently, many people are going to have their health and their lives restored because of the information and perspectives found in this book. Fortunately, the incorporation of complementary and alternative techniques into the hospital environment is a global trend, moving more rapidly in some countries and some cities than in others, but in an inexorable direction: toward a system that is more satisfying and comfortable for all concerned.

Carol Davis has obviously been inspired in her selection of contributors. Each is an expert in their field, and each has been meticulous in documenting the foundational concepts they present with thorough references to both the basic scientific literature and clinical trials. To the editor and contributors go much credit for the consistent quality and thoroughness found in each chapter. To me, the book is worth its price just for the reference lists at the end of each chapter. Taken together, these references constitute a precious compendium of the large and growing scientific base for complementary therapies. This is the kind of literature that enables physicians to feel more comfortable about directing patients into the hands of complementary therapists.

The editor is also to be commended for the remarkable chapters she has contributed. She has obviously delved thoroughly and thoughtfully into her chosen topics. Her wisdom and dedication and common sense are apparent from the way she has treated this whole subject from start to finish. For example, it is inspiring to read a chapter on the energetics involved in the very process of thinking about a patient, i.e. psychoneuroimmunology. The subject and her insights are of interest to all clinicians. It is also helpful to have a chapter on distant healing, a subject of increasing importance in medicine.

A consistent theme is the way energetic considerations bridge conventional and complementary therapies by bringing in the basic sciences that can clarify issues that have seemed mysterious in the past. The scientific mind is often baffled by phenomena that are outside of the normal educational framework. I have found that there are important subjects that the "man on the street" may understand more easily than the educated scientist or physician. While this may seem to be a trivial academic issue, it is important for all health care providers to have a common-sense language that resonates with patients of diverse backgrounds. The science related to energetics must clarify health care issues in a way that anyone can understand. Clear and compelling explanations are a big factor in getting these methods adopted by hospitals and other health facilities. It turns out that the physics and biophysics and cell biology related to healing are actually far more intuitively understandable than biochemistry, molecular biology, and pharmaceutics. Bringing energy into the equation provides a more complete picture of life and health that benefits everyone involved in medicine from any perspective.

In reading through the various chapters, I am struck by a repeated theme: an emerging picture of successes with patients who have not been helped by the best of conventional care. It is not that there are flaws in traditional diagnostic and treatment procedures. Instead, what emerges is that a tiny problem, in one focal area of the body, can compromise the entire organism. Whether it is an issue in the connective tissue or the psyche, for example, no amount of x-rays or MRIs or blood tests or exploratory surgeries will find the cause. It is here that the complementary therapies show inestimable value, both in terms of effectiveness and cost-effectiveness. A variety of comple-mentary tools, described here, can pin-point the source of a patient's discomfort; what is holding them back from living their life to the fullest. An observation of a subtle movement pattern, palpa-tion of a tiny disturbance in a deep layer of connective tissue, or identification of the physical or emotional consequences of a long forgotten trauma can make all the difference. Furthermore, as pointed out in an early chapter by the editor, locating the issue is often facilitated by a willingness to be guided by intuition; a willingness to give credence to a subtle sign. The condition may have an energetic basis, and may therefore be undetectable approaches that leave energetics out of the picture.

Recent biomedical research has shown us the reasons subtle energetic diagnosis and interven-tion can have profound effects for a patient. The discoveries center on the nature of inflamma-tion and its relationships with virtually every chronic disease. The public is increasingly aware of research showing a relationship between chronic inflammation and the most troublesome diseases, including virtually all of the so-called "diseases of aging." See, for example, the cover story for *TIME Magazine*, February 23, 2004: "The Secret Killer: The Surprising Link Between Inflammation and Heart Attacks, Cancer, Alzheimer's and Other Diseases." There is an enormous and rapidly growing literature on these "surprising links." Until recently, there has been little understanding of the mechanisms that create these links. Revealing the nature of the inflammation–disease connec-tion has profound implications for all branches of medicine, and can lead to a deeper appreciation of the complementary and alternative therapies because they are so successful for chronic issues.

There are at least three profound consequences to the veritable explosion of research on inflam-mation. The first is that it brings energetics into the most mainstream part of mainstream bio-medicine, since inflammation is best described as an energetic problem and is inexplicable without considering energetics. Chronic inflammation is a story of electrical charge, since it arises from the persistence of free radicals. These are highly charged toxic molecules that can only be neutralized by providing them with an electron. It is their lack of an electron that makes them so destructive to pathogens and that enables them to break apart damaged cells. There is only one way to prevent their destructive character from damaging healthy cells near a site of injury: provide electrons. This, of course, brings us to the realm of the physics and biophysics of energy.

A second consequence of the focus on inflammation concerns the mechanisms that enable inflammation to persist long after its vital life-saving processes have concluded. Little is said about mechanisms in the literally thousands of new articles that appear on the subject every year. The issue is so serious that a major biomedical research journal has put forward a call for hypotheses. In all of the excitement about the inflammation, some of the older literature has been forgotten. As a specific example, consider the studies of Hans Selye, the great Canadian endocrinologist who coined the term "stress," and whose classic investigations on that subject included studies of "inflammatory pockets" or "Selye pouches." From the study of artificial structures, Selye was able explore the nature of the stress hormones: the corticosteroids. He also showed how small remnants of uncompleted responses to injury could slowly leak toxic molecules into the tissue fluids that would gradually lead, over periods of years or even decades, to breakdowns in distant organs. As an example, he studied how an inflammatory pocket containing the bacteria that cause rheumatic fever can damage heart valves. These studies are described in Selye's classic book, *The Stress of Life* (1956, 1976, 1984).

A final consequence of biomedical attention to chronic inflammation concerns the question of how it can be reduced or eliminated. It is widely accepted that the best prevention is the regular consumption of antioxidants such as non-steroidal anti-inflammatory drugs (NSAIDs), vitamins C and E, dietary antioxidants such as turmeric, and so on. The most recent research, however, shows that while these molecules are highly effective in vitro, they are much less potent than we would like them to be in the living organism. From what we know about the inflammatory barricade, there is an obvious explanation for this. The inflammatory barrier the body establishes around a site of injury is designed to prevent leakage of free radicals into the surrounding healthy tissues.

The barricade also slows the entry of circulating antioxidants. The essential medical issue becomes "What do we do about this."

An answer to this vital question emerges from some interesting places. Bodyworkers and manipulative therapists of every tradition know about dense structures that can be palpated at various places in the tissues of a patient. For example, Ida P. Rolf, in her book *Rolfing*, stated that "in practically all bodies, on one muscle or another, small lumps or thickened nonresilient bands can be felt deep in the tissue. The lumps may be as small as small peas or as large as walnuts." Dr. Rolf reproduced Selye's picture of an inflammatory pouch formed after he injected air into a fascial sheath. "Some... injurious process no doubt gives rise to the lumpy knotting we have noted." Ask any physical or massage therapist or osteopath or chiropractor or other hands-on therapist about these densities and you will invariably get the same response. They often find these dense areas, and a little pressure or stretching or other manipulation makes them go away. On the basis of what we know about inflammation, it is likely that these therapists are, whether or not they realize it at the time, correcting or preventing current or future health issues. It seems likely that they are helping complete old injury repair processes that have bogged down for whatever reason. The consequences in terms of treatment of chronic disease and prevention are obvious. The hands-on manipulative therapies have an indispensible role in treatment and prevention; they are effective and cost effective complements to high-technology diagnostic tools and pharmacological approaches. What we are discussing here is one common denominator to the complementary therapies described in this book: the mechanisms by which they can resolve an issue that was simply undetectable by all of the best diagnostic tools and therefore untreatable because its cause could not be determined.

An understanding of the causes and treatments of chronic inflammation has come from a surprising line of investigation. This is the inquiry into the consequences of walking barefoot on the earth. Many people know that walking barefoot in the grass or on the beach feels good, but until recently there has been no explanation of why this is so. Researchers are now examining what happens to our physiology when we make barefoot contact with the earth. The results are revealing that the earth is a source of antioxidant electrons that cannot be accessed when we wear shoes with electrically insulating rubber or plastic soles. The barefoot person can absorb the earth's electrons through a low resistance acupuncture point on the ball of the foot known as Kidney 1. Many schools of bodywork teach the importance of holding this point for a minute or so as the final step in a treatment, and we now know the reason for doing this. The studies of the barefoot phenomena are also revealing why a highly inflamed patient will literally "drain" the therapist who touches them. The patient is drawing electrons from the therapist. This helps the patient feel better, but can leave the therapist feeling depleted. Most therapeutic schools teach the importance of washing the hands in cold running water after a treatment. We now know why this helps: they are restoring their reservoirs of electrons by connecting to the grounded water system. This fascinating research can be accessed by searching the World Wide Web for "the barefoot revolution."

These are just a few examples of the science that is demystifying the various therapies described in this book. This science is increasing at a rapid rate. Moreover, it is a fascinating and exciting kind of science as it enables the observations of complementary therapists to be integrated with the more familiar physiological and biochemical models. This is the book that will foster greater cooperation between all branches of medicine, and that will lead to a brighter future for many patients.

James L. Oschman, PhD
President—International Society for the Study of Subtle Energy and Energy Medicine
Author of *Energy Medicine: The Scientific Basis*

SECTION I

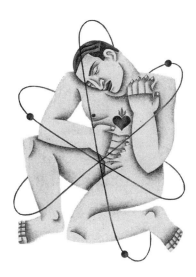

INTRODUCTION

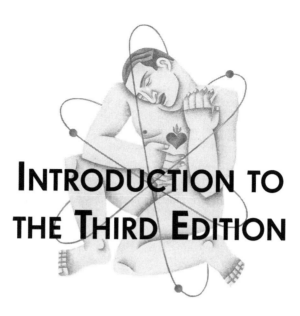

INTRODUCTION TO
THE THIRD EDITION

Carol M. Davis, DPT, EdD, MS, FAPTA

At this writing, we are well on our way through the first decade of the 21st century. This text was first conceived 15 years ago during the summer of 1993 in Sedona, Arizona. I took a leave of absence for 10 weeks from the University of Miami to read about quantum physics and complementary therapies, to see if I could figure out more about what the science behind "energy" approaches to healing might be.

Any layperson who says they truly understand quantum physics is probably not telling you the whole truth. The more I read, the more I understood, kind of, but could not find the words to explain it. Nonetheless, I did acquire a more complete grasp of the new science of psychoneuroimmunology, or mind/body medicine, and I realized that this new body of knowledge could also be envisioned as part of the new basic science of holistic therapies, those therapies that were aimed at producing positive changes not just physically, but mentally, emotionally, and spiritually as well. So I settled for a chapter on psychoneuroimmunology as the basic science chapter for the first edition of this text, which was really a kind of cop-out, but the best I could offer at the time. The book itself was not much more than a catalogue of the various holistic therapies that were being used by physical and occupational therapists and nurses in rehabilitation in the 1990s, but it got the message out that physical and occupational therapists and nurses were experiencing success in using holistic approaches with their patients, and patients were very pleased with their outcomes. And I kept on reading quantum physics! That first edition was published in 1997, although I first started it in 1993. Many of my colleagues felt that to publish such a text would be to diminish the professional status of physical therapy, which was struggling for recognition within medical science. The main thrust of the major peer-reviewed papers discouraged therapies that could not be proven to be efficacious with the gold standard of reductionism, the randomized controlled trial with placebo. However, I felt the outcomes that I was experiencing with my patients using myofascial release were too powerful to wait for a definitive mechanism of action, and therapies such as T'ai Chi and biofeedback had sufficient evidence, so I just decided to move forward with a whole group of approaches that were being used at the time.

Soon the evidence of efficacy for some of the various therapies began to accumulate, as the National Institutes of Health (NIH) agreed in 1997, after the results from a consensus conference on acupuncture, that the randomized controlled trial was not the only way science should proceed, particularly with energy-based therapies. I recognized that the text could become more than a catalogue, it could become a textbook that gave the evidence for treatments when it was available, and my understanding of quantum physics and systems theory also was expanding. So a group of authors agreed to write descriptions of the approaches they were using and agreed to review the literature and comment on the quantity and quality of the evidence. In addition, I took the leap, and a second basic science chapter was added to try to describe what might be happening on a quantum level to bring about the changes that people were reporting upon using these various therapies.

Now, here we are in 2008. The science of quantum physics is expanding and being interpreted and offered to laypeople on a regular basis, for example, in the *New York Times* Science section and in *Newsweek* and *Time* magazines. Public broadcasting stations on radio and television regularly feature programs on the latest quantum physics theories that impact our day-to-day lives. The science of quantum physics is expanding to all branches of science, from mathematics to chemistry and to biology and psychology. We are learning that quantum energy, heretofore thought to be too miniscule to affect the macroscopic universe, makes up 96% of all that is. What we experience in our world is only 4% of the total of our universe and in that 96% of dark matter and dark energy, quantum particles in wave form are impacting our reality as we know it. We benefit from quantum technology with cell phones and digital televisions and computers and MP3 players. Time to write a new basic science chapter. While we are at it, let's have the authors of the chapters on therapies update the evidence section of their chapters with the latest data on outcomes.

So, here it is—the third edition of *Complementary Therapies in Rehabilitation: Evidence for Efficacy in Therapy, Prevention, and Wellness*. The main changes you will see—in addition to the new science chapter featuring vibrational medicine, photons, and fascia—are in the evidence sections of each of the therapies. The various professionals reviewed the literature for updated evidence which appears in that section of most of the chapters. My thanks to the authors who were very excited and pleased to contribute. What an exciting time we live in! It is fun to keep up with the science and deeply meaningful to be involved with my patients in this particular approach to healing. We all benefit as the world becomes more understandable as it really is, not as we were imagining it all along.

CHAPTER 1

ENERGY TECHNIQUES AS A WAY OF RETURNING HEALING TO HEALTH CARE

Carol M. Davis, PT, EdD, MS, FAPTA

Some days, it gets very frustrating for me to treat patients in this new century. Doesn't it for you? I mean, I came into physical therapy in the 1960s to help people with movement problems to heal... to get better. I loved the challenge of each new patient and loved trying out all the skills I learned. I loved finding out that what I learned actually produced positive outcomes! I spent good time with my patients and I helped people and they got better and they thanked me! I was very happy. I thanked them! I had found a career that would serve me well and one that I could serve in proudly.

What happened to those days? What happened to health care as the century ended and the new one began? Slowly, over time, all of us were being asked to see more patients in less time. As proficient as I was with my interviews and treatments and home programs, I still lagged behind by the end of the day. Very behind. Moreover, the people in charge expected something different from me than I was prepared to give. Eventually, I got called into the office. "Look, Carol, you're just not carrying your load here. We have a certain amount of units we need to fulfill to break even with the current capitation and reimbursement system, and you've got to be more efficient. We don't want you to give up your wonderful rapport with patients, but just be aware of the time you're spending and speed it up a little. Actually, speed it up a lot. Oh, and remember, get their insurance coverage right away, because if they're Universal, we have to get approval before you even talk to them. So don't waste a session you're not going to get paid for."

In the late 20th and early 21st centuries, the economics of health care had taken over. Service shape-shifted into business, and a sea of change overtook my profession. Reluctantly, I seized an opportunity to go back to teaching full-time. I never got the hang of speeding up listening to people's stories. I was not inefficient; in fact, I actually developed clinical mastery over 25 years of practice. However, what was being asked of me and of my colleagues and students—of all of us—was to stop being health professionals devoted to being worthy of the trust that people in need placed in us, and to start earning enough money for our practices to stay alive. Meanwhile, while our calling seemed to abandon us, I read in the newspaper that many of those in charge of reimbursing us for our service were pocketing huge sums of money (a large share of which was rightfully ours) paid by the public to ensure that the service we provided was adequately reimbursed.

What exactly is a *professional* compared to a person in business who provides a needed service? Put simply, the hallmark of a profession—whether medicine, law, or theology—is to help people solve a particular problem or prevent problems from happening. We become educated with a body of knowledge and an art of being present with clients and patients with that knowledge, to have the capacity to decide if, indeed, we are qualified to help them. We are educated to listen carefully to help the person describe the problem, and then we name it, or diagnose. Professionals have what it takes to develop a sufficient and up-to-date treatment for the problem, carry out that treatment with skills especially learned as our craft. We have what it takes to decide how long a person should be in our care to benefit, and how to help the person take over the treatment process for him- or herself. We have the knowledge and virtue to charge a just and reasonable amount for our services. In other words, our aim in service is not to use our patients for our economic gain, but to charge fairly for the service we provide.

This is the foundation of all of the professions—the moral bedrock. Inherent in the description of what we do that distinguishes us from those in business to provide a service are two factors: the person who comes to us has a problem that he or she cannot seem to solve without our help, and the critical element in solving this problem hangs on the relationship we establish with that person as we assist in solving the problem. I maintain that we in medicine and health care have allowed every one of those processes to be taken away from us. It feels as if we have given up our power to a different purpose. That purpose, I believe, was intended to force us to become more fiscally accountable, as at the turn of the century the percentage of the annual gross national product in the United States that was going to health care was curving upward like a hockey stick. We needed to find a way to reign in the costs.

I am convinced that we have thrown the baby out with the bath water. In our attempts to control cost, and yet still stay alive as a profession to be able to see patients and help them, we've sold our souls to the unit, to the demand of quantity over quality. How will we ever pull ourselves out of this deep rut in which we find ourselves? How can we get back on track, help the pendulum to swing back to the middle, into balance? No one in health care is happy with the way it is now except for those who are profiting.

How Can We Tip the Pendulum to Swing Back to a Spirit of Healing in Rehabilitation?

There is a real and fundamental need for a shift in health care away from the business emphasis and back to sincere, professional helping and healing. How do we work to tip the pendulum so that the shift can come sooner? My belief is that all of us who practice health care can relate to what we call, for want of a safe word, a "sixth sense." You can't have practiced health care for long without experiencing a kind of clinical intuition that is not seated in our left brains, but comes from deep inside us, very often at the most opportune moments, and very often in a way we cannot even describe, let alone try to tell someone about. It's a shared mystery that we all acknowledge, for which we are very grateful, but also keep somewhat private. For this is an applied science we practice, and this right-brained intuition is universally seen as nonscientific and certainly not based in fact. Yet most of us, when we've been around long enough, learn to trust it, and even find ourselves quieting down and going inside to ask for help from that voice, especially when we find ourselves stumped with what to do next. We've learned that to access it, we need to get quiet, go inside, and listen carefully.

I don't know about you, but sometimes I sure would like to claim that the brilliance that comes from this sixth sense is really mine, but deep in our hearts we know that the information of clinical intuition comes from somewhere beyond us. Some may claim it as "forgotten knowledge" learned long ago and filed away for just this moment when needed. But most of us realize that there is a transcendent quality to this awareness and feel humbly grateful for it, for it never leads us astray, and we and our patients benefit from it enormously.

When I am listening carefully as my patient tells me her story, I find that the more I can move out of my left brain and into a deep listening (even if I only have 10 minutes to listen), then the better my response is going to be to what I hear. In short, I believe that the way we find our way out of this health care fiasco is by way of this inner core of our practice. The way out lies not in our rational left brains alone. We can't use logic and rationality alone to figure out how to move ourselves to a new place in our professions. The way out, I maintain, is once again, each and every time, to become present to our patients from our hearts, and to emphasize the mind-body connection with each of our patients. This does not mean we ignore the specialized knowledge we worked so hard to attain. By no means. The storehouse of knowledge remains at the ready for when we need it to make sense out of what we are experiencing. But when we listen solely from the rational left brain and our hearts are not in the listening, our patients feel treated like problems, like depersonalized sources of information. When we listen from our hearts as well, we become more efficient and more personally involved. We "get it" sooner, and we recognize what questions we must ask to get the priorities of this particular patient right, to weed out the chaff and focus in on the kernels that will be critical to our being effective. When we practice so that we incorporate mind and body in our therapy, we stimulate the whole of the patient to be engaged in the healing process. Then health care becomes what it is meant to be—a process of individualized care for the purpose of healing.

I practice outpatient physical therapy, and I have studied a manual complementary therapy, myofascial release, as taught by John F. Barnes, PT, which helps me tremendously to treat musculoskeletal and neuromuscular problems with movement effectively. When I relax and go inside, as I have been taught, I believe that I gain access to the universal energy that is all around us. In my mind, I actually picture this source energy that we cannot see flowing into my body through my head and up from the floor through the bottoms of my feet. (Of course, no one can see energy any more than we can see velocity. What we see is the product or the work that the energy does in the form of heat or pressure or vibration.) I state an inner intention that this healing energy that is available to us all will flow through me and out my hands and into my patient to release any blockages to flow, to bring about the highest good. I sit at the head of my patient who is lying supine, and I place my hands under the occiput, and then I go inside and just wait. Eventually, I will pick up a rhythmic movement under my hands that feels a little like a balloon filling up and then deflating slightly, and then filling again and deflating, about 6 or 8 times a minute. This, I've learned, is the cranial rhythm. When I first was invited to experience the cranial rhythm by John Barnes in 1989, I doubted that I would feel anything. When I finally felt it, I experienced a movement different than I'd ever imagined and so realized that I could not be making this experience up. In other words, when I quieted myself and brought the focus of my attention to down inside my body and let go of my left brain's need to figure this experience out, I was able to discern this gentle cyclic rhythm of flow.

After a few minutes, I scan the person's body/mind, and I listen for any information that might come to me from my sixth sense about where to start with my myofascial release that might differ from where my left brain perceived the problems to be while I was previously carrying out my interview, postural, functional, and movement examination.

🗂 Case Example

Mrs. R. was an 82-year-old retired social worker who had received physical therapy for the past 10 years for a kyphoscoliosis and osteoporosis and osteoarthritis. She walked with a rolling walker and a twinkle in her eye. She was very motivated to keep active, as she realized that to sit still would be the death of her. Already her kyphosis was measured with my goniometer at a 30-degree angle at its peak at about T5. She had lost several inches in height, and her pain ranged between 4 out of 10 on good days to 8 out of 10 on bad ones. In spite of this, she walked for 1 hour with her walker each day. She came to me because her pain was lingering in the range of 8 out of 10 every day, and she felt her legs becoming weaker, and she was less able to function around her house doing dishes, taking her walks, cleaning the house, and so forth. She wondered if I might know of some exercises that would help strengthen her legs. She had been told that nothing could be done for her kyphosis. She had a plate inserted at the lumbosacral junction years ago, followed later with Harrington rod surgery. The rods became too painful to bear, so she had them removed 2 years later. The surgical scar went from her occiput to her sacrum.

I told her that I believed that I could help her with exercises, not only for her legs, but for her back and her arms as well. I also thought I might be able to help her to straighten up a little more. At least I was willing to see if the total of that kyphotic curve was bony, or if some of it was soft tissue and amenable to release. Also, I was anxious to release the tight anterior fascia around her rectus abdominus, iliopsoas, and diaphragm.

She was a little skeptical, but she agreed to let me try. She informed me that she had been a hospital social worker, had been married to a physician, and that her son-in-law was chief of a division at the National Institutes of Health, and that no other physical therapists ever told her about fascia or releases; they simply gave her some good exercises and sent her on her way. Now and again she was able to receive some heat and some paraffin for her arthritis in her hands, but never any releases of any sort.

I completed my examination of her posture and balance, and then I had her lie supine (with pillows) on the treatment table. I sat at her head, and I asked her to bring her attention to her breathing. As she breathed normally, I asked her to scan her body and tell me what she felt. She said she felt my hands on her head moving slightly, and that it felt good. Other than that, she could feel nothing else, except for the pain in her back. I moved one hand to her sternum, gently tractioning toward her chin, and I gave traction at the occiput with my other hand for about 5 minutes, achieving some release and lifting. I released her pectorals for another 5 minutes and then went to her diaphragm. As I placed one hand on top of her abdomen just below her rib cage and the other under her back to do a transverse plane release, she said, "Oh, I feel the heat coming out of your hands. It feels like I have a hot pack on." I invited her to assist me by maintaining her attention on breathing so that her stomach inflated before her upper chest, and to just relax and stay focused inside her body rather than on her thoughts. I invited her to go on a vacation in her mind. I find this helps patients get out of the left brain "work" mode and get into their bodies.

Next, I released her iliopsoas bilaterally, fingers pressing gently down on that strap muscle that tightens up so to keep us forward flexed at the hips, and then I asked her to turn over on her stomach. I placed my hands to either side of her kyphotic curve and I took the slack out and placed a slight tension toward her pelvic rim, and I just waited. Soon the fascia under my hands began to feel like it was "melting" like soft butter, and rather dramatic releases began to occur. I followed the release to the fascial barrier as the melting feeling abruptly stopped, and then I patiently waited at the barrier for the next release. Sweat was beading under my eyes and I felt heat under my hands, but I was not working hard. A lot of energy was being released from the fascia around her stuck rib cage. Soon she said, "Oh! I can feel myself getting taller! I'm straightening out under your hands. My feet are moving farther down on the table. I can feel myself letting go and getting taller."

I finished up with some work on her cervical area and her thorax in rotation and extension as she sat on the side of the table. Then I gave her some exercises for pelvic mobility, back and shoulder extension, cervical rotation, and straight leg raises with ankle cuff weights. As she stood up at the side of the table she said, "I feel so different. I have never felt like this before after physical therapy. I feel energized, and light and taller."

She got dressed and as she walked out of the treatment room with her walker she declared to everyone in the office, "Look at me! Just look at me! I'm taller. I feel like I could walk forever!"

Mrs. R. said that the feeling of being taller translated functionally in her home to being able to reach higher in her cupboards and to being able to see herself in the mirror. I wanted to take a systematic look at what exactly was happening with Mrs. R. that resulted in outcomes that surprised her so dramatically, so I decided to do a case study with her. I pulled out the Polaroid grid camera, and my students and I took before and after photos and measured height, Timed Up and Go, balance standing on one foot, forward reach, vital capacity, pain level, and quality of life with an instrument called the SF-36. After 2 weeks of treatment of three 45-minute sessions of myofascial release followed by 15 minutes of exercise, we noted positive change in most measures. Pain was reduced to 2 to 3 out of 10, very bearable for her. We videotaped an interview with her at the conclusion of 2 weeks, and her report of her improvement focused on what she felt with the energy work, both during the releases on the treatment table and for up to 48 hours later.

I would have hoped for, even expected, eventual positive change in all measures with exercise alone, except perhaps height and posture. My question was, "What part did the myofascial release, the energy work, play on our positive outcome?" I don't know for sure. Mrs. R. served as her own control, having experienced physical therapy without energy work for years. Were our outcomes simply a result of the positive rapport we developed? I imagine that the way we are with our patients, not just what we do, has a lot to do with our outcomes. I suspect we will come to discover that even our interactions can, in part, be analyzed to be helpful by way of our positive expectations, our compassion for our patients that may translate into bioenergetic forces that assist with healing. Science is moving rapidly forward in documenting the effects of intention, compassion, and empathy in interpersonal exchanges.

Of all of the factors we tested for change in Mrs. R., the most dramatic was her exit interview in which she described the effect of the myofascial release on her energy level, and her perception of how she felt at home following treatment compared to years of physical therapy without myofascial release. After 2 to 3 days, gravity would again seem to take over, and she could feel herself shrinking, but her pain level maintained at a 2 to 3/10 and she was able to walk more comfortably and function around her house without having to lie down in the middle of the morning and afternoon.

Although Mrs. R. tells quite a dramatic story, her positive outcomes parallel those of all the patients I treated with myofascial release in our faculty practice. In fact, at the same time, I was treating another older woman with a remarkably similar kyphoscoliosis who walked with a rolling walker. She had not had the surgeries that Mrs. R. had, but had experienced several years of traditional physical therapy. My students and I repeated the single case design with her and got similar results. Once again, as we videotaped her exit interview, she remarked that the difference she felt with physical therapy that included myofascial release was a feeling of being able to stand taller and feel more energy. Functionally, that meant she could stand at the sink and wash her dishes without having to lean on her elbows to hold herself up so that she could breathe. This positive effect, again, lasted 2 days or so. Occasionally, I would treat a patient who was unable to experience the releases as they happened, but that was very rare.

What does this have to do with the crisis in health care and how we find our way out of this rut we are in?

Energy Medicine as a Way Out of the Crisis in Health Care

I believe that we are all surrounded not just by air, but by a healing energy field that is available to us when we let it in. David Bohm first wrote about this in the 1930s.[1] Science is confirming that people are like crystals, made up of a vibrating matrix of life that is capable, like the crystals in a radio receiver, of resonating with the energy of the earth. James Oschman,[2] in his book,

Energy Medicine, goes into great detail reporting the properties of the living matrix, and central to the vibrational energetic function in the body/mind is the connective tissue, the fascia. As John Barnes[3] wrote in his book on myofascial release, fascia surrounds every cell in the body, extending into each cell forming a cytoskeleton. It is responsible for our being able to maintain vertical posture in gravity.[4] Fascia determines our shape and architecture, and some believe it acts as the "copper wire"—the conduction mechanism to transmit bioenergy—the ch'i of our body/minds, the flow that is responsible, in part, for homeostasis, for self-regulation, for our ability to stay in remarkable balance, to heal ourselves and maintain our healing state as our natural state.[2,5] Every cell in our body/mind is encased in this conducting tissue made up of collagen, elastin, and a central, more fluid polysaccharide layer. It is more accurate to visualize each cell embedded in the fascia, like shells in the wax of a candle, than it is to visualize fascia simply surrounding each cell.

According to the research, Oschman reports that "gravity, pressure, tension, muscle pull, each movement on our bodies causes the crystalline lattice of the connective tissue (fascia) to generate bioelectronic signals that are precisely characteristic of those tensions, compressions and movements. Thus, the connective tissue fabric is a semiconducting communication network that can carry the bioelectronic signals between every part of the body and every other part."[2] Perhaps the fascia serves as the pathways for body energy, or ch'i. Perhaps the fascia forms the elusive meridians described in traditional Chinese medicine. Western science has been slow to accept the concept of meridians because they cannot be dissected in cadavers, but neither can a major part of the distal lymphatic system, also responsible for life-sustaining flow. Even though we cannot "see" the air traffic route a plane takes from Miami to Frankfurt, I hope that the captain has filed a flight plan nonetheless, accurately reporting the coordinates she intends to take.

The fluid nervous system, described so artfully by Candace Pert in *Molecules of Emotion*,[5] also contributes to this flow of communication. The three types of natural chemicals that make up this communication system include the neurotransmitters (serotonin, dopamine, norepinephrine, acetylcholine, histamine, glycine, gamma-aminobutyric acid [GABA], and many more), steroids (cortisol, testosterone, estrogen, progesterone), and peptides. The largest category, which regulates life processes with secretions such as insulin and growth hormone, helps regulate the emotions with the endorphins and include many other peptides that are not yet named. When we add the flows of nerve stimulation, blood, and lymph to bioenergetic and neurochemical flows, we can begin to see how important "keeping the channels open" is to the healthy functioning of the body/mind. We hypothesize that if fascial restrictions close channels, flow would be interrupted and dysfunction and disease can result. Multiple sclerosis, we know, results from the interrupted flow of nerve stimuli due to a degeneration of the myelin sheath. Parkinson's disease results from an inadequate amount, and therefore diminished flow, of dopamine. Immune system functioning is very dependent on the emotions, as is being described by the science of psychoneuroimmunology and psychoendocrineimmunology.[5] Aerobic exercise has been shown to positively effect the secretion of neurotransmitters that help prevent mood disorders and depression.[6] Fascial tightness is responsible for myalgias, diminished lung function, trigger points, carpal tunnel syndrome, and a whole host of musculoskeletal disorders.[4] Envision also what would happen if the fascia surrounding the vital organs of the chest or pelvis become tightened. Diminished flow of and to cardiac, lung, gastrointestinal, and pelvic organs would severely disrupt the balance of the body/mind needed for optimum function and could contribute to many of the pain syndromes and organ dysfunction of chronic illness.

What we have yet to learn from science, however, is the exact mechanism of healing action that results from this flow of ch'i, energetic, and chemical communication. We do, however, know the various causes of connective tissue dysfunction: trauma, scarring, infection, dehydration, habitual postures, repetitive motion injuries, and quite possibly the wear and tear of daily life in gravity along with the postures that attend our varying emotions as we struggle through life.

It becomes clear that, as health care professionals, whatever we can do to assist with energy flow very likely will be facilitative to our goals of treatment, wellness, and prevention, as all of these events are continuous with balance and self-regulation. As manual therapists, what science has demonstrated is that, when we are calm and centered, removed from functioning in our left brains and focusing attention into our bodies, we can open ourselves up to receive the vibrations from the earth's energy.[2] These electromagnetic signals from the core of the earth are thought to be picked up by the pineal gland and melatonin cells (magnetite-bearing tissue in the brain), conducted over the fascia perineural system throughout our body/mind, amplified somewhere in the body up to 1000 times, and finally projected out our hands into the body/minds of our patients.[2] This is termed Schumann resonance after the scientist who explored the connection of our brainwaves with the energy of the earth.[7] Through the process of entrainment, the therapist who is calm and centered, intending to bring about the highest good, can transmit this energy to patients, as described by Zimmerman[8] in his studies of therapeutic touch practitioners. If the patient is also in the right state to receive this energy, the entrainment can extend to him or her. How this results in healing is still in question. We believe that the vibration of the energy affects the system positively in two ways. With the pressure of our hands in gravity over the fascial tensegrity system, a piezo-electric effect takes place wherein mechanical pressure is converted to chemical energy, and the polysaccharide layer between the collagen and elastin of the fascia changes from a stiffer gel into a more fluid soluble state, "releasing" the structure of the tightened fascia in such a way that results in what may be a more permanent release than what we see with traditional stretching of soft tissue. A tensegrity system, described first by Buckminster Fuller, is characterized by "a continuous network (tendons, ligaments, fascia) supported by a discontinuous set of compressive elements."[2] Heidemann's work[9] with tensegrity provides a conceptual link between the structural systems and the energy-information systems described above. "The body as a whole and the various parts, including the interiors of all cells and nuclei, can be visualized as tensegrity systems... Mechanical energy flows away from a site of impact through the tensegrous living matrix. The more flexible and balanced the network (the better the tensional integrity), the more readily it absorbs shocks and converts them to information rather than damage..."[2] Flexible and well-organized fascia and myofascial relationships enhance performance and reduce the incidence of injuries.[2]

Even more impressive, the contribution of the tensegrity system to optimum function is, in part, due to the fact that the entire system is a vibratory continuum. When a tendon on a model of the system is plucked, the entire system vibrates. Molecules do not have to be touching to receive the vibratory stimulus from our hands on the surface.

Returning Healing to Health Care

If we are all surrounded by a healing energy field, as Oschman and before him physicists such as David Bohm[1] maintained, and if we are a living tensegrous system that vibrates continuously, and if we as health professionals have the capacity to assist our patients through energy medicine techniques to maintain the connection with the healing energy surrounding us to prevent the disruption of the flows that ensure self-regulation and the natural state of wellness, then our role as healers becomes clear. The crisis in health care becomes obsolete. What patients require from us is to assist them in opening up to the vibrations, the connections that contribute to energy flow. We do that by including as a part of our treatments complementary and alternative therapies to enhance the flow of ch'i and restore balance and wellness. We also strive to foster relationships with each patient characterized by rapport, empathy, active listening, and a true desire that they be able to open up to the energy that is available to them to heal themselves. Finally, and perhaps most important, practitioners must practice those techniques that keep their channels open and flowing as well.

This is the future of health care that restores the healing process to our medical profession. It is not only possible, it is probable that these changes will occur rapidly, for they have already begun. There is good science to support this dream of what can be. Once again, patients will be served by us in ways that make us excited to be involved in the healing process and grateful for each day and each interaction. Vibration is the key phenomenon to watch develop in this new science. We must be aware of the power of our thoughts in vibrating reality to us. The intention of the health care practitioner must be carefully focused on the most optimum outcome available for each patient.

In Chapter 21 of this book, Susan Morrill Ramsey reports the latest science on the power of consciousness as creative at a distance. Larry Dossey asked in a recent editorial, "Can the thoughts and intentions of health care professionals affect their patients physically, nonlocally, at a distance? Should they be considered as factors in the therapeutic relationship that develops between a health care professional and her client?"[10] Indeed, we need not be certified in a complementary therapy to support the holistic healing of our patients. Simply providing quality care with the intention that our patients heal and be able to open up to receive the healing energy vibration that surrounds us all is what is required for the new, healing health care. What a pleasure it will be to practice in the coming years of this century.

References

1. Bohm D. *Wholeness and the Implicate Order.* London: Routledge and Kegan Paul; 1980.
2. Oschman JL. *Energy Medicine—The Scientific Basis.* Edinburgh: Churchill-Livingstone; 2000.
3. Barnes JF. *Myofascial Release: The Search for Excellence.* Paoli, PA: MFR Seminars; 1990.
4. Simons DG, Travell JG, Simons LS. *Myofascial Pain and Dysfunction.* 2nd ed. Baltimore, MD: Williams and Wilkins; 1999.
5. Pert C. *Molecules of Emotion.* New York, NY: Scribner; 1997.
6. LaPerrier A, Antoni M, Fletcher MA, Schneiderman N. Exercise and health maintenance in HIV. In: Galantino ML, ed. *Clinical Assessment and Treatment of HIV/Rehabilitation of a Chronic Illness.* Thorofare, NJ: SLACK Incorporated; 1992:65-76.
7. Konig HL. ELF and VLF signal properties: physical characteristics. In: Persinger MA, ed. *ELF and VLF Electromagnetic Field Effects.* New York, NY: Plenum Press; 1974:9-34.
8. Zimmerman J. Laying-on-of-hands healing and therapeutic touch: a testable theory. BEMI currents. *Journal of the Bio-Electro-Magnetic Institute.* 1990;24:8-17.
9. Heidemann SR. A new twist on integrins and the cytoskeleton. *Science.* 1993;260:1080-1081.
10. Dossey L. The dark side of consciousness and the therapeutic relationship. *Alternative Therapies.* 2002;8(6):12-16,118-121.

SECTION II

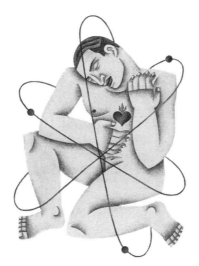

THE SCIENCE
THAT SUPPORTS
COMPLEMENTARY
THERAPIES

CHAPTER 2

PSYCHONEUROIMMUNOLOGY
THE BRIDGE TO THE COEXISTENCE
OF TWO PARADIGMS

Carol M. Davis, DPT, EdD, MS, FAPTA

Introduction

In 1971, Herbert Benson and colleagues published results of research that seemed to point toward a mind-body link and coined the term *relaxation response*.[1,2] At the same time, Robert Ader and Nicholas Cohen were researching the phenomenon of anticipatory nausea resulting from the effects of chemotherapy on patients.[3] Patients began to become sick just thinking about the drugs long before they took them. They were aware of Pavlov's dogs salivating to the sound of the bell (research published in 1928),[4] and that was really all that they were looking for—a laboratory model to confirm that similar conditioning was what was also happening to their patients. They gave rats cyclophosphamide along with saccharin-sweetened water. Then, when they took away the chemotherapy and gave the sweetened water alone, they looked to see if the rats vomited. When they did, they indeed had their laboratory model of "learning" by conditioning that seemed to be occurring in Ader's patients.

Ader realized, however, that the chemotherapy not only caused nausea in patients, it also depressed their immune systems, lowering patients' resistance to infectious disease. What he did not anticipate is that when the rats were given the sweetened water alone, not only did they develop nausea, the rats also "learned" by conditioning to depress their immune systems. This biochemical result seemed to provide powerful evidence, using reductionistic research methods, that the mind and the body are not able to be separated.[5] Somehow, the mind (which is still thought to reside in the nervous system) "told" the immune system to become suppressed in the absence of the chemotherapeutic immune-suppressive agent.

Interestingly, Ader and Cohen make the point in the second edition of their landmark text[3] that the effects on conditioning were observed and reported as early as 1896 by Mackenzie,[6] who provoked an allergic response in a patient with asthma by showing the patient an artificial rose. Later, Osler repeated this observation. However, science had no theory that would substantiate such a response, for the mind "had no influence on the body." Anyone can see how valuable a contribution they made by publishing their results, no matter what the prevailing theory of science would accept or reject.

Subsequent research over the past 20 years has demonstrated, again with rigorous science, that there is a continuous dialogue between the mind and the nervous and immune systems that suggests the emotions can affect the immune system in both positive and negative ways. With his results, Ader coined a term to describe a new basic science of mind/body medicine, health care, and research: *psychoneuroimmunology* (PNI),[3] psycho (from the mind or psyche), neuro (via the brain or neurons), immunology (to the immune system).

Two pathways of communication have been identified between the mind and the body: the autonomic nervous system (sympathetic and parasympathetic) and the nonadrenergic noncholinergic nerves (NANC). Felten et al[7] maintain that these pathways innervate bone marrow, thymus, spleen, and mucosal surfaces where immune cells develop, mature, and encounter foreign substances. "Each [of the two nerve systems] communicates with the immune cells directly through the release of chemical messages which range from adrenaline, noradrenaline, and acetylcholine to small proteins called neuropeptides... and cause an inflammatory or anti-inflammatory effect on the immune system."[7]

This foundational challenge to Cartesian separatist thought opened the way for reductionistic methods to be used to verify holistic principles, and the beginning of an important bridge was formed, which may span the seemingly uncrossable void to link reductionism and holism into coexistence.

Application of Psychoneuroimmunology

With regard to the initial studies that tested the application of PNI to patient care, in 1991 the *New England Journal of Medicine* reported that rates of both respiratory infection and clinical colds increase in a dose-response manner with the increase in degree of psychological stress.[8] In 1992, David Spiegel, a psychiatrist at Stanford Medical School, published his research conducted in 1989 that suggested that breast cancer patients randomly placed in weekly support groups lived markedly longer than control patients assigned only to regular care.[9] These studies have been followed by countless more,[3] and now research departments in the nation's major medical centers that are investigating hypotheses based on the science of PNI compete successfully for National Institutes of Health (NIH) grants. Among the most important to rehabilitation is the research that investigates the effects of massage[10] and exercise[11] on the immune systems of those with chronic and fatal diseases such as HIV and AIDS.

At the encouragement of Senator Thomas Harkin, a congressional mandate created the Office of Alternative Medicine in 1992 to investigate and approve proposals for research on alternative methods of healing. Although roadblocks and criticisms from the prevailing science bias against alternative approaches made the initial 2 years of this office quite difficult,[12] the office seems to be establishing itself at last. Scientists at NIH did not want to add possible "legitimacy by association" to researchers who had no formal education in reductionistic methods. They felt that practitioners of holistic approaches were using their association with NIH to promote illegitimate research, but in the end they realized that they had no choice but to accept the congressional mandate.[12]

In spite of the fact that proposals seldom could be reviewed for the usual NIH standards of the quality of the principle investigator's "track record," nor for "scientific merit," in 1996 the office awarded selected research centers a total of $9,744,535 in grant funds. In a rather critical article found in the June 18, 1996 *New York Times National,*[12] the following institutions were listed as recipients:

1. The University of Virginia School of Nursing (use of magnets to relieve pain)

2. Kessler Institute for Rehabilitation (use of Chinese herbs with neurological problems including stroke)

3. Columbia University (Chinese medicine and women's health)

4. University of Texas Health Science Center at Houston (alternative cancer therapies)

5. Beth Israel Hospital in Boston (conventional therapy for low back pain vs acupuncture and massage)

6. Minneapolis Medical Research Foundation (alternative therapies for addiction)

7. Bastyr University in Seattle (survey of 1500 to 2000 people with AIDS to determine alternative therapy use and results)

8. University of Maryland School of Medicine (alternative medicine effects on bone and muscle pain)

9. University of California-Davis (survey alternative practitioners, including Native Americans, on use of therapies to treat patients with asthma)

10. Stanford University (alternative therapies such as massage and the use of support groups to enhance the quality of life of older people)[12]

Interactions between the mind or psyche and the neural and immune systems have been shown to have relevance in a broad range of diseases, such as cancer and arthritis; viral infections, such as HIV; and other autoimmune diseases, but knowledge of just how these systems interact is still not conclusive.

Black's study, reported in December 1995 in *Scientific American*,[13] reveals how the brain and the immune system interact via hormones, neurotransmitters, and cytokines traveling through blood and nerves. This bidirectional chemical communication is regulated by corticotropin-releasing factor, which is stimulated by thoughts and emotions or immune activation to affect the hypothalamic-pituitary-adrenal axis. Stress, in particular, compromises immunity. Stressful life events have been linked with susceptibility to infection, reactivation of herpes virus, and with cancer and HIV progression. Effects on depression, as well as other clinical aspects, are also under study.[13]

The positive effects of exercise, massage, therapeutic touch, and manual therapies on the immune system securely places both alternative therapies and PNI research in rehabilitation.[10,11] These therapies are listed among the "alternative therapies" in the *Chantilly Report of the National Institutes of Health*[14] and are placed in categories as follows:

1. Mind-body interventions—psychotherapy, support groups, meditation, imagery, hypnosis, biofeedback, dance and music therapies, art therapy, prayer, and mental healing

2. Bioelectromagnetics application to medicine—thermal applications of nonionizing radiation: radio frequency (RF) hyperthermia, laser and RF surgery, and RF diathermy; nonthermal applications of nonionizing radiation for bone repair, nerve stimulation, wound healing, etc

3. Alternative systems of medical practice—70% to 90% of all health care worldwide. Popular health care, community-based health care, professionalized health care, traditional Asian medicine (including acupuncture, Ayurveda), homeopathy, anthroposophically extended medicine (elements of naturopathy plus homeopathy), naturopathic medicine

4. Manual healing methods—touch and manipulation, osteopathy, chiropractic, massage therapy, biofield therapeutics (healing touch, therapeutic touch, and SHEN therapy)

5. Pharmacological and biological treatments—drugs and vaccines not yet accepted in mainstream medicine (antineoplastons, cartilage products, ethylenediaminetetraacetic acid [EDTA], immunoaugmentive therapy, 714-X, Coley's toxins, MTH-68, neural therapy, apitherapy, iscador, biologically guided chemotherapy)

6. Herbal medicine—folk remedies that rely on botanical knowledge of the effects of herbs on the body

7. Diet and nutrition in the prevention and treatment of chronic disease—perhaps the best-known example is Dean Ornish's program for heart disease that emphasizes nutrition, yoga, meditation, guided imagery or visualization, as well as exercise

The Integration of Reductionism With Holism

It appears from the most recent literature that holistic practices and reductionistic medicine and health care finally are coming together, and many holistic practices do lend themselves to verification with reductionistic methods, but some clearly do not. Meanwhile, the public and health care professionals are continuing to explore the benefits of complementary and alternative therapies. Most important, because of the reductionistic results revealed by PNI, biomedical research is finding it more difficult to ignore the mind-body connection.

While research is being conducted and these two explanatory paradigms struggle to coexist, nurses and physical and occupational therapists are utilizing various complementary therapies in their practices and are experiencing what they and their patients describe as success, even when traditional approaches such as exercise and mobilization have not helped. This text was created to help reveal the variety of efforts in this area. The chapters in this text may make it more difficult for those who would dismiss complementary therapies out-of-hand as nonscientific and not appropriate for professionals to use because the results cannot be duplicated in controlled studies.

The accepted belief among holistic practitioners with regard to interrater reliability is that holistic methods have the intention to affect not just one system, but all body systems, by influencing the patient's vital life force in a positive way through the manipulation of the body's energy system. In spite of numerous studies, the very existence of body energy is still questioned by most reductionists.[15] However, holistic practitioners believe that once the bioelectromagnetic field is altered by one therapist, another therapist with his or her own energy field will not be able to locate the same energy field response from the patient, as it has already been affected by the first researcher.[16]

That does not mean we should ignore the need to understand and test alternative approaches to help make them complementary in rehabilitation. The most common complaints of those who chose "nonconventional" therapies in Eisenberg's 1990 study[17] were chronic conditions often treated in outpatient physical therapy departments, such as musculoskeletal pain, headache, arthritis, and back pain, as well as insomnia, depression, and anxiety, which often accompany chronic musculoskeletal conditions.

Just as Dr. Mackenzie reported the inexplicable finding of his patient's allergic response to an artificial rose in 1895,[6] practitioners must continually document and publish systematic observations of methods, clinical decision making, the patient's descriptions of the effects of treatment, and subsequent outcomes when alternative and complementary therapies are used.

Professionals Best Suited to Transform Alternative Therapies into Complementary Therapies

Clearly, doctorally and postdoctorally prepared scientists, rehabilitation professionals, psychologists, physicians, and exercise physiologists are most adequately prepared to conduct the scientific studies that will go a long way to allow us to offer the greatest number of safe and tested alternatives to the greatest number of patients at the most reasonable cost. We will then be working toward a truly sustainable health care system.[1] However, many postbaccalaureate prepared health professional clinicians and teachers also have the appropriate educational background suited to conduct systematic studies and tests, to prepare indepth case studies, and to contribute to a central data bank designed to report the outcomes and adequacy of those therapies not easily explored by controlled reductionist research.

Likewise, most professional-level health practitioners are well educated in the theoretical foundations and the art of treatment, and can rather easily expand their knowledge and art to utilize alternative therapies and make them complementary for their work. For example, psychologists, art and music therapists, ministers, priests, and rabbis are well positioned to apply selected appropriate mind-body interventions listed in the NIH *Chantilly Report*.[14] Physical and occupational therapists, as well as nurses and massage therapists, are—or should be—well educated to perform alternative massage methods. As this text illustrates, physical therapists can rather easily extend their traditional education in touch and exercise to incorporate the approaches of therapeutic touch and other touch therapies such as Jin Shin Do, Rolfing, Qi gong, and the Rosen method. Physical therapists often are well suited to have interest and desire to undertake the years of training required to develop the art and skill needed to be certified as Feldenkrais and Alexander practitioners. Indeed, many have done this, as well as have taken necessary training to apply the Trager approach, T'ai Chi, and so on.

Some physical therapists have also extended their professional education to be qualified to conduct research on alternative therapies.[18] For example, at Emory University, Steven Wolf, PhD, PT, FAPTA was awarded a National Institute on Aging FICSIT (Frailty and Injuries: Cooperative Studies of Intervention Techniques) grant to study the effects of T'ai Chi on balance in older people.[18] As the authors of this text reveal, even more physical and occupational therapists have studied specific alternative approaches in order to make them complementary to their practice. Mind-body approaches such as yoga, T'ai Chi, and those aspects of traditional Chinese medicine, acupuncture, acupressure, polarity, reflexology, and Touch for Health, which are proposed to act to "balance" the vital energy and assist in pain control and in the prevention of disease, are all being practiced by physical therapists.

Exercise (along with diet, nutrition, and herbal medicine) and improved medications that mimic the body's own immune system defenses have become the foundation of the treatment plans that turn what once were rapidly fatal diseases, such as AIDS, into chronic diseases with which one can live many years.[11] Physical therapists seem best prepared to prescribe exercise for ill persons whose disease has affected many systems. In contrast, exercise physiologists and sports medicine personnel have entered the exercise area with an emphasis on exercise prescription for prevention and wellness.

Therapeutic Presence: Holistic Principles in Action

Embracing a new theory of care that is diametrically opposed to the system that we are trying to reform carries many risks. For example, believing that all illness is a metaphor and that we are all 100% in control of our health is as absurd as believing we are passive victims of germs and our genetic heritage, and there is nothing we can do except follow the physician's orders.[19] Even before being validated, even against the advice of some medical scientists, alternative therapies are routinely being integrated with conventional therapies as complementary to facilitate healing, and the valuable aspects of holism cited above are being applied universally in health care. If people have consistently reported over a long period of time that a treatment works to help relieve symptoms, thus they feel better and their symptoms are indeed relieved, then this outcome measure of personal anecdote should be considered one type of evidence of efficacy, whether or not the treatment fits the qualifications of accepted research design.[20]

Just as this text illustrates, based on the teachings of such ancient practices as traditional Chinese medicine and Ayurveda, and based on the recordings kept by more recent systems of thought such as homeopathy and naturopathy, the alternative approaches based on holism are being applied with increasing frequency as complementary to conventional practice.

Holistic Application of Traditional and Complementary Treatments

PNI has helped to show that healing is facilitated not only by the alternative approach itself, but also by way of the principles of therapeutic presence, or the holistic nature of how health professionals are with their patients. The characteristics of one who uses oneself as a therapeutic agent with the patient reflect the philosophy of holism.[21] Cancer surgeon and holistic physician Bernie Seigel continually points out how important the doctor-patient relationship is to the recovery from cancer.[22]

John Carmody, a marathon athlete recovering from leg surgery for his incurable multiple myeloma, wrote in the journal *Second Opinion*[23] that the first of his two postoperative physical therapists responded to his fatigue from surgery and two crushed lumbar vertebrae with great insensitivity, "You just have to push through the pain... it's mainly a question of your will to get better." He goes into rather lengthy detail documenting the physical therapist's callousness and indifference to him, not only to his weakness, but to his fear of never being able to walk again. For example, her response to his request for help in positioning his hands and feet to get up off the bed to use his walker was, "It doesn't matter. Just get on with it. Push off the bed and start walking." Finally, he responded to her continual insinuations that he was a rather clumsy coward with an outburst, an attack on her to "back off," accusing her of patronizing him and showing a severe lack of sympathy for his unique situation as a patient. He was an athlete with pain from his treatment for incurable cancer, but more than that, he was a productive writer and a person able and willing to benefit from needed instruction. Yet, she never seemed to relate to those unique characteristics in him. She treated him as if he were a "thing," a noncompliant complainer.

When this therapist was replaced by a second clinician, his perceptions of the first therapist's insensitivity and nastiness were confirmed. His second physical therapist acknowledged his pain and instructed him to breathe through it as a way to assist relaxation and pain control. She took the time to show him where he should place his hands to take his weight as he rose from the bed to begin walking with the walker. She spoke to him gently and encouragingly, and conveyed optimism, telling him she knew he could do this, it would just take time. This gentle and personal approach got him over his hopeless hump and soon he progressed, first to using crutches and, eventually, to a welcome discharge home.

At home, as he exercised he heard the voice of the second therapist encouraging him and, as he felt stronger, he added swimming and other challenges for increasing his strength and function. She had facilitated hope, and he was motivated to recover because she had spoken to him, connected with him in his uniqueness, and had believed in him and encouraged him by her very presence.[23] The positive effects of compassion on the patient's healing response illustrate PNI, no matter whether the employed treatment is traditional or complementary.

What are the roots of compassion? What allows some of us on some days to be able to extend ourselves to our fellow humans who happen to be our patients, but not on others? What forces interfere with the capacity to respond with sympathy or empathy to patients? And why is it important to be able to be therapeutically present? Isn't just satisfying our contract to "teach and fix" enough?[24]

Therapeutic presence is the capacity to, at the least, sympathize with patients or enter into "fellow feeling" and interact from the space of genuinely shared emotion.[25] This demands that professionals feel with their patients and respond to them in a way that acknowledges the "feeling with"—the interconnection.[26] Biomedical ethicists suggest that our moral obligation as health care professionals mandates that patients, as people, should never feel dehumanized or treated as "things" separate from the human race.[27] According to our codes of ethics and the writings of medical ethicists, we are morally obliged to act in certain ways that reflect what it means to be professional, to respond to fellow human beings who place trust in us because of their vulnerability in times of need.[27,28]

In other words, part of medical and health care education should be devoted to developing self-awareness of the behaviors that we bring with us into our professional education that interfere with communicating interest in and rapport with our patients. These behaviors are based on the appropriate values and attitudes of the mature healing professional so that competent practitioners can know how to display morally responsible caring to patients, even on days when their lives are out of balance and stressful. Patients deserve response not only with proficient knowledge, but with well-advised care and compassion suited to the uniqueness of each person and his or her problem.[21,27,28]

Crossing Over in Empathy—Holistic Integration

Therapeutic presence describes a connection with patients that is based on the principles of holism, of interconnectedness, that makes an uncomfortable wall, a separateness, impossible. In contrast to sympathy, empathy is a unique interaction that actually involves the experience of "crossing over" into a "shared moment of meaning" that is deeply felt and makes it impossible not to experience the impact of one's actions on the patient, both negative and positive.[24,29] Any health professional or patient who has experienced the emotional "at-oneness" felt with the crossing-over moment in empathy, where one is so identified with the other that for a brief millisecond, you forget that the other is separate from you, has experienced the interconnectedness of holism.[24] Sympathy is not, as many would believe, harmful for patients.[25,26] Indeed, it is encouraging and helpful for patients to feel as if a health care professional has walked with them on their journey for a while and that the feelings shared were more than simply acknowledged, they were "fellow feelings" resulting from a strong bond or connection. *Pity* is harmful in that it is sympathy with a feeling of being worthier than the one pitied, so it distances the patient with a "poor you" attitude that again depersonalizes the patient.[24,26]

Therapeutic presence, or using oneself to make a warm and encouraging connection with the patient, is based on the important acknowledgment that the mind and feelings of the patient are inseparably linked with the patient's physical body, and that the patient's feelings, emotions, and beliefs are just as critical in patient recovery as exercise, medications, and rest.[21]

Carmody comments from the patient's perspective[23]:

> [R]easonable patients—the majority—know full well that medicine is fallible, uncertain, and very human. What healers risk in meeting their patients as their equals in humanity is little compared to what they stand to gain. For both the efficacy of their treatments and their growth as human beings, health care professionals will be wise to take down as many barriers as they can, give away as many distancing privileges as possible. [Health professionals] who have been sustaining me are alike in their ability to create a sense of "we." We patients and healers are sharing a joint venture, even a joint (somewhat macabre) adventure. This sharing can make us free. I feel free to ask about any problem and express any emotion, positive or negative. They, I hope, feel free to speak truthfully, to be playful or somber as the moment dictates. In a word, we have all become friends, and also joint apprentices to a basal truth: All of us are simply people. Our lives are short. None of us has ever seen God, let alone been mistaken for God.

This interconnectedness stands in sharp contrast to the rigid boundaries of allopathic medicine where health care workers are taught to work "on" patients. I am not suggesting that the important boundaries that must exist between patient and therapist to ensure therapeutic objectivity be dissolved. Many have written on the dangers of the miscommunications that can be harmful to therapist/patient effectiveness when helper/helpee boundaries are ignored.[24] Patients should never feel obligated to help their practitioners, nor, as Carmody felt, should they ever feel as if their helpers are concerned only with the physical—with their leg, blood count, or urine output. Patients have the right to believe that their health care practitioner is concerned about them as unique human beings with special rights, patients' rights, always acknowledging the inextricable interaction of mind and body. The meaning that a patient attributes to his or her experience of illness or injury has very much to do with his or her past history and very personal hopes for the future. To ignore this in patient care is to ignore the uniqueness of the person and risk the necessary cooperation of the patient in the goals that are set for care. To ignore this is to fail to maximize the positive effects of the mind on the body.

Patients need professionals to be clearly worthy of their trust, both in the knowledge and skill they bring to their problem as well as in the relationship that is formed.[28] What Carmody asks for, and what holism suggests, is that the professional recognize the importance of patient autonomy. Autonomy is the moral responsibility that professionals do all possible so that the patient can remain in charge of his or her own problem. With this in mind, the most relevant perspective, for both patient and professional, is to acknowledge that they both need each other, not only to be able to fulfill their unique missions, but also in order to grow, develop, and change. In this way, patients take on a more equal status in the interaction, practitioners consult with them at every choice point, and always follow the moral tenets of informed consent. This important moral attitude serves to lift self-esteem and help patients to feel autonomous and adult in a culture that can be very unfamiliar and frightening. This preservation of one's self-esteem can be an important mind/body advantage in the healing process of the patient and in preserving the quality of the moments that practitioners spend with their patients.

Applying Holistic Principles in Health Care

Whether employing traditional or complementary therapies, *The Heart of Healing*[1] suggests that there are several ways in which medicine and health care can change to reflect therapeutic presence, the compassionate use of oneself as a partner to the patient in the process of examination and treatment, which actualizes the finest ideals of holistic practice. What is suggested is that health care should reflect the following changes:

1. A commitment to treat people, not diseases. Instead of asking, "What is wrong with this person, and how can it be fixed?" we will ask, "Who is this [unique] person, and how can he or she be helped to achieve maximum health?" Depending on the nature of the problem, once evaluated carefully, patients might be better served by a psychotherapist, a physical therapist, a bodyworker, or biofeedback for chronic headache.

2. A reassessment of the appropriate use of technology. Twenty-eight percent of the $70 billion spent by Medicare in 1985 went to people during their last year of life, and 30% of that $70 billion was spent during the last month of life alone.

3. A new openness to complementary therapies. The survey published by Eisenberg and associates[17] seemed to show that patients who were educated carefully chose the benefits and risks of trying "nonconventional" therapies. Unfortunately, an editorial in the same issue of the January 1993 *New England Journal of Medicine* deprecated many of the alternative treatments that Americans had chosen. "Many of the relaxation techniques, massage therapies, special diets, and self-help groups could be considered to be lifestyle choices more than therapeutic interventions," the editorial stated. Other therapies were singled out as being "patently unscientific," including chiropractic, herbal medicine, homeopathy, and acupuncture—although the editorial did grant that such therapies are sometimes recommended by, or even delivered by, physicians.[17] At the very least, since the mid 1980s, research in PNI has strongly concluded that lifestyle choices are therapeutic interventions.

4. A new view of prevention. Even though more Americans are exercising and have quit smoking than ever before, prevention still lags behind in insurance reimbursement and in money for health care. Money for infant, child, and maternal health programs for the poor dropped steadily in the 1980s. This drop in funding has led to higher rates of prematurity and related developmental disorders, such as cerebral palsy and mental retardation. The

savings gained in cutting money for prenatal programs is dwarfed by the costs of caring for premature babies.[1]

The new health care system should be directed not only toward preventing disease and integrating alternative approaches that help the body to heal itself, it should also be concerned about the whole, the world community, and preventing social conditions that foster disease and poor health.

Integrative Medicine

No system of medicine or health care has all of the answers. Conventional or Western medicine and health care do some things very well. "But conventional medicine manages crises so well that it tends to treat every condition as if it were a crisis."[30] Andrew Weil, a graduate of Harvard Medical School, has developed a new medical school residency curriculum at the University of Arizona that teaches what he terms integrative medicine. He maintains that if we would apply allopathic medicine only to crisis cases, then money would be saved and harm would not be done to the body's own ability to heal in the attempt to eliminate symptoms of a disease. He suggests that[30]:

Allopathic medicine and health care are appropriate for approximately 10% to 20% of all health problems, and that for the other 80% to 90%, where there is no emergency and where there is no need for strong measures, there is time to experiment with other methods, alternative therapies that are cheaper, safer, and ultimately more effective because they work with the body's healing mechanisms rather than working against them.

Weil's new 2-year fellowship for family and internal medicine physicians has the main goal to "emphasize the body's own healing system and healing potential so that doctors and patients will work from the premise that people can get better, that the body can heal itself, and that we should explore all available methods and ideas out there that can facilitate the process."[30] The fellowship begins with a course in the philosophy of science, "to train doctors to know what science is, what are its appropriate uses, and how to interpret scientific research." The next didactic area of study is the history of medicine, including traditional Chinese medicine and Ayurvedic medicine, placing a great emphasis on mind/body interactions. Fellows will also be instructed in the spirituality of medicine, emphasizing experiences of death and dying, and the birthing process. Finally, they will be required to master the universally useful approaches of interactive guided imagery, successful for stress-related illness, and the techniques of two of the following three alternative health care systems: osteopathic manipulation, medical acupuncture, and homeopathy.

Eventually, nurses and other practitioners will be invited into the program, and a long-term goal is to develop an integrative medical clinic devoted to patient care and research on patient outcomes. Patients will be matched for age and condition, one will be followed by the conventional medical clinic and the other by the integrative medical clinic. In this way, Weil hopes to collect the data that will start to turn around the resistance for funding of alternative therapies and therapy for prevention from insurance agencies and other funding sources. Fellows were accepted in June 1996 at the University of Arizona, Tucson.[30]

Because health care and medicine occupy a central place in our culture, Weil hopes that the changes in the care of people will spill over into other social systems and professions, and that the principles of holism will begin to be viewed as preferable to the current linear and fragmented way that we interact with one another in society and in the world.[30]

Conclusion

Healing and medical care were once synonymous in medicine, even in the United States, but are no longer.[1] The focus of medicine and health care in the 21st century has been on correct diagnosis of symptoms and on curing symptoms with the one best "magic bullet" available. High technology and reductionistic science have served us well in crisis medicine and in the cure of infectious disease. In the early 21st century, we may remember that one of the definitions of millennium is "a thousand years of peace and prosperity."[31] Current information, much more now than the wake-up call of the 1991 data from Eisenberg's study,[17] has indeed forecasted that consumers will find a way to be served by a health care system that returns the emphasis of care to the whole body's ability to heal itself, even as they receive the benefits of allopathic medicine.[12] Weil comments that this is one of the true benefits of capitalism. Neither consumers nor providers in business are bound by an ideology. Where the market goes, business goes, and consumers are helping to drive a rapidly changing health care system "market."[30]

What seems necessary is a form of medicine and health care that combines the best of allopathic medical care and holistic treatment. This text is offered as support to assist in beginning this paradigmatic shift. The shift is indeed occurring, with or without cooperation, and it would be in their best interest for health care practitioners, researchers, and teachers to be aware of how this shift is affecting their practice, and what research and credentialing methods are needed to help ensure the safety of patients.

When people are ready to acknowledge that it is far more important to link who we are in health care and what we do with healing and service with doing good for fellow members of our community rather than with just being part of a business whose job is to correctly diagnose a disease based on symptoms and then treat that disease alone, we will begin moving into our rightful place in society as health professionals.[1] When medical scientists agree to be flexible about what constitutes acceptable rigor or merit in research and minimize their suspicion of alternative approaches because these approaches appear to allow the body to heal itself by influencing all systems for the good (thus, these approaches fail to fit the criteria of rigorous science),[32] then we will see an even greater advancement of a health care system that more adequately meets the needs of citizens at less cost.

What is being asked for, and demanded by many, is health care based on the principles of holism that emphasize healing over curing, and that is safe, that is supported by systematic research whenever possible, and that is less costly and toxic. This new health care will bring to the world the safest, most cost effective, and most flexible system possible both for prevention and healing. What it means to help someone, really help a person, will then become clear to many of us for the first time.

References

1. Institute of Noetic Sciences, Poole W. *The Heart of Healing*. Atlanta, GA: Turner Publications; 1993.
2. Wallace RK, Benson H, Wilson AF. A wakeful hypometabolic physiologic state. *Am J Physiol*. 1971;221(3):795-799.
3. Ader R, Cohen N. The influence of conditioning on immune responses. In: Ader R, Felten DL, Cohen N, eds. *Psychoneuroimmunology*. 2nd ed. San Diego, CA: Academic Press; 1991:611-646.
4. Pavlov IP. *Lectures on Conditioned Reflexes*. New York, NY: Liveright; 1928.
5. Ader R, Cohen N, Felten D. Psychoneuroimmunology: interactions between the nervous system and the immune system. *Lancet*. 1995;345:99-103.
6. Mackenzie JN. The production of so-called "nose cold" by means of an artificial rose. *Am J Med Sci*. 1895;91:45-57.
7. Felten SY, Felten DL, Olschowka JA. Nonadrenergic and peptide innervation of lymphoid organs. *Chem Immunol*. 1992;52:25-48.
8. Cohen S, Tyrrell DAJ, Smith AP. Psychological stress and susceptibility to the common cold. *N Engl J Med*. 1991; 325:606-611.
9. Speigel D, Bloom JR, Kraemer HC, Gotteil E. Effect of psychosocial treatment in survival of patients with metastatic breast cancer. *Lancet*. 1989;888-891.
10. Galantino ML, McCormack GL. Pain management. In: Galantino ML. *Clinical Assessment and Treatment of HIV/ Rehabilitation of a Chronic Illness*. Thorofare, NJ: SLACK Incorporated; 1992:104-114.
11. LaPerriere A, Antoni M, Fletcher MA, Schneiderman N. Exercise and health maintenance in HIV. In: Galantino ML. *Clinical Assessment and Treatment of HIV/ Rehabilitation of a Chronic Illness*. Thorofare, NJ: SLACK Incorporated; 1992:65-76.

12. Kolata G. In quests outside mainstream, medical projects rewrite the rules. *New York Times National.* 1996; CXLV(50,462):A1,14.

13. Black PH. Psychoneuroimmunology: brain and immunity. *Scientific American.* 1995:16-25.

14. Alternative Medicine: Expanding Medical Horizons. Report to the NIH on Alternative Medical Systems of Practices in the United States. Pittsburgh, Pa: US Government Printing Office, Superintendent of Documents; 1992.

15. Rubik B. Energy medicine and the unifying concept of information. *Altern Ther Health Med.* 1995;1:34-36.

16. Hanten WP, Dawson DD, Jwata M, et al. Craniosacral rhythm: examination of interexaminer and intraexaminer reliability of palpation and relationships between the rhythm and cardiac and respiratory rates of the subject and examiner. *Phys Ther.* 1996;76(5):S5.

17. Eisenberg DM, Kessler RC, Foster C, et al. Unconventional medicine in the United States. *N Engl J Med.* 1993;328: 245-252.

18. Reynolds J. Profiles in alternatives. *PT Magazine.* 1994;2(9):52-59.

19. Borysenko J. The best medicine. *New Age Journal.* 1990;47:102-103.

20. Cassidy CM. Cultural context of complementary and alternative medicine. In: Micozzi MS, ed. *Fundamentals of Complementary and Alternative Medicine.* New York: Churchill Livingstone; 1996.

21. Davis CM. *Patient Practitioner Interaction: An Experiential Manual for Developing the Art of Health Care.* 2nd ed. Thorofare, NJ: SLACK Incorporated; 1994.

22. Seigel B. *Love, Medicine and Miracles.* New York, NY: Harper and Row; 1986.

23. Carmody J. The case: Bad care, good care, and spiritual preservation. *Second Opinion.* 1994;20(1):35-39.

24. Davis CM. What is empathy and can empathy be taught? *Phys Ther.* 1990;70(11):707-715.

25. Schleler M. *The Nature of Sympathy.* Hamden, CT: Anchor Books; 1970.

26. Wyschogrod E. Empathy and sympathy as tactile encounter. *J Med Phil.* 1981;6(1):25-34.

27. May WF. *The Physician as Healer/Images of the Healer in Medical Ethics.* Philadelphia, PA: Westminster Press; 1983.

28. Pellegrino ED. What is a profession? *J Allied Health.* 1983;12(3):168-176.

29. Stein E. *On the Problem of Empathy.* 2nd ed. The Hague, Netherlands: Martinus Nijhoff/Dr. W Junk; 1970.

30. Weil A. The body's healing systems/the future of medical education. *J Alt Comp Ther.* 1995;1(1):305-309.

31. *Webster's II/New Riverside Dictionary.* Boston, MA: Houghton Mifflin; 1984.

32. Harris S. How should treatments be critiqued for scientific merit? *Phys Ther.* 1996;76(2):175-181.

QUANTUM PHYSICS AND SYSTEMS THEORY
THE SCIENCE BEHIND COMPLEMENTARY AND ALTERNATIVE THERAPIES

Carol M. Davis, DPT, EdD, MS, FAPTA

Complementary and alternative therapies, also referred to as holistic therapies or energy medicine, are becoming more commonly researched in refereed journals since the initiation of the National Institutes of Health (NIH) Center for Complementary and Alternative Medicine and their awarding of grants. Few would disagree with the fact that more and more patients and clients are turning to holistic therapies as an adjunct to allopathic therapies. A recent issue of the *Journal of the American Medical Association*[1] reported increased use of alternative therapies because patients felt that this approach to healing was more consistent with their ideas about health and the body. But credible published research on the effectiveness of holistic therapies lags behind public acceptance, largely because these therapies and their mechanisms of action do not lend themselves for study by way of the gold standard of medical research—the randomized controlled trial. As a result, one may hear the opinion that complementary and alternative therapies should not be used because they are not science based, that is, they have not been proven to be effective according to the rules of medical science.

Most assuredly, when we stray from the reductionist model for verifying efficacy, we open ourselves to criticism and accusation of exploitation of patients as well as unscientific (even unsafe) practice. This chapter will review the current controversy over the use of complementary and alternative therapies as illustrated in the debate over noncontact therapeutic touch in a 1998 issue of the *Journal of the American Medical Association*.[2] Furthermore, it focuses on an explanation of the scientific theories behind holistic, energy-based therapies, specifically quantum physics, and systems theory. Mind/body health, central to the function of complementary therapies, will be described through the works of current scientists, and then citations of research that found clinical efficacy of the use of complementary therapies will follow. The chapter concludes with recognizing this paradigm shift in the foundations of medical science, from reductionism to holism, as a vehicle for the possible return of the concept of healing to health care, a service profession that is more commonly now referred to as an industry or business and, as such, has been largely criticized of late to be profit oriented and competitive.

The Struggle for Legitimacy: The Controversial Therapeutic Touch Article

In 1999, the American media took the opportunity to exploit the controversy over complementary therapies by highlighting the results of a sixth-grader's science fair project that was rewritten by her parents and submitted to the *Journal of the American Medical Association.* The article "launched an assault" on the alternative healing practice of noncontact Therapeutic Touch (TT).[3] It concluded that the failure of 21 experienced TT practitioners to detect the energy field of the investigator (the sixth grader who hovered her hands over one of the practitioner's hands) must mean that the beneficial claims of TT are groundless and further professional use of this therapy would be unjustified, and patients or clients should "refuse to pay" for this therapy. Subsequently, the article was judged to have serious methodological flaws.[3,4] Leskowitz[3] has published a full analysis of this critique, but in sum, judgment about this article concluded that the peer-review process for the journal apparently was altered; not only was there was no primary physician input, but several methodological flaws were cited. The authors' objectivity should have been questioned by virtue of their membership in the controversial organization, Quackwatch. The article claims logically inconsistent conclusions. The only logical conclusion that can be drawn from the experimental method was that the purported energy field of the hand of the experimenter could not be detected accurately by those sitting behind a screen exposing their hands to the test. No clinical treatments were given; thus, to conclude that TT is an ineffective therapeutic process because a purported mechanism of action was not found to be accurate is a huge leap. (For example, aspirin was used for decades successfully with its mechanism of action only becoming understood in the 1970s.) No mention was made of the possible effect of the mother's admitted skepticism on the energy field of the young experimenter. (Ambient electromagnetic fields are thought to be easily inhibited by several factors,[5-7] especially the intention of the participant.) An incomplete statistical analysis was offered (less than 50% of the correct answers were reported, so study results could not have been truly random) and a perfunctory literature review dismissing more than 800 documented studies on TT claiming inadequate validity, but failing to set standards for validity, round out the criticism of this controversial article.[3]

It is becoming more clear that attacks against holistic approaches simply because they do not lend themselves to proof of efficacy by the randomized controlled trial no longer carry blind acceptance from the community of professionals. That is not to say that holistic approaches should be exempt from careful study. The threat of patient exploitation is increased when there are unsubstantiated claims of patient benefit for new therapies. However, most holistic therapies are not new. They have been practiced as mainstream in other parts of the world for centuries and are now making their way into Western medicine as the limitations of traditional health care in the West, especially for patients with chronic illnesses and pain, become more frustrating for patients and practitioners alike.

The Paradigm Shift: Reductionism Enhanced by Holism

Chapter 1 describes the emergence of the science of mind/body medicine and health care, which is a more holistic view than that of reductionism. In truth, science never stands still. The current perspective that many in Western medical science tenaciously hold onto—the reductionist approach to the search for scientific truth, or cause and effect (instituted in the 17th century by French philosopher Rene Descartes and later perfected by the great mathematician Sir Isaac Newton) alone—is inadequate to explain some of the most compelling exceptions to current scientific theory. In the 1600s, science was inhibited by the prevailing view that illness and disease were the result of a capricious and punitive God. In an attempt to perfect the study of cause and effect,

Descartes declared that only that which could be perceived, the physical or material, would be studied, and the nonmaterial or ephemeral would fall under the purview of the church. Eventually this view led to the linear, reductionistic model of science, where that which is being studied is reduced to its smallest unit (ideally a molecule), and the structure that it may influence is reduced to its smallest unit (ideally a single cell type or even a part of the cell such as a receptor) to try to eliminate the effects on the outcome of the research of interfering variables or chance. Efforts then concentrated on perfecting our ways of perceiving that which exists in solid form, from the microscope and stethoscope to the tremendous advances in medical technology of the 20th century. At the same time, with this linear and reductionistic theoretical framework, there has been an unsuccessful shift toward finding the "magic bullet" to cure disease. The pharmaceutical industry has dominated health care, and its research and development efforts have helped drive up the cost of health care. With these and other events happening over the past decades, the 20th century ended with a crisis in health care with private insurance corporations making major medical care decisions with profit for stock holders and CEOs foremost, and managed competition coming under more intense criticism for patient abuse and neglect. The profession of medicine has never been under more intense disfavor.

Studying the macroscopic—the material world only—and ignoring nonmaterial reality (such as motivation, consciousness, and the role of the transcendent or faith in illness) fails to explain the profound effects of the invisible, the nonmaterial, or what we cannot perceive. Important exceptions to theory that lie outside the explanatory power of Newtonian physics currently are accumulating and can no longer be tossed aside as interesting "outliers." For example, reports and studies revealing the spontaneous remission of space-inhabiting tumors,[8] extrasensory perception, clinical intuition,[9] the power of prayer to help people heal,[10] and the impact of loving touch on premature infants[11] are extremely important and relevant examples of events that Newtonian physics and Cartesian logic cannot explain. The search for truth, for plausible explanations of what is happening in these instances recorded in studies of health care and healing, can no longer rely on the validity of the "scientific facts" generated largely by the randomized controlled trial and grounded in traditional Newtonian physics.

Holistic Approaches and Body Energy: The Importance of Flow

Holistic approaches, or complementary and alternative therapies, have in common what the World Health Organization refers to as[12]:

> ...care wherein people are viewed in totality within a wide ecological spectrum and which emphasizes the view that ill health or disease is brought about by an imbalance, or disequilibrium, of a person in his or her total ecological system and not only by the causative agent and pathogenic evolution.

The totality of the person is often referred to in holistic health as incorporating not just the body, but four quadrants of need and function: the physical (body and movement), the intellectual (brain and mind), the emotional (feelings), and spiritual (desire to know the nature of self, purpose for living, questions relating to the transcendent aspect of life). Complementary and alternative therapies focus on impacting all four quadrants of meaning and function and emphasize the scientifically validated link between the mind and body.[5,13-17] In contrast to reducing the variables, or finding the magic bullet, these therapies are administered to impact the whole of the person in an effort to help a client or patient recover from illness and/or injury (and to stay healthy) by facilitating the person's flow of natural energy, or ch'i. Holistic theory, the foundation for medicine and health care practiced in most areas of the world outside of the West, suggests that ch'i is responsible for health and homeostasis when it is free flowing and balanced. In other words, a human's natural state is to be "healed," and the body/mind can, and does, heal itself continuously.

The evidence that people heal themselves continually is the foundation of the rationale for the double-blind, placebo-based clinical trial. Blocks to ch'i interfere with health and render the body/mind vulnerable to succumbing to pathogens, or biochemical imbalance. These blocks to the flow of natural energy can occur from disruptions in each of the four quadrants of need and function. In sum, rather than "fixing" the ill or injured, facilitating self-healing is the goal of holistic practice.

The Controversy of Ch'i

The concept of the body emitting an energy (ch'i) has been accepted in traditional Chinese medicine for centuries, but in the West is controversial, in part because it has been impossible to identify the structure of the pathways of the energy flow, referred to as meridians. Likewise, it has been difficult to measure "whole body" energy, in contrast to the measurement of energy produced by the work of various body organs, such as muscle energy (EMG), cardiac energy (EKG, ECG), and brain energy (EEG). However, the work of Valerie Hunt[18] seems to be moving the scientific community toward the acceptance of recording body energy—or more accurately, the body/mind—in valid and reliable ways. Hunt has succeeded in constructing an experimental environment that successfully filters out interfering energy from the earth's core and surroundings. It is accepted in Western medicine that many lymph channels cannot be isolated, yet the flow of lymph is not questioned. Like airline travel routes that exist on a map but cannot be "seen," meridians have been charted on the map of the human by the Chinese and used successfully in the manipulation of body energy for the health and healing of people using acupuncture and acupressure for centuries. Recently, a consensus conference at the NIH on the published research on acupuncture issued a recommendation that body energy, as described in the research as ch'i, be studied more diligently.[19]

Scientific Foundations of Complementary Therapies

How can clinicians explain the documented positive outcomes and what they observe is happening with patients when holistic therapies are applied? If traditional Newtonian physics fall short in offering theoretical explanations, where can we turn for a more comprehensive approach to the description of reality? The current view is that the results from holistic therapies are more adequately explained by Einstein's quantum physics and by systems theory from the biological sciences.

To explain, one must start with the basic structure of all matter, seen and unseen. Atoms are often referred to as the "building blocks" of all that we know as real. The Periodic Chart of the Elements categorizes all discovered atoms according to their atomic weight, or the number of electrons they have revolving around the nucleus. Newtonian physics states that what is real is solid and is made up of atoms joining together to form molecules that, in turn, form solid discrete bits of matter with clearly differentiated boundaries. What is real is thus relegated solely to matter that we can perceive with our senses, but quantum physics developed by Einstein, Plank, Bohr, and others tells us that just because we cannot perceive a part of all that is real (the nonmaterial, the nonlocal, the invisible) does not mean that it does not exist and is not present interacting in meaningful ways with what we do perceive.

Atoms make very strange building blocks because the relative space between the nucleus and the orbiting electrons is very vast. The power of the electron charge seems to make it "feel" very dense. It was the behavior of the electron rather than the entire atom that interested quantum physicists. Einstein, Plank, Bohr, Bohm, and others were interested not just in the atom and molecule, but in the function of the subatomic particles that make up the atom, specifically of electrons, what their properties were, and how electrons interacted to form substances.

Most uniquely, quantum physics takes into account the role of the nonmaterial, especially consciousness, in the physical world.[20] In traditional materialistic theory, the invisible consciousness of the examiner is considered separate from any part of what is being examined, whereas in holistic theory that is grounded in quantum physics, this separation is not thought to exist. The subject being examined is affected by the examiner in ways that cannot be perceived directly. Foundational to mainstream traditional "objective" science is the theory that the knower and the known are thought to exist in completely separate domains; the boundaries of solid mass clearly separate matter into discrete parts. However, electrons and subatomic particles do not appear to be composed solely of solid matter. Electrons under certain circumstances behave as if they are solid particles, but under other circumstances disappear into invisible waves. Also, in some experiments, electrons are observed to take instantaneous jumps from one atomic orbit to another, with no intervening time and no journey through space—an impossible feat for a solid particle.[21] Quantum physics maintains that the behavior of subatomic particles has everything to do with the qualities of solid matter, as they form the building blocks of matter. However, quantum physics has experimentally shown that there is no such thing as "solid" matter, only what appears to be solid because our brains "interpret" what we see as solid.

The Copenhagen interpretation of quantum physics maintains that there is no such thing as strict causality because precise predictions for individual subatomic particles are impossible. There is no such thing as locality, for once two or more subatomic particles have interacted, they are instantaneously connected, even across astronomical distances; what is done to one is immediately reflected in the other, faster than any communication over distance could account for. Finally, if all subatomic particles are connected nonlocally, then any view that holds that particles can be reduced or separated and isolated is untenable.[21] Not all physicists accept the Copenhagen interpretation as valid, but several experiments in the 1980s produced results that confirmed these predictions consistently.[6,22,23]

These results, however, do not invalidate materialism altogether. In the everyday world of macroscopic objects, the mechanistic theories of Newtonian physics are approximately correct, which is why much of health care has been able to rely on it so successfully. At the fundamental, subatomic level, there is a totally different world-view that incorporates both macroscopic and microscopic realities, where the traditional laws of space and time do not apply. Many physicists now argue that the nature of reality is that it is composed primarily not of discrete physical particles, but of probability waves that are a function of intelligence alone.[22] Thus, the world is made up of wave/particles, and our brains interpret the vibration of the particles (1044 times per second) as solid, much in the same way that our brains translate 24 still frames per second into the motion of a movie; interpret the individual notes and rests of a symphony into the melody; and interpret the flash of red, blue, and green electrons on a special screen as a moving television picture. From the quantum perspective, the "perception of our brains" creates the sharp edges of the world we see. However, as anyone who is color blind will tell us, we each see the world as it is displayed on our individual retinas and interpreted by our individual perceptions, in spite of the fact that we share common cultural agreements about what constitutes, for example, the green of grass or the blue of sky.

Systems Theory

Holistic theory holds that the whole is always more than the sum of the parts. Quantum physics, with its wave/particle nature of electrons, makes this possible. Everything that is known of reality is an inextricable part of a larger system, from the smallest part of the universe, the electrons of the atoms of the DNA of, for example, the mitochondria, which is part of the system of the cell, which is part of the system of the blood, which is part of the circulatory system, which is part of the body/mind of the person, who is part of a family system, which is part of the community, which is located in a city, in a state, in a country, in a hemisphere, in an ecology system on the planet, and the planet is part of the solar system, which is part of the cosmos, and so on. Nothing that is made up of molecules with shared electrons can be isolated from that with which it interrelates. One cannot truly know the nature of water by studying hydrogen or oxygen alone. One must study what happens when the electrons of two hydrogen atoms and one oxygen atom interrelate, share orbits, and interact with each other to form the larger system of water. To reduce the water to its one oxygen atom, then experiment with that oxygen atom and conclude that the outcome of the experiment impacted water would be a false conclusion.

Holism holds that the same is true for the human. We cannot reduce a person to a cell or to one system alone, study the impact of a variable on the part of the system, and then truly know how the entire system was affected without collecting data on the outcome to the entire system. Since there are so many systems and so many variables, this has proven to be too difficult, so science has simply adopted reductionism as its best attempt to determine cause and effect, and acted as if the human can be separated into parts to be studied. The difficulties of this stretch of the imagination can be profoundly experienced, for example, in the various toxic side effects of medications.

Holistic therapies use whatever the human being offers in the moment of therapy as the focus of attention (eg, pain, headache, fascial restrictions, fatigue, malaligned posture), and by way of the manipulation of the energy of the client and the practitioner, these therapies attempt to influence the whole of the person by unblocking energy that is blocked or imbalanced, restoring length to soft tissue and homeostasis. The myofascial release practitioner, for example, attempts to lengthen tight fascia and balance the craniosacral rhythm; the noncontact TT practitioner balances the energy flow around the body; the Feldenkrais practitioner attempts to help the person analyze and feel alternatives to habitual ways of moving, thus providing greater choice of efficient posture and movement, and opening up the mind to consider movement and position in space in a totally new way. We do not yet know how this takes place, nor how to measure the mechanism of action between the practitioner and client or patient. Current science is attempting to craft a new paradigm for energy medicine, in part by measuring the energy output from the hands of healers and describing the effects of that energy,[24] through careful study of what happens to ch'i during the administration of therapy[18] and careful study of the nature of electron interaction and how electrons interrelate with each other.[24-27] The research cited here is just a small portion of what can be found in the literature and is offered as a starting point for the reader who is interested in this area of inquiry.

Research Evidence

A review of the literature and reading the chapters in this text reveal that in the past 10 years there has been a quantum leap in researching the effectiveness of complementary and alternative therapies. In 1998, the Office of Alternative Medicine at the NIH was upgraded to the Center for the Study of Complementary and Alternative Medicine, and several universities and health centers now compete for funding, for example, on the efficacy of therapeutic touch and manual therapies, massage, acupuncture, and magnets. Psychoneuroimmunology (PNI) is an established research unit at many medical universities, and the outcomes of this research have impacted dramatically, for one example, the treatment of patients with AIDS. Substantial bodies of evidence exist, for example, on biofeedback, acupuncture, and the use of botanicals. T'ai Chi as a treatment modality is receiving a good deal of attention among those interested in falls prevention.[7] Much of this research is published in European languages such as French and German, but one issue of *Physical Medicine and Rehabilitation Clinics in North America* (August 1999) was devoted to reporting the evidence on the use of holistic therapies. Several texts have been published[28-31] including the text *Complementary and Alternative Medicine: An Evidence-Based Approach*,[32] written by the former director of the Office of Alternative Medicine, which summarizes much of the research up until 1999. Several journals (peer reviewed and not) now report various levels of research in complementary and alternative therapies, including *Advances in Mind/Body Medicine* (Fetzer Institute), *Subtle Energies and Energy Medicine* (International Society for the Study of Subtle Energies and Energy Medicine), *Journal of Alternative and Complementary Medicine/Research on Paradigm, Practice and Policy* (Mary Ann Liebert, Inc, publishers), *Alternative Therapies in Health and Medicine* (Innovision Communications), *Noetic Sciences Review* (Institute for Noetic Sciences), and the *Journal of Consciousness Studies/Controversies in Science and the Humanities* (Imprint Academic of the United Kingdom).

Conclusion

This chapter began with the report of a recent, rather contentious episode in the history of the development of medical science wherein a rather poorly written research article in a major medical journal came up with less than well-founded conclusions criticizing one complementary therapy. Holistic approaches are unique and do not lend themselves to the randomized controlled trial for proof of efficacy. In 1997, the Council on Scientific Affairs of the American Medical Association suggested that "physicians should evaluate the scientific perspectives of unconventional theories for treatment and practice, looking particularly at potential utility, safety, and efficacy of these modalities."[33] Whereas reductionistic theory is based on traditional, linear, competitive views of reality that stress exclusion and win-lose strategies, holistic theory is circular and oriented toward inclusion and win-win strategies. The fact that noncontact TT has resulted in positive outcomes for thousands, as documented in the literature, does not mean that it should take the place of traditional forms of therapy, some of which have been shown to be efficacious by traditional science. Nontraditional, holistic therapies are being investigated as they are being practiced, with the hope that once shown to be helpful they will be accepted as complementary to traditional forms of therapy. In this way, complementary and alternative therapies will help expand the current medical science paradigm to include the manifestations of quantum physics-energy medicine. Perhaps, then, in the West there can be a return to a focus on what helps patients to heal, rather than on dividing up treatment times into appropriate units for billing purposes and referring to this as "therapy."

Holistic therapies, based on quantum physics and systems theory, emphasize evaluation and treatment of the whole person and application of whatever treatment modalities that help people to return to their natural state of healing, facilitated by enhancing the flow of body energy, or ch'i. Perhaps in the 21st century, observations will be refined to be able to more clearly explain the positive benefits of healing energy, even as it is manifested in careful listening and nurturing touch. For now, one can practice holistically even with empathic listening skills. The growing body of evidence in holistic complementary and alternative therapies represents the growing edge of the science of health care, and the subtle but powerful shift to a new paradigm of medical science that incorporates both traditional Newtonian physics and quantum physics will undoubtedly yield rich rewards for patients and practitioners alike. This text is an attempt to help stimulate that positive change.

References

1. Astin JA. Why patients use alternative medicine: results of a national study. *JAMA*. 1998;279:1548.
2. Rosa L, Rosa E, Sarner L, et al. A close look at therapeutic touch. *JAMA*. 1998;279:1005.
3. Leskowitz E. Un-debunking therapeutic touch. *Alternative Therapies*. 1998;4(4):101.
4. Achterberg J. Clearing the air in the therapeutic touch controversy. *Alternative Therapies*. 1998;4(4):100-101.
5. Pert CB. *Molecules of Emotion*. New York, NY: Scribner; 1997.
6. Rarity JG, Tapster PR. Experimental violation of Bell's inequality based on phase and momentum. *Physical Rev Let*. 1990;64:2495.

7. Wolf SL, Barnhart HX, Ellison GL, et al. The effect of Tai Chi Quan and computerized balance training on postural stability in older subjects. *Phys Ther.* 1997;77(4):371.

8. Chopra D. *Quantum Healing: Exploring the Frontiers of Mind/Body Medicine.* New York: Bantam Books; 1989.

9. Schulz ML. *Awakening Intuition: Using Your Mind-Body Network for Insight and Healing.* New York, NY: Harmony Books; 1998.

10. Dossey L. *Healing Words: The Power of Prayer and the Practice of Medicine.* San Francisco, CA: Harper; 1993.

11. Field T, Schanberg S, Scafidi F, et al. Tactile/kinesthetic stimulation effects on preterm neonates. *Pediatrics.* 1986; 77(5):154.

12. World Health Organization. *Traditional Medicine.* Washington, DC: WHO Publications; 1978.

13. Ader R, Cohen N. The influence of conditioning on immune response. In: Ader R, Felten DL, Cohen N, eds. *Psychoneuroimmunology.* 2nd ed. San Diego, CA: Academic Press; 1991:611.

14. Pert CB, Ruff Mr, Weber RJ, et al. Neuropeptides and their receptors: A psychosomatic network. *J Immunol.* 1985; 35:2.

15. Pert CB. Healing ourselves and society. *Presentation to the Elmwood Symposium* (unpublished). Boston, MA; 1989.

16. Pert CB. The wisdom of the receptors: neuropeptides, the emotions and bodymind. *Advances.* 1986;3(3):8.

17. Wallace RK, Benson H, Wilson AF. A wakeful hypometabolic physiological state. *Amer J Physiol.* 1971;221(3): 795.22.

18. Hunt VV. *Infinite Mind: The Science of the Human Vibrations of Consciousness.* Malibu, Calif: Malibu Publishing; 1989.

19. National Institutes of Health. Acupuncture consensus statement and literature review. *The Integrative Medicine Consult.* 1999;1(3):23.

20. Stapp HP. *Mind, Matter and Quantum Mechanics.* New York, NY: Springer-Verlag; 1994.

21. Sharman HM. Maharishi Ayurveda. In: Micozzi MS, ed. *Fundamentals of Complementary and Alternative Medicine.* New York, NY: Churchill-Livingstone; 1996:244.

22. Aspect A, Grangier P, Roger G. Experimental tests of realistic local theories via Bell's theorem. *Physical Rev Let.* 1990;47:460.

23. Aspect A. Bell's inequality test: more ideal than ever. *Nature.* 1999;398:188.

24. Rubik B. Energy medicine and the unifying concept of information. *Alternative Therapies.* 1995;1(1):34.

25. de Quincey C. Old roots of a new science: historical review. *Noetic Sciences Review,* 1993;Winter:30.

26. Schwartz GE, Russek LG. Dynamical energy systems and modern physics: fostering the science and spirit of complementary and alternative medicine. *Alternative Therapies.* 1997;3(3):46.

27. Walleczek J. Bioelectromagnetics and the question of "subtle energies." *Noetic Sciences Review.* 1993;Winter:33.

28. Davis CM. *Complementary Therapies in Rehabilitation: Holistic Approaches for Prevention and Wellness.* Thorofare, NJ: SLACK Incorporated; 1997.

29. Horstman J. *Arthritis Foundation's Guide to Alternative Therapies.* Atlanta, GA: Arthritis Foundation; 1999.

30. Micozzi MS. Characteristics of complementary and alternative medicine. In: MS Micozzi, ed. *Fundamentals of Complementary and Alternative Medicine.* New York, NY: Churchill-Livingstone; 1996:5.

31. Micozzi MS, ed. *Current Review of Complementary Medicine.* Philadelphia, PA: Current Medicine; 1999.

32. Spencer JW, Jacobs JJ. *Complementary and Alternative Medicine: An Evidence-Based Approach.* St. Louis, MO: Mosby; 1999.

33. Dickey NW. Foreword. In: Spencer JW, Jacobs JJ, eds. *Complementary and Alternative Medicine: An Evidence-Based Approach.* St. Louis, MO: Mosby; 1995:x.

CHAPTER 4

ADVANCES IN THE SCIENCE OF ENERGY MEDICINE

VIBRATION, PHOTONS, AND THE ZERO POINT FIELD

Carol M. Davis, DPT, EdD, MS, FAPTA

Introduction

This is a time of paradox in medical care in that two different things can both be true. Many of us, ourselves or our loved ones, have faced frightening critical illness, but thorough the miracles of chemotherapy and/or surgery have survived that life-threatening event and moved on to live healthy lives. We are so grateful for the medical research in cancer and infectious diseases that has allowed loved ones who would have died even 10 years ago to live. Likewise, more and more people are taking responsibility for their own health, quitting smoking, eating less trans fats, and getting more regular exercise. These are wonderful signs that indicate that modern medicine is helping us to live in more healthy ways.

However, it is also true to say that health care professionals today practice *disease management* more than *health care*. In spite of the fact that many health care insurance plans reimburse for an annual physical exam, it is still far easier to obtain third party reimbursement for therapy related to treating disease than for fostering health and healing.

It is also true that many health professionals are not happy with the way politics and business has co-opted the profession that they spent many years preparing for in order simply to serve. Service has too often yielded to business and profit, and there is great unhappiness and a deep desire for meaningful change.

Patients and clients are growing more discontented with a health care system that emphasizes the idea that good health is elusive, not a natural state of balance, and the pathway to long life and happiness lies in pharmacology. Medicine and surgery have both saved lives and also let the public down repeatedly, and thousands of people die each year of the side effects of medication, of iatrogenic diseases caught while being hospitalized and of medical malpractice mistakes.

With this growing backdrop, as people read and become more informed, they are claiming health as a natural state, realizing that the body/mind is meant to be healthy, and maintaining life-long health involves a process of unifying mind, body, and spirit. Energy medicine practices, or complementary therapies, are now commonly viewed as a healthier alternative to pharmacology and traditional medicine, particularly for chronic illness.

Yet, medical establishment leaders and government-supported medical researchers are slow to embrace energy-based therapies. Some of the reasons for this are undoubtedly political. Further, because the research on energy-based therapies often must wander from the gold standard randomized controlled trial, as energy is a very elusive subject to pin down, traditional medical science rejects energy-based therapies as unproven. You can only measure energy by the work it does, indirectly. It does not lend itself to validation and reliability measures that are the hallmark of reductionism. How do you research something you cannot measure? Many scientists still say you cannot, and dismiss bioenergetic therapies and the hypotheses on which they are based as pseudoscience, all the while acknowledging the limitations of traditional medicine.

But the train has left the station. People are turning to energy-based therapies over traditional health care in ever-increasing numbers because of their positive effects. More and more young scientists are publishing their hypotheses about the mechanisms of action of bioenergy therapies, based in an unfolding discovery of quantum physics, the physics of subatomic particles, and how they affect us and the world we live in. We are living in a major paradigm shift regarding our understanding of how the universe really "works" and the reality of what we perceive with our five senses.

The Mystery of Photons

Quantum physics is a mystery, difficult to read and understand, even by the most talented of scientists. Yet, more and more we are learning that the mysteries of this world of invisible waves has a major impact on the world we perceive as solid.

Adult learning theory states that adults need to be able to integrate new ideas with what they already know if they are going to keep—and use—new information. Information that conflicts sharply with what is already held to be true, and thus forces a re-evaluation of the old material, is integrated more slowly. Information that has little conceptual overlap with what is already known is acquired slowly.

Quantum physics asks us to believe in forces that are too small to see or hear or feel or touch directly, but quantum physicists are, in greater numbers, writing and speaking about how they have determined that our universe really works, and how quantum events, particularly the action of subatomic photons, little packets of light, are affecting our body/minds every moment of every day. This new information is difficult to integrate because it diverges sharply with what we believe to be true from what we see and experience in the real world. Yet, science reminds us that the evidence is now incontrovertible that this real world as we know it constitutes only 4% of all that is; 96% of all that is, is "dark" to us, dark or un-seeable energy and matter.[1,2] How do we access it if it is dark? How do we discover what effects this 96% of "all-that-is" has on us as human beings, and on the world as we know it? That discovery is happening in wondrous ways now, as the new science unfolds.

The Unfolding Awareness of What Constitutes the "New Science"

The new science, sometimes referred to as "noetic" science, is becoming more refined as each year passes in this new century. In the first edition of *Complementary Therapies in Rehabilitation*, published in 1997, we presented the science of "psychoneuroimmuniology," or mind/body science, as a key feature of the new science—science that was diverging from traditional Newtonian physics that emphasized reductionism and measurement of parts of a whole to determine cause and effect. Spurred on by the outbreak of HIV and the recognition that exercise as a treatment had a measurable positive effect on both body and mind, on both the immune system and on mental state such as depression, psychoneuroimmunology bridged the body/mind dichotomy that had been practiced in reductionistic science and medicine since the 1600s. With this work, and the discoveries of National Institutes of Health (NIH) researcher Candace Pert,[3] we recognize that the mind and body were inseparable parts of one whole, and that the mind is not found in the cranium, but is located throughout the entire body in various communication systems that inform each and every cell of what is happening to the whole, and that emotions and thought, activities of the mind, had a direct effect on all the cells of the body. The details of how that cell-to-cell transmission takes place remained mysterious, but we knew from Pert's work that the molecules of emotion were being transmitted, in part, by endocrine, neurotransmitter, and neuropeptide molecules, and perhaps other unknown messengers.

In the second edition of this text, published in 2004, we introduced quantum physics and systems theory as the sciences that offered more of a sound theoretical base to the understanding of what might underlie the mechanism of action of energy-based, holistic complementary therapies. We went into as much detail as we could understand about the relevance of electron and subatomic particle action to the physiology of mind and body, and the importance of recognizing that the whole is more than the sum of all the parts.

Now, in this third edition, many more advances have been made in bringing the knowledge of how the universe really "works" to the understanding of possible mechanisms of action in health and healing, illness and disease, and how complementary therapies that impact people in all areas of need and function—physically, intellectually, emotionally, spiritually, and socially—really work. The new science—science that is holistic rather than reductionistic and based on enfolding Newtonian physics into quantum physics—is undergoing a wave of new discoveries that relate directly to the health of people and the health of the earth and the entire universe.

The New Science and How It Relates to the Old Science

Cellular biologist Bruce Lipton summarized the path from reductionism to holism.[4] To understand nature and the human experience, we must transcend the "parts" aspect that was focused upon in reductionism, (to understand the whole, divide it into as many small parts as possible and study all of the parts, and then you will understand the whole) and look more toward the integration and coordination of all parts of the universe, both material and immaterial, into a larger whole. This revisioning of conventional science to a new or noetic science will, Lipton believes, "rescue us from extinction."

Lipton states that conventional or traditional science can be seen as hierarchical, with basic scientific theories supporting, or giving foundation to upper level knowledge (Figure 4-1). At the base of all traditional scientific understanding is *mathematics*, the laws of which are absolute, certain, and indisputable. Built upon our understanding of math is *physics* and built upon physics are the laws of *chemistry*. The laws and science of chemistry support the next tier, *biology*, and biology supports the final top layer—*psychology*.[4]

The new science is expanding our understanding on all 5 of these levels. For example, our growing understanding of the laws of mathematics is enhanced by the disciplines of *fractal geometry* and *chaos theory*. Fractal geometry informs us that all that we can see and know in the physical universe is derived from the integration and interconnectivity of all the parts, often turned back on themselves in common patterns that repeat over and over from the branching of tributaries of a river, to the branching of veins in a leaf, and capillaries in a section of living tissue. Most important, in the larger view, cooperation and harmony seem to trump the old dictum of survival of the fittest as the predominant descriptor of how the universe organizes itself. Chaos theory proves that

Figure 4-1. Traditional scientific understanding.

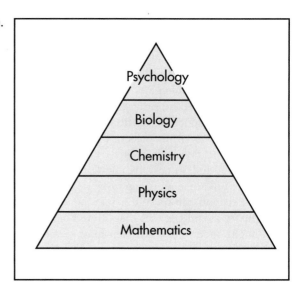

ultimately, if one waits long enough, there is underlying order in even the most chaotic of events, and, more important, small changes have huge impact in nature when we take a longer, larger view. To prematurely interrupt a process as it unfolds to its order, even for the noblest of reasons, can result in the kind of devastation that we are experiencing in the growing disaster of the warming of the atmosphere, the steady decline in colonies of honeybees, the extinction of so many species of plants and animals that sustain a balanced and ordered planet. We acted as if the earth were a "thing," ours to manipulate for our own advancement, not as if the earth were a balanced, living entity that would suffer globally from our manipulations.

The changes in our understanding of *physics* emerge out of our mounting awareness of the *nature of mind, or consciousness, as non-local.* Books on the nature of consciousness, *The Field: The Quest for the Secret Force of the Universe,*[5] *The Law of Attraction*[6] and the *Secret,*[7] have caught the attention of those who are both excited and terrified to contemplate that we may actually be able to effect, even to create, what happens to us day to day by what we pay attention to, what we think about, and what we observe. Consciousness studies unfold the concept that thought is, indeed, matter in wave form, and that the universe is made up of far more than the 4% of matter that we can experience with our five senses. People are beginning to consider what Einstein, Planck, Bohr, Bohm, and Heisenberg wrote about in the first half of the 20th century as having practical validity in their lives—that the universe is not a bunch of solid physical parts, but is instead an entanglement of vibrating energy waves a small portion of which our senses interpret as hard matter, and that the observer of all of this actually creates what is observed out of wave form. Lately, exciting theory has been offered regarding the invisible energy field that surrounds us, and how our interaction with this field at the quantum level affects our health and our vibrational balance.[8]

The third level, *chemistry*, is expanding its theoretical base by focusing on the true nature of solid matter (ie, the atoms that are made up of nuclei and spinning subatomic electrons and other particles such as photons). These subatomic particles turn out not to be solid at all, but to be made up of vibrating strings or immaterial energy vortices such as quarks. As such, vibrational chemistry concerns itself with *"the role of vibration in creating atomic bonds and driving molecular interactions."* We know that chemical reactions that take place regularly in our bodies can be influenced by vibration, be it from free radical action from the food we eat, or from vibration of our cell phones or from our thoughts. The idea that how we think about the food we eat can actually affect how the body digests that food is the stuff of vibrational chemistry.[4]

The new *biology* rejects the theory that, if we understand fully all of the parts, down to the smallest cells, the whole will be made clear. *Noetic biology posits that all that is physical is energetically entangled with and influenced by the vibrational space that surrounds us, the zero point field.*[8] In addition, the new biology endorses Lovelock's hypothesis that *"the Earth and the biosphere represent a single living and breathing entity known as Gaia."*[9] Noetic biology also endorses the science of *epigenetics*, the recognition that underlying the genetic code of the DNA is another force that is influenced by vibration, thought, perception of the environment, etc and, in fact, vibration actually dictates the "on-off" function of the genes. In other words, perception and consciousness, bioenergetic vibrations, trump genetic determinism.[10]

Finally, *energetic psychology* focuses on the idea that our perceptions control our lives; that the life we experience evolves from the *vibration of thought and the meanings we give to our thoughts and perceptions.* Physiochemical processes are placed in a wider context of the role of energy fields and how our subconscious gets programmed by our thoughts. The focus then lifts from stopping with a pharmaceutical management of body chemistry and analytical analysis of repeatedly going over "what went wrong in our lives," to teaching people how to evaluate the nature of their thinking, and then, in the moment, choose thoughts that are more resonant with relief, with decreased resistance and with gratitude. The attention shifts from emphasizing the negative to helping people describe and create experiences for themselves and for their children that enhance joy and appreciation. With the choice to change a thought comes a change in the entire body chemistry and mood. Practicing hope and optimism results in a happier, less stressful, and longer life.[11]

Bioenergetics: The New Science of Healing

Bioenergetics has been termed the "new science of healing."[10] We now know that we are vibrating, bioenergetic beings, but in our mechanistic tradition we have treated illness as a chemical imbalance, resolved by adding or altering body chemistry to restore balance. As a result, we have searched for remedy almost exclusively in the use of pharmaceuticals to alter natural chemistry, or surgery to repair and replace diseased or damaged "parts" without a diligent effort to understand the concomitant effects of either practice on the whole of us—physical, intellectual, emotional and spiritual aspects.

The Paradigm Shift:
Chemical to Vibrational or Bioenergetic

What if all illness were perceived not as a chemical imbalance primarily, but as a *vibrational imbalance*, resulting from an alteration in the natural healthy frequency of vibration of cells that then upsets the chemical balance and harmony in our living systems? How would this change our view of meaningful interventions for pain and illness?

James Oschman, both a new scientist and an excellent reviewer of new science states[13]:

> *From observing the successes of many different kinds of energy therapists, I have come to the radical conclusion that there is only one kind of problem that arises in the human body, one way to diagnose that problem, and one way of treating it. The common denominator is energy. All of those conditions we refer to as diseases stem from an energetic imbalance located somewhere in our body. And all of our successful treatments come from correcting that imbalance... The common denominator to all chronic disease is inflammation, caused by free radicals which are fundamentally electronic and energetic in nature.*

He goes on to say that energy therapists have one intention—to effect the imbalance in energy, to affect the "local density of electric polarization, and this affects inflammation,"[13] whether by manual therapies, cold laser or pulsed electromagnetic fields therapy.

Inflammation, the production of free radicals, is responsible for the body's being able to heal itself. These unstable molecules lack one or more electrons, and to restore electrical balance, the molecule must steal an electron from another molecule, thus destroying bacteria, viruses and cellular debris. Problems arise when free radicals persist after they have done their clean up job, turning acute inflammation into chronic disease, and free radicals attack normal cells, proteins, DNA and lipids. The body needs an antioxidant defense to scavenge the free radicals and render them harmless, and then restore damaged molecules.[14-16]

Electromagnetic healing devices such as low level laser and pulsed electromagnetic field therapy introduce electrons into the system, which are the ultimate antioxidants. The energy field that is emitted from the hands of skilled holistic manual therapists may be accomplishing the same effect.[13]

The Possible Interaction of the Body/Mind With the Surrounding Zero Point Field

Mark Comings, a new science theoretical physicist and engineer has long been studying the nature of what we know as energy, and how living systems engage with energy. In a recent article, Comings suggests the following:[16]

> Nobel Prize physiologist and biophysicist A.V. Hill, and later, physiologist D.R. Wilkie, proved that the amount of energy that is needed to drive muscle contraction exceeds the amount of energy produced by the mitochondria. Where does that extra energy come from? Researchers do not yet know. One path of discovery would be to investigate other chemical processes within the body that might be contributing to this energy. Another, perhaps "deeper," path would be to ponder the possible contribution of energy from the space that surrounds us, from the quantum vacuum state or the zero point field, that is not a vacuum at all, but is filled with energy.

So-called "empty" space is enormously full of energy. "Space is, in fact, a very energy dense medium filled with radiant potential to degrees that far exceed, by many orders of magnitude, the energies constituting matter."[17] This subtle energy matrix that surrounds us, which we move about in, much like the water that surrounds swimming fish, influences our physiological and biological systems in ways that are just beginning to be understood. It all has to do with the science of bioenergetics and vibration.[8,6,17]

We know that living organisms are literally efflorescing with biophotons which are more and more being understood to be fundamental to their functioning. Even in the darkest of dark environments, living organisms give off light, photons from within. Comings offers this:[16]

> Looking at life in the context of the "quantum plenum," or energetic space that surrounds us, we can say that because space is also itself radiating an enormously intense flux of vacuum photons, they must be pervading and thus somehow influencing living systems in fundamental ways that are not yet comprehended. Perhaps all this work going on in biophotonics needs to be contextualized within the pre-existing radiant flux of vacuum photons... or what I would prefer to call "plenum photons"... a large flux of which characterize the nature of space at a fundamental level.

We are on the threshold of a quantum shift in understanding how the body/mind interacts with low frequency electromagnetic activity in the atmosphere which encompasses everything and may influence how we think and function. Physicist EA Rauscher says this:[17]

> I started out as a skeptic about the concept that such low intensity and low frequency fields could affect humans and animals so profoundly. Magnetic and electromagnetic fields emitted from the earth are fundamentally related to life, which evolved on this planet. Certain frequencies affect brain waves of humans, and canines, one of which is one of the main frequencies that is emitted by photon interactions with the upper atmosphere ...around 9.4 Hz... the brain wave frequency of a relaxed state of mind.

The Role of Fascia in Quantum Communication

Oschman emphasizes the importance of the fascia in healthy functioning of the mind/body.[18,19] He maintains that biological communication systems (nervous system, circulatory system, endocrine system, immune system) do not adequately explain what we observe in outcomes, particularly the speed with which a human can respond to various stimuli. He suggests that there is a high speed, body-wide energetic communication system that includes the nervous, circulatory, and immune systems, but also includes all the other systems in the body. He calls this energetic system the "living matrix" and suggests it is made up of the crystal lattice of fascial cells that surround each and every cell in the body/mind.[18] Fascia, rather than being an insulator, has been found to be a superconductor of energy.

James Oschman views intuition as, "an emergent property of a very sophisticated semiconducting liquid crystal matrix that is capable of storing and processing a vast amount of subliminal or non neural information…" including how to hit a baseball. He maintains that "since research has shown it is impossible to hit a baseball,"[18] that is, there is just not enough time between the instant a pitcher releases a ball and the moment it crosses the plate for a hitter to spot it, react to it and swing the bat in time to meet it, some other kind of link between sensation and action must exist. Oschman suggests that this link can be found in the primordial matrix of consciousness within and around cells, the fascial semiconductor matrix. We must rely on intuition to hit the ball.[19]

Consciousness, intuition, a split second response to sensation that exceeds the speed of 20 meters/second of the nervous system, result from sub atomic particle communication along the fascial matrix.[20]

From a quantum view of the function of photons in human physiology, it might be suggested that health at a basic, vibrational level results from balance, resonance, and homeostasis perpetuated by the transmission of energy from the DNA by way of invisible photons. Illness then may result from imbalance, loss of communication from the photons, and the loss of healthy vibration as a result of blockage in photon communication brought on by blocks in the photon pathways (the fascia).

Fascial restrictions may result from a solidifying of the ground substance in fascia when it dehydrates. When this occurs, fascia has lost the ability to conduct photons because of lack of hydration, much like wood sap dehydrated turns to resin, and resin dehydrated under pressure turns to amber. Manual therapists practicing energy-based myofascial release thus may rehydrate the fascia by releasing the restrictions by way of a piezo-electric effect, which would normalize the vibrational communication system and eliminates pain and imbalance, as the flattened fascial cells, and the cells that they surround, "plump up" and vibrate for their own healing.[19]

Fascia is the tissue that composes the living crystal matrix that may serve as the container of the mind. Candace Pert's research on neuropeptides revealed that the molecules of emotion and their receptors can be found everywhere in the body, on every kind of cell.[3] They are not confined to the nervous system. The mind is not in the brain.[3,8] Mind is a whole body phenomenon. The subconscious can be found in the entire body. At the moment of physical or emotional impact, energy gets trapped in the fascia which then dehydrates and causes a restriction. Fascial restrictions can be caused by absorption of energy in auto accidents, absorption of energy in deep fear and grief, as a result of scars and inflammation, habitual postures, and repetitive motion injuries, and the simple wear and tear of life in gravity over the years. This energy stays trapped in the fascia until it is released by manual energy techniques such as myofascial release. Once the energy is freed from the tissue, other energy-based therapies can assist the healthy vibrational flow to restore health and healing, reduce pain, and restore balance to all flows: endocrine, breath, blood, lymph, neurotransmitter, neuropeptides, hormone, and steroids.

According to a most recent peer-reviewed journal article on energy medicine[21]:

> *A normal cell has an electrical potential of about 90 millivolts. An inflamed cell has a potential of about 120 mv. and a cell in a state of degeneration may drop to 30 mv. By entraining the electrical fields of the cells within its range to the magnetic pulses emitted by a pulsed electromagnetic machine, cells can be brought back into a healthy range.*

Perhaps one day instead of relying on pharmaceuticals to change the chemistry in our body minds for re-balancing, we will instead find a way to use vibrations that resonate with the natural vibrations of the DNA in our cells, and thus empower our cells to heal. With stem cell transplants, vibrational interventions from devices such as low volt laser and pulsed electromagnetic devices, and the healing power of bioenergetic transmission from the hands of those therapists whose intention is to boost natural healing energy, we may be able to offer health and healing in ways that minimize negative side effects, and find ourselves returning to a more natural state of balance and homeostasis, and self regulation that is confirmed and supported by the healing energy that is all around us.[21] That is something worth hoping for.

References

1. Reiss AG, Strolger LG, Tonry J, et al. Type 1a supernova discoveries at z>1 from the Hubble Space Telescope: Evidence for past deceleration and constraints on dark energy evolution. *Astrophysical Journal.* 2004;607:665-687.
2. Boyd, RS. "Dark energy" still baffles astronomers. *Miami Herald.* September 27, 2007:7a
3. Pert C. *Molecules of Emotion.* New York: Scribner; 1997.
4. Lipton B. Toward a new noetic science: embracing the immaterial universe. *Shift.* Dec 05-Feb 06;9:8-12.
5. McTaggart L. *The Field: THe Quest for the Secret Force of the Universe.* New York, NY: Harper-Collins; 2002.
6. Hicks J, Hicks E. *The Law of Attraction.* Carlsbad, CA: Hay House; 2005.
7. Byrne R. *The Secret.* New York, NY: Atria Books; 2006.
8. Laszlo L. *Science and the Akashic Field.* Rochester, VT: Inner Traditions; 2004.
9. Lovelock J. *The Ages of Gaia: A Biography of Our Living Earth.* New York, NY: WW Norton; 1988.
10. Jaenisch R, Bird A. Epigenetic regulation of gene expression: how the genome integrates intrinsic and environmental signals. *Nature Genetics.* 2003;33:245-254.
11. Scioli A, Samor CM, Lapointe AB, et al. A prospective study of hope, optimism and health. *Psychol Rep.* 1997;81:723-733.
12. Smith K. Bioenergetics: the new science of healing. *IONS Shift.* 2006;10:11-13,34.
13. Oschman, J. Breakthrough in subtle energies and energy medicine. *Bridges.* 2003;14(4):5.
14. Challem J. *The Inflammation Syndrome.* Hoboken, NJ: John Wiley and Sons; 2003
15. Ingber DE. Mechanobiology and diseases of mechanotransduction. *Ann Med.* 2003;35:1-14.
16. Comings M. The quantum plenum: the hidden key to life, energetics and sentience. *Bridges.* 2007;17(1):4-13,20.
17. Rauscher E. Science, mysticism and the new tomorrow. *Bridges.* 2007;17(1):1,14-19.
18. Oschman JL. *Energy Medicine in Therapeutics and Human Performance.* Edinburgh: Butterworth-Heinemann; 2003:58.
19. Oschman JL. The intelligent body. *Bridges.* 2005;16(1)11-13.
20. Slater-Hammel AT, Stumpner RL. Batting reaction time. *Research Quarterly.* 1950;21:353-356.
21. Feinstein D, Eden D. Six pillars of energy medicine: clinical strengths of a complementary paradigm. *Alter Ther Health Med.* 2008;14:44-54.

SECTION III

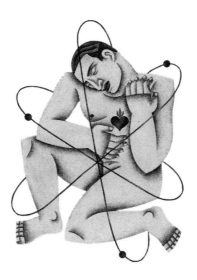

BODY WORK

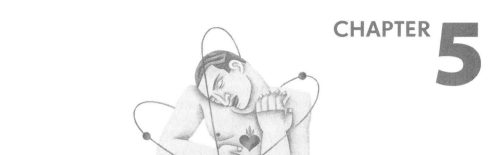

CHAPTER 5

THERAPEUTIC MASSAGE AND REHABILITATION

Janet Kahn, PhD, MT

Introduction

This chapter is about the contributions of therapeutic massage in the rehabilitative process. Massage plays a central role in the emerging picture of integrative health care. In a national survey of US adults' use patterns of complementary and alternative medicine (CAM), Eisenberg et al reported that massage was one of the three most commonly used CAM modalities between 1990 and 1997. It is estimated that American adults make more than 100 million visits to massage therapists annually, virtually all paid for out of pocket.[1] They must be getting something that they value. What is it? And should the health care system itself also be valuing massage and incorporating it more frequently into rehabilitation care?

To discuss massage and rehabilitation meaningfully requires a closer look at the concept of rehabilitation. Therapeutic massage can play a meaningful role in an individual's rehabilitation from injury, illness, repetitive strain, and the like. Just as importantly, however, massage has the potential, along with many of the modalities described in this book, to rehabilitate the current culture—a culture that in viewing people as machine-like in their employment; has created jobs that produce repetitive strain syndromes because they are not planned around the realities of human bodies; a culture that is so confused about touch that we have an epidemic of inappropriate touch and have responded to that epidemic by banning touch in schools (and in certain professions) rather than engaging in re-education about it; a culture that teaches "physical education" in public school without imparting much, if any, information about one's body, and which includes instructions to overrule the signs from the body that an activity or position is painful and to press on anyway. This is a culture in need of rehabilitation—in need of re-understanding the opportunities and limitations of human embodiment. Massage can be tremendously helpful in this regard.

Thinking About Therapeutic Massage

It is estimated that there are between 200,000 and 260,000 massage therapists in the United States today. While all offer healing through touch, there can be wide variation in their methods. Some massage therapists practice within a Western mechanistic framework of anatomy and physiology, while others practice within an energy-based Eastern view. Even with this variation, however, massage therapists share a view of the integrity of the human being. This has been beautifully stated by Deane Juhan, author of *Job's Body*[2] who said, "The skin is no more separated from the brain than the surface of a lake is separate from its depths... the two are different locations in a continuous medium... The brain is a single functional unit, from cortex to fingertips to toes. To touch the surface is to stir the depths."

When thinking about contemporary practice of therapeutic massage in the United States, it is helpful to keep at least two things in mind. First, massage is an ancient healing practice (or more accurately an array of practices) that is newly emerging as a health care profession and struggling, with real ambivalence, to meet the demands of that status. Second, to understand massage in the United States of the 21st century, it is helpful to see it as a modality with important roots in at least three separate streams—sports and fitness, medicine, and the various wellness and human potential movements of the past 4 decades.

History

In grasping its ties to medicine, it is important to remember that massage is not, in and of itself, a whole system of medicine, but rather has been an integral component of virtually every form of medicine that humans have ever devised. The Asian roots of massage reach to the origins of both Chinese and Ayurvedic medicine. Massage appears in the ancient medical texts of China, Japan, and Tibet. Its use in many countries has continued uninterrupted to the present time. In its earliest recorded forms and in contemporary Asian practice, massage therapy has been used both for the promotion of well-being and for treating (if not curing) the injuries and ailments that inevitably arise over the course of a lifetime.

In contrast to the Asian experience, the inclusion of therapeutic massage in Western medicine has been erratic. Both Greek and Roman practices included it. We find specific prescriptions for rubbing, friction, chest-clapping, and so forth in the writings of Hippocrates, Galen, and Celsus.[3] Massage was used to treat injuries such as sprains and dislocations, as well as to alleviate weariness. Alexander the Great is known to have traveled with a personal triptai (ie, massage therapist) for just that purpose. Massage was also used to prepare athletes before competition and to help them in postgame recovery. During the Middle Ages, classical writings about medical uses of massage were destroyed. Nonetheless, massage continued as part of folk practice and was reintroduced as a medical treatment during the Renaissance. The French surgeon Ambrose Pare (1517-1590) wrote of massage as a treatment for both postoperative healing and joint stiffness. An important figure in developing therapeutic massage as we know it today is Per Henrik Ling (1776-1839), who developed a system of passive and active movements he named "medical gymnastics," later known as the Swedish movement cure.[4] In the 19th century, these medical gymnastics were used to treat respiratory ailments including asthma and emphysema, gastrointestinal problems including constipation and incontinence, and nervous conditions such as neuralgic pain and epilepsy.

While Ling is often credited with bringing a scientific base to massage by grounding it in the study of anatomy and physiology, the Dutch physician Johann Mezger (1838-1909) systematized the work by grouping all known methods into four categories of soft tissue manipulation: gliding, kneading, friction, and percussive strokes. Mezger's enthusiastic students had much to do with the reintroduction of massage into medical settings in the late 19th and early 20th centuries.

Interest in massage in the United States heightened during World War I when Americans became aware of the rehabilitation work available for soldiers (and civilians) among the allied nations. The Reconstruction Department of the United States Army was initiated in 1918 and included both physiotherapy and occupational therapy. Mary McMillan, a prominent figure in the development of physical therapy in England and founder of physical therapy in the United States, served as chief aide at Walter Reed Hospital, taught special courses in war-related reconstruction at Reed College Clinic during World War I, and was director of physiotherapy at Harvard Medical School from 1921 to 1925, during which time she wrote her text, *Massage and Therapeutic Exercise.* McMillan defined the five major strokes of Western massage as effleurage, petrissage, tapotement, friction, and vibration.

While massage continued to be an important part of physical therapy treatment through World War II, its use declined after that time. Increasing availability of potent pharmaceuticals, as well as reliance on technology in the fields of both physical therapy and nursing, rendered the relatively labor intensive, and therefore costly, massage a less frequently prescribed treatment throughout the late 1940s and 1950s.

In the 1960s, renewed interest in massage came less through medicine and more through the human potential movement. The field of therapeutic massage and bodywork benefited tremendously from opportunities that arose at Esalen Institute and other gathering places of the human potential movement, from the intermingling of bodyworkers and psychotherapists. Here, through an exploration of the links between mental and bodily ease and distress, notions of wellness were expanded and new modalities such as Rolfing, bioenergetics, and Aston patterning were developed. This deepened exploration of the relationship between human structure and consciousness, which had begun earlier in Europe, is likely the greatest American contribution to the field.[5] It brought attention to the relationship between practitioner and client in creating and maximizing therapeutic effects,[6,7] an aspect of healing still in need of systematic investigation.

Contemporary Practice of Therapeutic Massage in the United States

In this chapter, the term *therapeutic massage* refers to the vast array of massage and bodywork modalities in use today because most massage therapists are trained in, and employ, multiple approaches. Thousands of massage therapists are trained in methods, some of which are described in other chapters of this book, including myofascial release, neuromuscular therapy, craniosacral therapy, Rolfing, Hellerwork, Reiki, polarity, reflexology, Trager, and to a lesser extent Alexander technique and Feldenkrais method, as well as in classical Swedish massage. The field encompasses work with the soft tissues of the body (muscle, fascia, ligaments), the lymphatic system (manual lymph drainage and Swedish massage), as well in which where the focus is largely energetic, whether within a framework of energy meridians (eg, Shiatsu and Tuina) or within a more Western concept of an energy field (eg, Reiki, Therapeutic Touch, and polarity therapy).

A single massage treatment may incorporate many kinds of strokes performed with a variety of intentions. Both the technique and the intention are important. Physically speaking, massage therapists glide, knead, tap, compress, stretch, roll, shake, vibrate, apply friction in various ways, and simply hold while bringing our own attention and that of the client to the area we are holding. Through these strokes, we engage not only the musculoskeletal system, but also the circulatory, lymphatic, and nervous systems. Slow, gliding strokes of Swedish massage engage the parasympathetic nervous system and induce a generalized relaxation response at the same time that they increase the circulation of fluids and relax the muscles themselves.[6] The various forms of therapeutic or orthopedic massage are applied with a greater attention to anatomic specificity, targeting specific muscles, ligaments, or fascia in response to the practitioner's assessment of the cause of the client's pain or dysfunction.

Massage therapists take a holistic view of the client and his or her condition. Our assessment includes a thorough history to help us understand not only this "incident" of injury or pain, but also the full story of what this client's body/mind has experienced, including any injuries or accidents, periods of unusual emotional or physical stress, as well as the "usual" stresses the client may experience at work or home (eg, physical stresses of work such as lifting or computer use, as well as psychological stresses). Physical examination includes both observation and palpation. We observe the client's posture seated and standing, his or her movement in walking, both active and passive range of motion, and his or her physical holding patterns in both the face and the body. All of these give us strong clues about the experience of being in that body and about primary and secondary pain patterns. Once the client is on the massage table, the assessment continues as we notice, again through observation, how the person and his or her body lies on the table, and whether there are areas of vasomotor reaction. Through both observation and palpation we can detect myofascial restrictions, chronic holding patterns of muscular tension, scar tissue and adhesions, and skin temperature indicating areas where energy and/or blood is not flowing efficiently and/or areas of hyperthermia.

This initial assessment allows the therapist to form a preliminary view of what is happening and to create an initial treatment plan. Therapeutic massage, however, is an ongoing dance of constant treatment and assessment. More is learned as we see how the tissue, and the client as a whole, respond to each stroke.

Case Example

I worked with a client who was scheduled for carpal tunnel surgery. Massage was her "last ditch" attempt to avoid the surgery. As I put my hands on the area of her trapezius, I found a particular pattern of nonresponsiveness in the tissue that I have learned from my experience can be the result of a reaction to caffeine. I asked, and the client informed me, that she consumed an average of 4 to 5 cups of coffee, 3 to 5 cans of cola, and a bit of chocolate virtually every day. There are clients who could do that with nonproblematic effect on the muscles, but for this client, as for a significant percentage of people, it created extreme chronic tension in the shoulders and neck, leading to nerve impingement and diminished use of her hands that mimicked carpal tunnel. A combination of myofascial work and Swedish massage on the upper extremities, with significant decrease in her caffeine consumption, rendered her able to return to quilting, gardening, and computer use without surgery.

The Skills and Mindset of the Massage Therapist

The fact that all of the physical work of massage takes place within the context of the practitioner/client relationship is of utmost importance. Embedded in this relationship is both the specific intention the practitioner is holding for that session, as well as the overall view the practitioner holds of her own role and the role of the client in the healing process. It also includes the quality of the rapport that is established between them.

The rehabilitation of both the client and the culture begins with the view of integrity, of body-mind unity, that the practitioner holds, as described in the previous quote from Juhan. The understanding that when we touch the surface (the skin), we stir the depths is profound. This statement is true at many levels, including the level of the neurotransmitters and the information they provide about how we are, even at the level of the psyche and soul itself.[8] Awareness of our potential to touch at this depth prompts a sense of reverence that many massage therapists experience as we work, and to which clients readily respond. Tracy Walton has described it this way[9]:

By touching a body, we touch every event it has experienced. For a few brief moments we hold all of a client's stories in our hands. We witness someone's experience of their own flesh, through some of the most powerful means possible; the contact of our hands, the acceptance of the body without judgment, and the occasional listening ear. With these gestures, we reach across the isolation of the human experience and hold another person's legend. In massage therapy, we show up and ask, in so many ways, what it is like to be another human being. In doing so, we build a bridge that may heal us both.

Within this overall unfolding relationship, the practitioner holds a conscious intention toward one or more of the following, which will guide the treatment: to promote relaxation or comfort, to promote increased body-mind integration through kinesthetic awareness or somatoemotional repatterning, and/or to promote physiological or structural change (eg, increased circulation, reduction of muscular or fascial hypertonicity). Table 5-1 presents many of the massage and bodywork modalities clustered under these three headings of intention. Although not exhaustive in scope, this framework organizes a number of the terms familiar to the public and acknowledges that many modalities can be used for more than one of the intentions listed.

Being able to work with intention, both large and small, requires a number of skills. Andrade and Clifford[10] have conceptualized what they refer to as intelligent touch, which they see as comprised of five distinct abilities:

1. Attention, which they describe as "the capacity to focus on the sensory information that the practitioner receives primarily, but not exclusively, through her hands."[10] This would include the ability to detect meaningful variations in tissue temperature, texture, and tension as described above, as well as the learned ability to detect information specific to a particular modality, such as the cranial rhythm that is a source of critical information about the craniosacral system and the health of the dura.

2. Discrimination is described as a refinement of the ability that comes with increasing familiarity with the feel of tissue over time and the clinical implications of the variations we find.

3. They describe identification both as the ability to know what you are touching based on a thorough knowledge of anatomy, as well as skill in knowing the implications of what you are feeling in terms of identifying healthy and dysfunctional tissue conditions.

4. These authors have given the name inquiring touch to what has been identified previously as the continual dance of treatment and assessment, and they consider this constant inquiry to be a hallmark of a good clinician.

5. Finally, they describe intention as an important clinical skill, with the therapist's overall intention being "to produce as close to the ideal tissue response as possible, given the constraints of the client's characteristics and the clinical setting."

Effective communication is another essential skill of the massage therapist. In addition to the hands-on work of massage, we also talk. Education is an important aspect of many massage treatments and encompasses everything from a reminder to breathe when the client seems to be forgetting, to an exploration and analysis of the client's work situation from the placement of the video screen and mouse, to proper sitting, standing, and lifting posture. Client education may also include suggestions for visualization during therapy, or simply information about the body/mind so that the client can work in harmony with him- or herself and attune to, and thus enhance, the treatment.

Shapiro and Schwartz[11] also offer important reflections on intention, which they refer to as the how and why of paying attention. The effects of our attention will be most beneficial, they suggest, when the attention has such "mindfulness qualities" as acceptance, nonjudging, patience, gentleness, generosity, and the like. These qualities echo the previous words that Walton used to describe what the massage therapist brings to the client: "...the contact of our hands, the acceptance of the body without judgment, and the... listening ear." At its best, massage therapy offers the client a direct experience of these qualities through the presence and contact of the therapist, and encouragement to offer them to oneself.

Table 5-1

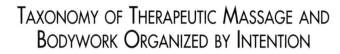

TAXONOMY OF THERAPEUTIC MASSAGE AND BODYWORK ORGANIZED BY INTENTION

TO PROMOTE RELAXATION OR COMFORT:

Swedish massage
Esalen massage
Craniosacral therapy
Trager psychophysical integration
Reiki
Polarity
Energy balancing
Therapeutic touch

TO PROMOTE KINESTHETIC AWARENESS, NEUROMUSCULAR EFFECTIVENESS, OR SOMATOEMOTIONAL REPATTERNING:

Craniosacral therapy
Aston patterning
Rolfing
Alexander technique
Feldenkrais method
Trager psychophysical integration
Myofascial release
Rubenfeld synergy
Hellerwork
Muscle energy techniques (MET)
Proprioceptive neuromuscular facilitation (PNF)

TO PROMOTE PHYSIOLOGICAL OR STRUCTURAL CHANGE:

Swedish massage
Neuromuscular techniques
Myofascial techniques
Rolfing
Trager psychophysical integration
Sports massage
Lymphatic drainage
Reflexology
Oriental massage
Muscle energy techniques (MET)
Proprioceptive neuromuscular facilitation (PNF)

In addressing the why of attention, Shapiro and Schwartz encourage an awareness of larger contexts in which the system, or a symptom, exists. In this way, we encourage clients not only to reduce tension in the neck muscles, but through the breath and other means to ease the whole body, and through the heart to ease the tension with which they regard themselves and others. Just as the neck is part of the larger body, so too are we part of a larger social body. Our ability to bring ease, a lessening of constriction, to our corner of the world will have benefit throughout.

Offering this sort of accepting attention to our clients is a form of deep intimacy. This is as true in the many forms of bodywork that are done with the client fully clothed as it is in practices done with the client naked and draped. Helping clients learn to bring such nonjudgmental attention to themselves offers them a beautiful exercise in self-intimacy. This is an important aspect of our much-needed social rehabilitation.

The Skills and Mindset of the Client

The physical aspect of massage is often a part of a larger healing process. If, for instance, a massage therapist is treating someone who has frequent headaches, his or her goals will be to relieve the immediate symptoms (headache pain), to ascertain and begin to address the myofascial patterns that produce frequent headaches, and to enlist the client in his or her own long-term care. The therapist's job is to help the client become aware of personal patterns—postural, dietary, emotional—that may contribute to the headaches. The therapist will also want to help clients discover the physical early warning signs of an approaching headache. If, for instance, the headaches are caused by chronic tension in the muscles of the neck and/or jaw, one may be able to avert a real headache by noticing slight increases in the tendency to clench the jaw, hunch the shoulders, constrict the breath, jut the chin, and so forth. By noticing and addressing these early shifts, a client can undo minor tension before it culminates in an excruciating headache. Part of the massage therapist's job, then, is to help clients learn how to pay attention to themselves. This attunement to the self, to one's own body and emotions, and the ability to constantly and gently release tension and adjust posture, breath, and attitude toward ease is a critical step toward lasting and creative rehabilitation for the client as well as for the culture. It is lasting because it is a skill that can be applied again and again. It is creative because it is a skill that can be applied to new situations. If one learns attunement to address one's headaches, it can be used later to attune to an injured limb, or to the holding of breath that leaves one feeling anything less than optimal, to the rush of adrenaline that follows a near miss in traffic, and so forth.

Again, Shapiro and Schwartz have coined the term *intentional systemic mindfulness* to describe the gentle loving attention a person can learn to bring to him- or herself for healing and simply for good living.[11] Self-regulation is the process through which any system, whether an organism or an organization, maintains itself as functional within changing circumstances. Feedback loops, both positive and negative, allow the system to take in and use information about itself and the environment it is in. Enhanced attention clearly will lead to more effective self-regulation, and therapeutic massage has the capacity to increase one's awareness both through the educational methods just described in the example of the client with headaches and, importantly, because massage can give the client the felt experience of an alternative to the usual state. This experience of newfound relaxation, absence of pain, shift in posture, and the like can be used as a homing device, providing the client with a home base in contrast to which the pain or tension can be recognized and attended to. In sum, enhanced or conscious attention, Schwartz has said, leads to connection, which in turn leads to self-regulation and then to order and health.[12]

The Importance of Space and Other Gifts of Massage

Clients often express a sense of timelessness during a massage. In sharp contrast with much of life, massage gives us a chance to quiet our minds, tune into our bodies, and experience the subtlest of sensations. Under these circumstances, our sense of time changes. As time opens up, so does space. When muscles relax they become longer, broader. On the cellular level, more space is created or, more accurately, found, since its potential is always there. As space opens up, so does time. We live in an era when people complain frequently about a lack of time and/or space. We experience our lives as crowded. Even when they are crowded with people and activities we love, we experience the crowding itself as discomfort, as pain. We can re-establish a sense of well-being at any moment by bringing our attention back into the body and finding/creating space there. We can do this with the help of a massage therapist who helps create space within our tissues. We can do this ourselves by bringing breath directly into the tissues and creating space that way.

Space is possible, unmanifested potential. With possibility comes choice. Addiction can be viewed as the absence of choice. It is a response or a reaction to a stimulus or circumstance without conscious thought or purposeful decision about what to do. When the phone rings we can answer it automatically, or we can take a moment to decide whether we want to talk on the phone at this moment. When food is put before us, we can eat it because it is there, or we can take a moment to notice whether we are hungry, and, if so, whether this is what we want to eat. We can only make these choices, however, if we notice that there is a moment, a space in time, in which to make a decision. The absence of noticing this space is reaction, much like an automatic reflex. It is easier to notice space in time when we are living in a more spacious environment within our own body. This is one of the gifts that massage can offer.

The Accumulating Evidence of Massage

As an emerging health care profession, therapeutic massage has a relatively small, though growing, body of scientific evaluation. The early research in particular, while invaluable in pointing out important directions of inquiry, is often of limited enduring utility due to methodological limitations, including small sample size, lack of randomization, inability to ensure reproducibility of the therapy, absence of a meaningful comparison or control group, and inadequate blinding.[13,14] Meta-analyses are limited by heterogeneity in the massage interventions themselves, duration of individual treatments, extent of the total intervention, and the outcomes assessed.[15,16]

While some of these issues arise in the early literature of many professions, due in part to low funding levels, there are some particular design issues that arise in the massage research literature. For instance, many studies include cointerventions that make it impossible to evaluate the specific effects of massage. Others have evaluated massage delivered by individuals who were not fully trained massage therapists and/or were following treatment protocols that did not reflect common (or adequate) massage practice. Haraldsson et al, in a review of trials for massage and neck pain said, "Most studies lacked a definition, description, or rationale for massage, the massage technique or both. In some cases, it was questionable whether the massage in the study would be considered effective massage under any circumstance."[17] The field is still without any literature on best practices for particular conditions rendering it impossible to know if the best practice was tested in a trial. Similarly, there are no known attempts to establish optimal dosage. In addition, it should be said at the outset that few theories exist and virtually none have been tested about the mechanism of action for the effects that we see. With those provisos in mind, and acknowledging that the quality of massage research is steadily improving, we can consider the available literature.

Systematic Reviews Involving Massage Therapy

A search of Medline and the Cochrane Library yielded over 170 systematic reviews that included massage research. Few were relevant to our purposes. While an important 1999 review on the clinical effectiveness of massage was summarized by the authors with the comment that, "the lack of scientific rigor of the studies retrieved was the most outstanding finding of the search,"[18] the evidence has improved since then. A 2004 review by the same lead author said massage has "shown a significant promise in the treatment of musculoskeletal conditions"[19] specifically citing back pain. In addition, a 2005 review reported that "Massage seems more beneficial than sham treatment for chronic nonspecific LBP [low back pain] but effectiveness compared with other conventional therapies is inconclusive."[20] The benefits from massage that were noted included both reduction in pain and increase in function. The back pain literature will be discussed below.

One review examined four studies relevant to whether therapeutic massage as an adjuvant to routine nursing care could improve critically ill patients' ability to cope with the intensive care unit (ICU) experience.[21] The massage interventions varied across studies from 1 to 17 minutes, and the only randomized controlled trial (RCT) utilized patients with quite different reasons for being in the ICU. Nonetheless, the authors concluded that massage "could be profoundly beneficial to critically ill patients on a general level."

While a 1998 review of nonpharmacologic strategies for managing cancer pain[22] yielded only one small RCT involving massage, much more research has been done on massage for cancer pain since then. The early study was a nonblind, randomized trial by Weinrich and Weinrich with two arms: massage and conversation control.[23] Their single outcome measure was a visual analogue scale (VAS) of pain administered at baseline, post-treatment, 1 hour post, and 2 hours post. The subjects were 28 hospitalized cancer patients, mean age 61.5, paired by medication prior to randomization. The treatment was a 10-minute Swedish back rub administered by a nursing student. While the authors concluded that men had immediate short-term pain relief (p=0.01) from massage, it should be noted that males in the treatment group indicated twice the pain level of females in the treatment group prior to receiving massage. Thus, pain intensity could easily be at least as relevant as gender in determining the effect of treatment. While this study was hardly conclusive, it suggested that massage might be an effective treatment for cancer-related pain.

Since that time, dozens of studies have been conducted evaluating massage as a treatment for symptoms of cancer including pain, anxiety, and nausea. The largest of these, an outcome study rather than an RCT, was an evaluation of pre and post massage data from 1290 cancer patients receiving massage at the facilities of Memorial Sloan Kettering.[24] Both inpatients and outpatients were included, all of them completing pre- and post-VAS evaluations of their pain, anxiety, nausea, fatigue, and depression levels. Results were strongly positive with reduction of all symptoms for both inpatients and outpatients. For the outpatients, who received somewhat longer massages, the improvement lasted through the 48-hour follow-up period of this study. A 2005 review on the topic concluded,[25]

> *Conventional care for patients with cancer can safely incorporate massage therapy, although cancer patients may be at higher risk of rare adverse events. The strongest evidence for benefits of massage is for stress and anxiety reduction, although research for pain control and management of other symptoms common to patients with cancer, including pain, is promising.*

A 2000 review evaluating evidence for a number of complementary and alternative medicine modalities in relation to end-of-life symptoms of pain, dyspnea, and nausea located only three studies of massage.[26] Two were case series and the third was the Weinrich and Weinrich study already mentioned. A review focusing on CAM therapies for treating multiple sclerosis included three relevant RCTs—one on soft tissue manipulation,[27] one on Feldenkrais awareness through movement,[28] and one on reflexology.[29] The variation in these treatments illustrates one of the challenges in the field. While all three studies were deemed methodologically weak, they do show enough promise to warrant further investigation. The first two studies showed treatment group improvements in reducing anxiety, stress, and depression. The reflexology group showed significant improvement in multiple sclerosis-related symptoms including paraesthesia, urinary symptoms, muscle strength, and spasticity.

A review of studies on low back pain, conducted in 1999, yielded four RCTs, all with small sample sizes and other limitations.[30] Two of the studies included massage only as a control condition for investigations focused on other modalities, and little attention was actually given to the massage treatment. One of the studies found massage to be superior to no treatment, two found massage as effective as spinal manipulation, and one found massage to be inferior to spinal manipulation. These findings are fairly positive given the minimal attention paid to designing the massage intervention. Not surprisingly, the authors concluded that more research was needed. Happily some has been done, and these more recent and more carefully designed studies are discussed below. Remaining reviews either were not directly relevant to rehabilitation issues, or covered uses of massage only in combination treatments that did not allow a real look at the value of this modality alone.

Patterns of Massage Usage

In 1999, Cherkin et al conducted a survey of licensed acupuncturists, chiropractors, massage therapists, and naturopathic physicians.[31] They gathered systematic data from practitioners in two states for each of these four modalities, gathering information on the practitioners themselves, their clients, and the purposes for which clients came for care. Data from massage therapists were collected in Washington and Connecticut, states that are similar in that both had statewide licensure and different in that only Washington had mandated insurance coverage for massage. Information from more than 2000 visits to these massage therapists indicates that 63% of the visits were for musculoskeletal concerns. Back pain was the largest subcategory (20%), followed by neck (17%) and shoulder (8%) complaints. The second most common reason for visits was wellness/relaxation (19%), which, if coupled with visits for reduction of stress and/or anxiety (5%), accounted for nearly one in four visits. We will examine the literature for both of these uses, as each in it own way is relevant to successful rehabilitative efforts

Massage for Musculoskeletal Pain

It is only in recent years that researchers have turned their attention to the issue of massage for musculoskeletal pain. Ernst's 1999 systematic review of studies on back pain[15] located only four clinical trials in which therapeutic massage was employed as a single therapy intervention, and each of these was considered to have serious methodological problems. The author concluded that while there was some suggestion that therapeutic massage may be an effective treatment for low back pain, the paucity and quality of data precluded any confident estimation. More research was encouraged. A 2002 review by Furlan et al[32] examined eight trials for back pain that included a massage treatment arm. Four examined massage only as a control group and were not designed to evaluate massage as a potentially effective intervention, and one compared two German forms of "massage" not typically practiced in the United States (Teil massage and acupressure using a metal roller), mostly for patients with herniated discs.[33]

Among the remaining three studies, the most rigorous was a carefully conceived study by researchers in Seattle[34] who randomized 232 subjects with persistent low back pain to either massage, acupuncture, or self-care education (via booklet and video). Both acupuncturists and massage therapists were given treatment parameters that provided reasonable definition to the treatments while allowing practitioners to use their best clinical judgment in treating their clients within those parameters. Massage therapists were limited to soft tissue manipulation (eg, no energy balancing) and could not utilize Asian techniques that would be too similar to acupuncture. Within those limitations, they could employ a host of techniques including Swedish, neuromuscular, and myofascial strokes. This was an important innovation in research design since compared to more rigid protocols, it more nearly approximates the kind of patient-tailored mixed-technique massage one might receive in many therapists' offices. Outcomes included functionality as measured by the Roland Disability Scale, bothersomeness of symptoms, disability, satisfaction with care, and cost of care. In the short term (at 10 weeks/end of treatment), massage had a significant effect on symptoms (p=0.015) and function (Roland) (p=0.01), and reduced reported use of pain meds. At 42 weeks post-treatment, massage benefits persisted and subjects showed 30% to 45% lower annual low back pain care costs than did the other groups. Thus, the massage treatment resulted in both immediate and sustained relief, surpassing the effects of both acupuncture and self-care.

While the Cherkin study demonstrated that massage offered relief that lasted well beyond the period of treatment, it did not, however, shed any light on why this is true. Perhaps it is because the treatments designed by the practitioners actually addressed not only the symptomatic issues of pain, but also the underlying causes of it. Perhaps the pain relief was sustained because the educational suggestions regarding exercise and posture allowed the clients to stave off any subsequent episodes of low back pain. It will require further research to shed light into that black box, as well as to confirm the finding through replication.

Another study on low back pain, conducted by Michelle Preyde,[35] also offered an important innovation. Investigators compared what they call comprehensive massage therapy (CMT), comprised of soft tissue manipulation (STM), and exercise with posture education (E&E), with each of those components delivered individually, thus offering some insight into what might be contributing to the effect of therapeutic massage treatments for low back pain. They randomized a convenience sample of 98 patients with subacute low back pain to one of the three conditions listed above or to a sham laser treatment. Subjects were given six sessions within a 1-month time period. The STM was a 30- to 35-minute treatment utilizing primarily friction and trigger point massage. The education component was 15 to 20 minutes of training in specific stretching techniques. The CMT included somewhat shortened versions of each of these treatments. Post-treatment and at a 1-month follow-up, the CMT group had significantly better scores on functionality and pain than either E&E or sham laser (p<0.05), and better than SMT on pain intensity at post-treatment only. The SMT group had significantly better scores than E&E or sham laser on functionality (p<0.05) post-treatment. All of the CMT subjects reported that pain levels decreased in intensity from baseline to post-treatment. At follow-up, 63% of CMT subjects reported no pain, compared with 27% in SMT, 14% in E&E, and 0% in sham laser. By itself, the exercise and posture training offered noticeable but nonsignificant help in pain reduction and function. There were no group differences in range of motion. In summary, while both CMT and STM produced significant improvements over exercise alone and the sham laser control, the comprehensive form was stronger, particularly in producing effects that endured 1 month post-treatment.

The final study of low back pain and massage was a small (24 subjects) two-armed RCT comparing massage therapy and progressive muscle relaxation, conducted by Hernandez-Reif[36] and colleagues at The Touch Research Institute of the University of Miami. This was a weaker study both because of the small sample size and because the assessors were nonblinded. Nonetheless, the other larger studies, perhaps, give credence to their finding that massage therapy was more effective than progressive muscle relaxation in reducing low back pain. In summary, all three RCTs conducted since the Ernst review indicate that therapeutic massage could be an effective treatment for people with low back pain.

Cherkin's survey of massage therapists[31] indicated that 17% of patients come for relief of neck pain. The most recent systematic review of studies on massage for neck pain[37] examined 19 trials, 12 of which they deemed to be of low quality. Finding that results were inconclusive in 14 of the trials using massage as part of a multimodal intervention and in the six trials evaluating massage alone, the authors concluded that "No recommendations for practice can be made at this time because the effectiveness of massage for neck pain remains uncertain." Echoing an earlier publication by Haraldsson et al[17] they say that "the credentials of those delivering the massage was frequently missing so there was no guarantee that 'professional' massage had been tested in these studies." A second weakness, underpowering, could not be overcome through aggregation of the data because the populations and treatments were too heterogeneous. Haraldsson's review had concluded that massage was safe for people with this chronic neck pain, but that the data did not indicate that it was more effective than the treatments to which it was being compared. There was a broad array of such treatments across the included studies.

Two relevant studies have been made available since that review. Sherman et al compared massage with self-care education for the treatment of chronic neck pain.[38] In this RCT, 64 patients with neck pain of at least 3 months duration were randomized to receive massage (up to 10 massages over 10 weeks) or a self-care book. Data were collected at 4, 10, and 26 weeks on outcomes that included dysfunction (Neck Disability Index [NDI]), a 0 to 10 symptom bothersomeness scale, and medication usage. They found that massage recipients were more likely than the self-education subjects to experience a clinically significant improvement on the NDI (48% vs 18% of controls; RR=2.7; 95% CI=1.2 to 6.5) and on the bothersomeness scale (55% vs 25% of controls; RR=2.2; 95% CI=1.1 to 4.5) at 10 weeks (end of treatment). At 26 weeks, the difference in function remained, though at a reduced level. There was no longer a significant difference in symptom bothersomeness. There was a difference between the groups in medication usage, with increased usage among the book group participants from 63% at baseline to 77% at 26 weeks, and somewhat decreased usage among the massage recipients (56% at baseline, 53% at 10 and 26 weeks). While a single small study is hardly definitive, this does suggest that massage is likely to provide some relief for those with chronic neck pain.

A Finnish study on neck pain compared traditional bonesetting, standard physiotherapy, and massage.[39] Neck pain intensity (VAS), perceived disability (NDI), and neck spine mobility measurements were used as outcomes. Data were analyzed using time (pre and post) by group (TBS, PT, and M), two-way analysis of variance for repeated measures. The implications of this study are difficult to evaluate for a number of reasons. First, all three treatments included some form of massage, bonesetting being described as "...a soft and painless manual mobilization of the extremities and spine... [designed] to relax the muscles and to correct body asymmetry" and physiotherapy being a combination of exercise therapy, massage, and stretching therapy. Second, the treatments differed in length averaging 45 minutes for the physiotherapy, 1 hour for the massage, and 90 minutes for the bonesetting. Additionally, while all subjects received 5 treatment sessions, the intervals between sessions were somewhat variable across subjects, rendering the total treatment period variable. Given these challenges, it is perhaps most notable that neck pain and NDI scores decreased significantly in all three groups from baseline to 1 month post-treatment ($p<0.001$). Bonesetting was found to have more long-lasting effects and to produce a greater sense of satisfaction among subjects.

Perlman et al investigated the effects of 8 weeks of massage on pain and other symptoms associated with osteoarthritis (OA) of the knee.[40] Adults (n=68) with a diagnosis of OA of the knee and a prerandomization score of 4 to 9 on the Western Ontario & McMaster Universities OA Index (WOMAC) and pain VAS (eg, 0=no pain, 10=worst pain ever) were randomized to massage or to a delayed intervention control. A standardized protocol of full-body Swedish massage was administered twice weekly in the first 4 weeks to build a loading dose, then once weekly for the next 4 weeks. The massage therapy group demonstrated significant improvements in the WOMAC Global Score (-21.15 ± 2.46 mm; $p<0.0001$), Stiffness (-21.60 ± 26.99 mm; $p<0.0001$), Physical Function domains (-20.50 ± 22.50 mm; $p<0.0001$) and Pain (-17.62 ± 31.06 mm; $p=0.0023$) at 8 weeks (end of treatment) as well as decreased pain (VAS) and time to walk 50 feet ($p<0.05$). At 16 weeks (8 weeks post-treatment), improvements seen in the massage therapy group generally persisted. The authors conclude that massage seems to be an efficacious treatment for OA of the knee.

Two recent studies have examined massage as a treatment for postoperative pain. The first involved 605 male veterans (mean age, 64 years) who underwent major surgery between February 1, 2003, and January 31, 2005 at a Department of Veterans Affairs hospital in either Ann Arbor or Indianapolis.[41] This very well-designed RCT involved three arms-usual care, Usual care plus a 20-minute Swedish back massage, or usual care plus 20 minutes of nonmassage attention (eg, conversation) delivered by a massage therapist, for up to 6 days following the operation. The massage group was found to have significantly better outcomes than the control group on short-term pain intensity (p=0.001), pain unpleasantness (p<0.001), and anxiety (p=0.007). Importantly, massage recipients experienced a faster rate of decrease in pain intensity (p=0.02) during the first four postoperative days. The authors found this quite notable stating[41]:

> *Perhaps the most important observation from this study is the immediate (short-term) effects of massage on pain intensity, unpleasantness, and anxiety. These significant reductions were most pronounced on the first postoperative day. A 1-point (1-cm) reduction in the pain score (of a possible 10) on a VAS in the acute postoperative setting may sometimes require the administration of several small (eg, 1-mg) boluses of parenteral morphine, depending on the individual. This suggests that massage may be a very potent pain reliever in some patients.*

The second study on postoperative pain was a two-armed trial with 180 subjects, comparing usual care with usual care plus massage and acupuncture.[42] While this RCT also found significantly greater decreases in pain and depression among the treatment group, it is impossible to disentangle the specific effects of massage from the contributions of acupuncture or the synergetic effect of the two.

Another aspect of musculoskeletal pain that has been explored in one study is the use of massage to ease myofascial pain. Hong et al[43] examined four commonly used treatments for myofascial trigger point pain—deep tissue massage, stretch preceded by flouri-methane spray, heat applied via hydrocollator, and ultrasound with heat—and a control of sham treatment. Subjects were 84 adults with myofascial pain recruited from a pain control clinic, plus 24 subjects who had experienced no chronic pain for at least the prior 6 months. The primary outcome measure in this trial was a pain threshold measurement via pressure algometer of an active trigger point in the upper trapezius. The measurement was taken pre- and post-treatment. The massage treatment consisted of 10 to 25 minutes of compression on palpable taut bands with stretch. The ultrasound treatment was 1.2 to 1.5 watt/cm^2 for 5 minutes. The spray and stretch was flouri-methane spray applied in the usual method of physical therapy. The hydrocollator pack was applied for 20 to 30 minutes. While it could be argued that a weakness in this design is the noncomparability in time spent in each of the four treatments, the counterargument is that each treatment was applied in the customary manner of current practice. All four manual medicine modalities showed significant improvement over controls (p<0.05 for ultrasound and p<0.01 for other massage, hydrocollator, and spray and stretch). Inter-treatment comparison showed massage to be more effective than any of the other approaches (p<0.05). This study then indicates that massage may be an effective treatment for myofascial pain. One primary contribution of this study is the use of an objective measure of pain.

Massage and Pain Mechanisms

As we consider the question of "mechanism of action" two features of massage are important to keep in mind. First, all massages are not the same and the effects of different treatments may be prompted by different mechanisms. Second, a massage treatment is a complex mix of tissue manipulation, human connection, verbal cuing for cognitive reframing, an ongoing therapeutic relationship, and a host of nonspecific effects including both patient and practitioner expectations. Part of the power of massage may be its ability to affect a number of these simultaneously.

There are competing theories about why massage is effective in reducing pain. Field has suggested that pain reduction is one result of a cascade of effects set in motion by shifts in stress hormone levels.[44] Many of her studies report significant postmassage increases in serotonin levels and decreases in epinephrine, norepinephrine, and cortisol. However, Moyer's later meta-analysis of relevant data contradicted one aspect of Field's findings, indicating that cortisol levels were not significantly reduced.[45] Moyer did find evidence of significant reductions in heart rate and blood pressure, which had been reported by Meek[46] and Fakouri,[47] but not by Reed.[48]

Others have suggested the gate control theory of pain as an explanatory model, or that massage works as a superficial analgesic. One would not expect these explanations to account for pain relief sustained well beyond the period of treatment, which we have seen in some of the studies reviewed above. Braverman and Schulman,[49] in reviewing massage effects for rehabilitative contexts, cited evidence that massage can prompt increased joint mobility, improved connective tissue pliability and mobility, and enhanced immune system function in addition to the reduction in stress hormones already cited.

More efficient use of muscles and concomitant reduction of strain and overuse through improved postural alignment is one explanation that massage therapists often offer to explain why massage is effective in relieving musculoskeletal pain. This explanatory model would be applicable to both immediate relief and long-term improvement. Some of the improved postural alignment is achieved through purposefully stretching the connective tissue in areas that the therapist finds to be inappropriately constricted. Connective tissue is notoriously pliable and can become "remodeled" via many forms of mechanical stress including overuse, underuse, or simply unusual use such as repetitive motions.[50] Connective tissue change can prompt alterations in the muscle(s) with which it is associated. For instance, shortening of muscle fibers due to immobilization has been shown to be preceded by shortening of the associated connective tissue which responds more quickly to the lack of movement.[51]

In a very promising paper, Langevin and Sherman offer a pathophysiological model of low back pain that incorporates data on tissue remodeling as well as on pain-related behavior.[52] They reference literature indicating that some people in pain, fearing that movement will cause more pain, limit their physical activity, and/or alter their movements in ways that over time can become repetitive misuse.[53,54] Massage therapists see clients every day who have developed inefficient and painful ways of moving, often involving distortions that were employed originally to protect an injury that may have long since healed. Langevin and Sherman hypothesize that "...dynamic and potentially reversible plasticity of perimuscular connective tissue plays a key role in the pathophysiology of LBP as well as in the mechanism of therapies utilizing mechanical forces (eg, massage, chiropractic manipulation, acupuncture)."[52] Clearly this hypothesis is not limited to back pain, but could pertain to other musculoskeletal pain as well.

Finally, re-evoking the quote from Juhan cited near the beginning of this chapter about the inseparability of the skin and the brain, Kerr et al have offered a possible explanation grounded in neural plasticity.[55] They suggest that what they call touch healing therapies may be effective in chronic pain treatment through four features that jointly encourage neural plasticity, particularly the reformation of the somatosensory cortical map. These four features, any and all of which can be present in a massage treatment, are light tactile stimulation, a behaviorally relevant and relaxed context, repeated sessions, and directed somatosensory attention. It is known that chronic pain is sometimes centrally maintained, meaning that it can persist even when there is no remaining damage to the tissue, thus no present time nociception to account for the pain sensation. Cortical dysregulation has been associated with centrally maintained pain.[56-58] Studies have indicated that remodeling is possible in the somatosensory maps of adults.[59] Body maps of chronic pain patients have shown enlargement in the areas related to the painful body regions.[60-62] Taking all this into account, Kerr et al hypothesize that touch healing "modalities work to renormalize somatotopic maps via a therapeutic plasticity mechanism."

In sum, there are a number of models that might explain how massage is effective when it is, as well as why it is not, when it is not. The recent models offered by Langevin and Sherman, as well as by Kerr and colleagues, are appealing in that they offer multifactorial explanations that could apply to a multidimensional form of treatment. They remain to be tested.

Massage, Stress, and Wellness

Relaxation, stress relief, and anxiety reduction are primary reasons for visits to massage therapists. Dozens of small investigations, many conducted at the Touch Research Institute, indicate that massage offers immediate reductions in stress and anxiety in a variety of situations. The five studies presented here, while not exhaustive, will offer some evidence of this range.

The first of these, chronologically speaking, was a 1998 study by Field et al, exploring the possible use of massage to ease the debridement process for burn victims.[63] Twenty-eight adult burn patients, recruited consecutively upon admission for debridement at a burn center, were randomized to either standard care (SC), which included physical therapy, or SC plus massage. The massage consisted of daily administration of a 20-minute Swedish massage to face, torso, limbs, and back for 1 week. The treatment was given just prior to morning debridement. Outcomes, taken pre- and post-treatment on the first and last days, included a state/trait anxiety inventory (STAI), three pain measures, and a number of observational measures completed by staff. The massage group was found to have significant pre- to postimprovement in state anxiety, pulse, observed affect, vocalization, and signs of anxiety. Longer-term outcomes (change from first to last day) included significant decrease in anger, depression, and all three pain measures. SC subjects showed only a decrease in pulse pre- to post-treatment, and a decrease on one pain measure from day 1 to the last day. While our confidence in the findings is weakened by the investigator's use of nonblinded observers, it nonetheless points out a potentially important avenue of inquiry and use of massage in rehabilitation. That is, massage appears to have the potential to ease patients' experience of medical treatments that, while helpful and/or necessary, are difficult to endure.

Ahles et al conducted a related study,[64] investigating the potential use of massage for patients undergoing autologous bone marrow transplant (BMT). Thirty-four adults scheduled for autologous BMT at a large teaching hospital were enrolled in a nonblinded randomized comparison of (SC versus SC plus massage. In this study, massage consisted of up to nine 20-minute Swedish massages that included strokes to shoulders, neck, and head. They averaged three massages per week for 3 weeks. Anxiety, depression, and mood were assessed at baseline, midtreatment, and predischarge; nausea, pain, and fatigue were assessed pre- and post-massage. While the massage group demonstrated significant improvements immediately post-treatment, in diastolic blood pressure, distress, nausea, and state anxiety, no significant effects over time were found.

In a second study, Field explored the potential for two treatments—therapeutic massage and a combination of yoga and progressive muscle relaxation—to ease depression among clinically depressed adolescent mothers.[65] Thirty-two depressed adolescent mothers, just postdelivery, were given half-hour massages (standardized Swedish protocol) or relaxation therapy (yoga plus progressive muscle relaxation) twice weekly for 5 weeks. Both treatments proved effective in significantly reducing subjects' state anxiety. However, only the massage also significantly reduced behavioral ("fidgitiness," $p<0.01$) and physiological (pulse and heart rate) signs of anxiety, as well as reducing depression ($p<0.05$). Staff observational reports of behavior indicated that the massage group had improved affect ($p<0.001$) and cooperation ($p<0.005$). The combination of self-report, observational, and physiological data is a strength of this study, and their converging results are encouraging in suggesting that massage is beneficial in reducing anxiety and depression with this population.

A study by Hernandez-Reif et al on massage for children with cystic fibrosis[66] is representative of many studies done at the Touch Research Institute that measured general indicators of relaxation/stress reduction (eg, self-reports on STAI, saliva cortisol levels, etc) as well as some measure particular to the condition under study. In this case, peak airflow was measured. While the value of the study is diminished by its small sample size (n=20) and lack of blinding, it still offers helpful information. The massage treatment in this study was a 20-minute evening massage given by parents to their children for 30 evenings. The fact that all but one family completed this regimen indicates the possibility of the use of parentally administered home-based massage in pediatric applications, should the research show it is warranted. The comparison group received 20 minutes of reading with the parents. The results of this study indicated a reduction in anxiety for both parents (p<0.05) and children (p<0.05), as well as improved mood for children (p<0.05) postmassage on the first day. There was also a significant reduction in anxiety for parents and children from day 1 to day 30 in the massage group (p<0.05). Importantly, there was an increase in peak air flow for children in the massage group from day 1 to day 30 (p<0.05). These data support further study, which should include more rigorous design. Data indicating a reduction of parental anxiety mirrors other studies indicating benefit from giving massage, especially for parents.

Many adults, of course, experience great stress in their workplace. Hodge et al investigated the potential of seated massage as an effective workplace stress reduction intervention.[67] In this study, 100 employees, both male and female, ages 25 to 60, working in a large teaching hospital were randomized to one of two conditions. The treatment group received a 20-minute massage twice weekly for 8 weeks, done seated, clothed, with shoes off. The protocol was a blend of light to medium pressure circular motions to the upper body, acupressure to the face and chest, and foot reflexology. Control group subjects were offered a quiet room in which to take their 20-minute break. Outcome measures included a range of psychological, physiological, and organizational outcomes assessed via previously validated instruments. Findings indicate that compared with those in the control group, subjects receiving massage had lower anxiety (state p=0.009, trait p=0.04), were less depressed (p=0.05), and experienced improved emotional control (p=0.05). There was also a decrease in sleep disturbance for massage subjects on 12-hour shifts (p=0.02), although there were no significant differences between groups on a multidimensional measure of fatigue. Significant improvements were also noted in heart rate and blood pressure for massage subjects compared with the controls, and for massage subjects pre- and post-treatment. Interestingly, the massage group had significant improvement in cognition scores (p=0.000), as assessed by the Symbol Digit Modalities Test. Work satisfaction scores remained constant for the massage group, but decreased for the control group.

Hodge's study is the largest and latest of three published studies to explore the use of massage to reduce workplace stress. Earlier studies by Field et al[68] and Shulman and Jones[69] also indicated that seated massage is an effective tool for this widespread problem. Shulman and Jones included measurements taken 2 and 3 weeks after the completion of the intervention. While the stress reduction had somewhat diminished since the end of treatment, it was still significant. Field et al had compared seated massage with a rest break. Interestingly, they included a measure of brainwave activity that indicated that, although subjects receiving both massage and the rest break experienced increased frontal delta power (indicative of increased relaxation), only the massage group also showed the decreased frontal alpha and beta powers that are indicative of enhanced alertness. This runs counter to the idea some hold that subjects would emerge from massage in a relaxed, but somewhat vegetative state—perhaps "too relaxed" to return to work effectively. It suggests instead that massage induces something like the state of meditation—relaxed and alert. This interpretation was supported by the finding that the massage subjects were able to complete a set of math computations more quickly and more accurately than the control group. This finding, which will not surprise those who have come to massage via the human potential movement, suggests that we would do well to conduct studies investigating the potential of massage to enhance various aspects of human functioning.

Numerous studies, then, indicate that massage is effective in reducing stress in children, adolescents, and adults. This seems to be true for those diagnosed with clinical depression and anxiety, as well as healthy subjects. Data presented support the notion that this aspect of massage can be useful in easing medical procedures, workplace stress, and in home-based pediatric applications.

Regulation and Information

A good review of regulatory issues for therapeutic massage and other CAM professions has been provided by Eisenberg et al in an article published in the *Annals of Internal Medicine*.[70] Briefly, regulation of individual massage practitioners has been quite uneven in the United States. In the absence of coherent governmental regulation, the American Massage Therapy Association (AMTA), a nonprofit professional organization, initiated the National Certification Board for Therapeutic Massage and Bodywork (NCBTMB) in 1992. NCBTMB administers the National Certification Exam (NCE)—a psychometrically valid multiple-choice test measuring subjects' mastery of a core body of knowledge concerning anatomy and physiology (both Eastern and Western), pathology, treatment techniques and decisions, business practices, and professional ethics. Eligibility requirements to sit for the exam include completion of a minimum 500 hours of accredited instruction. Certification must be renewed every 4 years, including documentation of 50 hours of continuing education. The NCE is required for licensure in 32 states, and other states, will accept it. Much more recently the Federation of State Massage Therapy Boards formed and is also offering an exam that is now accepted for licensure by 11 states. This exam also covers anatomy, physiology, kinesiology, pathology, client assessment and treatment planning, contraindications and special populations, and ethical and legal issues.

Governmental regulation of therapeutic massage is inconsistent. Thirty-eight states and the District of Columbia regulate massage therapy via licensure. The trend in licensure legislation is toward two requirements: successful completion of a minimum 500-hour program and a passing grade on the one of the two certification exams. In states without licensure, regulation is handled by smaller jurisdictions or not at all. This regulation varies widely, with some local requirements having been created as antiprostitution legislation and having little to do with legitimate therapeutic massage.

Accreditation and Training

There are more than 1200 massage schools in the United States. The majority of these are for-profit proprietary institutions, licensed as businesses by their local jurisdictions. Only a small fraction of these massage schools are accredited by a nationally recognized accrediting agency. Most of these are accredited as vocational schools, although this is changing as more colleges establish massage programs and more massage schools become accredited as, or affiliated with, colleges. Since most accreditation is institutional, giving little attention to specifics of the instructional program in massage, the Commission on Massage Therapy Accreditation (COMTA) was initiated in the 1980s to provide meaningful program accreditation. COMTA received official recognition by the US Department of Education (DOE) in July 2002. To date, a total of 90 massage schools have received COMTA accreditation. DOE recognition, combined with COMTA's shift from hours-based to competency-based standards beginning in March 2003, are likely to have a notable positive effect on massage education in the United States. This change would be most welcome since the current situation is one of great inconsistency in the academic training and clinical experience of even licensed massage therapists in North America.

Summary

Massage is a therapeutic modality employed around the world and across time. Nonetheless, the literature investigating its effects is modest at best. Widespread use of therapeutic massage for both wellness and treatment of injury and/or pathology requires that more attention be given to investigations of this modality and to bringing greater coherence in training and regulation. Heterogeneity of clinical techniques requires detailed descriptions of research interventions so that clinical applicability can be clear. Research attention should be given to those applications for which consumers most often seek therapeutic massage, particularly musculoskeletal pain and injury. Future research should also seek to measure and give meaning to those outcomes that clients report as important, but for which objective measures do not yet exist. These could include particular aspects of well-being such as groundedness, centeredness, increased happiness, and comfort with oneself. The potential contributions of distinct aspects of therapeutic massage treatments should be disentangled through research, including soft tissue manipulation, educational interventions, and the therapeutic presence and intention of the practitioner. Far from being the nuisance that placebo or nonspecific effects were once thought to be, these practitioner/client issues may be at the heart of the healing process. Finally, inquiry is also sorely needed into the mechanisms of demonstrated effects.

References

1. Eisenberg DM, Davis RB, Ettner SL, et al. Trends in alternative medicine use in the United States, 1990-1997. Results of a follow-up national survey. *JAMA.* 1998;280:1569-1575.
2. Juhan D. *Job's Body: A Handbook for Bodywork.* New York, NY: Station Hill Press; 1987.
3. Tappan FM, Benjamin PJ. *Tappan's Handbook of Healing Massage Techniques.* 3rd ed. Stamford, CT: Appleton and Lange; 1998.
4. Kleen EA. *Massage and Medical Gymnastics.* New York, NY: William Wood & Co; 1921.
5. Johnson DH. *Bone, Breath & Gesture: Practices of Embodiment.* Berkley, Calif: North Atlantic Books; 1995.
6. Downing G. *The Massage Book.* New York: Random House; 1972.
7. Murphy M. *The Future of the Body: Explorations into the Further Evolution of Human Nature.* Los Angeles, CA: Jeremy Tarcher; 1992.
8. Pert C. *Molecules of Emotion.* New York, NY: Touchstone Books; 1997.
9. Walton T. The health history of a human being. *Massage Therapy Journal.* 1999;37:70–92.
10. Andrade C, Clifford P. *Outcome-Based Massage.* Baltimore, MD: Lippincott, Williams & Wilkins; 2001:11.
11. Shapiro S, Schwartz G. Intentional systemic mindfulness: an integrative model for self-regulation and health. *Adv Mind Body Med.* 1999;15:128-134.
12. Schwartz GE. Psychobiology and health: a new synthesis. In: Hammonds BL, Schweirer CJ, eds. *Psychology and Health: Master Lecture Series.* Vol. 3. Washington DC: American Psychological Association; 1984.
13. Field TM. Massage therapy effects. *Am Psychologist.* 1998;53(12):1270-1281.
14. Crawley N. A critique of the methodology of research studies evaluating massage. *Eur J Cancer Care (Engl).* 1997;6:23-31.
15. Ernst E. Massage therapy for low back pain: a systematic review. *J Pain Symptom Manage.* 1999;17(1):65-69.
16. Ernst E. Abdominal massage therapy for chronic constipation: a systematic review of controlled clinical trials. *Forsch Komplementarmed.* 1999; 6(3):149-151.
17. Haraldsson BG, Gross AR, Myers CD, et al. Massage for mechanical neck disorders. *Cochrane Database Systematic Reviews.* 2006, Issue 3. Art. No:DC004871 DOI:10. 1002/14651858.DC004871, pub3.
18. Ernst E, Fialka V. The clinical effectiveness of massage therapy—a critical review. *Forsch Komplementarmed.* 1994; 1:226-232.
19. Ernst E. Musculoskeletal conditions and complementary/alternative medicine. *Best Practice & Research Clinical Rhematology.* 2004;18(4):539-556.
20. van Tulder WM, Furlan AD, Gagnier JJ. Complementary and alternative therapies for low back pain. *Best Practice & Research Clinical Rheumatology.* 2005;19(4):639-654.
21. Hill CF. Is massage beneficial to critically ill patients in intensive care units? A critical review. *Intensive and Critical Care Nursing.* 2003;9:116-121.

22. Sellick SM, Zaza C. Critical review of 5 non-pharmacologic strategies for managing cancer pain. *Cancer Prevention & Control.* 1998;2(1):7-14.

23. Weinrich SP, Weinrich MC. The effect of massage on pain in cancer patients. *Appl Nurs Res.* 1990;3:140-145.

24. Cassileth BR, Vickers AJ. Massage thereapy for symptom control: Outcome study at a major cancer center. *J Pain Symptom Manage.* 2004;28(3):244-249.

25. Corbin L. Safety and efficacy of massage for cancer. *Cancer Control.* 2005;12(3):158-164.

26. Pan CX, Morrison RS, Ness J, et al. Complementary and alternative medicine in the management of pain, dyspnea and nausea and vomiting near the end of life: A systematic review. *J Pain Symptom Manage.* 2000;20(5):374-387.

27. Hernandez-Reif M, Field T, et al. Multiple sclerosis patients benefit form massage therapy. *Journal of Bodywork and Movement Therapies.* 1998;2(3):227-231.

28. Johnson SK, et al. AS controlled investigation of bodywork in multiple sclerosis. *J Altern Comp Med.* 1999;5(3):237-243.

29. Siev Ner I, et al. Reflexology treatment relieves symptoms of multiple sclerosis: a randomized controlled study. *Focus Altern Complement Ther.* 1997;2(4):196.

30. Ernst E. Massage therapy for low back pain: a systematic review. *J Pain Symptom Manage.* 1999;17(1):65-69.

31. Cherkin D, Deyo RA, Sherman KJ, et al. Characteristics of visits to licensed acupuncturists, chiropractors, massage therapists and naturopathic physicians. *J Am Board Fam Pract.* 2002;15(6):463-472.

32. Furlan AD, Brosseau L, Imamura M, Irvin E. Massage for low-back pain: a systematic review within the framework of the Cochrane Collaboration Back Review Group. *Spine.* 2002;27(17):1896-1910.

33. Franke A, Gebauer S, Franke K, Brockow T. Acupuncture massage vs Swedish massage and individual exercise vs group exercise in low back pain sufferers—a randomized controlled clinical trial in a 2 x 2 factorial design. *Forsch Komplementarmed Klass Naturheilkd.* 2000;7(6):286-293.

34. Cherkin D, Sherman KJ, Deyo RA, et al. A randomized trial comparing traditional Chinese medical acupuncture, therapeutic massage and self-care education for chronic low back pain. *Arch Int Med.* 2003;138(11):898-906.

35. Preyde M. Effectiveness of massage therapy for subacute low-back pain: a randomized controlled trial. *CMAJ.* 2000;162(13):1815-1820.

36. Hernandez-Reif M. Lower back pain is reduced and range of motion increased after massage therapy. *Int J Neuroscience.* 2001;106:3-4.

37. Ezzo J, Haraldsson BG, Gross AR, et al. Massage for mechanical neck disorders: a systematic review. *Spine.* 2007;32(3):353-362.

38. Sherman KJ, Cherkin DC, Hawkes RJ, Miglioretti DL, Deyo RA. Randomized trial of therapeutic massage vs. self-care book for chronic neck pain. *Alt Ther Health Med.* 2006;12(3):63.

39. Zaproudina N, Hanninen O, Airaksinen O. Effectiveness of traditional bonesetting in chronic neck pain: randomized clinical trial. *Journal of Manipulative and Physiological Therapeutics.* 2007;30(6): 432-437.

40. Perlman AI, Sabina A, Williams A-L, et al. Massage therapy for osteoarthritis of the knee: a randomized controlled trial. *Arch Intern Med.* 2006;166:2533-2538.

41. Mitchinson AR, Kim HM, Rosenberg JM, et al. Acute postoperative pain management using massage as an adjuvant therapy: a randomized trial. *Arch Surg.* 2007;142(12):1158-1167.

42. Mehling WE, Jacobs B, Acree M, et al. Symptom management with massage and acupuncture in postoperative cancer patients: a randomized controlled trial. *J Pain Symptom Manage.* 2007;33:258e266.

43. Hong C-Z, Chen Y-C, Yu J. Immediate effects of various physical medicine modalities on pain threshold of an active myofascial trigger point. *J Musculoskeletal Pain.* 1993;1(2):37-53.

44. Field T. Presentation made at: First International Symposium on the Science of Touch; May 2002; Montreal, Quebec.

45. Moyer CA, Rounds J, Hannum JW. A meta-analysis of massage therapy research. *Psychol Bull.* 2004;130(1):3-18.

46. Meek SS. Effects of slow stsroke back massage on relaxation in hospice clients. *Image J Nurs Sch.* 1993;25:17-21.

47. Fakouri C, Jones P. Relaxation Rx: slow stroke back rub. *J Gerontol Nurs.* 1987;13(2):32-35.

48. Reed BV, Held JM. Effects of sequential connective tissue massage on autonomic nervous ystem of middle-aged and elderly adults. *Phys Ther* 1988;68(8):1231-1234.

49. Braverman DL, Schulman RA. Massage techniques in rehabilitation and medicine. *Phys Red Rehabil Clin N Am.* 1999;10(3):631-49.

50. Cummings GS, Tillman LJ. Remodeling of dense connective tissue in normal adult tissues. In: Currier DP, Nelson RM, eds. *Dynamics of Human Biologic Tissues: Contemporary Perspectives in Rehabilitation.* Philadelphia, PA: FA Davis; 1992:45-73.

51. Williams PE, Goldspink G. Connective tissue changes in immobilised muscle. *J Anat.* 1984;138(Pt 2):343-350.

52. Langevin H, Sherman K. Pathophysiological model for chronic low back pain integrating connective tissue and nervous system mechanisms. *Medical Hypotheses.* 2007;68:74–80.

53. Hurwitz EL, Morgenstern H, Chiao C. Effects of recreational physical activity and back exercises on low back pain and psychological distress: findings from the UCLA Low Back Pain Study. *Am J Public Health.* 2005;95(10):1817-1824.

54. Swinkels-Meewisse IE, Roelofs J, Oostendorp RA, Verbeek AL, Vlaeyen JW. Acute low back pain: pain-related fear and pain catastrophizing influence physical performance and perceived disability. *Pain.* 2006;120(1-2):36-43.

55. Kerr CE, Wasserman RH, Moore CI. Cortical plasticity as a therapeutic mechanism for touch healing. *J Altern Complement Med.* 2007;13(1):59-66.
56. Treede R, Kenshalo DR, Gracely RH, Jones AK. The cortical representation of pain. *Pain.* 1999;79:105-111.
57. Price D. Central neural mechanisms that interrelate sensory and affective dimensions of pain. *Molecular Interventions.* 2002;2:392-403.
58. Flor H. Cortical reorganization and chronic pain: implications for rehabilitation. *J Rehabil Med.* 2003;41:66-72.
59. Pascual-Leone A and Torres F. Plasticity of the senorimotor cortex representation of the reading finger in Braille readers. *Brain.* 1993;116:39-52.
60. Flor H, Braun C, Elbert T, Birbaumer N. Extensive reorganization of primary somatosensory cortex in chronic back pain patients. *Neuroscience Letters.* 1997;224:5-8.
61. Flor H, Elbert T, Knecht S, et al. Phantom-limb pain as a perceptual correlate of cortical reorganization following arm amputation. *Nature.* 1995;375:482-484.
62. Maihofner C, Handwerker HO, Neundorfer B, BIrklein F. Patterns of cortical complex regional pain syndrome. *Neurology.* 2003;61:1707-1715.
63. Field T, Peck M, Krugman S, et al. Burn injuries benefit from massage therapy. *J Burn Care Rehabil.* 1998;19:241-244.
64. Ahles TA, Tope DM, Pinkson B, et al. Massage therapy for patients undergoing autologous bone marrow transplantation. *J Pain Symptom Manage.* 1999;18(3):157-163.
65. Field T, Grizzle N, Scafidi F, Schanberg S. Massage and relaxation therapies effects on depressed adolescent mothers. *Adolescence.* 1996;31(124): 903-911.
66. Hernandez-Reif M, Field T, Krasnegor J, et al. Children with cystic fibrosis benefit from massage therapy. *J Pediatr Psychol.* 1999;24(2):175-181.
67. Hodge M, et al. Employee outcomes following work-site acupressure and massage. In: GJ Rich, ed. *Massage Therapy: The Evidence for Practice.* St. Louis, MO: Mosby; 2002.
68. Field T, et al. Massage therapy reduces anxiety and enhances EEG pattern of alertness and math computations. *Int J Neurosci.* 1996;86(3-4):197-205.
69. Shulman KR, Jones GE. The effectiveness of massage therapy intervention on reducing anxiety in the workplace. *Journal of Applied Behavioral Science.* 1996;32(2):160-173.
70. Eisenberg DM, Cohen MH, Hrbek A, et al. Credentialing complementary and alternative medical providers. *Ann Intern Med.* 2002;137(8):660-664.

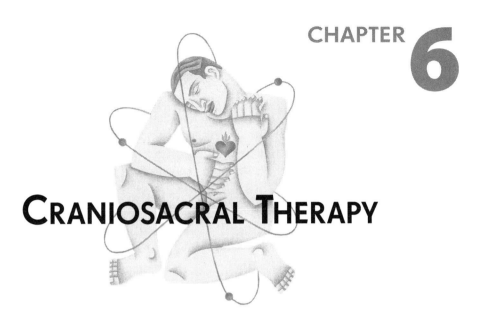

CHAPTER 6

CRANIOSACRAL THERAPY

Deborah A. Giaquinto-Wahl, MSPT, ATC

Craniosacral therapy is a manual therapy technique that utilizes the craniosacral system to promote self-correction and healing within the body. This is truly a profound technique that looks at the human body as an integrated whole. The craniosacral system includes the bones of the cranium, sacrum, underlying meningeal membranes, all other structures that connect to the meninges, and the cerebrospinal fluid (CSF). A therapist can utilize the bones of the cranium and sacrum are used as bony handles to access the underlying dura and release any restrictions within the system. When restrictions are released, the organism (person) functions more efficiently. Dr. John Upledger, the founder of craniosacral therapy, once phrased it as follows: "It's like removing stones from a river so flow is not impeded." The CSF has an intimate relationship with the brain and spinal cord, and is encased within the dural system. This dural system connects either directly or indirectly to every muscle, joint, tendon, and organ in our body. Therefore, one can see that a restriction within the craniosacral system can be far reaching and may show symptoms anywhere throughout the body.

Two belief systems must be in place in order to be cohesive with Upledger's work: 1) that cranial bones connect by jointed articulations that are mobile throughout life, and 2) that there is an ongoing rhythmical motion of the underlying dural membrane caused by the production and reabsorption of CSF, which is transmitted to the bones.

The history of craniosacral therapy begins in the early 19th century with the father of osteopathy, Dr. A. T. Still. He believed that the body is a self-regulating, self-correcting system. He also believed that the body works as a unit and that the body structure is intimately related to its function. If the system is structurally out of balance, it will constantly and inherently try to seek homeostasis.

In the early 1900s, an osteopath by the name of William G. Sutherland, a student of Dr. Still's, was very interested in nature's design of the human skull. Similar to most Western medicine practitioners, he was taught that the bones of the human skull calcify when full growth has been reached. When Dr. Sutherland examined the skull, he realized that the cranial sutures were actually joints and, consequently, reasoned that there had to be movement between the bones. He saw that "some cranial bones were beveled like the gills of a fish, indicating articular mobility for a respiratory mechanism."[1] Using himself as a case study, and with the aid of various ingenious devices he created, Sutherland screwed down portions of his skull, creating restrictions within himself, and then noted the changes that occurred.[1-3] As a result of the magnitude of the responses he experienced from this self-experimentation and self-correction, Sutherland concluded that freeing up the restrictions along the cranial sutures and allowing proper movement could improve overall function. The birth of cranial osteopathy was thus established.

Other than the osteopathic community, very few practitioners in the Western world believed that the cranial bones moved after childhood until the work of Dr. John Upledger had evolved. In the early 1970s, Dr. Upledger worked with a team of physicians and researchers from Michigan State University. Their objective was to determine the validity of Sutherland's work with cranial manipulation and to determine if the cranial bones really did or did not move. They also wanted to learn the composition of the intra-articular suture material. Using electron microscopy, Upledger and the Michigan State team determined that the intra-articular suture material contained blood vessels, nerves, and connective tissue.[4-7] These findings were more conducive toward dynamic mobility versus bony fusion of the cranial bones.

To determine if cranial bones move, the Michigan State team also studied the cranial movement of live primates. Fastening antennae into the parietal bones of monkeys and through the use of radio waves, they were able to observe a rate and amplitude of movement between the cranial bones at 6 to 12 cycles/minute.[5] Another study published by Thomas Adams, PhD, entitled "Parietal Bone Mobility in the Anesthetized Cat,"[8] reported findings of a rhythmic motion other than the cardiac and respiratory rate in cats at approximately 11 cycles/minute[8] (using strain gauges across the parietal bones of cats). Wallace and colleagues observed intracranial pulsations at a rate of 9 cycles/minute in human brain and membrane tissue with the use of ultrasound.[9] With all these studies, it now seemed realistic that Sutherland's premise of cranial manipulation held true. But what was actually causing cranial bone movement? Two theories predominate: the stretch receptor mechanism[1] and the arachnoid granulation body theory.[2]

Stretch Receptor Mechanism

What was previously known anatomically was that the meningeal membrane has an intimate relationship with the skull and connects at various points along the spinal canal. Referred to as the intracranial membrane system, it is made up of a vertical membrane system formed by the falx cerebri and falx cerebelli and continues down to form a strong, dense circle of tissue around the foramen magnum (Figure 6-1). The horizontal portion of the intracranial membrane system is created by "leaves" that run laterally off the falx cerebri superiorly and the falx cerebelli inferiorly, forming a bilayered horizontal membrane, the tentorium cerebri and the tentorium cerebelli, respectively. We also know that CSF is housed below the dura mater within the subarachnoid space and is formed within the ventricular system of the brain. Prior to the Michigan State research, Sutherland believed that the keystone of all cranial bone motion was movement at the sphenobasilar joint. He believed that there was a contraction and expansion of the ventricular system and that this tensile motion caused movement at the sphenobasilar joint,[3] an external pumping action by the brain if you will.

Although Upledger's research confirmed the bulk of Dr. Sutherland's model, Upledger postulates that there is actually an internal pump as well as volume/pressure receptors that are responsible for the volume changes of the CSF. He theorizes that it is the volume change of the CSF within the intracranial membrane system that causes the movement of the cranial bones. Upledger and his colleagues have posed the "pressure stat" model, explaining the craniosacral rhythm, the movement of CSF, and their relationships to the movement between the cranial bones. This model is a semiclosed hydraulic system in which CSF is constantly being produced and reabsorbed within the container of the meningeal system. Physiologically, what happens is that the CSF drains at a

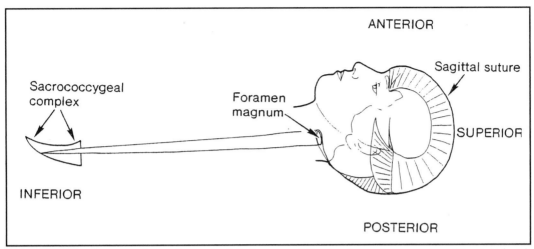

Figure 6-1. Anterior-posterior and superior-inferior axes of the dural membrane system. (Reprinted with permission from Upledger JE, Vredevoogd JD. *Craniosacral Therapy.* Seattle, WA: Eastland Press; 1983:70.)

constant rate through the arachnoid villi of the sagittal suture and at the anterior straight sinus through arachnoid bodies, then is reabsorbed back into the venous system. By way of electron microscopy and cadaver dissection, pressure-sensitive receptors within the sagittal suture ground material have been located along with nerve tracks that run down to the choroid plexus of the lateral ventricles. Theoretically, these pressure receptors could signal the choroid plexus to increase production of CSF once a low threshold has been reached. When enough CSF has been produced, the meningeal membranes expand to the point of triggering stretch receptors in the sagittal suture, signaling the choroid plexus to stop production of CSF. The CSF continues to be reabsorbed through the arachnoid villi until the low threshold is reached; sense receptors in the suture will again send signals to the choroid plexus to produce CSF. This dynamic theory poses that CSF is produced at a rate twice that of the constant reabsorption, and that when an upper threshold is reached, the production is turned off by an internal homeostatic mechanism.[3]

Arachnoid Granulation Body Theory

Another feedback mechanism that would support the rhythmic flow of CSF within the craniosacral system is one that involves the arachnoid granulation body. This body projects into the floor of the straight sinus at its angle of union with the great cerebral vein and contains a sinusoidal plexus of blood vessels that, when engorged, serves as a ball-valve mechanism. The increasing backpressure from the engorged vessels may affect the secretion of the CSF by the choroid plexus of the lateral ventricles.[3] Both theories support the hypothesis of the pressure-stat model and its ability to be the driving force of craniosacral motion.

Impact of Restrictions in the Craniosacral Flow

Upledger and colleagues maintain that with sufficient education and training, a skilled practitioner can locate and evaluate the quality of a person's craniosacral rhythm anywhere on the body. This rhythm is interrupted when restrictions occur. How do these restrictions occur within the system, how do these restrictions affect the patient, and what can practitioners do about it?

There are two types of trauma that can cause restriction in the system: *direct* and *indirect*. Direct trauma affects the structures of the cranial system such as a bone, a suture joint, or the membrane itself. It can occur from any of several events like a birthing injury, a direct blow from a fall or auto accident; a fracture, a surgical procedure, a tumor or a cerebrovascular accident.

An indirect trauma eventually affects the craniosacral system but it does not initiate there. Indirect trauma may result from repetitive motion injuries, poor sitting or standing postures or any habits of movement or position that pull the body out of its correct anatomical alignment. An old injury elsewhere on the body may work its way back into the CS system through the fascia disrupting its rhythm and flow.

The body's fascial system, as described in detail in Chapter 7, plays a large role in both direct and indirect traumas that result in restrictions to the craniosacral flow. Remember that fascia is a fibrous collagenous web of connective tissue that runs through the entire body, covering every muscle, organ, osseous structure, and cell in the body. If one uses the metaphor of a wax candle with seashells embedded in it, the seashells would be every cell, every organ, every muscle, bone, and nerve in the body, and the wax would represent the fascia. Anatomically, fascia runs primarily in a longitudinal direction within the sagittal plane from the top of the cranium to the plantar fascia of the feet in one continuous web of connective tissue. Horizontal diaphragms or planes of fascia also exist, creating compartments that facilitate integrity and stability, and allow our visceral organs to stay in place. Without these horizontal fascial planes, gravity would take over and our kidneys would drop into our pelvic bowl or our lungs would continually expand laterally and drop into the abdominal cavity. The horizontal fascial planes are located at the base of the occiput, at the level of the hyoid bone in the throat, at the thoracic inlet, the respiratory diaphragm, and the pelvic floor. The fascia of the dura surrounding the cranium and the spinal cord forms the dural sheath within which the craniosacral fluid flows and rhythm takes place.

Fascia is connected to the meningeal system through the dural sheaths as they exit the spinal column. With trauma, the fascial system can be disrupted. Since fascia is so ever-present, adhesions can form and extend their influence in a multitude of patterns and directions anywhere in the body. Consequently, it is feasible that an injury to the knee could present with symptoms in the cranium in the form of headaches or tinnitus. In either case, there is no direct line of neuromuscular or osseous connection to the knee itself. With this model in mind, practitioners must learn to look at the fascial system as a whole unit instead of simply focusing on the site of the symptom or injury.

An excellent clinical example of the need to explore the larger whole body system for the cause of a particularly symptom can be found in the example of Mary Clark, a US Olympic diver, whose career came to a complete standstill due to problems with vertigo. Her balance was affected so severely that she was unable to stand on the platform, let alone compete as a diver. She had tried many traditional medical remedies with no results, until she was examined and treated by Dr. John Upledger. He assessed her craniosacral system and concluded that her vertigo problem was most likely stemming from an old knee injury. He palpated the lines of fascial pull which coursed from her knee to her temporal bone, actually pulling the lateral bone of her head into an anterior torsion. The ear canal running through the temporal bone was affected, and her symptoms presented as vertigo. Releases in the fascial system allowed the temporal bone to realign, and the vertigo problem was resolved.[5] Miss Clark was able to return to diving competition, and ultimately won the bronze medal in platform diving in the 1996 Olympic Games.

Upledger's Protocol in Evaluating and Treating the Craniosacral System

Craniosacral practitioners release fascial adhesions through diaphragm release techniques and release membrane restrictions by mobilizing the separate bones of the cranium. The cranial bones directly adhere to the cranial membranes. Upledger has devised a sequential protocol to evaluate and treat the craniosacral system. After he has assessed the craniosacral rhythm along different areas of the body, his *first step* is to induce a "still point" somewhere on the patient's body.[3] Usually performed at the base of the cranium or at the level of the sacrum, a still point occurs when the practitioner intentionally manually impedes the flow of craniosacral fluid, bringing the system to complete rest. This action balances the autonomic nervous system and enhances relaxation. While in this state of "pause," the system has a chance to self-correct and reorganize. Typically, the practitioner will find the cranial rhythm to be stronger and more fluid after a still point induction, because such manual interference in the system forces new pathways and breaks through old restrictions.

Step two of Upledger's protocol addresses the horizontal fascial diaphragms located at the level of the pelvis, the respiratory diaphragm, the thoracic outlet (inlet), the hyoid, and the cranial base better known as the suboccipital region. Most longitudinal fascial fibers can be accessed through these horizontal diaphragms. The practitioner is basically treating by mobilizing the tissues found between one hand on the top of the body and the other underneath in the area of the horizontal plane. For example, at the level of the pelvic diaphragm, we could be addressing not only fascial restrictions under the skin, but also problems with the lumbosacral-coccygeal complex and/or the urogenital system. Symptoms such as urinary frequency, prostate, and vaginal problems that might be emanating from restrictions in the fascia surrounding the organs and cells in that area would be addressed.

The respiratory diaphragm located at the transition area of T12-L1 posteriorly and just below the xyphoid process anteriorly encompasses the diaphragm muscle. Naturally, any breathing problems, rib excursion, esophageal, stomach, inferior vena cava, pancreas, liver, spleen, transverse colon, adrenal, and associated spinal segment problems could all receive benefits from the release in hypertonicity of the respiratory diaphragm.

The thoracic inlet is named for the blood, lymph, and CSF that course through this area into the thoracic cavity from the head.[1] This fascial diaphragm is located at the level of C7-T1 posteriorly and at the clavicular/sternal manubrium level anteriorly. If restricted, this area potentially can back up fluid into the cranium. Between this area lies a myriad of structures that could potentially be affected by hypertonicity of the transverse fascia and, thus, reduce normal craniosacral fluid flow. The plural dome, the shoulders and scapula, the clavicle and first rib, the arms, the hyoid musculature, the sternocleidomastoid, the upper trapezii, the scalene and platysma muscles, the jugular veins, subclavian arteries and veins, and the thyroid and parathyroid glands all lie within this region. One can see how a forward head with rounded shoulder posture might place severe fascial strain on these structures and cause symptoms in several locations, including a full-blown upper quadrant syndrome of neck pain, weakness in the rotator cuff muscles, subdeltoid bursitis, and paresthesias in the fingers of the hand.

The hyoid diaphragm is exactly that—above and below the hyoid. Fascial strain in this area can affect the hyoid musculature, which is important for chewing and swallowing activities. This horizontal plane is commonly compromised with a whiplash-type injury, and restrictions are associated with temporomandibular joint disease (TMJ), tinnitus, and ear infections.

The occipital cranial base is the area where the suboccipital muscles lie at the base of the skull, between the occiput, atlas, and the axis vertebrae. The dural tube directly connects to the foramen magnum and to the posterior surface of the vertebral bodies of C1 and C2. Lesions are common in this area and can severely and directly compromise the craniosacral system. With a whiplash injury, the suboccipital structures get jammed together and the condyles of the occiput can be pushed forward on the superior articular facets of the atlas. This area must move freely in order for the atlas to rotate properly on the axis. Freeing the cranial base is also beneficial for the tissues involved with the jugular foramen. Besides freeing up backpressure from the jugular vein, the glossopharyngeal, the vagus, and the spinal accessory cranial nerves run through the foramen. Release here can benefit the patient neurologically.[3]

After all of the above horizontal diaphragms are released, *step three* in Upledger's protocol calls for releases of the sacrum from the lower lumbar spine and from the ileal or innominant bones.

Obviously, any tissue trauma from sprains or strains of the lumbar spine and the sacroiliac joint can be addressed with this technique. Disc problems and problems with structures innervated by sacral nerve roots—the colon, rectum, gluteus, piriformis, and resulting leg-length discrepancies—can also be addressed by releasing the sacrum. The craniosacral system has a direct dural attachment to bones at the level of S2, so restrictions to it can directly have an adverse affect on the flow of the system. This can release, not only at the level of the lumbosacral spine, but all the way up to the head and neck. The dural tube is meant to glide freely within the vertebral canal, and the occiput and sacrum are designed to move in synchrony with one another. After freeing up the sacrum, one can perform a "dural tube traction" at the sacral end.

Step four is a dural tube "rock and glide" which while holding both the sacral and occiput ends of the dural tube we rock the tube back and forth "flossing" the dural tube within the spinal canal. The rock and glide is useful for both treatment and assessment of the dural tube within the spinal canal because a trained therapist can feel between his or her hands where further craniosacral restrictions reside and pinpoint which segments are locked up within the system. If the therapist feels the tube is clear at the proximal end until he or she gets down to the level of T6, and then is clear again from the distal end up to about T11/L1, the therapist can ask him- or herself, "Is the restriction residing within the tube directly under T6? Is it just outside the dural tube in the surrounding soft tissue or joint, or is it further away somewhere in the viscera or fascia causing a drag at the level of T6?" Once the restriction is accurately located, the therapist can utilize other modalities, such as joint mobilization and myofascial release, to free up these two levels and completely clear the dural tube from one end to the other.

In addition to using joint mobilization, muscle energy techniques, position and hold, or soft tissue/myofascial release techniques to free up these restrictions, Upledger reintroduced a technique first conceptualized by Sutherland called the "V-spread" technique, which also incorporates a technique called "direction of energy." Both are incredibly powerful techniques for tissue healing and reorganization. The therapist simply spreads two fingers across the suture line or the facilitated segment he or she wants to mobilize and, with the other hand usually on the opposite surface of the body, sets his- or her intention to where he or she wants the energy to go. With compassion, energy is directed from one hand through the tissue toward the V-spread until a release is felt. Signs of a release might include heat, pulsation, and/or a softening that is perceived between the therapist's two fingers (Figure 6-2). Although the mechanism of action at the cellular level remains a mystery, the intentional focus of energy into the body has been scientifically determined to result from biomagnetic emanations from the practitioner's hands.[10] In the near future, I am sure scientific technology will advance to the point where instrumentation can quantifiably measure the results we are seeing. Not to disregard the unexplainable now, it serves us well to remember that Dr. Fritz Hoffman created aspirin to help his father's arthritic pain in 1897. We did not have the sophistication in science until the 1970s to discern the prostaglandin response. Simply put, it worked well and he used what worked.

After freeing up the dural tube, *step five* focuses on addressing and correcting restrictions in the cranial bones themselves. Each bone connects to other bones and to different cranial membranes. Opening up the frontal bone anteriorly and the parietal bones superiorly, the therapist connects to the falx cerebri and the vertical membrane system. The frontal bone sits anteriorly over the cerebral cortex; therefore, decompressing this bone may have positive effects on headaches, head trauma, and frontal sinus problems. We have seen some children with cerebral palsy have an overlap of the frontal suture, and freeing it up can result in profound reductions in spasticity.[3] Since the horizontal plate of the frontal bone contributes to the orbit and nasal cavity, decompression here could positively affect eye pain and olfactory issues, as well as sinus drainage.

Step six is a parietal bone release. The parietal bones lie directly over the cerebral cortex. This step actually allows the practitioner to take pressure off the brain itself. The parietal lift assists in releasing bony restrictions from the frontal, temporal, sphenoid, and occipital bones. The sagittal suture runs between the parietals, and the falx cerebri runs vertically and lies directly on the

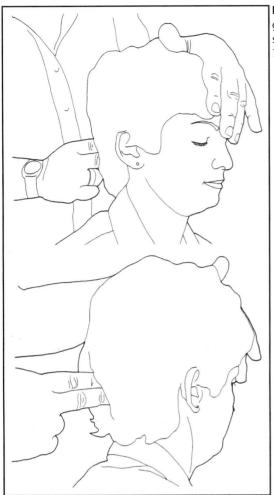

Figure 6-2. Finger placement for direction of energy release of falx cerebri. (Reprinted with permission from Upledger JE, Vredevoogd JD. *Craniosacral Therapy*. Seattle, WA: Eastland Press; 1983:73.)

undersurface of these paired bones. Utilizing the superior lift technique, a skilled practitioner can mobilize and release restrictions of the falx cerebri, move through the falx cerebelli and continue caudally releasing the dural tube itself. This technique is excellent for improving fluid exchange within the ventricular system. Signs and symptoms such as headaches, sinus problems, transient ischemic attacks, memory loss, and difficulties with motor planning can be addressed with this technique. A newborn with a forceps delivery should be treated with a parietal bone release as soon as possible after birth, as the parietals are often the surface that the forceps grab onto for the extraction.

Steps seven and *eight*, releasing the temporal bones laterally and the sphenoid bone in the anterior-posterior directions, we address restrictions of the tentorium cerebri and tentorium cerebelli (also known as the horizontal membrane system). Cranial nerves III (oculomotor), IV (trochlear), and VI (abducens) run between the layers of the horizontal membrane system and dysfunctions associated with eye movement may be addressed with these techniques.[11] Even strabismus has been corrected with this technique.[3] A skilled therapist uses the temporal bones as bony handles to laterally distract the membrane. Compression of the temporals utilizing another technique can release fascia connected to osseous and soft tissue structures that attach to the temporal bone and mastoid process. Since the sternocleidomastoid, splenius capitus, rectus capitus, longus capitus, and temporalis muscles all attach to the temporal bones, practitioners would do well to evaluate for restrictions in the temporal bones for symptoms of neck and shoulder pain, whiplash injuries, and TMJ problems. Attention should then be brought to the mandible once temporal bones have been cleared.

As a personal note, many times in the clinic I have found the upper cervical vertebrae of my clients to be out of alignment, and until I release the cranial base and temporal bones, the client's symptoms will not completely dissipate.

With regard to the involvement of cranial nerves V (trigeminal), which is important for the muscles of mastication, VII (facial) for facial expression and sensation of part of the tongue, and IX (glossopharyngeal), for speech, swallowing, and the tongue—all three exit at the level of the brainstem and, thus, can be affected by the orientation of the temporal bones.[11,12]

The jugular foramen, just lateral to the petrous portion of the temporal bone, is an important structure, and adverse tissue tension around it can increase backpressure up into the head and sinuses. Tension here can also disrupt neural activity for the cranial nerves that run through it. The vagus nerve that innervates so many structures can go into vagotonia and cause all kinds of problems as a result of abnormal tissue tension around the jugular foramen. The auditory canal actually runs through this bone, so any problems with balance, hearing, tinnitus, and chronic ear infections may be reflective of the position of the temporal bones and their mobility. Clinically, children with autism often seem to have had a history of very severely compressed temporal bones bilaterally.[3,4] In children with dyslexia, craniosacral therapists often find the right temporal bone compressed; and in children with dyscalcula (disability with respect to using mathematics), the left temporal bone is compressed.[3,5]

Step eight is a release of the sphenoid, the final cranial bone to be released for freeing up the entire horizontal membrane system (Figure 6-3). A technique of compression and decompression is used. Sitting at the head of the supine client, the practitioner places the tips of the fingers gently on either side of the temple just lateral to the eyes. The initial movement is in the direction of ease, thus "unlatching the stuck door" before opening it, which is a gentle compression downward towards the surface on which the client is lying. Once fully compressed, the practitioner reverses the direction of the gentle pressure to an upward direction. Upledger maintains that 85% of all sphenoid dysfunction can be addressed with this simple technique of compression followed by decompression.[5]

Once in a while, the sphenoid (which lies behind the eyes and nose and attaches to the side of the face just lateral to the eyes) jams superior or inferior to the occipital bone. These lesions are more severe and need to be addressed independently, but much of the side-bent, torsioned, or lateral strains to the sphenoid can be addressed with the simple compression/decompression technique described above. If not, "normalizing each of the sphenobasilar dysfunctions is achieved by stabilizing the occiput and moving the sphenoid into its greatest range of motion (the named direction of dysfunction) and allowing for release," then moving into the direction of the restriction.[12] Since the sphenoid is the only bone within the cranium that is connected to all other bones, it can be affected by many restrictions. The sphenoid, however, is typically not the source of the primary problem since the sphenobasilar joint is a syncondrosial joint having no capsule or fluid, just a cartilaginous bar between the bones. Any restriction here is often a compensatory problem stemming from fascial pull originating somewhere else in the body. Releasing the sphenoid is effective in treating such symptoms as headaches, migraines, sinusitis and allergy problems, pituitary problems, visual problems, learning dysfunctions, sacral dysfunction, coccyx compression, TMJ dysfunction, and even depression. One very interesting clinical picture is what Upledger has termed the "unhappy triad." Many times in the presence of endogenous depression, compression at vertebral level L5-S1, the occipital cranial base, and at the sphenobasilar synchrondrosis can be identified.

After all cranial bones have been released we move to *step nine*, which is balancing the mandible in relation to the cranium. A compressive then decompressive force (as done with the sphenoid) is used to release any tension at the temporomandibular joint and along the client's mandible.

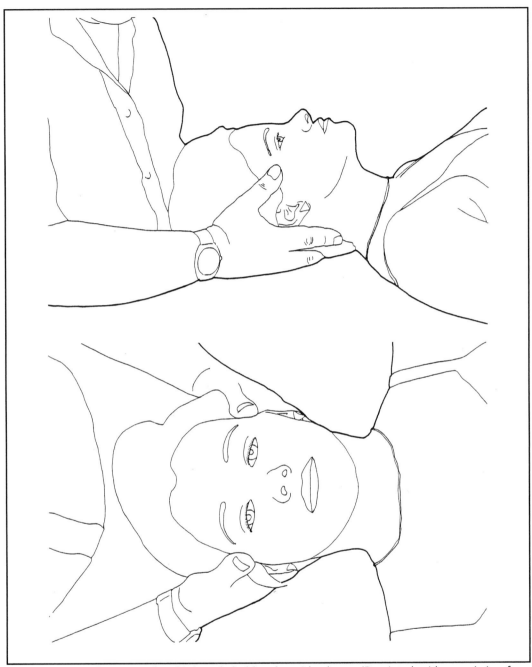

Figure 6-3. Hand position for third vault hold, sphenoid release. (Reprinted with permission from Upledger JE, Vredevoogd JD. *Craniosacral Therapy.* Seattle, WA: Eastland Press; 1983:100.).

The therapist places each hand lengthwise along each side of the mandible, and use a very gentle relaxed force to compress the mandible upward to its endpoint. Once complete, the therapist gently induces a slight downward pressure of not more than 5 g until full release has occurred. Many TMJ patients have been treated with great relief using this technique.

The final and *tenth step* of Dr. Upledger's protocol is an induction of another still point which is typically done at the head. This allows the patient's system to realign and integrate the work that has been done during the session.

Contraindications to Craniosacral Therapy

Craniosacral therapy should not be used whenever changes in intracranial fluid pressure would be detrimental to the patient, such as in the presence of intracranial hemorrhage, an acute cerebrovascular accident, or an aneurysm.[1] It is also not recommended to induce a still point using a CV-4 technique at the head of small children (under 8 years old), as a therapist could compress vulnerable structures not yet matured in the growing child.

Evidence of Efficacy of Craniosacral Therapy

A review of the recently published studies of craniosacral therapy is disappointing both in terms of measurable outcomes and with regard to reliability. J. L. Oschman[10] describes in detail the origin of the biomagnetic pulses that emanate from the hands of those practitioners who have an intention to use that energy to heal. "Practitioners of therapeutic touch and related methods produce strong biomagnetic fields that are not steady in frequency… (but) are within the same range of frequencies that biomedical researchers are finding effective for jump starting healing in a variety of soft and hard tissues."[10] Medical research is moving toward discovering the cellular mechanism of action when practitioners use energy in their healing practices, as do craniosacral therapists. It has been hypothesized that, during the manual therapy session, an ideal arrangement for entrainment of the biological rhythms of the patient and therapist takes place.

The experience of the energy of the therapist entraining with the energy of the client presents difficulty when one wishes to study the effects of an energetic therapeutic technique, for as soon as the energies of the client and therapist "connect," the total of the energy field shifts to incorporate the sum of the two energies. This may be the origin of the difficulty in establishing interrater reliability and validity in traditional research trials.

Martin Green and colleagues[13] from the University of British Columbia reviewed craniosacral therapy "as an intervention with a scientific basis." Seven databases were screened in February of 1999 by two reviewers using accepted standardized criteria for the evaluation of scientific studies. Topics explored included the correlation of craniosacral interventions and health outcomes, the reliability of craniosacral assessment, and the pathophysiology of the craniosacral system. Thirty-three studies were identified. Seven of the studies were categorized with the lowest grade of evidence using the Canadian Task Force on Preventive Health Care rating system. Four of the five studies that examined agreement by practitioners on craniosacral assessment findings reported low reliability with intraclass correlation coefficients (ICC) ranging from 0.02 to 0.20 across these studies. Nine of the studies found support for minute movements that may occur between the bones of the adult cranium. Eleven studies supported the idea that CSF may flow in a pulse-like manner. No evidence was found supporting ability to manipulate the cranial sutures or that manual techniques actually affect the flow of CSF. Not surprisingly, in the studies that were examined, the authors concluded that, "research was not able to definitively demonstrate a causal relationship between restrictions or misalignments of the cranial bones and health outcomes."[13]

J. S. Rogers and colleagues at the University of North Carolina[14] published the results of a study that examined simultaneous palpation of the craniosacral rate at the head and feet of clients, examining intrarater and interrater reliability and rate comparisons. Twenty-eight adult subjects were divided in half by a curtain as they lay supine on a treatment table, with an experienced craniosacral examiner at the head and another at the feet. The examiners' findings were recorded with the activation of a silent foot switch that was depressed when no signal was present, and activated by lifting the foot at the beginning of the flexion phase of the craniosacral rhythm. Intrarater reliability measures were taken with examiner A at the head, examiner A at the feet, examiner B at the head, and examiner B at the feet. Interrater reliability measures were compared at the head and the feet. Interrater ICCs were 0.08 at the head and 0.19 at the feet. Intrarater ICCs ranged from 0.18 to 0.30. Craniosacral rates measured at the feet and the head were not identical. Just as was reported in the review article mentioned above, the results indicate the craniosacral rhythm cannot be palpated reliably. One reason for the discrepancies may be explained by, as stated earlier, entrainment. Because the scientific evidence and hypotheses surrounding the theory of entrainment are not well known, the authors made no mention of the idea and the possible effect of the examiners' energy fields on what was being measured. Another reason for differences in rate between examiners listening at the head and feet simultaneously is that patient injury may cause differences on the CSF rhythm within the same body.

As one can see, a lot of these recent studies are not well favored with craniosacral therapy but if one looks at the clinical evidence it becomes more difficult to argue its effectiveness. When an autistic child moves from being withdrawn and unable to communicate effectively with others to being able to sit and eat socially at the dinner table with cranial therapy being the only intervention, one must take notice. Another great example of cranial sacral therapy's effectiveness is when it was used in the cases of conjoined twins. Two Italian girls treated in Cleveland, Ohio, and the two Egyptian boys treated in Dallas, Texas, both have received the benefits of craniosacral therapy. It has been documented that in 2002, prior to having surgery and before craniosacral treatments were implemented, the Egyptian boys, both conjoined at the head, were lethargic, subdued, and unable to play or touch their feet. One of them had difficulty feeding and moving his bowels. After extensive craniosacral therapy, and still prior to surgery, the children were playful, eating, moving their bowels, interacting socially, and had progressed to some weight bearing on their feet leaning on a theraball. Even their primary physician from Cairo who was initially "skeptical" couldn't deny the results.[15] On October 12, 2003, Dr. Kenneth Slayer performed a successful surgery and separated the conjoined twins with the help of a team of physicians. The boys continued to participate with craniosacral therapy even after surgery and are thriving.

Conclusion and a Personal Note

This chapter describes craniosacral therapy in terms of its structure, its anatomy and physiology, the basic techniques of practice, the types of clinical problems it can help, and the rationale behind how symptoms are relieved. I was attracted to this approach because, coming from a strong science background, it expanded the knowledge I had as a traditional physical therapist. After beginning instruction from Upledger and associates, I found that I was able to use the basic tools effectively with patients in my physical therapy clinic. I was quite conservative during my introduction to this therapy, as I was fearful as to what the rehabilitative population was willing to accept. As a result, I do not feel I have completely given the work its just due in what it can accomplish, not only for our patients, but for ourselves as practitioners. I've learned that craniosacral therapy is so much more than tissue releases. It has changed the way I look at the body, the way I work with my clients, and the way I walk in the world today. Traditionally, as physical therapists, we were taught to look at the body as a compilation of muscles, nerves, joints, bones, and the resulting biomechanics of motion. Traditionally, We were instructed to evaluate patients with the idea in mind of what we could do to "fix" their problems. This old way of thinking puts the burden of responsibility on the shoulders of the therapist, because our role is to perform and help "heal" this patient. Through craniosacral therapy, both as a patient myself and as a therapist, I have come to realize that: 1) it's not that simple, and 2) with this new perspective, the burden and responsibility in patient/client care is actually much easier than I have made it in the past. The cross is theirs to bear, but we can help. We can help them get clear on what is happening for them and support them as they work through their injury. We as therapists are there to aid the client in their healing process. They, as the client, are responsible for their own healing process. Thank goodness the body has a beautiful innate ability to heal and move towards wholeness.

Experience in practice teaches us that we are more than muscles, nerves, joints, and bones. We are whole living human beings with aspects that are not often considered in patient care, such as energy fields, beliefs, perceptions, and emotions, and we all have spiritual connections. The "trauma" or "disease" that brings us to treatment in reality can be physical, mental, emotional, or spiritual in nature and in origin. There is really no way to separate out the aspects of ourselves that are difficult to measure from that which we can see and measure. If some part of us is out of balance, our body-mind intelligence will do what it can to re-establish homeostasis. If homeostasis cannot be achieved, according to the theories of energy medicine, disease and disharmony eventually manifests.

Upledger describes how trauma can enter the body and form what he calls "energy cysts." Either an injury by force or trauma or a negative experience "enters" the body and, depending its severity and how often it is repeated, as well as the emotional state of the patient at the time of injury, the body-mind can either dissipate the trauma, "wall it off," or isolate it in order to minimize the problem.[3] This formation of an energy cyst decreases the patient's natural flow of body energy, "life force," or vitality. It also affects the patient's craniosacral rhythm. Thus, energy cysts form the "stones in the river" to the craniosacral flow described earlier in the chapter. Through whole body evaluative techniques and treatment by way of somatoemotional recall and release, we are able to dissipate these cysts.

Many patients will present with problems that have eluded all of the traditional therapists they have seen and often have been told that their symptoms are "all in their head." It has been my experience and the experience of thousands of practitioners and patients that craniosacral therapy very often unlocks those elusive symptom puzzles and thus enables us to more adequately help our patients.[3]

When I say that with the craniosacral therapy approach and techniques my burden and responsibility as a therapist is much easier than I have made it in the past, I mean that I have learned to shift my perspective from being the only active agent, the "healer," the therapist that will "fix your problem" to that of a "facilitator" in my clients' healing process. In the past, I would leave the clinic feeling emotionally and physically drained by the end of the day, giving 110% of myself trying to remove the restriction, fix what I thought the problem was, and many times it seemed to me that I was working much harder than my client in this process. Upon learning and practicing craniosacral therapy regularly, I have come to see that the task of therapy is really not about me and what I need to do "to" the patient. Instead, it is a listening process and a co-creation of a different, more balanced energy field within the patient as fascial restrictions are located and released. Although I continue to struggle in letting go of old ways and old belief systems, I have seen that if I can step back and hold a supportive space for my clients, if I can get out of my own way and theirs, if I can set my own agenda aside and follow their body tissue where they need to go instead of where I think they "should" go, then the therapy session flows with much more ease and grace, and the client and I feel much better at the end of a treatment.

I'm not saying turn it all over and let it fly, because I also realize that the more I study, the more I understand how the body-mind works, the more detailed my knowledge of the anatomy becomes, and the more skilled the palpation in my hands becomes, the more accurate and specific my energy can be toward the problem. This results in a quicker more effective treatment for the client.

When helping a client or patient release the physical manifestations of the emotional component of an injury, the therapist needs only to hold a supportive, safe place for the patient to let go of that which no longer serves them and their healing. Of course, there is a always a critical place for psychotherapy in healing emotional issues that sometimes accompany the clients in rehabilitation, and every good therapist should have access to a mental health professional to refer to when necessary. We are in the 21st century and health care, specifically physical therapy and rehabilitation, have entered a new era of healing. It is time we as clinicians read the science behind energy medicine, broaden our minds about approaches to patient care that facilitate balance and the flow of body energy, and take appropriate responsibility for learning, practicing, and researching complementary therapies that are effective for our patients. Craniosacral therapy has proven to me over and over again that it is an invaluable tool. In time, the science will catch up to what craniosacral practitioners and their patients have experienced for decades and provide us with a description of just how this technique results in the healing process. Meanwhile, as practitioners, we need to be documenting our treatments and results, and publishing for the benefit of all.

References

1. Magoun HI. *Osteopathy in the Cranial Field*. 2nd ed. Denver, CO: Sutherland Cranial Teaching Foundation, Cranial Academy; 1996.
2. Feely RA. *Clinical Cranial Osteopathy*. Meridian, OH: The Cranial Academy; 1988.
3. Upledger JE, Vredevoogd JD. *Craniosacral Therapy*. Seattle, WA: Eastland Press; 1983.
4. Upledger JE. *Your Inner Physician and You*. Berkley, CA: North Atlantic Books; 1997.
5. Upledger JE. *Craniosacral I Study Guide*. Palm Beach Gardens, FL: Upledger Institute Publishing; 1997.
6. Retzlaff EW, Upledger JE, Mitchell D. Beggert. Structure of the cranial bone sutures. *J Am Osteopath Assoc.* 1976; 75.
7. Retzlaff EW, Upledger JE, Mitchell, Beggert. Nerve fiber and endings in cranial sutures. *J Am Osteopath Assoc.* 1978;77.
8. Adams T, et al. Parietal bone mobility in the anesthetized cat. *J Am Osteopath Assoc.* 1992;92(5).
9. Wallace, Avant, McKinney, Thurston. Ultrasonic measurement of intracranial pulsations at 9 cycles/min. *J Neurol.* 1975:10.
10. Oschman JL. *Energy Medicine: The Scientific Basis*. New York, NY: Churchill Livingstone; 2000.
11. Schultz RL, Feitis R. *The Endless Web Fascial Anatomy and Physical Reality*. Berkley, CA: North Atlantic Books; 1996.
12. Kandel ER, Schwartz JH. *Principles of Neural Science*. 2nd ed. New York, NY: Elsevier; 1985.
13. Green C, Martin CW, Bassett K, Kazanjian A. A systematic review of craniosacral therapy: biological plausibility, assessment reliability, and clinical effectiveness. *Contemporary Therapies in Medicine*. 1999;7:201-207.
14. Rogers JS, Witt PL, Gross MT, Hacke JD, Genova PA. Simultaneous palpation of the craniosacral rate at the head and feet: intrarater and interrater reliability and rate comparison. *Phys Ther.* 1997;78:1175-1185.
15. International Alliance of Healthcare Professionals. Craniosacral therapy improves health of conjoined twins. *Events and Press*. March 2007.

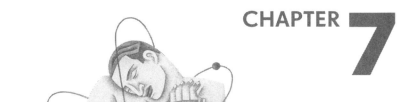

CHAPTER 7

MYOFASCIAL RELEASE
THE MISSING LINK IN TRADITIONAL TREATMENT

John F. Barnes, PT

Introduction

Myofascial release is a whole-body, hands-on approach for the evaluation and treatment of the human structure. Its focus is the fascial system. Physical trauma, an inflammatory or infectious process, or structural imbalance from dental malocclusion, osseous restriction, leg-length discrepancy, and pelvic rotation may all create inappropriate fascial strain.

Fascia, an embryologic tissue, reorganizes along the lines of tension imposed on the body, adding support to misalignment and contracting to protect the individual from further trauma (real or imagined). This has the potential to alter organ and tissue physiology significantly. Fascial strains can slowly tighten, causing the body to lose its physiologic adaptive capacity. Over time, the tightness spreads like a pull in a sweater or stocking. Flexibility and spontaneity of movement are lost, setting the body up for more trauma, pain, and limitation of movement. These powerful fascial restrictions begin to pull the body out of its three-dimensional alignment with the vertical gravitation axis, causing biomechanically inefficient, highly energy-consuming movement and posture.

Janet Travell's[1] detailed description of the myofascial element has taught us that there is no such thing as the muscle we have identified in traditional anatomy and physiology. A smooth fascial sheath surrounds every muscle of the body, every muscular fascicle is surrounded by fascia, every fibril is surrounded by fascia, and every microfibril down to the cellular level is surrounded by fascia. Therefore, it is the fascia that ultimately determines the length and function of its muscular component, and muscle becomes an inseparable component of fascia. The implications of this important fact have been largely ignored in Western or traditional health care.

Fascia

The fascia is a tough connective tissue that spreads throughout the body in a three-dimensional web from head to foot functionally, without interruption. It has been estimated that if every structure of the body except the fascia were removed, the body would retain its shape. As described by

Scott[2] and by Oschman,[3] the fascia serves a major purpose in that it permits the body to retain its normal shape and thus maintain the vital organs in their correct positions. It also allows the body to resist mechanical stresses, both internally and externally. Fascia has maintained its general structure and purposes over the millennia. These functions are evident in the earliest stages of multicelled organisms, in which two or more cells were able to stay in contact, communicate, and resist the forces of the environment through the connective tissue.[2]

Fascia covers the muscles, bones, nerves, organs, and vessels down to the cellular level. Therefore, malfunction of the system due to trauma, poor posture, or inflammation can bind down the fascia, resulting in abnormal pressure on any or all of these body components. It is through that process that this binding down, or restriction, may result in many of the poor or temporary results achieved by conventional medical, dental, and therapeutic treatments.[4]

As Travell[1] has explained, restrictions of the fascia can create pain or malfunction throughout the body, sometimes with bizarre side effects and seemingly unrelated symptoms that do not always follow dermatome zones. It is thought that an extremely high percentage of people suffering with pain, loss of motion, or both may have fascial restriction problems. Most of these conditions go undiagnosed, however, as many of the standard tests, such as radiographs, myelograms, computerized tomographic scans, and electromyograms do not show the fascia. If we cannot see it, we cannot look for restriction with our eyes.

Touching patients with skilled hands, however, can be one of the most potent ways of locating fascial restrictions and effecting positive change. Touching patients through mobilization, massage, and various forms of exercise and movement therapy, coupled with the gentle, refined touch of myofascial release and the sophisticated movement therapy called myofascial unwinding, creates a sensorimotor interplay. This experience of contact and movement is the very experience we need to reprogram our biocomputer, the mind-body, the basis for learning any new skill. Those practicing myofascial release use the skin and fascia as a handle or lever to create new options for enhanced function and movement of every structure of the body. Myofascial release helps remove the straightjacket of pressure caused by restricted fascia, eliminating symptoms such as stiffness, pain, and spasm. Then, through its influence on the neuromuscular and skeletal systems, it creates the opportunity for patients to "learn" new enhanced movement patterns. Manipulation and myofascial release both are highly effective treatments when they are accomplished with skilled hands and mind. They are designed to be used together to enhance the total effect. Joint manipulation is specific, attempting to improve the motion and function of a particular joint. Myofascial release, however, is a whole-body approach designed to discover and rectify the fascial restrictions that may have caused the effect or symptoms.

Discovering Fascial Restrictions

The skin has many ways of perceiving the universe. It is the largest organ of the body, covering approximately 18 square feet and weighing about 8 pounds, that is, 6% to 8% of total body weight.[5,6] It has about 640,000 sensory receptors that are connected to the spinal cord by over half a million nerve fibers. The tactile fibers vary from 7 to 135 per square centimeter.[5-7] The tactile surface of the skin is the interface not only between the body and our world, it is the interface between the mind's thought process and our physical existence.[7] This is also the interface by which therapists can facilitate incredible changes in the patient through the amazing plasticity of the central nervous system and the brain. Embryologically, both the skin and the nervous system are produced by ectoderm. When considering the connection of mind and body, we might ask, is the skin the outer surface of the brain or is the brain the deepest layer of the skin?[7,8]

Touch by itself can be powerfully therapeutic.[5] It can also serve as a powerful diagnostic tool by itself and through its role in proprioception. In general, of all the senses, the proprioceptive sense is least understood by most people; thus, it is seldom consciously used. However, when this sense is developed through the awareness and use of the more holistic right brain, rather than the logical left-brain "knowing," proprioceptive input opens up vistas of untapped intuitive potential for clinicians in both evaluation and treatment. The development of our proprioceptive sense also allows us to detect the quality and quantity of the often unnoticed very fine motion that is inherent in our bodies. As this approach is developed and refined, it is discovered that when we quiet our mind and body, and gently touch the patient with both hands, for example, on the dorsum of the feet, our proprioceptive senses help us in our evaluation by feeding us information as if our hands were moving like a mirror image to the patient's movement, thus detecting the subtle motions occurring in the patient's body that we cannot see or feel any other way. This activity, when practiced and honed, allows us to discover fascial restrictions and feel when they release. The informed touch of myofascial release also allows us to feel the motion that will take the patients' bodies into the three-dimensional position necessary for more total structural release or, as for many, for bringing disassociated memories to a conscious level, as will be discussed later in the chapter.

Myofascial Release: The Blending of Current and Emerging Explanatory Paradigms

A paradigm is a theoretical model that provides a way of describing, believing, and understanding what we consider to be real.[9] A paradigm "shift" changes our models of reality, our concepts, and logic and can create anxiety, fear, and anger in those persons deeply entrenched in the status quo. For others, it represents an opportunity for growth. Fear paralyzes some, while for others it provides the stimulus and motivation to move to higher and deeper levels of understanding, awareness, and achievement. The current paradigm or theory upon which Western medicine is based (reductionism) is becoming less and less adequate as it fails to explain such common phenomena as spontaneous remission of tumors, how the mind and emotions affect the physiology of the body, extrasensory perception, and other observed and documented occurrences.

The current paradigm that drives medicine and health care therapy and research springs from the centuries-old "either/or logic" of Aristotle. In it, everything is isolated, individual, and separate. There is no "middle ground" or shades of gray. This kind of thinking makes one theory wrong because another is right, or one person wrong because another is right.[10] Such thinking is exclusionary; it does not acknowledge connectedness among individuals or allow for the possibility of the coexistence of explanatory models.

Based on the logic of Aristotle, the universe, as perceived by Isaac Newton and René Descartes, is a giant machine that functions precisely, logically, sequentially, and correctly. This model of classic physics, which is the basis of our current paradigm, is informed by reductionistic research, which carefully allows for only one correct solution to a problem. In the field of medical science, theory based on this model and its research have reduced human illness to the "biochemistry of disease," completely losing sight of the fact that the disease or dysfunction is part of a whole person. That this model "has reached its limits and has crossed into absurdity" is obvious.[3,10] The emerging explanatory paradigm (holism) places priority on describing connectedness, relativity, complexity, multiple possibilities, and a nonlinear mind-body unity. The practice of myofascial release has to do with wholeness, connectedness (connective tissue), the wave and particle theory of atoms, and the subatomic realm of quantum physics.

Both systems theory and quantum physics, in part, describe the awareness and facilitation of interwoven, nonlinear systems in the universe where the whole is greater than, and makes sense of, the parts.[11,12] This theory contrasts reductionism, where the parts make sense of the whole because the whole is nothing more than the total of all the parts.[3,10] This paradigm shift requires a change of perspective and represents a "breakthrough in science. It connects living biological systems to physics and shows nature to be much more than just mechanical. The whole universe is alive and participating."[10]

Traditionally, medical education teaches that emotions are totally separate from the structure of the body. The body is essentially a machine, and when a part breaks down, it is to be medicated, surgically altered, or have some form of therapy directed at it and it alone. For years, this Cartesian viewpoint or model has been accepted as true, and patients were treated accordingly, even though logic and our experience tells us it could not be true.

Myofascial release is a logical expansion of the very roots of the health professions. It incorporates quantum theory and systems theory into practice, but it does not necessitate the dismantling of traditional health care or physical therapy. Rather, myofascial release represents a powerfully effective addition of a series of concepts and techniques that enhance and mesh with our traditional medical, dental, and therapeutic training.

A Close Examination of the Anatomy and Physiology of Fascia

The fascia is generally classified as superficial or lying directly below the dermis—deep, surrounding and infusing with muscle, bone, nerves, blood vessels, and organs to the cellular level, or deepest, the dura of the craniosacral system, encasing the central nervous system and the brain.

At the cellular level, fascia creates the interstitial spaces. It has extremely important functions in support, protection, separation, cellular respiration, elimination, metabolism, and fluid and lymphatic flow. It can have a profound influence on cellular health and the immune system. Therefore, trauma or malfunction of the fascia can set up the environment for poor cellular efficiency, necrosis, disease, pain, and dysfunction throughout the body.[13]

Molecular Structure of Fascia

Connective tissue is composed of collagen, elastin, and the polysaccharide gel complex, or ground substance.[3,14] These form a three-dimensional, interdependent system of strength, support, elasticity, and cushion.

Collagen is a protein consisting of three polypeptide chains that line up to form fibrils in such a way as to ensure that there are no weak points that could give way under tension. Collagen fibers thus contribute strength to fascial tissue and guard against overextension.

Elastin, another protein, is intrinsically rubber-like. Its fibers are laid down in parallel with an excess length of collagen fibers in places where elasticity is required, such as skin and arteries. This combination absorbs tensile forces. Tendons, specialized for pulling, mainly contain these elastocollagenous fibers.

The polysaccharide gel complex, mainly composed of hyaluronic acid and proteoglycans, fills the spaces between fibers. Hyaluronic acid is a highly viscous substance that lubricates the collagen, elastin, and muscle fibers, allowing them to slide over each other with minimal friction. Proteoglycans are peptide chains that form the gel of the ground substance. This gel is extremely hydrophilic, allowing it to absorb the compressive forces of movement. Cartilage, which acts as a shock absorber, contains much water-rich gel.

As long as the forces are not too great, the gel of the ground substance is designed to absorb shock and disperse it throughout the body. If fascia is restricted at the time of trauma, the forces cannot be dispersed properly and areas of the body are then subjected to an intolerable impact, and injury results. Injurious forces do not have to be enormous; a person who lacks sufficient "give" can be severely injured by minor forces.[3,4,14]

Realizing this, we can explain the sports and performance injuries that recur despite extensive therapy, strengthening, and flexibility programs. An athlete with fascial restrictions will not efficiently absorb the shocks of continued activity. Thus, the body absorbs too much pressure in too small an area, and during performance the body keeps "breaking down." This same effect takes place over time from the microtrauma of discrepancies of leg length due to weight bearing on a continuously torsioned pelvis. Each step sends imbalanced forces throughout the body, which then tries to compensate through muscular spasm and fascial restrictions, ultimately producing symptoms.

Myofascial release techniques are performed to reduce these symptoms of pain, spasm, and malalignment. In addition to increasing range of motion, the enormous pressure of the fascial restrictions is eliminated from pain-sensitive structures, alleviating symptoms, restoring the normal quantity and quality of motion, and restoring the body's ability to absorb shock without compensatory injury.

The Functions of Fascia

The fascia, as mentioned earlier, is particularly significant in supporting and providing cohesion to the body structures; thus, its functions are varied and complex. Functional, biomechanically efficient movements depend on intact, properly distributed fascia. Fascia creates a plexus to support and stabilize, thus enhancing the body's postural balance. Appropriately, loose fascia permits movement between adjacent structures, which are free of friction due to the presence of bursal sacs. In addition, loose tissue contains a fluid that serves as a transport medium for cellular elements of other tissues, blood and lymph. In this manner, fascia also supports a nutritive function.[15]

Fat is stored in the superficial fascia. This layer also provides a covering that helps conserve body heat. The deep fascia is an ensheathing layer. It maintains physiologic limb contour and enhances venous and lymphatic circulation. In combination with intermuscular septa and interosseous membranes, the deep fascia provides additional surface area for muscle attachment.[3,15]

Structurally, the planes in connective tissue allow passage of infectious and inflammatory processes. The presence in the tissue of histiocytes, however, offers a defense against bacteria. These phagocytes also remove debris and foreign matter from fascia. In addition, connective tissue neutralizes or detoxifies both endogenous (produced under physiologic conditions) and exogenous (introduced from outside the body) toxins. Finally, its fibroplastic qualities permit fascia to assist in healing injuries by depositing collagenous fibers by way of scar tissue.[15]

In addition to the structural function of fascia, recent research by Langevin[16] at the University of Vermont and by Ingber[17] at Harvard has identified the role of fascia as a whole body communication network. Fascial cells, responsive to mechanical forces, seem to generate three categories of signals: electrical, cellular, and tissue remodeling.[16] Ingber's work reveals that mechanical distortion of fascial cells profoundly affects the cells' behavior that can "switch cells between distinct gene programs (eg, growth, differentiation and apoptosis)." By way of tensegrity and solid-state mechanochemistry, fascial cells may "mediate mechanotransduction and facilitate integration of chemical and physical signals that are responsible for control of cell behavior."[17(p.811)]

Myofascial Release Effect on Collagen

Collagen comes from the ancient Greek word that means "glue-producer." The feeling one perceives during myofascial release treatment is rather like stretching glue. The therapist follows this sensation with sensitive hands as it twists and turns, barrier through barrier, until an increased range of motion is accomplished.

A therapist cannot mechanically overstretch the collagenous aspect of the fascia. Although we are as yet unable to prove it, the improvements seen after myofascial release are probably due to a stretching of the elastic component, a shearing of the cross-links that can develop at the nodal points of the fascia, and a change in the viscosity of the ground substance from a more solid to a gel state. This change in viscosity increases the production of hyaluronic acid and increases the glide of the fascial tissue. Also observed regularly is what appears to be a positive effect on the spindle cells, the Golgi tendon organs of the musculotendinous component, and the tone of the peripheral, autonomic, and central nervous systems.[3,4]

Thus, to separate fascia from its influence on muscle and their influence on each other is impossible. In other words, we have been evaluating and treating an illusion. Anatomical and scientific reality demand that we consider both muscle and fascia as inexorably linked as one. Understanding their integrated characteristics, we use this more accurate information to inform our evaluation and treatment. My experience has shown that medicine, modalities, muscle energy techniques, mobilization, manipulation, temporomandibular joint appliances, massage, and flexibility and exercise programs affect *only* the muscular and elastic components of the fascial system. Only myofascial release, with its emphasis on using bioenergy and the piezoelectric effect that occurs as we sustain the release, barrier after barrier, affects the total fascial system. This is why it is important to add myofascial release techniques to our current treatment regimens. Otherwise, we are only treating part of the problem and part of the patient. The inclusion of myofascial release allows the conscientious health professional to offer patients a truly comprehensive approach.

Myofascial Release Techniques

The myofascial skeletal system, with its combined ability to provide both compressive forces by hydrostatic pressure and tensile strength, creates a space truss system that realistically replaces the post and lintel or lever model.[3,4] Pierce[18] refers to this principle of natural construction as minimal inventory/maximum diversity. In the spine, post or columnar loading as support of the body has only limited use. In certain species, in certain positions, and when it converts to a lever, it is highly energy consuming and an unlikely support system in nature. D'Arcy Thomson[19] suggests that trusses can be a model for structural support in vertebrates. Trusses have clear advantages over post and lintel construction as a structural support system for biologic tissue. Trusses have flexible, even frictionless, hinges with no coupled moments about the joint, and the support elements are in tension and compression only, with no bending moments. Loads applied at any one point are distributed about the truss as tension or compression, rather than local loading as levers, as in post and lintel construction. There are no levers in a truss. The truss, being fully triangulated, is inherently stable and cannot be deformed without producing large deformations of the individual members, even with frictionless hinges. Only trusses are inherently stable with freely moving hinges. Any structure that has freely moving hinges and is structurally stable is a truss. Vertebrates, having stable structural configurations, in spite of essentially frictionless hinges, must therefore be constructed as trusses. The tension elements of the body—the soft tissues, muscles, ligaments, and connective tissue—have largely been ignored as supporting members of the body frame and have been viewed only as the stabilizers or motors. In loading a truss, the elements that are in tension could be replaced by flexible materials such as ropes, wire, muscles, or other soft tissues.

It is imperative that our structures have the ability to respond appropriately to our gravitational field as it plunges down through us. Ideally, we should be balanced around the vertical axis of this constant gravity; otherwise, imbalance almost always shortens the body and increases the expenditure of energy. Myofascial release, along with therapeutic exercise and movement therapy, improves the vertical alignment and lengthens the body, providing more space for the proper functioning of osseous structures, nerves, blood vessels, and organs.

Due to an injury to the lumbosacral area, patients have been known to experience distant symptoms such as occipital headaches, upper cervical pain and dysfunction, feelings of tightness around the thoracic area, lumbosacral pain, and tightness and lack of flexibility in the posterior aspect of the lower extremity. It is this author's belief that, during trauma, or with the development of a structural imbalance, a proprioceptive memory pattern of pain is established in the central nervous system. Beyond the localized pain response from injured nerves, these reflex patterns remain to perpetuate the pain during and beyond healing of the injured tissue, similar to the experience of phantom limb pain. Also in operation is the psychosomatic mode of adaption, which is part of Selye's general adaptation syndrome.[20]

Once fascia has tightened and is creating symptoms distant from the injury, all of the appropriate, traditional localized treatments will produce poor or temporary results because the imbalance and excessive pressure from the myofascial tightness remain untreated. Myofascial release techniques are therefore performed in conjunction with specific symptomatic treatment. It is believed and observed that the gentle tractioning forces applied to the fascial restrictions will elicit heat from a vasomotor response that increases blood flow to the affected area, which will enhance lymphatic drainage of toxic metabolic wastes, realign fascial planes, and most importantly, reset the soft tissue proprioceptive sensory mechanism. This last activity seems to reprogram the central nervous system, enabling the patient to perform a normal, functional range of motion without eliciting the previous pain patterns.[21]

The goal of myofascial release is to remove fascial restrictions and restore the body's equilibrium. When the structure has been returned to a balanced state, it is realigned with gravity. When these aims have been accomplished, the body's inherent ability to self-correct returns, thus restoring optimum function and performance with the least amount of energy expenditure. A more ideal environment to enhance the effectiveness of concomitant symptomatic therapy is also created.

The therapist is taught to find the cause of symptoms by evaluating the fascial system. Visually analyzing the structure of the human frame, palpating the tissue texture of the various fascial layers, and observing the symmetry, rate, quality, and intensity of the craniosacral rhythm make up this evolution process. The technique requires continuous re-evaluation during treatment, including observation of vasomotor responses and their location as they occur after a particular restriction has been released. This provides instantaneous and accurate information, enabling the therapist to proceed intelligently and logically from one treatment session to the next, to the ultimate resolution of the patient's pain and dysfunction. Detailed systematic documentation of this information will assist us in compiling the data for further qualitative research needed to explain and predict patient outcomes.

When the location of the fascial restriction is determined, gentle pressure is applied in its direction. It is hypothesized that this has the effect of pulling the elastocollagenous fibers straight. When hand or palm pressure is first applied to the elastocollagenous complex, the elastic component is engaged, resulting in a "springy" feel. The elastic component is slowly stretched until the hands stop at what feels like a firm barrier. This is the collagenous component. This barrier cannot be forced; it is too strong. Instead, the therapist continues to apply gentle sustained pressure, and soon the firm barrier will yield to the previous melting or springy feel as it stretches further. This yielding phenomenon is related to viscous flow; that is, a low load (gentle pressure) applied slowly will allow a viscous medium to flow to a greater extent than a high load (quickly applied) pressure.[3,22] The viscosity of the ground substance has an effect on the collagen, since it is believed that the viscous medium that makes up the ground substance controls the ease with which collagen fibers rearrange themselves.[22] As this rearranging occurs, the collagenous barrier releases, producing a change in tissue length.[3]

It is important to keep in mind the properties of fascial tissue. Viscoelasticity "causes it to resist a suddenly applied force over time. Creep is the progressive deformation of soft tissues due to constant low loading over time. Hysteresis is the property whereby the work done in deforming a material causes heat and hence energy loss."[23] The therapist follows the motion of the tissue, barrier to barrier, until freedom is felt. The Arndt-Schultz law also explains how the gentle, sustained pressure of myofascial release can produce such consistent changes and improvements. The law states that there is a therapeutic window of effectiveness, where weak stimuli increase physiologic activity, but very strong stimuli from the same source can inhibit or abolish activity.[24]

The development of one's tactile and proprioceptive senses enhances the "feel" necessary for the successful completion of these techniques. We were all born with the ability to feel the releases and the direction in which the tissue seems to move from barrier to barrier. When first learning myofascial release, students perform the techniques mechanically. With a little practice, they discover the feel and move to a more artful or higher level of achievement.

No prior knowledge of mobilization or manipulation is required to learn the concept and techniques of myofascial release. The procedures should be combined with neuromuscular technique (muscle energy), joint mobilization, and manipulation by skilled practitioners. However, since it is usually fascial restrictions that created the osseous restrictions in the first place, releasing the fascia first is often the desired order of treatment.

The biomechanical, bioelectrical, and neurophysiological effects of myofascial release represent an evolutionary leap for our professions and our patients. This is a total approach incorporating a physiologic system that, when included with traditional therapy, medicine, or dentistry, acts as a catalyst and yields impressive, clinically reproducible results.[3,4]

Myofascial Cranial Techniques

Application of myofascial release to the cranium is most effective when light pressure is used. Once you have learned to "read the body," more pressure may be indicated at times. Practitioners are taught to start lightly on the mechanical level. Through time and experience, their awareness and sensitivity increases to the point where treatment on the head or body flows in a dynamic fashion.

Direct and Indirect Cranial Techniques

Many people performing cranial therapy use a direct technique. Although some start out this way, trial and error teaches an indirect technique is usually far more productive for lasting results. It is nontraumatic and extremely effective.

With the direct technique, the therapist aligns each cranial bone according to how it appears in an anatomy book. This is a logical solution. The problem with direct technique is that it does not pay attention to the fascial system. It is the fascial system, firmly attached to the cranial bones by the endosteum, that determines the three-dimensional position of the cranial bones and, eventually, their function. Indirect technique uses the fascial system as a handle or lever to realign the cranial bones, or other osseous structures, into their correct physiological position so that they achieve maximum function. This technique avoids the guesswork of mimicking pictures of anatomic structures or the need to use the arbitrary statistical average approach. Rather, it is truly physiologic therapy that allows the body to self-correct.[3]

A helpful way of viewing the differences between traditional direct and indirect myofascial cranial techniques is to imagine a screen door with a stuck latch. Direct technique is the equivalent of trying to pull forcefully against the latch to get the door open. If we use force in treatment, the body's protective mechanism responds by pulling back. If we then tug a little harder, the body pulls back to an even greater degree. Indirect technique is the equivalent of gently closing the stuck screen door a little more and then opening it. It will almost always open easily and nontraumatically. Applying this concept to the body or head, one exaggerates the lesion (shuts the screen door a little more) and then decompresses (unlatches the screen door).

A still point, or a feeling of complete stillness that results from shutting down of the craniosacral rhythm, occurs at that position. "The craniosacral system is characterized by rhythmic, mobile activity which persists through life... It is distinctly different from the physiological motions which are related to breathing, and different from cardiovascular activity as well... The normal rate of craniosacral rhythm in humans is between 6 and 12 cycles per minute."[25]

During the still point, a reorganization of the neuromuscular system occurs and the holding or bracing patterns change.[4] A new balance or reference point is found and a positive therapeutic event involving structural, emotional, and intellectual improvement occurs. This change or release then allows us to decompress. As with other forms of myofascial release, we allow our hands to follow where the tissue wants to go, barrier to barrier, until all is released and balanced.

It seems that confusion about what techniques (direct or indirect) to use has arisen because we were taught to differentiate between flexion and extension,

> **Personal Example**
>
> My experience has shown that while a direct technique is excellent as a last resort or finishing technique, especially when the dysfunction is primarily an osseous restriction, it is usually most effective to start with an indirect technique. Therefore, myofascial cranial techniques start with compression—exaggeration of the lesion—followed by decompression. It seems that when we compress lightly and follow the body part three-dimensionally where it wants to go (the direction of ease), we will reach the exact position where the body must be in order to release itself.

side-bending and rotational lesions, and how to correct them mechanically. The problem with this lies in the realization that, in vivo, there is no such thing as a strictly flexion or extension lesion or a strictly side-bending or rotational lesion. These are simply linear labels of the most predominant part of the lesion. Although they are convenient teaching tools, they are illusions. In life, all lesions are three-dimensional, having a component of either flexion or extension, side-bending, and rotation. No machine or person is intelligent enough to figure out what degree of any of these dimensions is necessary to find the exact position for the body to release. Only the wisdom of the body's self-correcting mechanism can do this. Quieting the mind and following where the fascia or the body wants to go naturally (as in myofascial unwinding) will take the therapist exactly into the degree of flexion or extension, side-bending, and rotation that the individual needs, barrier to barrier, until the individual is released and balanced.

Cranial therapy is, by nature, gentle and thus has virtually no serious side effects. Because of its potent influence on intracranial fluid dynamics, however, the following are considered definite contraindications:

1. Acute intracranial hemorrhage: therapy may prolong the duration of hemorrhage by interrupting clot formation.

2. Intracranial aneurysm: treatment may induce leak or rupture.

3. Herniation of the medulla oblongata: a life-threatening condition.

4. Recent skull fracture: the techniques are best avoided.

5. Acute systemic infections: therapy is generally avoided; however, cranial compression and a distraction-induced still point may help reduce fever.

Myofascial Unwinding: The Body Remembers

To ask how the mind communicates with the body or how the body communicates with the mind assumes that the two are separate entities. The research of Popper and Eccles confirms this.[26] My research and experience with myofascia have shown that they seem to respond as a single unit or two sides of the same coin. Mind and body act as if they are different aspects of the same spectrum, immutably joined, inseparable, connected, influencing, and intercommunicating constantly. Myofascial release techniques and myofascial unwinding seem to allow for the complete communication of mind with body and body with mind, which is necessary for healing. The body remembers everything that ever happened to it, and Hameroff's research[27] indicates that the theory of quantum coherence points toward the storing of meaningful memory in the microtubules, cylindrical protein polymers that we find in the fascia of cells. Mind-body awareness and healing are often linked to the concept of "state-dependent" memory, learning, and behavior, also called deja vu.[20] We have all experienced this, for example, when a certain smell or the sound of a particular piece of music creates a flashback phenomenon, producing a visual, sensorimotor replay of a past event or an important episode in our lives with such vividness that it is as if it were happening at that moment. Based on the work of Hameroff and colleagues[25] and my experience, I would like to expand this theory to include position-dependent memory, learning, and behavior, with the structural position being the missing component in Selye's state-dependent theory as it is currently described.[28]

My experience has shown that during periods of trauma, people form subconscious indelible imprints of the experience that have high levels of emotional content. The body can hold information below the conscious level, as a protective mechanism, so that memories tend to become dissociated or amnesiac. This is called memory dissociation, or reversible amnesia. The memories are state (or position) dependent and can therefore be retrieved when the person is in a particular state (or position). This information is not available in the normal conscious state, and the body's protective mechanisms keep us away from the positions that our mind-body awareness construes as painful or traumatic.

It has been demonstrated consistently that when a myofascial release technique takes the tissue to a significant position, or when myofascial unwinding allows a body part to assume a significant position three-dimensionally in space, the tissue not only changes and improves, but memories, associated emotional states, and belief systems rise to the conscious level. This awareness, through the positional reproduction of a past event or trauma, allows the individual to grasp the previously hidden information that may be creating or maintaining symptoms or behavior that deter improvement. With the repressed and stored information now at the conscious level, the individual is in a position to learn which holding or bracing patterns have been impeding progress and why. The release of the tissue with its stored emotions and hidden information creates an environment for change.

Neurobiological research into the nature of neuronal activity during a specific mental event remains inconclusive.[29] Taylor[30] suggested that content inherent in consciousness may only be relevant when compared to previous memory. The meaning of an input is given by the degree of overlap such an input has to past inputs. Korb[31] has written about how inputs can have meaning, and the reader is referred to that research.

Selye's classic works[20,28] are concerned with the phenomenon of state-dependent memory, learning, and behavior, the general class of learning that takes place in all complex organisms that have a cerebral cortex and a limbic-hypothalamic system. Pavlovian and Skinnerian conditioning are specific varieties of state-dependent memory and learning.[20]

Memory and learning in all higher organisms take place by way of two internal responses:

1. A memory trace forms on the molecular-cellular-synaptic level.[32,33]

2. There is an involvement of the amygdala and hippocampus of the limbic-hypothalamic system in processing and encoding the memory; recall of the specific memory trace may be located elsewhere in the brain.[7,34]

The limbic-hypothalamic system is the central core to Selye's general adaption syndrome. The neurobiology of the three stages of the syndrome—the alarm reaction, the stage of resistance, and the stage of exhaustion—help explain the observed outcomes of myofascial release and myofascial unwinding and illustrate the mind-body integration.

The hormones that are responsible for the retention of memory, epinephrine and norepinephrine, are released during the alarm stage just before the trauma by the activation of the sympathetic branch of the autonomic nervous system. The state or position the person is in at the moment of trauma is encoded into the system as the person progresses into the second stage, the stage of resistance. At that point, the system adapts and develops subconscious strategies to protect itself from further trauma, fear, or memories by avoiding those three-dimensional positions the body is in at the time of the insult. The emotions also communicate this mind-body information by way of the neuropeptides. This creates a vicious cycle of interplay among the endocrine, immune, and autonomic neuromyofascial systems and the neuropeptides.

If this cycle continues for too long, the person enters the third, or exhaustion stage, in which the body's defense mechanisms expend enormous amounts of energy, thereby depleting one's reserve and perpetuating or enlarging the symptom complex.

Selye[20] frequently described this type of resistance as being "stuck in a groove," something we have all experienced. When something familiar happens, we react subconsciously in a habitual pattern before we can consciously be aware of it to control it. For example, if you were injured in a car accident, every time you see a car coming too fast you tighten and brace against the possible impact. People replay these incidents and the automatic, habitual bracing patterns associated with them subconsciously until these hidden memories and learned behaviors are brought to the surface. Myofascial unwinding helps bring this information to a conscious level, allowing patients to re-experience it and let go, if they choose.

How is it that normal bodily movements or daily activities do not reproduce these memories, emotions, and outdated beliefs? I believe that these positions represent fear, pain, or trauma. In an attempt to protect oneself from further injury, it seems as if the subconscious does not allow the body to move into positions that re-enact the microevents and important microcognitions essential for lasting mind-body change. The body then develops further strategies or patterns to protect itself. These subconscious holding patterns eventually form specific muscular tone or tension patterns, and the fascial component then tightens into these habitual positions of strain as a compensation to support the misalignment that results. Therefore, the repeated postural and traumatic insults of a lifetime, combined with the tensions of emotional and psychological origin, seem to result in tense, contracted, bunched, and fatigued fibrous tissue.

A discrete area of the body may become so altered by its efforts to compensate and adapt to stress that structural and, eventually, pathologic changes become apparent. Researchers have shown that the type of stress involved can be entirely physical, such as the repetitive postural strain developed by a typist, dentist, or hairdresser or purely psychic, such as the muscle tightening associated with chronic repressed anger.[15]

More often than not, a combination of mental and physical stresses alters the neuromyofascial and skeletal structures, creating a visible, identifiable physical change which, itself, generates further stress, such as pain, joint restriction, general discomfort, and fatigue. A chronic stress pattern produces long-term muscular contraction which, if prolonged, can cause energy loss, mechanical inefficiency, pain, cardiovascular pathology, and hypertension.[15]

Therapist Technique Required to Facilitate Release

Working in reverse, myofascial release and myofascial unwinding release the fascial tissue restrictions, thereby altering the habitual muscular response and allowing the positional, reversible amnesia to surface, producing emotions and beliefs that are the cause of the holding patterns and ultimate symptoms. In order to allow this spontaneous motion to proceed without interference, it is important for the therapist to quiet his or her mind and feel the subtle inherent motions in the patient. Quietly following the tissue (myofascial release) or body part (myofascial unwinding) three-dimensionally along the direction of ease, the therapist guides the patient's movement into the significant restrictions or positions. With myofascial unwinding, the therapist eliminates gravity from the system, unloading the structure to allow the body's gravity-oriented righting reflexes and protective responses to temporarily suspend their influence. The body is then free to move into positions that allow repressed state or position-dependent physiologic or flashback phenomena to recur. As this happens within the safe environment of a treatment session, the patient can facilitate the body's own inherent self-correcting mechanism to obtain improvement.

When a significant position is attained, the craniosacral rhythm, when palpated, is felt to shut down into a still point. During this still point, a reversible amnesia surfaces, replaying all the meaningful physiologic responses, memories, and emotional states that occurred during a past traumatic event. Rossi describes this dissociation, or reversible amnesia, as a double-conscious state.[35] In other words, what is experienced and remembered at the time of the original incident or trauma and the meaning attached to it is dependent on the psychophysiologic state of the individual at the time that the experience took place.[27] The resulting dissociation, or block, between the conscious and subconscious minds may be the major source of many poor or temporary traditional physical therapy outcomes.[35]

Myofascial release and myofascial unwinding bring the tissue or support the body part into a position eliminating gravity as the patient moves spontaneously. This allows the individual to be more fully aware of his or her divided consciousness. Reactivating the original conditions and the resultant physiologic responses by influencing the fascia to release results in a flashback phenomenon, which brings the repressed memory to conscious awareness and then allows the patient to have the choice to change. No longer do patients habitually find themselves holding or stiffening to protect themselves from future pain or trauma. Genuine release of fear and emotion takes place simultaneously with physical fascial release and physiologic release of the associated stress hormones.

As a result of observing the outcomes of many patients who have benefited from myofascial release and unwinding, I have concluded that the myofascial release approach is more than just an assemblage of techniques. Instead, it helps create a whole-body awareness, allowing the health professional to facilitate more than just structural change, but also growth and the possibility for a more total resolution of restrictions, emotions, and belief systems that may impede patient progress physically, emotionally, and cognitively. Thus, this treatment is holistic in nature and complements traditional physical therapy based on reductionism.

Fascia's Old and New Explanatory Paradigms

Clinical evidence has demonstrated that restrictions in the fascial system are of considerable importance in relieving pain and restoring function.[4] Myofascial release becomes vitally important when we realize that these restrictions can exert tremendous tensile forces on the neuromuscular-skeletal systems and other pain-sensitive structures, creating the very symptoms that we have been trying to eliminate.[36]

The prevailing view of the skeleton is that it is a group of bones. The vertebrae are "stacked" one on top of the other, the rest of the bones are "hitched on" somehow, and the whole mechanism is moved by the muscles that attach to the bones. Because the function of the fascial system largely has been ignored or misunderstood, we have developed an erroneous view of how our bodies truly function. We also have developed techniques to treat this misunderstood or "fictional" body. When these techniques do not achieve our desired outcomes, we tend to blame the patient for having a poor attitude or for not complying.

Tensegrity

What is really happening in our bodies can be best explained by the term *tensegrity*, coined by the architectural genius Buckminster Fuller, as interpreted by Deane Juhan.[7] Juhan noted that the vertical position of the skeleton is dependent on tensional forces generated by the fascia, the tone and contractility of the muscular components, and the hydrostatic pressure exerted by fascial compartments. The osseous structures (bones) act as rigid beams whose position and motion are determined by the guy wires (myofascial elements) attached to them. The integrity of a tensegrity unit depends on the tensional force of these guy wires, not on the compressional strength or stable balance of the rigid beams. It is the relationship among the fascia, muscles, and osseous structures that constitutes the tensegrity units of the body.[3,7,37]

There is not a single horizontal surface anywhere in the skeleton that provides a stable base for anything to be stacked upon it. A stone mason did not conceive the design of our bodies. Weight applied to any bone would cause it to slide right off its joints if it were not for the tensional balances that hold it in place and control its pivoting. Like the beams in a simple tensegrity structure, our bones act more as "spacers" than as compressional members; more weight is actually borne by the connective system of cables than by the bony beams.[3,7]

From this viewpoint, one can readily appreciate how crucial it is for the fascial "cables" to be of the proper length throughout the system. An abnormally tight cable in the lumbar area will negatively affect the entire balance of the spine and cranium. Conversely, increased or imbalanced tension in the upper regions of the body will produce compensatory tensions throughout the lower aspects of the structure, adversely affecting proper alignment.[7] This more accurate view of the body necessitates an understanding of the function of the fascial system and requires a total reversal of perspective.

As I developed this myofascial release approach, it became obvious that more than muscles and fascia responded; the whole body was involved. Treating a musculoskeletal symptom in isolation was no longer possible. During myofascial release, the body did not react like an inert machine, but rather was responsive, almost plastic or moldable under the therapist's hands. The tissues seemed to hold a consciousness, or thoughts of their own.[27,30] As releases occurred, patients reported memories or emotions emerging that were connected to past events or traumas. As their fascial systems changed and the memories or emotions surfaced, patients felt better and their symptoms improved, even though they previously were unresponsive to all other forms of traditional care that were tried. Taylor[30] and others are conducting current research about the possible role of fascia in the phenomenon of the mind-body connection.

As noted, the traditional or Western focus of medical and therapeutic education and treatment was on symptoms. The word *symptom*, derived from Greek, means "sign" or "signal." Symptoms are not the actual problem, however, but signs of the problem and treating the symptom does not necessarily affect the cause or source of the signaling. Modern physiology suggests that symptoms are the body's adaptive responses to stress, imbalance, or infection. Viewed this way, effective therapy must facilitate a return to balance,[4] not just relieve symptoms. All of the holistic complementary therapies are based on this belief.

To discover the cause of the imbalance that is creating the distant effect (symptoms), we use the principles of both traditional mechanistic therapy and the newer, more general theory of the nonlinear whole-body. We treat the interconnecting system through relieving restrictions in the three-dimensional network of fascia utilizing a mind-body approach. The two viewpoints, together with their techniques, dovetail comprehensively to maximize our ability to promote healing. For example, we may begin with myofascial releases around the shoulder and neck and then move to traditional shoulder mobilization. For those interested in understanding both the Cartesian theory and the emerging "new" quantum theory, Rupert Sheldrake's *The Presence of the Past*[37] is an excellent resource, as well as Micozzi's text *Fundamentals of Complementary and Alternative Medicine,*[38] and James Oschman's highly regarded text, in which much of the previous material in this chapter is described in detail, *Energy Medicine: The Scientific Basis.*[3,39]

The exponents of the Cartesian dualistic vs the quantum systems theory viewpoints have continued to argue, each claiming to be right while the other is wrong. It is possible that many of their explanations are both "right" and simply represent different perspectives of the whole picture. In a practical sense, treating specific symptoms complements the more general whole-body myofascial release approach. The latter, the mechanistic and specific, highlights where the former, the holistic, might be most appropriately utilized, thereby making mobilization and exercise regimens even more effective. In other words, both traditional physical therapy and myofascial release are parts of the whole and can be used together to enhance the result. Treating both the cause and effect of symptoms often produces more lasting improvement.

However helpful the specific mechanistic approach, it is obviously time for us to change our erroneous and misleading view of the human as a machine. The medical, dental, and physical and occupational therapy professions continue to be based on Newtonian physics, which is 300 years old and was proven to be totally inadequate more than 50 years ago. Yet, the very foundation of our scientific training is based on this inadequate information. When a theory is created out of an inaccurate belief, many other assumptions based on the fundamental inaccurate belief also will be incorrect, leading us to misunderstand how our bodies actually function in vivo. Oschman goes into great detail about this in his text.[3]

Too many health professionals have become captivated by the obvious—the symptom—paying no attention to the possible cause: fascial restrictions. We have missed something so fundamental because the model we were taught and believed in, based on Newton and Descartes, was incomplete. Not only was the fascia of the body ignored, traditional mechanistic theory separated what we could see, the physical or the material, from what we could not see—nonmaterialistic feelings and emotions—and dictated that only the materialistic should be of concern. However, both scientific and anecdotal information have emerged stating that by including the fascial system in evaluating patients, we can treat the cause of the symptoms nontraumatically with consistently effective and permanent results.[3,4]

Application of Mind-Body Theories to Traditional Physical Therapy

An important component of the theory behind the mind-body connection is the ability for people to transmit natural bioelectrical currents along the endogenous electromagnetic fields of the three-dimensional network of the fascial system of another person.[3] Medical applications of exogenous bioelectromagnetics (like x-ray) are very common. Endogenous bioelectromagnetic fields, natural within all living beings, have only more recently been studied.[3,40]

Increasingly, medical researchers and experienced health professionals are beginning to view the body as a self-correcting mechanism with bioelectric healing systems. According to one author,[41] while some scientists are starting to explore the body's sensitivity to electromagnetic energy, those of the old school still choose to ignore the matter because it upsets their long-held theories. Such an attitude is unwarranted, however, and also may be unhealthy. It is known that electromagnetic fields "trigger the release of stress hormones... [and] can affect such processes as bone growth, communication among brain cells, and even the activity of white cells."[41]

Becker and Seldon[42] found naturally occurring direct-current signals that they called the *current of injury* (COI). These signals are thought to be transmitted by the sheaths of Schwann and glial cells that surround their neurons. Others, however, consider the body's healing currents to use the microcapillary systems. In this theory, the bioelectric circuits are turned on when membrane conductivity closes down, and the electric flow then takes the path of least resistance through the blood stream.[43] The mechanism has not been determined but, clearly, the body sends endogenous electromagnetic energy wherever its healing effects are required.[3,42]

When we use traditional physical therapy electromagnetic devices (exogenous), it is not clear if the body interprets the energy of many of our modalities and of our sometimes abrupt manual techniques as intrusive and, therefore, resists our efforts.[42] If this is the case, the body would likely recognize such resistance as important to its survival. Many therapeutic efforts to heal have, in fact, caused patients discomfort. This may begin to show why endogenous microcurrents and the gentle, sustained pressures used in myofascial release produce results when conventional modalities and other hands-on techniques have failed. If the body does not view these as intrusive, it is not compelled to resist. Instead, the techniques are accepted as assistive and allow the organism's self-corrective mechanisms to be facilitated.[3] This is not to say that conventional modalities, exercises, and hands-on techniques are not valuable; certainly they are. It means that to treat the body comprehensively, the approaches must be combined, as they enhance each other in a complementary fashion and produce consistent results.

Copper wire is a well-known conductor of electricity. If copper wire becomes twisted or crushed, it loses its ability to conduct energy properly. It is thought that fascia may act like copper wire when it becomes restricted through trauma, inflammatory processes, or poor posture over time. Then its ability to conduct the body's bioelectricity seems to be diminished, setting up structural compensations and, ultimately, symptoms or restrictions of motion.[3]

The diminution of our fascial system's ability to conduct energy may be due to melanin.[44] Melanin is present in copious quantities in the fascia, and neuromelanin is present in the neural structures and brain, which are encased by fascia all the way down to the cellular level. Melanin has superior conducting properties at room temperature and is synthesized in mast cells, also found in the fascia, which influence the immune system. As a superconductor, melanin may regulate firing of nerve cells. It seems centrally involved in the control of all physiologic and psychological activity.[3,44]

The neuromelanin-neuroglial system is the major site of mental organization.[3,44] The nervous system is made up principly of glial cells. These cells have electrical properties that appear to be responsible for the piezoelectric phenomenon. Piezoelectric behavior is an inherent property of bone and other mineralized and nonmineralized connective tissues. Compressional stress has been suggested to create minute quantities of electrical current flow.[3,42]

Myofascial release can restore the fascia's integrity and proper alignment and, similar to the copper wire effect, can enhance the transmission of our important healing bioelectrical currents. Just like untwisting a copper wire, myofascial release techniques seem to restore the fascia's ability to conduct bioelectricity, thus creating the environment for enhanced healing. Release techniques can also structurally eliminate the enormous pressures that fascial restrictions exert on nerves, blood vessels, and muscles.[3]

Fascial "Memory"

Another observed patient response from myofascial release techniques is also explained more thoroughly within the mind-body paradigm. Recent evidence and my experience have demonstrated that embedded in our structure, particularly the fascial system, lie memories of past events or trauma.[4] These stored emotions can produce lessons in literal or symbolic form from which the patient can discover blocks that may have been hindering his or her healing process. By using effective communication skills, the therapist often can facilitate the efforts of a psychiatrist or psychologist well-trained in counseling and help the patient discover the sources of blockage preventing full recovery.

It appears that not only the myofascial element, but also every cell of the body has a consciousness that stores memories and emotions.[3,45] Research findings suggest that the mind and body act on each other in often remarkable ways. With the help of sophisticated new laboratory tools, investigators are demonstrating that emotional states can translate into altered responses in the immune system, the complex array of organs, glands, and cells that comprises the body's principle mechanism for repelling invaders. The implications of this loop are unsettling. To experts in the field of psychoneuroimmunology, the immune system seems to behave almost as if it had a brain of its own. This is creating a revolution in medicine in the way we view physiology. More than that, it is raising profound and tantalizing questions about the nature of behavior, about the essence of what we are.[10]

The field of psychoneuroimmunology stems from the three classic areas of neuroscience, endocrinology, and immunology. Scientists have discovered a neuropeptide bidirectional network of communication between our body and mind by way of the emotions.[46]

Neuropeptides are information carriers composed of 50 to 60 chemical substances and their corresponding receptors, making or preventing something from happening.

Receptors are not fixed; they have been accurately described as looking like lily pads that have floated up from the depth of the cell. Like lily pads, their roots sink downward, reaching the cell's nucleus where the DNA sits. DNA deals in many, many kinds of messages, potentially an infinite number. Therefore, it makes new receptors and floats them up to the cell wall constantly. There is no fixed number of receptors, no fixed arrangement on the cell wall, and probably no limit to what they are tuned in to. A cell wall can be as barren of lily pads as a pond in winter or as crammed as one in full flower in June.[47]

The neuropeptides are the key to the biochemistry of the emotions that are not just in the brain, but also in the cells of the entire body. In other words, the mind is not confined to the brain. We are an integrated totality, a mind-body network of information flowing throughout every system and cell of the body.

A network, like a web or fish net, is different from a hierarchic structure, which has one top place. Theoretically, you can plug into a network at any given point and get to any other point. By viewing the three-dimensional fascial system as a network, we can begin to appreciate how releasing the tissue at any one point in the body affects other areas, such as the spindle cells of the muscles, the Golgi tendon organs, the circulatory system, the lymphatic system, the body's organs, and the position and function of the osseous structures. By way of the hormonal and neuropeptide systems, information is then sent to the peripheral, autonomic, and central nervous systems to allow physical and emotional change and reduce pain, thus improving the quantity and quality of motion.

Remember that the discovery of invisible bacteria that transmitted disease and the discovery of penicillin were important turning points in Western medicine. Both were greatly resisted as being impossible to be true. The paradigm shift that is now occurring due to the understanding and awareness of the importance of quantum theory to how we view the mind-body and the discovery of the inseparability of the mind from the body resulting in the network of communication within the mind-body concept are creating yet another revolution.[3,45]

It has been demonstrated over and over that when a fascial barrier is engaged in myofascial release or when a person reaches a significant position during myofascial unwinding, the tissue releases and a memory or emotion surfaces. This electrophysical event produces a positive change and improvement in the patient. Myofascial release and myofascial unwinding are not linear but result in a whole-body effect, capable of producing a wide variety of physical, emotional, and mental effects.

The fascial and neuropeptide systems have thus turned our view of how our bodies function upside down and inside out. This is good news, for our old view of the body as a mindless machine was embarrassingly inadequate. While advances in medicine, surgery, and electronics have accomplished marvelous things, much more can be done. A better understanding of the fascial system that surrounds and influences every other system and cell of the body, and how cells can communicate with the brain and central nervous system and vice versa, allows us to see the enormous value of myofascial release in positively affecting the whole person.

We have a physiologic basis for emotions, and emotions and structure cannot be separated no matter how hard we might try. The improvements in emotional tone and structure have been demonstrated consistently for years with the various forms of myofascial release.[4]

Evidence for Efficacy of Myofascial Release

The literature does not distinguish between energy-based myofascial release and the more traditional, mechanical manual therapy myofascial release practiced by some osteopaths, chiropractors, and manual physical therapists. Nonetheless, there is a paucity of published studies on myofascial release in particular, very likely due in part to the fact that for double-blind trials, you cannot blind subjects who are receiving manual therapy. Subjects know when they are touched. (One can, however, blind the pre- and post-test evaluators and compare results from an experimental group vs a control group.) Also, as soon as the therapist touches the client or patient with the intent to offer myofascial release, the energy of the system is affected by that touch, and the therapist and subject lock into an energetic cybernetic system between themselves, making inter-rater reliability very difficult to reproduce.[3] Having said that, a review of the current published and abstract literature reveals the start of a collection of evidence.

Sucher[48] reported clinical improvement of carpal tunnel syndrome in four patients following myofascial release with home stretching exercises. This clinical improvement was confirmed by magnetic resonance imaging demonstrating that the anterior-posterior and transverse dimensions of the carpal canal significantly increased after treatment, and nerve conduction studies showed reduction in distal latencies or increase in motor response amplitudes.[48]

Weiss[49] investigated the effectiveness of a manual therapy technique similar to or identical to myofascial release trigger point therapy for interstitial cystitis and urinary urgency/frequency. Forty-five women and seven men (10 of whom had interstitial cystitis and 42 who had urgency-frequency syndrome) received myofascial release manual trigger point therapy to the pelvic floor for one to two visits each week for 8 to 12 weeks. Results tabulated from a competed symptom score sheet indicated the rate of improvement. Of the patients with urgency-frequency syndrome with or without pain, 35 (83%) experienced moderate to marked improvement or complete resolution of symptoms. Seven of the 10 (70%) with interstitial cystitis reported moderate to marked improvement. Ten of the patients also underwent electromyography, and mean resting pelvic floor tension decreased from 9.73 to 3.61 microvolts. Positive results were maintained for up to 12 months as long as patients continued practicing stress reduction techniques, Kegel exercises, and other physical therapy exercises.

Parish and Hardy[50] from the University of Mississippi published an abstract of a presentation given at a national scientific conference. They examined the use of myofascial release and its effect on pain and overall feeling of health, and investigated whether any changes in self-perception persisted over time. Ten patients with a variety of pain-related diagnoses, including fibromyalgia, neck pain, and migraine headaches were treated an average of eight times over approximately a 1-month period. The authors do not delineate in the abstract of what is specifically consisted in the myofascial release treatments. Patient self-assessments were made four times with the SF-36 immediately before the first treatment, following the final treatment, 3 to 6 months, and 9 to 12 months following discharge. Student t-test for paired data indicated that the patients had "a significantly greater sense of health (p=<0.02) immediately following the period of myofascial release treatments." Benefits were also reported to be long-lived, "persisting through the 9- to 12-month survey."

Abstracts of two presentations at a national scientific session in 2001 were published in *Physical Therapy*. Bezner and colleagues[51] from Southwest Texas State University examined the effects of myofascial release techniques on pulmonary function measures. Forty women and 18 men (mean age of 26 years) with no pathology were randomly assigned to the control group or the experimental group. The experimental group (n=30) received myofascial release to the shoulder, chest, and abdomen for 10 minutes, while the control group (n=28) received therapeutic light touch to the same areas for the same amount of time. Pre- and post-pulmonary function measures were recorded prior to treatment, immediately following, and 1 week following treatment. Forced vital capacity, forced expiratory volume in 1 second, slow vital capacity, inspiratory volume, and expiratory reserve volume measures were compared by t-test. Results were that no differences were identified between the two groups. One might argue that, in the absence of pathology, myofascial release techniques would not affect already sufficiently lengthened fascia.

Keggereis and colleagues[52] from the University of Indianapolis examined the immediate and cumulative effects of a transverse plane myofascial release to the respiratory diaphragm. Thirty subjects from a community hospital chronic pain and rehabilitation program were randomly assigned to a treatment or control group. All subjects received one session of energy-based myofascial release to the diaphragm lying supine. All 30 subjects were evaluated for changes in heart rate, respiratory rate, blood pressure, rib cage expansion, and forced vital capacity 5 to 10 minutes post- treatment. Sixteen of the subjects were studied after four treatment sessions for the cumulative effect. Control group subjects received light touch only, with no attempt to "follow the release as it progressed through fascial barriers" as was done with experimental group subjects. Multianalysis of variance and post hoc multivariant tests were used on individual dependent variables." A significant immediate and cumulative effect existed in lowering respiratory rate for the treatment group ($p<0.05$) using within subjects multivariant testing. Significant differences were not found immediately or cumulatively for heart rate, blood pressure, rib cage expansion, or forced vital capacity."[52] The authors conclude that myofascial release may be clinically useful in lowering respiratory rate in patients with chronic pain. Variance in the results may have resulted from inconsistent rest periods following treatment at each session before measuring post-test results.

Davis[53] and her students at the University of Miami presented a paper at the June 2002 annual scientific meeting of physical therapists that examined the effects of myofascial release on the fascial restrictions limiting a golf swing.[49] Four men who were amateur golfers (handicap greater than 10) and two male professional golfers (handicap less than 10) underwent data collection on the golf course and in the clinic. The professional golfers were tested one time on the driving range to establish a best-practice benchmark for each of the variables. Of particular interest was the shoulder-hip relationship in rotation in the swing, named the X-factor by golf professionals. Each of the four subjects was videotaped swinging a golf club, and their X-factors were measured to compare with the measures obtained from the professionals. In addition, the four subjects underwent pretest and post-test measures of seated (static) thoracic rotation, dynamic shoulder and hip rotation, and swing speed measures. Each subject received 30 to 45 minutes of myofascial release from the same experienced therapist based on what limitations of fascia were found in each subject on examination. Subjects were given a home program to do daily and returned 2 weeks later for follow-up. A second treatment was given based on re-examination, and the home program was modified. Post-test measures were then taken following the second treatment. The researchers found a significant positive correlation ($R_{pre}=0.54$, $R_{post}=0.82$, $R_{diff}=0.79$) between seated thoracic rotation and swing speed. Significant or near significant differences were also obtained when comparing professional and pre-treatment amateur results for seated thoracic rotation ($p=0.02$) and X-factor ($p=0.07$). In sum, the researchers concluded that an myofascial release treatment program appears to play a role in improving certain identified soft tissue range of motion variables, such that amateur golfers' performance more closely approximates that of professionals'. One subject reported an inability to play more than eight holes of golf without back pain that persisted for several years. Following one treatment that included the use of wedges to derotate the ilia, he played 18 holes without pain. One year later, he reported he continued to play 18 holes without pain, and he was continuing with his home exercise wedging "sporadically."[53]

Davis and colleagues,[54] also examined the effects of myofascial release integrated with therapeutic exercise on two older women (one 78 years old, the other 82 years old) with severe kyphoscoliosis. Each subject received 2 weeks of treatment consisting of 45 minutes of myofascial release and 15 minutes of exercises either two or three times each week. Each subject walked with a rolling walker and had received exercises alone for her osteoporosis and osteoarthritis for several years previously. Thus, each served as her own control with regard to reporting any differences that she experienced with this treatment protocol compared to exercise alone. Pre- and post-test measures examined pain (VAS), range of motion, strength, balance (one leg stance and forward reach), quality of life (SF-36), functional mobility (Timed Up and Go), posture (Polaroid [Waltham, MA] grid pictures in four positions), vital capacity, and patient exit interview on videotape. Results were that postural changes by grid picture were evident in both patients. Both patients experienced decrease in pain (4.8/10 to 2.1/10 and 10/10 to 4/10) and an improved quality of life following the final session in 2 weeks of treatment. Patient A also improved in Timed Up and Go and range of motion. Patient B improved in vital capacity, Timed Up and Go, functional reach, and one leg stance. Most significant with regard to myofascial release was that both patients in separate exit interviews described being acutely aware of the feeling of energy and release of tight tissue under the therapist's hands during treatment, an experience that they had not ever felt before with physical therapy. In addition, both, unbeknownst to the other, described feeling energized and able to function with more energy and "pep" for an average of 2 days.[54]

Brtalik, LeBauer, and Stowe[55] from Elon University reported similar results in a yet to be published case study, myofascial release for and adult with idiopathic scoliosis helped decrease pain and increase quality of life. One woman subject with a double major curve with a Cobb angle of 45 degrees, following 6 weeks of two 60-minute mfr sessions a week reported significant decrease in pain by VAS (4.8/10 to 1.8/10) and improvement in her quality of life as measured by SRS-22, (3.82 to 4.45) and pulmonary function (UCSD SOB 9-4).

From the Czech Republic, the *Journal of Manipulative and Physiological Therapeutics* reported a study on the reduction of myofascial pain using myofascial release as described in this chapter on abdominal scars. Lewit and Olsanska[56] described results in 51 subjects undergoing myofascial release to abdominal scars. Treatment produced marked immediate results in 36 of the 51 cases.

In the April of 2007 issue of *Journal of Bodywork and Movement Therapies*, Russell[57] reported the effects of 3 weeks of Swedish massage along with myofascial release on a 35-year-old woman with restless legs syndrome (RLS). Forty-five minute massage treatments were given twice weekly with a space of 2 days. The subject kept a log recording hours of sleep; nocturnal waking; intensity and type of RLS symptoms; caffeine, alcohol, tobacco, and medication intake; and an estimate of her stress level. Frequency, intensity, and duration of symptoms were kept in the Functional Rating Index before, during, and after the study. Tingling sensations, urgency to move the legs, and sleeplessness were decreased after two treatments and continued to improve throughout the 3 weeks. It was conjectured that massage and myofascial release may have increased the natural release of dopamine which has been shown to improve symptoms of RLS.[57]

Several studies have been reported in the literature on the effectiveness of myofascial release on pelvic dysfunction in women and men. In 2001, Lukban et al[58] published the results of a pilot study in urology on the effect of myofascial release along with joint mobilization and muscle energy techniques on 16 women with interstitial cystitis, pelvic floor dysfunction and sacroiliac dysfunction[58]:

> *A comparison of pre- and post treatment Modified Oswestry scores revealed a 94% improvement in dyspareunia. Pretreatment Modified Oswestry scores ranged from 1 to 5, with a mean of 2.75. Post therapy scores ranged from 0 to 4, with a mean of 0.875. Nine of 16 patients were able to return to pain-free intercourse. A comparison of pre- and post-treatment O'Leary-Sant scores revealed a 94% improvement in symptomatology, with the greatest improvement seen in the indices of frequency and suprapubic pain, and less improvement in urgency and nocturia. Pretreatment O'Leary-Sant scores ranged from 5 to 29 with a mean of 15.75. Post treatment scores ranged from 1 to 20, with a mean of 8.5... Manual physical therapy may be a useful therapeutic modality for patients diagnosed with IC, high-tone pelvic floor dysfunction, and sacroiliac dysfunction. Intervention seems to be most useful in patients with primary complaints of urinary frequency, suprapubic pain, and dyspareunia.*

Wurn and associates[59] published an article on line in the NIH Medscape General Medicine in 2004 on the use of myofascial release to the pelvic floor and abdomen in increasing orgasm and decreasing painful intercourse in women with histories of infertility or abdominopelvic pain. Twenty-three of the 29 patients were available for follow-up and all had significant improvement pre to post test on all measures of sexual dysfunction at the p≤0.003 level of significance.[59]

Dr. Lee Learman,[60] in a review article on chronic pelvic pain published in *Johns Hopkins Advanced Studies in Medicine* in 2005 stated, "It is essential to address perpetuating mechanisms of pain. Patients with myofascial pain should be referred to physical therapists specializing in pelvic floor muscle work." Weiss, in the *Journal of Urology* in 2001,[45] described myofascial release as the effective intervention.[60]

Peters et al[61] published, "Prevalence of pelvic floor dysfunction in patients with interstitial cystitis" in the July 2007 issue of the journal *Urology*. They suggest that pelvic floor dysfunction may set off an inflammatory response to the pelvic organs, and that "myofascial release may be offered as the first line of symptoms."

Finally, Hartmann et al[62] published the results of a survey identifying current practice trends of physical therapists specializing in women's health in the January 2007 issue of the *Journal of Reproductive Medicine*. An Internet poll in mid-2005 directed to physical therapists treating localized, provoked vulvodynia revealed that greater than 70% indicated that they included myofascial release of the pelvic, girdle, pelvic floor, and associated structures along with exercise, joint mobilization, and neuromuscular re-education. Typical care was an hour long session once weekly for 7 to 15 weeks.[62]

Conclusion

Myofascial release techniques were discovered and are performed acknowledging that the existing view of the body as a machine is totally incorrect, and acknowledging that the fascia cannot be separated from each and every cell and structure that it surrounds. This approach starts with the belief that one must influence the patient's fascial restrictions in order to obtain and secure permanent recovery from the causes of pain, limitation of motion, and paresthesia secondary to postural or structural malalignments.

Fascia is not accessed by traditional mechanical methods such as joint mobilization modalities or traditional stretching methods. Fascia, instead, responds to the combination of the intentional application of endogenous bioelectromagnetic energy fields and the sustained mechanical pressure at the myofascial barrier from within the therapist, through the palms and fingers of the therapist's hands to soften the molecular structure of the fascia, and the gentle, sustained mechanical pressure of the therapist's hands at the myofascial barrier, facilitating a yielding or release of its barriers or restrictions.[3] The mind seems to store memories and experiences in restricted fascia, for upon the release of restrictions, patients commonly become transported back to an injurious experience and with similar emotion, relate the experience in detail. Once the trauma is completely experienced and the fascial restrictions have given way, healing can commence. We have yet to learn the cellular mechanism of the healing process, but it is believed that once restrictions are removed from the fascia, body energy, blood, lymph, neurotransmitters, neuropeptides, and steroids are free to flow, restoring balance, homeostasis, and overall health to the system.[3]

Traditional Western medical theory based on the philosophies of Sir Isaac Newton and René Descartes cannot explain these observed patient experiences and outcomes. However, the emerging new explanatory theory of mind-body holism, based on the quantum theory of the behavior and characteristics of atoms and molecules, offers explanations for these and many other "unexplainable" outcomes. The science of energy medicine is rapidly helping to answer many of the questions that have eluded us for decades.

Myofascial release is not offered to replace traditional physical therapy techniques, but to supplement and enhance them as a complementary approach in evaluating and treating patients with pain, restriction of motion, and structural symptoms. Success in the application of these techniques requires therapists to keep an open mind regarding holism and mind-body theory, and to develop themselves personally in such a way that their manual techniques and their attitudes and priorities in care reflect a centered, creative, artful attention to the patient's description of the problems and to the feedback they receive from the patient's mind-body as they apply their treatment. Touch must be applied with compassionate intention, focused awareness, and the conscious purpose to mechanically and bioenergetically release fascial restrictions and, thus, facilitate the reorganization of the mind-body neuromuscular system.

Our goals are to learn from each patient; to teach by example; and to remain attentive, creatively focused, sensitive, nonjudgmental, supportive, and compassionate in accepting the patient's story as authentic and treatable. We must then document our results in detail to start building a database from which we can publish our outcomes so that all may benefit.

Myofascial release offers a beginning into a new world of evaluation and care that is intelligent, based on sound theories, humane in its holistic approach, and effective when traditional mechanistic approaches to care have failed. The organization and publication of systematic and thorough documentation of qualitative and quantitative data is encouraged so we can share results with one another for the good of all patients.

References

1. Travell J. *Myofascial Pain and Dysfunction*. Baltimore, MD: Williams & Wilkins; 1983.
2. Scott J. Molecules that keep you in shape. *New Scientist*. 1986;111:49-53.
3. Oschman JL. *Energy Medicine: The Scientific Basis*. New York, NY: Churchill Livingstone; 2000.
4. Barnes JF. *Myofascial Release: The Search for Excellence*. Paoli, PA: MFR Seminars; 1990.
5. Montague A. *Touching: The Human Significance of the Skin*. New York, NY: Harper & Row; 1971:4.
6. Barnes JF. The significance of touch. *Physical Therapy Forum*. 1988;7:10.
7. Juhan D. *Job's Body*. Barrytown, NY: Station Hill Press; 1987.
8. Netter FH. *The CIBA Collection of Medical Illustrations: Nervous Systems*. West Caldwell, NJ: CIBA; 1983:197.
9. Kuhn TS. *The Structure of Scientific Revolutions*. Chicago, IL: University of Chicago Press; 1970.
10. Kurtz R. *Body Centered Psychotherapy: The Hakomi Therapy*. Ashland, OR: The Hakomi Institute; 1988.
11. Bohm D. *Causality and Chance in Modern Physics*. Philadelphia, PA: University of Pennsylvania Press; 1957.
12. Bohm D. *The Special Theory of Relativity*. Boston, MA; Addison Wesley; 1988.
13. Page L. *Academy of Applied Osteopathy Yearbook*. 1952:85-90.
14. Hall D. The aging of connective tissue exp. *Gerontology*. 1968;3:77-89.
15. Chaitow L. *Neuro-Muscular Technique—A Practitioner's Guide to Soft Tissue Mobilization*. New York, NY: Thorsons; 1985: 13-15.
16. Langevin HM. Connective tissue: a body-wide signaling network? *Med Hypotheses*. 2006;66(6):1074-1077.
17. Ingber DE. Cellular mechanotransduction: putting all the pieces together again. *FASEB J*. 2006;20(7)811-827.
18. Pierce P. *Structure in Nature as a Strategy for Design*. Cambridge, MA: MIT Press; 1978:xii-xvii.
19. Thomson D. *On Growth and Form*. London: Cambridge University Press; 1965.
20. Selye H. *The Stress of Life*. New York, NY: McGraw-Hill; 1976.
21. Barnes JF, Smith G. The body is a self-correcting mechanism. *Physical Therapy Forum*. 1987;27.
22. Jenkins DHR. *Ligament Injuries and Their Treatment*. Rockville, MD: Aspen Publications; 1985.
23. Twomley L, Taylor J. Flexion, creep, dysfunction and hysteresis in the lumbar vertebral columns. *Spine*. 1982;2:116-122.
24. *Dorland's Medical Directory*. 26th ed. Philadelphia, PA: WB Saunders; 1985.
25. Upledger J, Vredevoogd J. *Craniosacral Therapy*. Seattle, WA: Eastland Press; 1983:6.
26. Popper KR, Eccles JC. *The Self and its Brain*. Berlin, Germany: Springer; 1977.
27. Hameroff SR. Quantum coherence in microtubules: a neural basis for emergent consciousness. *J Consciousness Studies*. 1994;1(1):91-118.
28. Selye H. History and present status of the stress concept. In: Goldberger L, Breznitz S, eds. *Handbook of Stress*. New York, NY: Macmillan; 1982:7-20.
29. Searle JR. Minds, brains and programs. *Behavioral and Brain Sciences*. 1980;3:417-424.
30. Taylor JG. Towards a neural network model of the mind. *Neural Network World*. 1992;6:797-812.
31. Korb KB. Stage effects in the Cartesian theater: a review of Daniel Dermetts' "Consciousness Explained." *Psyche*. 1993;1(1).
32. Hawkins R, Kandel E. Steps toward a cell-biological alphabet for elementary forms of learning. In: Lynch G, McCaugh J, Weinberger N, eds. *Neurobiology of Learning and Memory*. New York, NY: Guilford Press; 1991:384-404.
33. Rosenzweig M, Bennett E. Basic processes and modulatory influences in the stages of memory formation. In: Lynch G, McCaugh J, Weinberger N, eds. *Neurobiology of Learning and Memory*. New York, NY: Guilford Press; 1984:263-288.

34. Siegel B. *Love, Medicine and Miracles.* New York, NY: Harper & Row; 1986.

35. Rossi EL. From mind to molecule: a state-dependent memory, learning, and behavior theory of mind-body healing. *Advance.* 1987;2:46-60.

36. Klebe RS, Caldwell H, Milani S. Cells transmit spatial information by orienting collagen fibers. *Matrix.* 1989;9:451-458.

37. Sheldrake R. *The Presence of the Past.* New York, NY: Times Books; 1994.

38. Micozzi MS. *Fundamentals of Complementary and Alternative Medicine.* New York, NY: Churchill Livingstone; 1996.

39. Oschman JL. *Energy Medicine in Therapeutics and Human Performance.* London:Butterworth-Heinemann; 2003.

40. USGP and National Institutes Of Health. *Alternative Medicine: Expanding Medical Horizons. Report to the NIH on Alternative Medical Systems of Practices in the United States.* Pittsburgh, PA: US Government Printing Office, Superintendent of Documents; 1992:48-50.

41. Cowley G. An electromagnetic storm. *Newsweek.* 1989;July:77.

42. Becker RO, Seldon G. *The Body Electric: Electromagnetism and the Foundation of the Life.* New York, NY: William Morrow; 1985.

43. Picker RI. Microcurrent therapy: "jump-starting" healing with bioelectricity. *Physical Therapy Forum.* 1989;July:27.

44. Barr F. Special issue: melanin as key organizing molecule. *Brain/Mind Bull.* 1983;12(13):1.

45. Pert CB. *Molecules of Emotion: The Science Behind Mind-Body Medicine.* New York, NY: Touchstone; 1997.

46. Ader R. *Psychoneuroimmunology.* New York, NY: Academic Press; 1981.

47. Chopra D. *Quantum Healing: Exploring the Frontiers of Mind/Body Medicine.* New York: Bantam Books; 1989.

48. Sucher BM. Myofascial manipulative release of carpal tunnel syndrome: documentation with magnetic resonance imaging. *JAOA.* 1993;93(12):1273.

49. Weiss JM. Pelvic floor myofascial trigger points: manual therapy for intesrstitial cystitis and the urgency frequency syndrome. *J Urology.* 2001;166:2226-2231.

50. APTA. *Section on Research Newsletter.* 33(1):13-14.

51. Bezner JR, Boucher BK, Hernandez M. *Phys Ther.* 2001;81(5):A46.

52. Kegerreis S, Worrell T, Perry D. *Phys Ther.* 2001;81(5):A46.

53. Davis CM, Schrodter BS, Klatt R. The effects of myofascial release treatment program on the musculoskeletal restrictions limiting the golf swing [abstract]. http://www.ptjournal.org/abstracts/pt2002/abstractsPt2002.cfm?pubNo=PL-RR-214-F. Accessed November 28, 2003.

54. Davis CM, Doerger C, Eaton T, Rowland J, Sauber C. Myofascial release (Barnes method) is complementary in physical therapy for patients with osteoporosis: two case studies. *J Geriatric Physical Therapy.* 2002:25(3):33

55. Personal communication with poster, Aaron LeBauer.

56. Lewit K, Olsanska S. Clinical importance of active scars: abdominal scars as a cause of myofascial pain. *Journal of Manipulative and Physiological Therapeutics.* 2004;6:399-402.

57. Russell M. Massage therapy and restless leg syndrome. *Journal of Bodywork and Movement Therapies.* 2007;11(2):146-150.

58. Lukban J, Whitmore K, Kellogg-Spadt R, et al. The effect of manual physical therapy in patients diagnosed with interstitial cystitis, high-tone pelvic floor dysfunction , and sacroiliac dysfunction. *Urology.* 2001;57:121-122.

59. Wurn LJ, Wurn BF, Roscow AS, et al. Increasing orgasm and decreasing dyspareunia by a manual physical therapy technique. www.pubmedcentral.nih.gov/articlerender.fcgi?artid=1480593.

60. Learman LA. Chronic pelvic pain—part 2: an integrated management approach. *Johns Hopkins Advanced Studies in Medicine.* 2005;5(7):360-366.

61. Peters KM, Carrico DJ, Kalinowski SE, Ibrahim IA, Diokno AC. Prevalence of pelvic floor dysfunction in patients with interstitial cystitis. *Urology.* 2007;70(1):16-18.

62. Hartmann D, Strauhal MF, Nelson CA. Treatment of women in the United States with localized provoked vulvodynia: practice survey of women's health physical therapists. *J Reprod Med.* 2007;52(1):48-52.

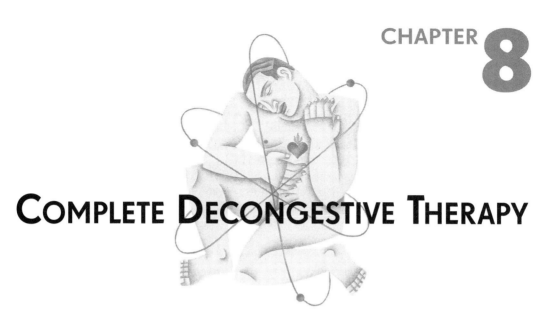

CHAPTER 8

COMPLETE DECONGESTIVE THERAPY

Barbara Funk, MS, OTR, CHT

Introduction

Manual lymph drainage (MLD) is one component of a comprehensive lymphedema management program termed *complete decongestive therapy* (CDT). Both occupational and physical therapists come from traditional training programs that include minimal background for the treatment of lymphedema disorders. Supplemental lymphedema training offered by specialists is needed to adequately ensure that treating therapists have the full knowledge base and manual techniques required for this management program. MLD gives therapists an opportunity to facilitate both the molecular and energetic flow in their patients through direct contact with the skin. James Oschman has said that "When you touch a human body, you are touching a continuously interconnected system composed of all the molecules in the body... Properties of the whole net depend upon integrated activities of all the components."[1]

Disease and disorders (such as lymphedema) limit the informational streams through the energetic circuits in the living organism.[1] CDT offers the therapist the latest methodology to encourage the continuous flow within the body, promoting self-regulation and homeostasis.

Function of the Lymphatic System

The structure and function of the lymphatic system represents the foundation of knowledge needed to apply the therapeutic techniques required in CDT. The lymph system is a component of the complex circulatory system as reflected in its embryological development and functionally offers an additional one-way route to return tissue fluids to the blood stream. Anatomically, the system has four ongoing processes: lymph production, lymph transport, lymph concentration, and lymph filtration.[2] The successful completion of these activities in conjunction with the blood vascular system provides for the optimal functioning and integrity of the extracellular and intracellular environment.

Three Basic Functions of the Lymph System

MAINTAIN FLUID BALANCE IN TISSUES

This function consists of removing excess fluid, bacteria, large proteins, and particulate matter away from the interstitial spaces and body tissues. The removal of substances from the interstitial spaces of high molecular weight such as protein is an essential function, without which death would occur within 24 hours.[3]

The extensive web of blood vessels and lymphatics travels intimately between the interstitium or tissue channels. It offers a route and mechanism to transmit all substances that go to and from the cells. The environment of the lymph system at all levels, superficial to deep, is intertwined and supported by the fascial system. John Barnes describes an extensive review of the fascial system.[4] On a cellular level, the fascia creates the interstitial spaces; on another level, it forms layers around the muscle influencing lymph circulation. It is through the proper functioning of this connective tissue that many of the body's physiological processes are supported, such as humeral and vascular profusion, lymphatic flow, bioelectric conduction[4] and energy balance.[5] The interstitial environment or connective tissue is composed of collagen fibers set in proteoglycan molecules forming the solid (gel phase) of the connective tissue and in fluid (sol phase) where there is minimal gel.[6] The polysaccharide gel complex fills the spaces between the collagen fibers; proteoglycans and hyaluronic acid compose the gel.[4] It has been postulated that the gel in the interstitium creates the structure to hold interstitial fluid in place. Gel dehydration does not occur due to the electrostatic charges that cause osmosis of water into its lattice (Donnan equilibrium).[2]

The fluid balance of the tissues is preserved by mutual regulation of the blood capillaries, the interstitial tissues, proteolytic cells, and the initial lymphatics.[7] It is a fine balance of the capillary filtration and capillary reabsorption. Factors that can shift the equilibrium are capillary (hydrostatic) pressure, interstitial tissue pressure, and colloidosmotic pressure in the capillaries and tissue fluids (Starling's flow mechanism).[8] The lymph minute volume (LMV) generally operates at 10% of its maximum transport capacity. This is important in maintaining homeostasis when there are shifts in the hydrostatic and oncotic pressures. However, as we will see, this large functional reserve and safety valve function is no longer adequate under certain circumstances, resulting in lymphedema. Under normal conditions, the venous capillaries reabsorb 90% of the fluid, and the lymphatics reabsorb the remaining 10%. This generates approximately 2 to 4 liters of liquid transported by the lymph system in 24 hours and between 80 and 200 grams of protein removed.[8]

MAINTAIN OPTIMUM FUNCTIONING OF THE IMMUNE SYSTEM

Through a process of lymph filtration, noxious matter such as bacteria, toxins, and dead cells are removed from the system. The filtering of foreign agents alerts the system to trigger through humeral and cellular support, antibodies, and lymphocytes that cause dissolution of these cells.[9]

TRANSPORTATION AND ABSORPTION OF 80% TO 90% OF FAT FROM THE INTESTINES

The lymphatics draining the intestines absorb through the central lacteals of the villi-emulsified fat principally in the form of fatty acids. These fatty acids or chylomicrons are transported by the lymphatics to the thoracic duct, eventually conveyed to the blood by the left subclavian vein.[9]

Organization and Structure of the Lymphatic System

Creating an internal image of the vast lymphatic system facilitates our intention and direction of the treatment process. With a three-dimensional respect and knowledge of the lymphatic structure, the therapist is best able to effectively influence the equilibrium of the system. The lymphatic system consists of organs and vessels that contain lymphoid tissue. These include lymph nodes, lymph vessels, the spleen, thymus, tonsils, and Peyer's patches (cells in the intestinal lining). Clearly, the lymph vessels and lymph nodes hold the greatest influence on lymphedema.

LYMPH VESSELS

Lymph Capillaries (Initial Lymphatics)

Lymph capillaries represent the most peripheral elements of the system as a valveless network. They originate in the tissue spaces and form a web-like plexus throughout the body. Their cell walls are composed of flat, overlapping endothelial cells with anchoring filaments. The filaments attach to the surrounding connective tissue and prevent the collapse of the initial lymphatic vessels. The vessel structure allows for the absorption of fluid, large particulate matter, and proteins. It is generally felt that absorption occurs through passive conduction into the endothelial junctions. Casley-Smith[6] also describes capillary pumping action as a potential process.

Precollectors

These vessels contain smooth muscle cells and valves. Like the lymph capillaries, they also function to absorb and transport lymph from the interstitium.[8] They are the connection between the initial lymphatics and the collecting vessels.

Lymph Collectors

These receive lymph flow from the lymph precollectors. They have a three-layered cell wall that contains valves that guarantee direction of fluid flow from distal to proximal, or to a regional lymph node. Valves are evident every 0.6 to 2.0 cm, as they are proportional to the caliber of the vessel. The segment between two valves is called a lymphangion. Lymphangion intrinsic contractions occur in normal conditions 6 to 10 times per minute and may increase 2 to 3 times this value when needed. During exercise conditions, both the amplitude and the rate of contraction increase, creating a functional reserve tenfold.

Lymph Trunks and Ducts

These represent the largest lymph vessels receiving lymph from the collectors. The trunks eventually empty into the ducts that return the lymph into the blood circulation at the left and right venous angles.

LYMPH NODES

Lymph nodes play an integral part in the defense mechanism of the body. There are an estimated 600 to 700 nodes in the body. They receive the lymph fluid and function as a biological filtering station for noxious matter, regulate the concentration of protein in the lymph fluid, and produce lymphocytes.[9]

The lymphatic system is structurally adapted to absorb and transport lymph through intrinsic contractions. The sympathetic nervous system and the lymph volume influence the frequency rate of contractions. If lymph volume increases (such as in conditions of physical exertion or inflammation), an increase in lymph time volume would be accomplished through increased pulsation frequency, as well as increased filling amplitude of the lymphangion. Lymph transport is also facilitated by contraction of skeletal muscles, arterial pulsation, respiratory changes, negative pressure in the central veins, and external pressure.[8] Later in this chapter, we will address how CDT directly influences these processes.

Definition and Causes of Lymphedema

Lymphedema is defined as an abnormal accumulation of protein-rich fluid in the interstitial tissues resulting in swelling in any body segment, most often the extremities. Lymphedema is a disease that represents a significant health problem influencing the lives of millions over the world.

The World Health Organization[10] estimates that parasites contribute to the edema of 90 million people, breast cancer to 20 million people, and primary lymphedema affects 2 to 3 million people.

In underdeveloped countries, filarial infection (parasites) is the major cause of lymphedema, whereas in industrial countries a substantial number result from cancer treatments. Petrek and Lerner report breast cancer therapy affecting more than 400,000 women in the United States.[11] According to the National Cancer Institute, occurrence is 50% to 70% after axillary treatment.[12]

The pathophysiology in lymphedema occurs when the lymph load (volume) exceeds its transport capacity.[13] Stagnation of fluid creates changes in the microcirculation and in the overall cellular health. Changes that may occur include chronic inflammation, increased lymphatic pressure and vessel dilation, and valvular incompetence. Reactive tissue changes include proliferation of connective tissue cells, fatty tissue deposits, fibrosis, skin thickening, skin erythema, and, in rare cases, the development of an angiosarcoma. Patients are often prone to repeated infections, cellulitis, erysipelas, and lymphangitis.[13] Reduced oxygen availability due to tissue congestion can lead to delayed wound healing.

As girth of extremities and respective quadrants (ipsilateral trunk) increases, additional manifestations are noted. Reports include limitations in joint range of motion, decreased functional performance, pain, paresthesias, and weakness in the affected extremity.[14-17] Psychological morbidity is documented in several descriptive and case control studies identifying common psychological problems such as anxiety, depression, sexual dysfunction, social avoidance, and exacerbation of existing psychological illness.[17-19]

Classification of Lymphedema

Lymphedema is divided into two classifications: *primary* (idiopathic) and *secondary* (acquired). Primary lymphedema develops without obvious cause due to malformation of the lymphatics (dysplasias). Onset may be at birth but most frequently develops around 17 years of age. Lymphedema praecox (occurs prior to age 35) accounts for 83% of the primary lymphedemas, whereas lymphedema tardum (occurs after age 35) represents 17% of the cases.[20] Secondary lymphedema can develop due to several known causes:

1. Post-cancer management (node dissection, radiation, and reconstruction)
2. Significant trauma to nodes and vessels (from an accident or self-induced)
3. Repeated infections, such as cellulitis
4. Postsurgical procedures, such as coronary bypass
5. Malignant tumor vessel blockage
6. Filarial infection

Lymphedema may be found in combination with other disorders such as obesity, chronic venous insufficiency, lipedemia, and rheumatoid arthritis.[8]

Stages of Lymphedema

Foldi et al[21] describe three stages of lymphedema, from mild to severe.

STAGE I: REVERSIBLE LYMPHEDEMA

+ Accumulation of protein-rich edematous fluid

STAGE II: SPONTANEOUSLY IRREVERSIBLE LYMPHEDEMA

+ Protein-rich edematous fluid
+ Connective and scar tissue

STAGE III: LYMPHOSTATIC ELEPHANTIASIS

+ Protein-rich edematous fluid
+ Connective and scar tissue
+ Hardening of dermal tissues
+ Papillomas of the skin

In addition to these three stages, there is a subclinical (latent) phase when tissue alterations occur but are not clinically detected by circumferential measures.[22] During this time, patients describe limb heaviness, pins/needles, and pain.[23] Early diagnosis and treatment improves the prognosis for treating lymphedema, avoiding more serious sequelae. During Stage I, pitting is evident; upon arising in the morning, swelling may not be present. In Stage II, the tissue has a spongy consistency with less pitting. Fibrosis and hardening are noted as girth increases.

Diagnosis and Evaluation of Lymphedema

Lymphedema is diagnosed clinically by medical history and physical examination.[24] Estimated volumetric measures are frequently used to quantify limb edema.[25] Limb volume is estimated by taking several circumferential measures at prescribed standard distances. High correlation has been made with limb volume to the gold standard of water displacement.[26,27] Calculating volume assessments using the truncated cone method is noted by Morgan et al.[28]

Lymphoscintigraphy, which allows the visualization of the lymphatic system, is a major diagnostic tool in the evaluation of lymphedema.[29,30] Computer tomography and magnetic resonance are additional imaging methods.[31]

Complete Decongestive Therapy

HISTORY

CDT was first introduced by Von Winiwarter,[32] who suggested lymphatic massage and bandaging for the swollen limb. Vodder (1930s) was instrumental in developing a soft touch manual therapy for intact lymphatics.[5] Kinmonth,[33] Kubik and Manestar,[34] and Foldi[3] all revealed in their research a greater understanding of the anatomy, physiology, and pathophysiology of the lymphatic system. This enlarged foundation of knowledge was instrumental in the further development of a system for lymphedema management.

The Foldis (Germany, 1980s) are credited with modifications to the original Vodder manual techniques[35] and the further extension of care creating CDT.[21] Additional variations in methods have been credited to other schools of thought, such as Casley-Smith,[36] Leduc,[37] and Vodder.[38] Dr. Robert Lerner first introduced CDT in the United States in the 1980s.[13] As one reviews the extensive international literature on lymphedema management, the nomenclature used to represent CDT may also include complex physical therapy, complex lymphedema therapy, and complex decongestive physiotherapy.

DESCRIPTION OF COMPLETE DECONGESTIVE THERAPY

This approach is noninvasive, safe, and offers the patient the management skills needed to control his or her chronic condition. CDT is a tetrad consisting of skin care, manual lymph drainage, exercise, and compression therapy. These four principle strategies were agreed upon by Foldi, Leduc, the Vodder School (Kasseroller), and Casley-Smith.[39] Before engaging any person in this multimodal program, physician clearance is needed to rule out any complications that would influence the partial or full utilization of program components. CDT should be part of a comprehensive program offering the individual support including medical management, nutritional guidance, psychological support, and rehabilitation. Lymphedema is a chronic disease that cannot be cured. Therefore, long-term follow-up and case management are integral components to ensure the highest levels of patient functioning over time.

TWO PHASES OF COMPLETE DECONGESTIVE THERAPY (FROM KLOSE AND NORTON[20])

Phase I: Treatment Phase

1. Meticulous skin and nail care
2. Manual lymph drainage
3. Compression bandaging
4. Remedial exercises

Phase II: Maintenance Phase

1. Compression garments (during the day)
2. Bandaging (at night)
3. Meticulous skin and nail care
4. Remedial exercises
5. Manual lymph drainage as needed

GOALS OF TREATMENT

1. Control lymph formation and improve drainage through existing lymphatics and collateral routes
2. Eliminate fibrotic tissue (stages II and III)
3. Avoid reaccumulation of lymph fluid
4. Protect against infections
5. Ensure long-term maintenance for improved arm size and shape by patient
6. Achieve rehabilitation goals. This may include pain reduction, increased range of motion, improved independence in activities of daily living, reduction of tissue and scar adhesions, normalization of postural imbalances, increased strength, and endurance

Components of Complete Decongestive Therapy

MANUAL LYMPH DRAINAGE

This specific massage technique is designed to control lymph formation and improve drainage through existing vessels and collateral routes.[40] The therapist provides this manual facilitation through proprioceptive methods but also through his or her conscious intent of opening the flow of both fluids and vital energy. Technique principles and treatment pathways have been described in detail by Vodder,[5] Foldi,[21] and Casley-Smith.[6] According to Foldi et al,[21] MLD is first applied to the contralateral quadrant of the trunk, enhancing lymphatic contractility and lymph flow through watersheds. Following truncal clearance, the root of the involved limb is addressed, followed by the proximal to distal components.

Guides for treatment pathways are given but do not represent a fixed procedure, as each individual presents with differing tissue characteristics. The instruction in self-massage varies.[20] A major determinant is the time allowed for the intensive phase of care, which is influenced by insurance coverage, patient availability, institution policies, and severity of the condition.

MLD may also be effective as part of a treatment plan for other conditions, such as post-traumatic edema, postsurgical edema, complex regional pain syndrome, scleroderma, and chronic fatigue.[20] MLD has an extensive influence on the human constitution and life quality of the cells. Its role in stimulating the parasympathetic nervous system affects growth, recovery, and restorative tissue changes. The light, changing pressures function to decrease pain sensation and increase the lymphangiomotoricity. MLD offers immunological support by both facilitating transport and deactivating pathogens. Its immediate effect is noted in its influence on the cellular environment by normalizing the function and composition of the connective tissue.

Additional rehabilitative techniques may also be beneficial for these patients. An example of this is the use of myofascial release techniques to relieve chest wall pain, fascial restrictions, and emotional holding patterns in the body.[4,41]

SKIN CARE

Skin care includes the eradication of bacterial and fungal infections prior to initiating care and the daily application of low pH skin lotion to reduce chances of infection. Patient education is paramount regarding the knowledge and observance of limb precautions.[42]

COMPRESSION THERAPY

Compression therapy is a vital component in lymphedema management. Low-stretch compressive wraps are applied to the limb after MLD sessions and worn until the following session. The compression wraps prevent the reaccumulation of evacuated fluid, limit blood capillary filtration, and improve striated muscle pump efficiency.[40] In addition, bandaging helps to soften and mobilize fibrotic tissue. These wraps provide high pressure during muscular contraction and low pressure at rest. All patients are instructed in self-bandaging techniques when practical. During the maintenance phase, adaptations to bandage techniques are created to facilitate patient independence.

At the end of the intensive phase, patients are measured and fit for elastic support garments. Limb swelling creates enlarged intercellular spaces and reduces tissue elasticity, requiring the application of elastic garments to support the limb contour.[6] Generally, the elastic garments are worn during the day and short-stretch bandages are used while sleeping. Elastic garments need to be replaced every 4 to 6 months because they lose their compression. All patients are instructed in the proper care and donning of their garments. Alternative nonelastic compression devices are available in situations where short-stretch bandages and elastic garments are not feasible. The circaid[43] and the Reid sleeve are a few examples[44] of alternative wrapping.

The intermittent pneumatic pump is one of the original treatment methods used with lymph-edema. The single or multiple chamber pump removes excess fluid from the interstitial spaces but does not influence protein reabsorption from the involved extremity.[37] Today, there is divided opinion on the therapeutic influence of the pneumatic pump and its role in CDT. Its adjunctive use is advocated in multiple case studies.[45-50] On the other hand, several authors feel the pump is potentially dangerous and ineffective in the treatment of lymphedema.[3,6,36,51-53] Warnings include formation of residual fibrotic bands at the root of limbs, increased incidence of genital edema, damage to superficial lymph vessels, and truncal edema.

REMEDIAL EXERCISE COMPONENT

Exercise is performed while wearing the non-yielding short-stretch bandages or elastic gar-ments. Muscular activity and exercises, both active and passive, facilitate lymph propulsion through the filling and distension of lymph vessels, hence increasing lymph flow.[40] Exercise pro-grams are individually determined for each patient. A standard course might include passive range of motion and isotonic and isometric aspects. Specific exercise routines have been advocated by Casley-Smith in Swedborg,[54] Morgan,[28] Miller,[55,56] and Klose and Norton.[20] Deep breathing exercises are emphasized because they create a negative intrathoracic pressure, enhancing lymph flow into the thoracic duct.

In addition to the four components of CDT, additional treatments may be dictated by the occupational and physical therapists' findings during the evaluation. Rehabilitation may focus on improving range of motion, strength, self-care skills, joint mobility, posture, adhesions, and pain management. Patient need for psychological and nutritional guidance is supported through refer-ral assistance.

Evidence of the Efficacy of Complete Decongestive Therapy

By way of introduction, all of the studies cited below for evidence of efficacy have been per-formed by highly acclaimed specialists in lymphedema management. The study descriptions, patient characteristics, treatment methods, and study results allow the systematic evaluation of intervention strategies for the individual with lymphedema. Volume estimations by circumferen-tial measures have been shown to be highly correlated (r=0.93 to 0.98) with water displacement. The types of studies are cohort. Statistical analyses for the studies include paired student t-test, descriptive, and measures of covariance.

CDT represents a multimodal intervention strategy recommended by several NIH consensus panels and is currently the most efficacious treatment of both primary and secondary lymphede-ma.[24,57-59] Treatment of lymphedema involves interstitial fluid mobilization and removal, as well as the reabsorption of stagnant proteins.[3,60] In addition, fibrosis reduction and limb recontouring may be needed in order to provide comprehensive and desired outcomes. CDT therefore is recom-mended as the initial conservative treatment for lymphedema.[28,48,61-64]

The Foldis annually treat 2500 patients with CDT.[65] Clinical studies by Foldi et al revealed CDT resulted in volume reductions in 95% of 399 patients; 50% reduction in 56% of the patients; 25% to 49% in 31% of patients; and 1% to 24% in 8% of the population; 89% sustained their results at 3 years.[3] Casley-Smith reported over 60% reductions in 618 lymphedematous limbs.[26] Boris et al treated 119 patients with CDT. Reductions averaged 62% in 56 patients with one affected arm, and 68% in 38 single-leg patients. After 36 months, follow-up reductions were 63% for the arm patients and 62% for the single-leg patients. Boris showed compliance significantly influenced outcomes.[53] Szuba et al prospectively analyzed 79 treated patients with moderate to severe LE. Duration of treatment 8±3 days. Mean short term reductions in upper extremities

44%±62%; lower extremities 42%±40%. After 38±52 days, reductions in upper extremities were sustained at 38%±56% and 41%±27 % lower extremities.[66] Ko et al treated 299 patients over a duration of 15.7 days. Lymphedema reductions averaged 59.1% upper extremities and 67.7% lower extremities. Follow-up at 9 months demonstrated compliant patient reductions (86%) at 90% for upper and lower extremities. Noncompliant patients lost 33% of their reductions. Incidence of infections reduced per patient per year from 1.10 to 0.65.[64]

Since the first edition of this book, several issues have been raised by health care practitioners in the field of lymphedema management proposing the need for future investigations into practice methods. Rising health care costs, fiscal restraints, inadequate availability of trained personnel, and delayed and misdiagnosed lymphedema are impacting the comprehensive service utilization of CDT. The complex biology of lymphedema impacts the chronicity of the disease. Early intervention may have the ability to forestall, minimize, or even eliminate the consequences of lymphedema.[67] Suggestions for future research opportunities include early intervention strategies as a preventive approach for high risk individuals; large randomized controlled trials to investigate the effectiveness and efficiency of CDT interventions, in both the individual components and in combination; and effect of treatment on disease progression.

Case Example

Mrs. B is a 58-year-old school teacher with a diagnosis of secondary lymphedema of the right dominant upper extremity. She had a radical mastectomy in 1995, followed by radiation therapy. During her hospital stay, she was briefly instructed in a home range of motion program. In 1997, Mrs. B had a cellulitis infection in her right arm, which is when her swelling began. Mrs. B was on antibiotics for 2 months and was then referred to the outpatient rehabilitation clinic. Her physician gave her medical clearance to participate in all components of the CDT program.

FINDINGS ON INITIAL EVALUATION

1. Restricted range of motion in the glenohumeral joint following capsular pattern
2. Postural imbalances
3. Paresthesias in axilla along the lateral border of the right chest wall, in the right index finger, and in the thumb
4. Reduced strength of the right upper extremity including grip and pinch
5. Self-care restrictions with dressing, hygiene, cooking, home maintenance tasks, and writing on a chalk board
6. Pain in the right chest extending to the cap of the shoulder (4 to 6/10)
7. Stage II lymphedema with swelling throughout the limb and anterior chest wall, greatest along the lateral border of the forearm. Pitting and fibrosis in the lower arm, soft tissue texture in upper arm and in digits. Total volume of the right upper extremity 3798.2 cm^3, compared to 2735.4 cm^3 on the left. This represents a 38% greater edema volume on the right
8. Myofascial restrictions (anterior and lateral chest wall, right lateral trunk, anterior throat, and lateral cervical regions)
9. Insurance plan and prescription dictate 12 visits within 30 days for lymphedema

TREATMENT PLAN

Mrs. B has typical rehabilitation issues regarding her musculoskeletal system in addition to her lymphedema condition. As joint immobility of the shoulder negatively influences the lymphatic flow as well as function, it is important that this be addressed as soon as possible. Initially, Mrs.

B was treated daily for 12 visits with a major focus on CDT. The second diagnosis related to the shoulder was added once the lymphedema management was under way, allowing authorization for nine additional treatment sessions.

PROGRAM

1. The patient received educational materials regarding the lymphatic system, limb precautions, written pictures, review of home exercises (passive range of motion, strengthening, deep breathing, aerobics), and materials regarding community support groups

2. Rehabilitation intervention: joint mobilization, neuromuscular training, myofascial release and scar mobilization, postural training, neural gliding, and functional strengthening

3. Self-care training/and adaptations

4. CDT

5. Daily MLD followed by compression wrap with short-stretch bandages. Exercises were performed with bandages. Mrs. B and her husband were trained in the bandaging process. Mrs. B received her elastic glove and sleeve, which she wore during the day by week 4. Compression bandages were worn while sleeping and in early morning during home exercises

DISCHARGE STATUS

Mrs. B has full range of motion of the right shoulder, with reduced pain reported 2/10 at ends of range. Strength is functional for activities such as dressing, hygiene, cooking, and leisure interests. Chalkboard writing activities were adapted by using an overhead projector. Continued gains in strength are anticipated over the next several months. As myofascial restrictions were reduced significantly, alterations in posture were normalized along with reduction in paresthesia of 90%. Limb volume reductions after the first 12 visits were 48.5%, and after total completion of the rehabilitation program were 68%. Tissue texture is soft throughout with minimal fibrosis at the lateral border of the ulna. Mrs. B has continued trying to reduce the fibrosis with her bandaging method and through a massage technique she has been shown. Numbness in the hand is no longer an issue as long as compression methods are utilized and swelling is controlled.

Mrs. B was instructed to continue daily exercises, use daytime elastic garment wear, and sleep with bandages. Due to insurance restrictions, Mrs. B is followed by her physician, who would initiate additional treatment if there were any significant limb changes. Mrs. B will need a prescription from her physician in 6 months for a new glove and sleeve.

Training in Complete Decongestive Therapy

Present programs vary in their comprehensiveness of treatment and, hence, partially in successful management. Effective lymph management is directly related to therapist training and experience, insurance availability, and patient compliance. General standardization of treatment and education of professionals would facilitate the consistency of treatment outcomes required for research and efficacy, and offer policy makers and insurance companies the needed information to favorably influence reimbursement. There is an urgent need to develop legislative advocacy groups to facilitate the care of individuals with lymphedema.

Licensure for certification in lymphedema management became available in Spring 2001 through the Lymphology Association of North America (LANA), a nonprofit corporation composed of health care professionals developing standards of qualification for individuals who treat lymphedema. Once lymphedema therapists are certified, they can utilize the acronym CLT-LANA. This is an important step toward qualifying care standards. Information regarding professional training programs that offer the didactic and manual training, a component of the certification, is available through the National Lymphedema Network (NLN).[68] The NLN, a nonprofit organization, is dedicated to making information on prevention and treatment of lymphedema available to the general public and medical community.

Conclusion

Lymphedema is a chronic condition requiring lifelong consideration. The disease now has several treatment options available that demonstrate efficacy for reducing edema volume, preventing reaccumulation of fluid, and reducing frequency of infections. Patients who participate in a CDT program with a qualified therapist have available to them the opportunity for greater functional usage of their limb(s), improved quality of life, and a sense of control in their disease management.

References

1. Oschman JL. *Energy Medicine: The Scientific Basis.* Philadelphia, PA: Churchill Livingstone; 2000.
2. Guyton AC, Hall JE. The microcirculation and the lymphatic system: capillary fluid exchange, interstitial fluid and lymph flow. In: Guyton AC, Hall JE, eds. *Textbook of Medical Physiology.* 9th ed. Philadelphia, PA: WB Saunders; 1996:183-197.
3. Foldi E, Foldi M, Clodius L. The lymphedema chaos: a lancet. *Ann Plast Surg.* 1989;22:505-515.
4. Barnes JF. *Myofascial Release: The Search For Excellence.* Paoli, PA: MFR Seminars; 1990.
5. Wittlinger H, Wittlinger G. *Textbook of Dr. Vodder's Manual Lymph Drainage. Vol 1. Basic Course.* 3rd rev. Heidelberg, Germany: Haug; 1982.
6. Casley-Smith JR, Casley-Smith JR. *Modern Treatment of Lymphedema.* 5th ed. Malvern, PA: Lymphedema Association of Australia; 1997.
7. Casley-Smith JR. The structure and functioning of the blood vessels, interstitial tissues, and lymphatics. In: Foldi M, Casley-Smith JR, eds. *Lymphangiology.* New York, NY: Schattauer; 1983:27-143.
8. Weissleder H, Schuchhardt C. *Lymphadema Diagnosis and Therapy.* 2nd ed. Bonn, Germany: Kagerer Kommunikation; 1997.
9. Guyton AC. Immunity and allergy. In: Guyton AC, ed. *Textbook of Medical Physiology.* 4th ed. Philadelphia, PA: WB Saunders; 1971:118-125.
10. World Health Organization. Worldwide incidence of lymphedema. *WHO Technical Report. Series 702.* Geneva, Switzerland: World Health Organization; 1984.
11. Petrek JA, Lerner R. Lymphedema. In: Harris JR, Lippman ME, Morrow M, Hellman S, eds. *Diseases of the Breast.* 2nd ed. Philadelphia, PA: Lippincott-Raven; 1996:896-903.
12. National Cancer Institute. *The Breast Cancer Digest: A Guide to Medical Care, Emotional Support, Educational Programs, and Resources.* 2nd ed. Bethesda, MD: Office of Cancer Communications, National Cancer Institute; 1984.
13. Lerner R. Chronic Lymphedema. In: Chang JB, ed. *Textbook of Angiology.* New York, NY: Springer-Verlag; 2000;1227-1236.
14. Maunsell E, Brisson J, Deschenes L. Arm problems and psychological distress after surgery for breast cancer. *Can J Surg.* 1993;36:315-320.
15. Sneeuw KC, Aaronson NK, Yarnold JR, et al. Cosmetic and functional outcomes of breast conserving treatment for early stage breast cancer. 2. Relationship with psychosocial functioning. *Radiother Oncol.* 1992;25:160-166.
16. Segerstrom K, Bjerle P, Nystrom A. Importance of time in assessing arm and hand function after treatment of breast cancer. *Scand J Plast Reconstr Hand Surg.* 1991;24:875-892.
17. Passik SD, Newman M, Brennan M, Tunkel R. Predictors of psychological distress, sexual dysfunction and physical functioning among women with upper extremity lymphedema related to breast cancer. *Psycho-Oncology.* 1995; 4:255-263.
18. Velanovich V, Szymanski W. Quality of life of breast cancer patients with lymphedema. *Am J Surg.* 1999;177:184-188.
19. Tobin MB, Lacey HJ, Meyer L, Mortimer PS. The psychological morbidity of breast cancer-related arm swelling. Psychological morbidity of lymphedema. *Cancer.* 1993;72:3248-3252.
20. Klose G, Norton S. *Course Manual for Manual Lymph Drainage (MLD), Complete Decongestive Therapy (CDT).* Red Bank, NJ: Klose Norton Training and Consulting, LLC; 2000.

21. Foldi E, Foldi M, Weissleder H. Conservative treatment of lymphedema of the limbs. *Angiology.* 1985;36:171-180.
22. Piller NB. Pharmacological treatment of lymph stasis. In: Olszewski W, ed. *Lymph Stasis: Pathophysiology, Diagnosis and Treatment.* Boca Raton, FL: CRC Press; 1991:501-529.
23. Clodius L. Secondary arm lymphedema. In: Clodius L, ed. *Lymphoedema.* Stuttgart, Germany: Georg Thieme; 1977:166-174.
24. Casley-Smith JR , Foldi M, Ryan TJ, et al. Summary of the 10th International Congress of Lymphology working group discussions and recommendations, Adelaide, Australia, August 10-17,1985. *Lymphology.* 1985;18:175-180.
25. Sitzia J, Stanton AW, Badger C. A review of outcome indicators in the treatment of chronic limb oedema. *Clin Rehab.* 1997;11:181-189.
26. Casley-Smith JR. Lymphedema therapy in Australia: complex physical therapy, exercise and benzopyrones, on over 600 limbs. *Lymphology.* 1994;27(Suppl):622-625.
27. Casley-Smith JR. Measuring and representing peripheral oedema and its alterations. *Lymphology.* 1994;27:56-70.
28. Morgan RG, Casley-Smith JR, Mason MR, Casley-Smith JR. Complex physical therapy for the lymphoedematous arm. *J Hand Surg (Br).* 1992;17(4):437-441.
29. Brennan MJ, DePompolo RW, Garden FH. Focused review: Postmastectomy lymphedema. *Arch Phys Med Rehabil.* 1996;77(3 Suppl):S74-80.
30. Mortimer PS, Bates DO, Brassington HD, Stanton AW, Strachan DP, Levick JR. The prevalence of arm oedema following treatment for breast cancer. *Q J Med.* 1996;89:377-380.
31. Hafez HM, Wolfe JH. Basic data underlying clinical decision making: lymphedema. *Ann Vasc Surg.* 1996;10:88-95.
32. Von Winiwarter A. *Die Elephantiasis, Deutsche Chirurgie.* Stuttgart, Germany: Enke; 1892.
33. Kinmonth JB. *The Lymphatics.* London: Edward Arnold; 1972.
34. Kubik ST, Manestar M. Some lymphological problems in anatomical view. Progress in lymphology. Proceedings of the VIIth International Congress of Lymphology, Florence 1979. Prague: Avicenum Czcechoslovak Medical Press; 1981:22-25.
35. Boris M, Weindorf S, Lasinski B, Boris G. Lymphedema reduction by noninvasive complex lymphedema therapy. *Oncology.* 1994;8(9):95-106, 109-110.
36. Casley-Smith JR, Casley-Smith JR. Other physical therapy for lymphedema: Pumps, heating, etc. In: Casley-Smith JR, Casley-Smith JR, eds. *Lymphedema.* Adelaide: Lymphedema Association of Australia; 1991:155-159.
37. Leduc A, Leduc O. Physical treatment of oedema. *European Journal of Lymphology and Related Problems.* 1990;1:8-10.
38. Kurz I. *Textbook of Vodder's Manual of Lymph Drainage.* Vol II. Heidelberg, Germany: Haug-Verlag; 1989.
39. Casley-Smith JR, Boris M, Weindorf S, Lasinski B. Treatment of the arm: the Casley-Smith Method. *Cancer (Am).* 1998;83(12Suppl):2843-2860.
40. Mortimer PS. Investigation and management of lymphoedema. *Vasc Med Rev.* 1990;1:1-20.
41. Barnes JF. Pain relief for cancer patients. *PT and OT Today.* 1996;4:18-19.
42. Thiadens SRJ. *Eighteen Steps to Prevention for the Upper Extremity/Lower Extremity.* San Francisco, CA: National Lymphedema Network; 1997.
43. Bergan JJ. Control of lower extremity lymphedema by semirigid support. *Natl Lymphed Net Newslett.* 1994;6:1-2.
44. Reid T. Reid sleeve for effective treatment for lymphedema. Abstract presented at: Lymphedema: The Problem and the Challenge—Second National Lymphedema Network Conference; September 19-22, 1996; San Francisco, Calif.
45. Wozniewski M. Value of intermittent pneumatic massage in the treatment of upper extremity lymphedema. *Pol Tyg Lek.* 1991;46(30-31):550-552.
46. Mirolo BR, Bunce IH, Chapman M, et al. Psychosocial benefits of postmastectomy lymphedema therapy. *Cancer Nurs.* 1995;18(3):197-205.
47. Zelikowski A, Haddad M, Reiss R. The "Lympha-Press" intermittent sequential pneumatic device for the treatment of lymphedema: five years of clinical experience. *J Cardiovasc Surg.* 1986;27:288-290.
48. Bunce IH, Mirolo BR, Hennessy JM, Ward LC, Jones LC. Post-mastectomy lymphedema treatment and measurement. *Med J Aust.* 1994;161(2):125-128.
49. Pappas CJ, O'Donnell TF Jr. Long-term results of compression treatment for lymphedema. *J Vasc Surg.* 1992;16(4): 555-562.
50. Richmand DM, O'Donnell TR Jr, Zelikowski A. Sequential pneumatic compression for lymphedema. A controlled trial. *Arch Surg.* 1985;112(10);1116-1119.
51. Boris M, Weindorf S, Lasinski B. The risk of genital edema after external pump compression for lower limb lymphedema. *Lymphology.* 1998;31:15-20.
52. Eliska O, Eliskova M. Are peripheral lymphatics damaged by high pressure manual massage? [comments]. *Lymphology.* 1995;28(1):21-30.
53. Boris M, Weindorf S, Lasinski B. Persistence of lymphedema reduction after noninvasive complex lymphedema therapy. *Oncology (Hunting).* 1997;11:99-110.
54. Swedborg I. Effectiveness of combined methods of physio-therapy for post-mastectomy lymphoedema. *Scand J Rehab Med.* 1980;12:77-85.
55. Miller LT. *Recovery in Motion: An Exercise Program to Assist in the Management of Upper Extremity Lymphedema.* Philadelphia, PA: LT Miller; 1992.

56. Miller L. The enigma of exercise: participation in an exercise program after breast cancer surgery. *Natl Lymphed Net Newslett.* 1996;8:15-16.
57. Consensus document of the International Society of Lymphology Executive Committee. The diagnosis and treatment of peripheral edema. *Lymphology.* 1995;28:113-117.
58. Harris SR, Hugi MR, Olivotto IA, Levines M. Steering committee for clinical practice guidelines for the care and treatment of breast cancer: 11. Lymphedema. *CMAJ.* 2001;164:191-199.
59. International Society of Lymphology The Diagnosis and treatment of peripheral lymphedema. Consensus document of the International Society of Lymphology. *Lymphology.* 2003;36:84-91.
60. Janbon C, Ferrandez JC, Vinot JM, Serin D. A comparative lymphoscintigraphic evaluation of manual lymphatic drainage and pressotherapy in edema of the arm following treatment of a breast tumor. *Journal Malaise Vascular.* 1990; 15:287-288.
61. Rockson SG, Miller LT, Senie R, et al. American Cancer Society Lymphedema workshop. Workgroup III: Diagnosis and management of lymphedema. *Cancer (Am).* 1998;83(12 Suppl):2882-2885.
62. Kirshbaum M. The development, implementation and evaluation of guidelines for the management of breast cancer related lymphoedema. *Eur J Cancer Care (Eng).* 1996;5:246-251.
63. Asdonk J. Effectiveness, indications and contraindications of manual lymph drainage therapy in painful edema. *Z Lymphol.* 1995;19(1):16-22.
64. Ko DS, Lerner R, Klose G, et al. Effective treatment of lymphedema of the extremities. *Arch Surg.* 1998;133:452-457.
65. Foldi M. Treatment of lymphedema [Editorial]. *Lymphology.* 1994;27(1):1-5.
66. Szuba A, Cooke J, Yousuf S, Rockson S. Decongestive lymphatic therapy for patients with cancer-related or primary lymhedema. *Am J Med.* 2000;109(4):296-300.
67. Rockson S. XX international Society of Lymphology Symposium on Bioelectrical Impedance Analysis in the Management of Lymphedema. Addressing the unmet needs in lymphedema risk management. *Lymphatic Research and Biology.* 2006;4(1):41-56.
68. National Lymphedema Network (NLN). *Resource Guide Training Programs.* Available at http://www.lymphnet.org/resource-a.html.

Bibliography

Brennan MJ, Miller LT. Overview of treatment options and review of the current role and use of compression garments, intermittent pumps, and exercise in the management of lymphedema. *Cancer (Am).* 1998;83(12 Suppl):2821-2827.
Foldi E. Massage and damage to lymphatics [Editorial: comments]. *Lymphology.* 1995;28(1):1-3.
Passik S, Newman M, Brennan M, Holland J. Psychiatric consultation for women undergoing rehabilitation for upper-extremity lymphedema following breast cancer treatment. *J Pain Symptom Manage.* 1993;8:226-233.
Schmid-Schonbein GW. Microlymphatics and lymph flow. *Physiological Reviews.* 1990;70:987-1028.
Smith RD. Lymphatic contractility—a possible intrinsic mechanism of lymphatic vessels for the transport of lymph. *J Exp Med.* 1949;90:497-509.

Additional Resources

Lymphology Association of North America (LANA). Available at www.sonnet.org/lana.
Medical Advisory Committee National Lymphedema Network. Choosing a lymphedema therapist. Available at www.lymphnet.org/choosing.html.
National Certification for Lymphedema Therapists. Available at http://www.snonet.org/ lana/main.html.
National Lymphedema Network. Resource guide. Available at www. lymphnet.org/resource-a.html.

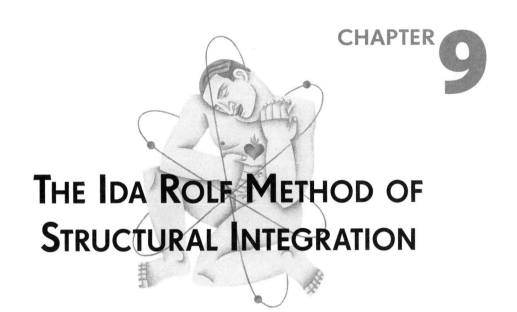

THE IDA ROLF METHOD OF STRUCTURAL INTEGRATION

Judith E. Deutsch, PT, PhD

D r. Ida Rolf, who was trained as a biochemist, developed the Ida Rolf method of structural integration in the late 1960s. Her theoretical framework and concepts supporting the method were first described in an article[1] and then elaborated on in the book she authored, *Rolfing: The Integration of Human Structures.*[2] Additional information about the approach can be gained from a book in which Dr. Rolf is interviewed about Rolfing.[3] The method is based on her personal interest with the human body and its response to use and injury, and especially its relationship to gravity.

Structural integration (SI) or Rolfing is classified by the National Center for Complementary and Alternative Medicine[4] as a manual body-based therapy (MBB). It is, like many of the MBB therapies, an approach to the examination and intervention of the body that focuses on the relationship between structure and function. In this chapter, the main ideas in Rolfing are described and the evidence that exists to support the approach is reviewed.

Background and Description of Structural Integration

Based on her observations of the human body, Dr. Rolf organized her approach around three main principles: 1) the role of gravity in shaping posture and movement, 2) the importance of the myofascial system as the organ that connects and supports all structures, and 3) the belief that structure (tissues of the human body) can be changed.[5] These principles guide the examination and intervention, which can be described as a 10-session process of soft tissue mobilization and movement education.

Dr. Rolf believed that the body was shaped or organized by the effects of gravity and that the fascia was the central organ in this process. The examination process in Rolfing is to view the body using a three-dimensional postural analysis referenced to a column of blocks. Each block represents a section of the body with the pelvis being the central block. This allows for descriptions of the segments of the body in all three planes using terms like rotations and obliquities. Because the fascial system supports posture, the examination also includes observing and describing the quality of tissues. For example, the practitioner observes if tissues appear tight or restricted in a particular area. Bony and soft tissue structures are also observed during movement. Specific movements are selected because they relate to the goals of a session. For example, in the first session the anterior chest is one of the main structures worked on, so the practitioner will observe the person's breathing. Thus, identification of deviations in posture and tissue restrictions serve to locate dysfunction and guide practitioners' interventions.

The 10 sessions of SI are sometimes referred to as a recipe.[3] To some extent, this is accurate because there is a systematic approach to each examination and intervention. Each session has a specific purpose, and the practitioner focuses on a set of soft tissue structures and then provides movement cues. For example, during the second session, practitioners focus on the alignment of the lower extremities and work primarily on the superficial soft tissue of the feet and legs, such as the retinaculum on the dorsum of the foot, the perimalleolar structures such as the peroneal tendons, the gastrocnemius muscles, medial and lateral collateral ligaments, the tibial crest, the Achilles tendon to the calcaneus, and the medial and lateral arches. Following this, the client is given movement awareness cues such as to "walk vertical" and attend to the weight distribution of the feet. While the elements of the second session would be recognized by all Rolfing practitioners, the intent and rendering of the session will vary depending on each client's needs.

The focus of each session, as well as the depth of the soft tissue work, is varied systematically. Sessions 1 through 6 alternate their emphasis on either the upper (odd numbered, 1, 3, and 5) or lower (even numbered: 2, 4, and 6) part of the body. In sessions 7 through 10, the work is done on large fascial planes that connect the upper and lower parts of the body. The depth of the work begins superficially in the first session, working on the fascia of the sternocleidomastoid in the neck, and moves to the deepest structures in the fourth session, such as the insertion of the adductors on the pubic ramus. The manual soft tissue work is performed with the intention of freeing the structures of adhesions so that they move freely. The focus of each session, the main structures that are worked on, and the depth of the work are summarized in Table 9-1. A more detailed description of the first six sessions can be found in the *Guild News*.[6,7] and of the entire series in the Journal of *Body Work and Movement Therapies*.[8-10]

While each session has a specific focus, certain structures are evaluated and worked on in each of the 10 sessions. A three-dimensional assessment of posture is always performed. The central structure of the body is the pelvis, so during each session a pelvic lift is performed. The pelvic lift is performed with the client supine and the knees flexed. One hand is placed on the sacrum with the fingertips resting on the lumbosacral junction. The second hand is placed on the subject's epigastrum to stabilize the trunk. A cranial traction force is applied using the hand on the lumbosacral junction to rotate the pelvis posteriorly.[11] There is evidence that using this pelvic lift increases parasympathetic tone and is therefore associated with a relaxation response.[11,12]

Sessions are typically performed with a week's rest in between. This is done to allow the body to reorganize itself with respect to gravity. After the 10-session process is completed, individuals may be re-evaluated if their symptoms persist. This is more likely to be the case if the person returns to habitual movement patterns and postures that created the original myofascial imbalance. Additional lessons are offered with a greater emphasis on movement re-education or to be used as tune-up sessions.[13]

Evidence of Efficacy: Validation and Outcome Studies

The literature that both describes and supports Rolfing is modest and varied, and will be reviewed chronologically. The first articles about Rolfing were published in 1973 in the psychiatry literature. Dr. Rolf described the assumptions underlying Rolfing and made a connection between imbalances in the structural system with disease, both physical and psychological.[1] An accompanying paper attempted to validate the assumptions of Rolfing by using electrophysiological and

Table 9-1

KEY ELEMENTS OF EACH STRUCTURAL INTEGRATION SESSION

SESSION	GOALS	DEPTH	KEY MYOFASCIAL RELEASE
1	• Establish a rapport with the patient • Increase movement with each breath of the thorax and ribs • "Horizontalize" the pelvis	Superficial	Rib cage and costal arch
2	• Restore the alignment between the calcaneus and the ischial tuberosities • Restore balanced movement between the hip, knee, and ankles • Direct attention to the relationship of the feet to the ground	Superficial	Peri-articular ankle retinaculum, plantar fascia, and lateral arch
3	• Lengthen the lateral line • Increase the space between the pelvis and the 12th rib • Release the shoulder and pelvic girdles	Superficial	Quadratus lumborum, 12th rib
4	• Reduce excessive rotation of the lower limb • Align the pelvis in all planes • Align the foot with respect to the spine	Deep	Medial retinaculum of the ankle, attachments of the adductors and hamstrings to the pubic ramus
5	• Lengthen the anterior thorax • Align the clavicles in all planes • Facilitate movement of the arm with proper scapular alignment • Facilitate movements of hip flexion	Deep	Psoas, pectoralis minor, rectus abdominus, and diaphragm

continued

Table 9-1 (continued)

KEY ELEMENTS OF EACH STRUCTURAL INTEGRATION SESSION

SESSION	GOALS	DEPTH	KEY MYOFASCIAL RELEASE
6	• Vertically align the lower limb • Align the pelvis, sacrum, and spine	Deep	Hip rotators sacrotuberous ligament, thorocolumbar fascia
7	• Align the head • Separate the fascia of the head and arms	Superficial to deep	Sternocleidomastoid, scalenes, masseter, occipital atlantic ligaments, deep cervical muscles, and cranial fascia
8 and 9	• Focus on either the upper or lower body • "Balance and relate the girdles" to the "dorsal lumbar hinge" • Relate the limbs to the spine	Varied	Mobility of fascial planes
10	• Integrate a functional whole • Maximize movement strategies and efficiency	Varied	Fascial planes across joints

Reprinted with permission from *Ortho Phys Ther Clin North Am*, 9(3), Deutsch JE, Derr L, Judd P, Reuven B, Structural integration applied to patients with chronic pain. 1059-1516. ©2000, with permission from Elsevier.

biochemical measures to quantify the effects of Rolfing on 15 healthy individuals.[14] Significant changes were found when comparing pre- and post-SI measures, suggesting that there was an effect for Rolfing. Using cluster analysis, the authors identified four groups of responders that correlated well with a blinded review by an SI practitioner characterizing the outcome of the patients. The authors concluded that they had provided preliminary evidence for relating the outcomes of SI to their prototypical model of an "open, receptive, efficient sensory information processor."[14] They argued that there was a connection between the muscular system and the sensory system.

A follow-up study was designed to examine energy in motor behavior using electromyography (EMG). Muscle activity was recorded using EMG on 13 individuals executing a variety of tasks before and after receiving 10 sessions of SI.[15] After receiving the 10 sessions of SI, subjects performed the same motor tasks with a shorter duration of muscle contraction and a greater force amplitude during the contraction. The authors interpreted this finding as evidence for subjects being able to overcome the resistances from inertia, gravity, and friction more rapidly, thus making their movements more efficient. Post-SI, subjects exhibited more sequential contraction and less co-contraction for all movements tested. This finding was interpreted as having the control of the movement accomplished by agonists by using either better recruitment of motor units or a change in frequency of motor unit firing. The authors also noted that this EMG pattern of firing was similar to the patterns identified of individuals who were in nonstressful situations, suggesting that SI may reduce stress. The authors also reported another interesting finding: decrease in neuromuscular excitation after SI for areas that were not related functionally to the motor task. The combined results of the specificity of muscle action with decreased overall motor activity post-SI can be interpreted as improved neuromuscular organization consistent with more efficient movement.[12] Finally, after SI, EMG patterns between static and rhythmic activities were performed with a clear distinction between isotonic and isometric contractions. The absence of random action potentials of EMG activity in between rhythmic activities is interpreted as a nonhyperactive neuromuscular system. The relationship between the observed EMG patterns of subjects post-SI and individuals who were not anxious was highlighted by the authors.

Clinical studies can be found in the pediatric and physical therapy literature published as early as 1981 through 2000. However, only three investigators have reported on the outcome of a complete 10-session process.[6-18] Only one of the studies, the effect of Rolfing on individuals with cerebral palsy, is prospective with detailed outcome measures.[16] The others are retrospective chart reviews about individuals with chronic fatigue syndrome[18] and chronic pain.[17] Two case reports have been used to document the effects of SI, one for an individual with a brain injury[19] and a second for individual with multiple sclerosis.[20] All found favorable outcomes when using SI both at the impairment and functional levels.

Cottingham, a physical therapist who is also a Rolfer, and colleagues published several articles on Rolfing between 1988 and 2000. Two of these articles were quasi-experimental design studies in which the effect of the pelvic lift (a standard part of an SI lesson) on autonomic nervous system function is reported.[11,12] These articles, along with the earlier work published in the 1970s, are the four that can be characterized as validation or mechanism studies. That is, the studies aim to support assumptions about the approach, such as the effect of soft tissue mobilization on increasing parasympathetic tone[11,12] and improved movement efficiency.[15] Cottingham also wrote case reports on an individual with low back pain[21] and an individual with amyotrophic lateral sclerosis (ALS) who received SI.[22] Interestingly, in the case report about the patient with low back pain, the authors attribute the positive outcome of the patient to the movement re-education component of the therapy and not the soft tissue work. In the case of the patient with ALS, the author reported an association with reports of well-being and the measured increases in parasympathetic tone.[22]

In sum, the literature supporting the efficacy of SI is quite modest. Most of the reported findings are positive and appear applicable to diverse patient populations. Literature based on the research designed to answer questions about the efficacy of SI is not strong. Therefore, the findings, while encouraging, are at best preliminary. It is interesting to note, however, that there have been no new studies contributed to the literature since 2000.

🗁 Case Example

A 71-year-old woman who had a right cerebral vascular accident (CVA) 3 months prior to receiving SI was referred for SI to reduce musculoskeletal and neuromuscular impairments that were interfering with balance and gait. The patient had a history of two previous left CVAs 3 months and 1 year prior, for which she had received both in- and outpatient services. Her medical history was also remarkable for coronary bypass graft surgery 3 years prior and a positive history of coronary artery disease, arrhythmias, hypertension, and borderline diabetes mellitus. Her personal goal for this outpatient referral was to "walk taller and with more energy."

Upon initial exam, the patient presented with bilateral loss of range of motion (ROM) and weakness in all hip and ankle musculature. She had residual right shoulder ROM loss from the previous strokes. Her sitting posture was flexed at the thoracic spine with a posterior pelvic tilt;

in standing her posture was flexed. Vital capacity, measured as an average of three trials with an incentive spirometer, was 950 cc. She ambulated at a speed of 0.45 m/s and exhibited shortness of breath. Her score on the Tinetti balance test was 14/28. It was determined that she may benefit from a full course of SI. The therapist's rationale for selecting SI was based on the assumption that reversing some of the ROM losses and postural deficits may have a positive impact on breathing and potentially improve the mechanics of walking.

She received six sessions of SI, which were not concurrent with physical therapy. She was unable to complete the 10 sessions because of inclement weather. She tolerated the sessions well. Upon completion of the six sessions, the following improvements were noted: ROM increases for both lower extremities (right > left), in particular the hip extensors, abductors, and internal rotators, with no remarkable change in range of the right upper extremity. There was no change in her strength. Posture upon observation was less flexed. Vital capacity increased 500 cc to 1450 cc. The Tinetti score increased by 2 points to 16/28 (still in the high fall risk category). Ambulation speed increased to 0.58 m/s, with a decrease in shortness of breath. The patient reported pain when reaching behind her back. The patient also reported feeling less shortness of breath when she walked, and a "little stronger," but she felt that otherwise she was unchanged.

Consistent with the therapist's prediction, the patient did make improvements with flexibility and posture and, in turn, had an improvement in respiratory capacity and walking. The appearance of new pain symptoms is interesting and may be attributed to a change in posture and available range without the appropriate mechanics to support movement in a new ROM. Since the patient remained in the high risk for falls category based on her Tinetti score, she was recommended for outpatient physical therapy to address balance and to increase endurance during ambulation. The SI intervention in this instance served to lay the groundwork for additional rehabilitation services and was likely a complement to physical therapy.

Acknowledgments

I wish to thank Patricia Judd, PT; Irene DeMasi, MA, PT; Barbara Reuven, PT; and Thomas Findley, MD, PT who have taught me much of what I know about structural integration.

References

1. Rolf IP. Structural integration: a contribution to the understanding of stress. *Confinia Psychiat.* 1973;16:69-79.
2. Rolf IP. *Rolfing: The Integration of Human Structures.* New York, NY: Harper & Row; 1977.
3. Feitis R. *Ida Rolf Talks.* New York, NY: Harper and Row; 1978.
4. National Center for Complementary and Alternative Medicine. Major domain of complementary and alternative therapies. Available at: www.nccam.nih.gov. Accessed November 4, 2003.
5. Oschman J. *The Origins, Theory and Practice of Rolfing in Aspen Research Institute Research on Rolfing and Related Topics.* 1981.
6. Urbanczik A. A tour of the first three sessions. *Guild News.* 1994;4:32-35.
7. Urbanczik A. A tour of the basic series: sessions 4, 5, and 6. *Guild News.* 1995;5:21-23.
8. Myers TW. Structural integration: developments in Ida Rolf's "recipe"—part 1. *J Bodywork Movement Ther.* 2004;8(2):131-142.
9. Myers TW. Structural integration: developments in Ida Rolf's "recipe"—part 2. *J Bodywork Movement Ther.* 2004;8(3):189-198.
10. Myers TW. Structural integration: developments in Ida Rolf's "recipe"—part 3, an alternative form. *J Bodywork Movement Ther.* 2004;8(4):249-64.
11. Cottingham JT, Porges SW, Lyon T. Effects of soft tissue mobilization (Rolfing pelvic lift) on parasympathetic tone in two age groups. *Phys Ther.* 1988;68:352-356.
12. Cottingham JT, Porges SW, Richmond K. Shifts in pelvic inclination angle and parasympathetic tone produced by Rolfing soft tissue manipulation. *Phys Ther.* 1988;68:1364-1370.

13. Kotzsch E. Restructure the body with Rolfing: deep massage that realigns the human form. *East West Natural Health.* 1993:35.

14. Silverman J, Rappaport M, Hopkins K, et al. Stress intensity control and the structural integration technique. *Confinia Psychiatrica.* 1973;16:201-219.

15. Hunt VV, Massey WW. Electromyographic evaluation of structural integration techniques. *Psychoenergetic Systems.* 1977;2:199-210.

16. Perry J, Jones M, Thomas L. Functional evaluation of Rolfing in cerebral palsy. *Develop Med Child Neurol.* 1981;23:717-729.

17. Deutsch JE, Derr L, Judd P, Reuven B. Structural integration applied to patients with chronic pain. *Phys Ther Clin North Am.* 2000;9(3):411-427.

18. Talty C, DeMasi I, Deutsch JE. Structural integration applied to patients with chronic fatigue syndrome: a retrospective chart review. *J Orthop Sports Phys Ther.* 1998;27(1)83.

19. Deutsch JE, Judd P, DeMasi I, Findley T. Structural integration: a description of the approach and application to a patient with a traumatic brain injury. *Phys Ther.* Submitted.

20. Deutsch JE, Judd P, DeMasi I. Structural Integration applied to patients with a primary neurologic diagnosis: two case studies. *Neurology Report.* 1997;21(5):161-162.

21. Cottingham JT, Maitland J. A three paradigm treatment model using soft tissue mobilization and guided movement awareness techniques for a patient with chronic low back pain: a case study. *J Orthop Sports Phys Ther.* 1997;26:155-167.

22. Cottingham JT, Maitland J. Integrating manual and movement therapy with philosophical counseling for treatment of a patient with amyotrophic lateral sclerosis: a case study that explores the principles of holistic intervention. *Alternative Therapies.* 2000;6:120-128.

SECTION IV

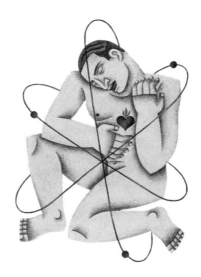

MIND/BODY WORK

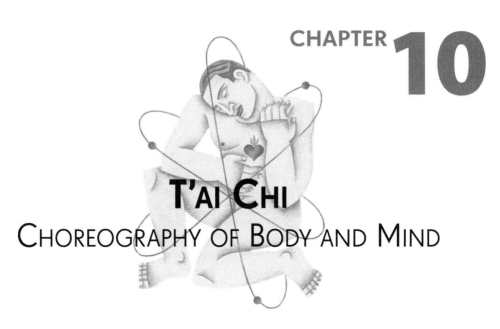

CHAPTER 10

T'AI CHI
CHOREOGRAPHY OF BODY AND MIND

Jennifer M. Bottomley, PhD, MS, PT

If there is light in the soul
There will be beauty in the person
If there is beauty in the person
There will be harmony in the house
If there is harmony in the house
There will be order in the nation
If there is order in the nation
There will be peace in the world

Chinese Proverb

Introduction

The use of T'ai Chi is an alternative therapeutic approach that can greatly enhance the practice of physical therapy. It is a form of exercise that recognizes the mind/body connection.[1,2] The movements are graceful, the tempo is slow, the benefits are great. It can positively augment physical therapy programs aimed at improving balance and posture, coordination and integration of movement, endurance, strength, flexibility, and relaxation.[1-13] T'ai Chi exercise has cardiovascular, neuromuscular, and psychological[7-12,14-17] benefits that are clinically observed. It is a form of exercise that allows the individual to assume an active role in obtaining maximal health and focusing on the prevention of disease, rather than the passive acceptance of illness as a consequence of life, aging, fate, or genetics. It is an exercise form that is particularly helpful in an elderly population because of its slow-controlled, nonimpact-type movement which displaces, thereby "exercising," the center of gravity. This exercise form incorporates all of the motions that often become restricted with inactivity and aging. It improves respiratory status, stresses trunk control, expands the base of support, improves rotation of the trunk and coordination of isolated extremity motions, and helps to facilitate awareness of movement and position.[3,5-8,10,18] Studies of elders participating in T'ai Chi programs have also indicated a significant improvement in self-reported well-being and quality of life measures.[14-18] Even in the frailest and most inactive elderly, studies have shown that T'ai Chi is effective for improving functional status and enhancing health-related quality of life measures.[19-21] An additional benefit is the interaction on a social basis, as most T'ai Chi is done in group settings.

What Is T'ai Chi?

T'ai Chi is an ancient physical art form, originally a martial art, where the defendant actually uses his or her attacker's own energy against him- or herself by drawing the attack, sidestepping the attacker, and throwing the opponent off balance. There are numerous forms of T'ai Chi[22] involving as many as 108 postures and transitions of controlled movement, each style with slightly different philosophical foundations. Family surnames came to be associated with the different styles of T'ai Chi that have been passed on from generation to generation (eg, Wu style, Yang style, Ch'en style, Chuan style). Each style is distinctive, but all follow the classic T'ai Chi principles.

T'ai Chi is a way of life that has been practiced by the Chinese for thousands of years. It is a Taoist philosophical perspective which forms the foundation of an exercise regime developed to balance mind and body. Unlike Western civilization which separates body from mind and allows spiritual development only in terms of religions and mystical beliefs, T'ai Chi integrates the connections between mind, body, and spirit in a quest for the highest form of harmony in life through the combination of exercise and meditation.[23-25] The Chinese conceived the human mind to be an unlimited dimension and focused on simplification of beliefs. They also viewed the human body as limitless in its physical capabilities. These beliefs were the keystones for the evolution of what we know as T'ai Chi Ch'uan today.[22]

Since ancient times, Taoist philosophy has been concerned with the question of how to reproduce and maintain the essential kind of energy required to prolong life and enhance creativity of the individual. The answer can be found in the T'ai Chi methods of Taoist meditation, in which a combination of movement, breathing, and mental concentration is used to purify the essential life energies, distill out its pure Yang aspect, the vital energy (ch'i), and transmit it through the eight body/mind channels to every cell in the body. The regular practice of these methods has been shown to result in longevity, good health, vigor, mental alertness, and creativity far beyond what is experienced by most people.[26]

In order to obtain the full benefit from the practice of T'ai Chi, it is essential to understand the principles underlying the methods. Hence, it is the aim of this chapter to not only describe the methods of meditation and exercise, but also to explain how they are based on the philosophy of Taoism.

The "spiritual" component of T'ai Chi is what makes many Westerners uncomfortable with this and other Eastern practices.[23-25] However, the concentration required to accomplish the rhythmic and coordinated movement patterns and integrate these motions with respiration in T'ai Chi induces a level of concentration that edges on meditation.[1,2,11] Movement is vital to preventing disability and maintaining health and well-being. The capability of cognitively understanding the movements is an essential element in the successful practice of the T'ai Chi exercise form. T'ai Chi requires practice (preferably throughout the life cycle) and commitment.[11,12] There would be a total lack of consistency and benefit from this exercise form if the mind/body connection was not made.

Philosophical Background of T'ai Chi

Behind every T'ai Chi movement is the philosophy of *Yin* and *Yang*. As described in chapters in Section IV, *Traditional Chinese Medicine*, the Yin-Yang principle has been the basis of the Chinese understanding of health and sickness since ancient times. Good health requires a balance between opposing forces within the body. If one or the other is too predominant, sickness results. It is the aim of Eastern Medical practices, including acupuncture, Qi Gong, and herbal medicine, to discover the source of the imbalance and restore the forces to their proper proportions. In the Western world, exercise concentrates on outer movements and the development of the physical body. T'ai Chi develops both the mind and body.[1,2] It embodies a philosophy that not only promotes health but can be applied to every aspect of life. T'ai Chi emphasizes the development of the whole person, promoting personal growth in all areas.[26]

T'ai Chi means "the ultimate" energy. This ultimate power is *ch'i*. According to the legendary theory of Yin and Yang, ch'i exercises its power creating a balance between the positive and negative energies of nature.[22] T'ai Chi's philosophical basis is directed toward improving and progressing towards the unlimited and immense interrelationship between the self and all other things in existence. T'ai Chi is guided by the theory of opposites: the *Yin* and the *Yang*, the negative and the positive. This is the *original principle* of Taoist thought.[27] According to the T'ai Chi theory, the abilities of the human body are capable of being developed beyond their commonly conceived potential. Creativity has no boundaries, and the human mind should have no restrictions or barriers placed upon its capabilities.

The fundamental principle of Taoist philosophy, the joining together of opposites, is the basis for the practice of T'ai Chi. The Taoist philosophy that underlies T'ai Chi exercise and meditation is a somewhat more complex in its application of the relationship between Yin and Yang within the body. It is not denied that a general balance is necessary to avoid illness, however, it is the aim of *meditation* to greatly *increase* the *Yang* and to reduce and *diminish* the *Yin*. One of the fundamental beliefs of Taoist philosophy is that the reason people become old and weak and eventually die is that they lack essential energy (ch'i) that sustains life.[22,26,28] Thus the goal of exercise is to greatly *reduce Yang* and to *increase* and *enhance Yin*.[26,28] The combined practice of meditation and exercise balances these opposing energies.

One reaches the ultimate level of health and physical and mental well-being through exercise and meditative means of balancing the opposing powers and their natural motions. *Yin*, the negative (yielding) power, and *Yang*, the positive (action) power. The theory is that the interplay and balance between opposite, yet complementary forces of equal strength promotes health. These two opposing manifestations have universal significance and apply to the phenomena of the cosmos as well as the operations of the human body. On the largest scale, heaven is Yang, while earth is Yin. Day is Yang, while night is Yin. Bright and clear weather is Yang; dark and stormy weather is Yin. On the scale of living things, the male is Yang, the female Yin. Spirit is Yang, body Yin. This opposition applies to the parts of the body and their functions as well. In the circulatory system, the arteries are Yang; the veins are Yin. Muscle contraction is Yang, relaxation is Yin. In breathing, exhalation is Yang; inhalation is Yin. In human activities, movement is Yang; rest is Yin.[29]

Hundreds of years ago, those who searched for a way to elevate the human body and spirit to their ultimate level developed the ingenious system known as T'ai Chi exercise. It has since proven to be the most advanced system of body exercise and mind conditioning ever to be created.[22,29] It makes intuitive sense from a clinical perspective to apply the idea of a natural harmony and a balancing of life forces to the integration of body and mind.

Historical Background of T'ai Chi

A systematic description of the relationships of Yin and Yang is found in the hexagrams of *I Ching*, the oldest and most important book of Chinese philosophy.[27]

One of the pioneers of the philosophy of Taoism was Lao Tzu.[22] He emphasized that "the soft overcomes the hard." Later, this idea permeated the practice of T'ai Chi Ch'uan. After Lao Tzu, the second great master of Taoism was Chuang Tzu.[30] To the philosophy of *soft over hard* he added the component of "breathing," not only as the process of the movement of air in and out of the lungs, but the process involving the whole body, including the circulation of oxygen to the extremities through the blood. In other words, the flow of ch'i, or vital energy. T'ai Chi Ch'uan was not actually developed until centuries after Chuang Tzu, though there is clear evidence that he was practicing methods of exercise coordinated with breathing,[31] which is the basis of T'ai Chi exercise.

Approximately 1700 years ago (3rd Century A.D.), a famous Chinese medical doctor, Hua-Tuo, emphasized physical and mental exercise as a means of improving health.[29] He believed that human beings should exercise and imitate the movements of animals to recover physical/cognitive abilities that had been lost to "civilization." Hua-Tuo organized a martial arts form called the Five Animal Games.[22] Since then, these exercises have become popular with the Chinese who wish to maximize their health through exercise.

Huang Ti, the so-called Yellow Emperor of 2700 B.C., practiced a form of exercise called *Tao Yin* with the aim of increasing his life span.[22] *Tao* means "guide" and *Yin* is translated here as "leading." These terms give a hint of how the exercise works: the movement of the limbs guide the circulation of the blood so that the tissues throughout the body can be repaired and cleansed more efficiently. The movement also leads the breath in and out of the lungs to nourish and energize the body through inhalation and rid the body of poisons through exhalation. Thus, movement is the foundation of a discipline that guides and leads the automatic bodily processes so that they will function efficiently.[26] The essential element of Tao Yin was the way in which the movements of the limbs were combined with breathing. Huang Ti's exercises were also known as T'u Na (t'u = exhale; na = inhale) exercises.[29] There is little doubt that Huang Ti's health practices, consisting of an alternation of movement and rest, and his form of exercise involving breathing in and out were direct applications of the Yin-Yang principle.

Ko Hung (325 A.D.), an alchemist, developed a series of 18 forms of "health exercise" to complete the evolution. Ko's system is only for health, not for self-defense.[28] He also combined exercise, breathing, and meditation.

These exercise forms were precursors of the methods of Taoist meditation and of the form of exercise known as T'ai Chi Ch'uan. Unlike movements of martial arts, which are generally strenuous and sometimes very quick, the movements developed in what we know as T'ai Chi Ch'uan today are done slowly, gently, and evenly from beginning to end, each posture unfolding with the same continuous rhythm. In this evolutionary way, the modified form of T'ai Chi became today's T'ai Chi Ch'uan, or the so-called T'ai Chi exercise. This is the T'ai Chi practiced publicly in China today.[22] It is the "T'ai Chi dance," also called the Chinese Ballet by some Westerners.[6]

Principles of T'ai Chi Ch'uan

An important insight to be attained through an understanding of Taoist philosophy concerns the way in which the practice of exercise, such as T'ai Chi Ch'uan and meditation should complement one another. The relationship between them manifests as a subtle interweaving of opposite tendencies. This relationship can be seen in the famous diagram known as the T'ai Chi T'u—Diagram of the Supreme Ultimate (Figure 10-1).

This diagram represents rest, the black portion which is called the "greater Yin," and the white portion representing movement is called "greater Yang." Within each figure there is a smaller circle of the opposite color. The black circle within the white figure is called the "lesser Yin" and the white circle within the black portion is called the "lesser Yang." This inner component represents the way in which each of the opposing forces, Yin and Yang, contains its opposite and continuously originates from its opposite. T'ai Chi, essentially a form of movement, is Yang—the white portion. Meditation, which involves quiet and rest, is Yin—the black segment of the T'ai Chi T'u. This distinction takes into account only the external aspects of theses activities. To perform T'ai Chi Ch'uan exercise effectively requires inner peacefulness and quiet while executing outwardly vis-

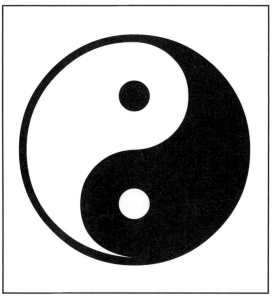

Figure 10-1. Yin and Yang. Diagram of the Supreme Ultitmate: T'ai Chi T'u.

ible movements. Conversely, the meditator uses breath and mental concentration to move the vital energy through the psychic channels while remaining externally at rest. Thus, the inner aspect of each of these practices is opposite to its outer aspect. In other words, just as the greater Yang contains the lesser Yin within it, the greater Yin embraces the lesser Yang. This diagram is a pictorial representation of how exercise and meditation grow out of one another as alternating practices. The movements of T'ai Chi Ch'uan tend to increase the Yang side of the Yin-Yang balance. When the Yang reaches a high point of energy and vitality, it generates the need to sit quietly...meditation, which precludes a more peaceful condition and increases the Yin side of balance. And this is cyclic. When Yin reaches its peak, it generates a need to increase the Yang once again. Thus, it is through the alternate practice of these two opposite methods that one can obtain the beneficial effects of this form of exercise/meditation: T'ai Chi Chaun.[26,28-31]

The traditional Chinese concept of the human body differs somewhat from the Western one. Physiological foundations are based in descriptions of ch'i, or vital energy. The body is hypothetically composed of eight energy (psychic) channels and has 12 meridians that run along the surface of the body. These channels and meridians form the basis of the highly sophisticated theories in acupuncture and acupressure.[24-26]

The eight channels systematically include all parts of the trunk and extremities. The *Tu Mo*, or channel of control, runs along the spinal column from the coccyx through the base of the skull and over the crown to the head to the roof of the mouth. The *Jen Mo*, or channel of functions, goes through the center and front of the body from the genital organs to the base of the mouth. The *Tai Mo*, or belt channel, circles the waist from the navel to the small of the back. The *Ch'eug Mo*, or thrusting channel passes through the center of the body between *Tu Mo* and *Jen Mo*, extending from the genitals to the base of the heart. The *Yang Yu Wei Mo*, is the positive arm channel, beginning at the navel, passing through the chest, and going down the posterior aspect of the arms to the middle fingers, while the *Yin Yu Wei Mo*, or negative arm channel, extends along the inner aspect of the arms from the palms and ending in the chest. Likewise, there are positive and negative channels for both lower extremities. The *Yang Chiao Mo* is the Positive channel that goes down the sides of the body, down the outer aspect of the lower extremity ending the soles. The negative channel is called the *Yin Chiao Mo*, and starts in the soles and extends upward on the inside of the legs through the center of the body to a point just below the eyebrows.[29] These energy channels are represented in Figure 10-2.

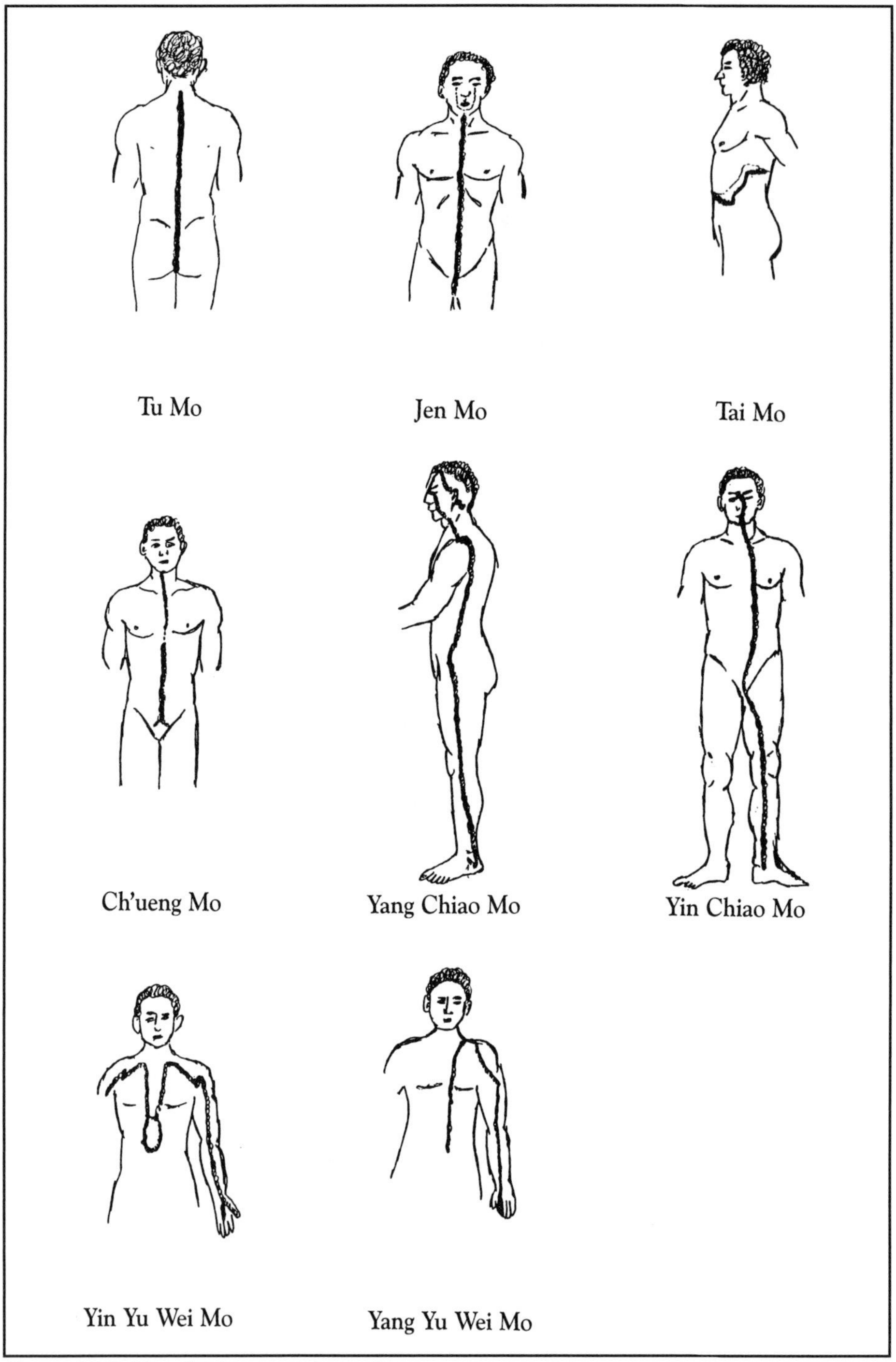

Figure 10-2. The eight energy channels.

Twelve "psychic centers" of the human body are identified in Taoist thought.[22,27,29] They are represented in the *I Ching*[27] by 12 Hexagrams which represent, not only the 12 pathways in the body, but also the 12 months of the year and the 12 times of the day (Table 10-1). According to Taoist thought the circulation of energy through these 12 psychic centers reflects the cyclic pattern of the universe that bring about the alteration of light and darkness as well as the changing

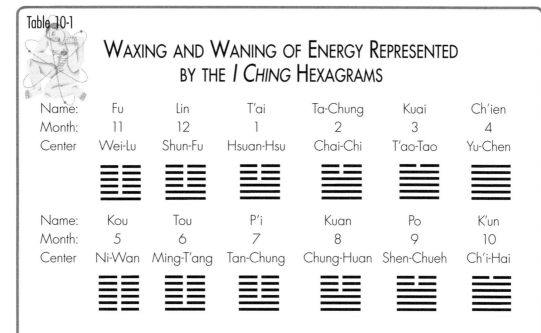

Table 10-1

WAXING AND WANING OF ENERGY REPRESENTED BY THE *I CHING* HEXAGRAMS

Name:	Fu	Lin	T'ai	Ta-Chung	Kuai	Ch'ien
Month:	11	12	1	2	3	4
Center	Wei-Lu	Shun-Fu	Hsuan-Hsu	Chai-Chi	T'ao-Tao	Yu-Chen

Name:	Kou	Tou	P'i	Kuan	Po	K'un
Month:	5	6	7	8	9	10
Center	Ni-Wan	Ming-T'ang	Tan-Chung	Chung-Huan	Shen-Chueh	Ch'i-Hai

Along the To Mo Centers: *Wei-Lu*=tip of the spine; *Shun-Fu*=slightly below the middle of the spine; *Hsuan-Hsu*=middle of the spine; *Chai-Chi*=slightly above the middle of the spine; *T'ao-Tao*=below the neck; *Yu-Chen*=back of the head; *Ni-Wan*=top of the head; *Ming-T'ang*=between the eyebrows.

Along the Jen Mo Centers: *Tan-Chung*=in the chest; *Chung-Huan*=above the navel; *Shen-Chueh*=in the navel; *Ch'i-Hai*=about 3 inches above the navel.

of the seasons.[29] Table 10-1 relates the 12 psychic centers to the twelve hexagrams that symbolize them, and indicates how the cycle reflects the times of the day and year and the center of the body that they represent.

According to Chinese astrologers the *Yang* movement begins with the eleventh month, which is identified with *fu*. This *Yang* movement increases through the twelfth month up to the fourth month as represented by the increase in solid lines in the hexagrams. At the fifth month, the *Yang* movement begins to decrease until it reaches the tenth month when *Yin* reaches complete dominance. The *Yin* movement is the opposite of the *Yang*.[26,27,29]

In addition to the psychic centers, there are 12 pathways of energy at the surface of the body called meridians (refer to Chapter 19). The 12 pathways take their names from the specific inner organs to which they correspond. The development of the T'ai Chi postures and movements are related to these meridians in the human body.[22,26,29] The transition from one posture to the next, combined with breathing, reflects the flow of energy through these meridians.

The importance of breathing techniques has long been stressed in Chinese medicine as a means of preventing illness, prolonging youth, achieving longevity.[32] The rationale behind this is that, besides oxygen, the air we breathe contains many other essential elements, such as iron, copper, zinc, fluorite, quartz, zincite, and magnesium,[22,26,28,29,32,33] and that the combination of exercise and breathing provides an efficient and effective method of taking these precious elements in and getting rid of wastes and poisons. It is believed that the breathing techniques of abdominal or "inner" breathing facilitates the flow of energy throughout the body. Inhalation "stores" energy while exhalation "releases" energy.[33]

The classic methods of T'ai Chi combine movement with breathing. The movements are performed to assist and guide the circulation of vital energy, *ch'i*, through the eight channels and 12 meridians. The mind consciously "lifts" the energy during inward breathing from the solar plexus region, which is considered the central energy source of the body.[22,28,29,33] During exhalation concentrated directing of the energy is from the solar plexus region toward the lower abdomen.[22,26,28,29,33] It is through this conscious directing of the energy that each of the eight channels is supplied with energy during the movement of T'ai Chi. It is hypothesized that in T'ai Chi exercise that the circulation of *ch'i* through the channels does not occur automatically as a result of the arm and leg movements combined with breathing. Rather, it is the mind's power of concentration that combines with the breathing to move the *ch'i* through the channels. The outer movements aid and guide the inner concentration. T'ai Chi is regarded as a method of "moving meditation."[28,29]

Both the movements of the limbs and the way they are coordinated with the breathing cycle constitute the T'ai Chi form of exercise. The movements are relatively simple, involving only the bending and unbending of the knees while the hands are lowered or raised. The movements are an effective way of directing the flow of energy through the channels. Several kinds of movement of the body and limbs during T'ai Chi exercise involve movements such as shifting the weight from one leg to another, rotating the body to the right or left, taking a step, moving forward or backward, and fine hand and foot movements, all put together and coordinated in more or less complicated combinations and sequences.

A T'ai Chi Routine

The mastering of the T'ai Chi exercise form requires the guidance of a knowledgeable teacher. However, the following is offered as a recommended routine for the elderly. This progression is an example of movement through a sequence of 45 classic T'ai Chi postures, diagrammed with their Chinese names. Each movement should be practiced several times until it can be performed fluidly. It is recommended that transition through each posture be built upon, so that the individual starts with the first 15 postures and gradually adds additional postures in the sequence until all 45 postures are perfected. Any exercise can be omitted if it presents difficulty for the individual. It is important to take note of the positions of the hands and feet and to keep the spine straight. For comfort, wearing loose-fitting clothing and slippers or aerobic sneakers is recommended. This author generally divides this exercise routine into three segments starting with double stance exercises (Figure 10-3A), progressing to single stance postures (Figure 10-3B), and cooling down with mostly double stance, stretching-type postures (Figure 10-3C).

Each T'ai Chi exercise session should be preceded by stretching. It is essential to stretch before a T'ai Chi workout in order to prevent injury and prepare for the best possible practice. Flexibility allows concentration on breathing, posit, pace, etc rather than on the limits of motion in poorly stretched muscles. General flexibility improves the effectiveness and benefits of T'ai Chi exercises.

To start the exercise routine, assume an erect standing posture. Turn your right foot out 45 degrees and sink down slightly on your right leg. Shift all your weight onto the right leg and extend your left leg, flexing your foot and crossing your hands in front of your chest (1. Salutation to the Budda). Step back onto your left foot, turning it out, and move your hands to waist level as you shift your weight to the left leg (2. Grasp Bird's Tail). Swing your arms to the right and press forward, shifting some of your weight to the right leg (3. Grasp Bird's Tail). Pivot left, shifting your weight to your right leg, bringing your left foot around and opening your arms (4. Single Whip). Step forward, leading with your right leg (5. White Crane Spreads Its Wings). Your right hand, elbow, knee, and toes should be in alignment. Slide your left foot forward and move your right arm parallel to the floor (6. White Crane Spreads Its Wings). Step back on your left foot as you

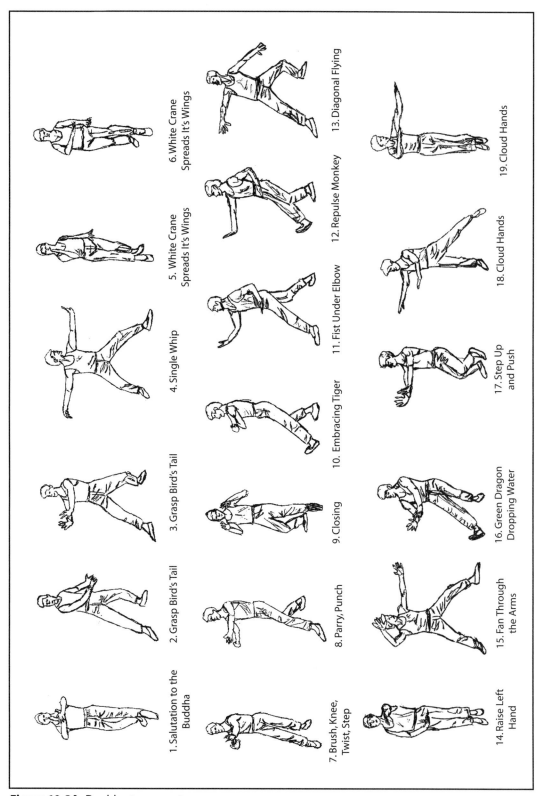

Figure 10-3A. Double stance postures.

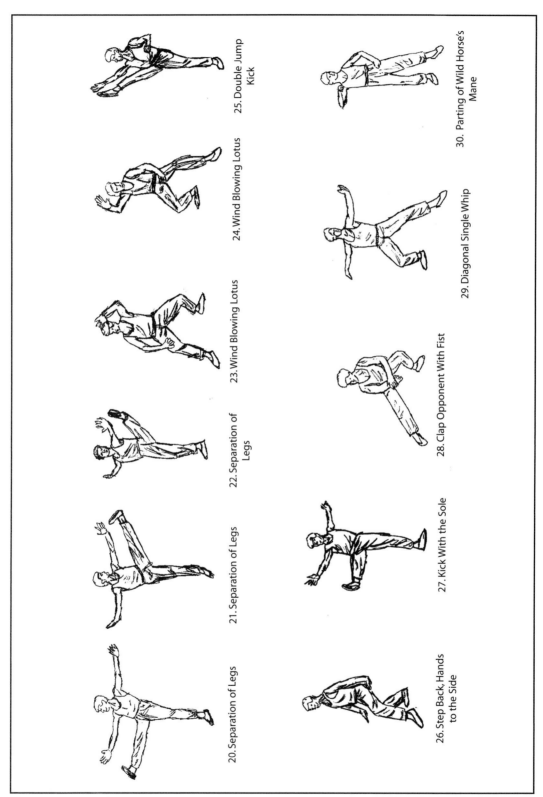

Figure 10-3B. Single stance postures.

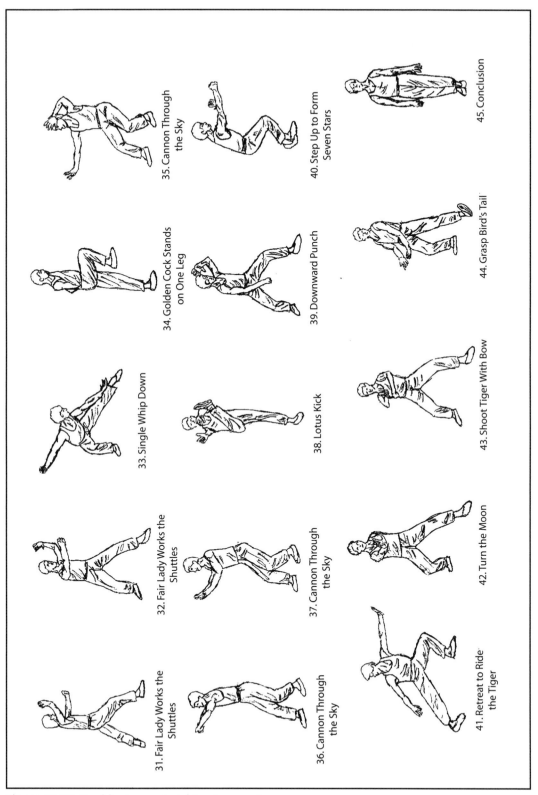

Figure 10-3C. Double stance, stretching-type postures.

raise your left hand and twist to the right (7. Brush, Knee, Twist, Step). Step back on your right foot (8. Parry, Punch); parry with your left arm and punch with your right. Rock back onto your right leg and bring your arms up (9. Closing). Pivot 90 degrees to the right, crossing your arms (10. Embracing Tiger). Slide forward, dropping your left hand to waist level and extending your right hand (11. Fist Under Elbow). Step back with your left foot and straighten your right leg and arm (12. Repulse Monkey). Pivot and step out, opening your arms (13. Diagonal Flying). Come forward, shifting your weight to your right leg, and extend your left arm (14. Raise Left Hand). Then pivot and step out with your left foot, moving your right hand up to your temple (15. Fan Through the Arms). Pivot right (16. Green Dragon Dropping Water). Step up, with knees bent, and push out with hands flexed (17. Step Up and Push). Pivot right, so that you face straight ahead, and extend your left leg out as your arms and torso rotate right (18. Cloud Hands). Rotate to the left as you bring your feet together (19. Cloud Hands). Rotate right and then left four times, ending in a single whip position (4. Single Whip). This ends the portion of exercise postures in which both feet are in contact with the ground. As this is mastered, progress to the single leg stance postures.

From the single whip position (4. Single Whip), rotate your torso right and kick your right leg straight out as you open your arms (20. Separation of Legs). Shift your weight to your right leg and kick with your left (21. Separation of Legs). Lower your left leg almost to the floor, turn your right foot out and kick again with your left leg (22. Separation of Legs). Drop your left leg back, shift your weight onto it and parry high and low with your arms (23. Wind Blowing Lotus). Pivot on your left foot and switch hand positions (24. Wind Blowing Lotus). Then pivot on your right foot, jump onto your left foot and kick your right leg—without straining—toward your extended right arm (25. Double Jump Kick). Step back on your right leg, drop your arms and shift backward onto your left foot (26. Step Back, Hands to the Side). Pivot in a full circle, coming around to stand on your left leg, and kick with your right (27. Kick With the Sole). Drop down on your left leg, keeping your right leg straight and your feet parallel; cover your right wrist with your left palm (28. Clap Opponent with Fist). Swing your right leg back and open your arms (29. Diagonal Single Whip). Step forward, moving your fists to your chest and hip (30. Parting of Wild Horse's Mane). This concludes the second segment of the exercise routine.

The third portion of this exercise routine starts with the Fair Lady Works the Shuttles (31. and 32.) by turning to one side. Parry with one hand and punch with the other. Then pivot 90 degrees to your left and punch and parry again. Repeat the 90-degree pivot, along with the punch and parry, two more times, bringing you full circle. Finish with a single whip position (4. Single Whip). Shift your weight to your right leg and extend your torso and left arm toward your left foot (33. Single Whip Down). Swing around to face left; shift your weight onto your left leg and raise your right leg (34. Golden Cock Stands on One Leg). Extend your right leg straight out and step forward. Turn and block your temple with your left hand as you move your right arm and leg forward (35. Cannon Through the Sky). Step onto your right foot. Bring your arms out in loose fists, as though you were punching an opponent's ears (36. Cannon Through the Sky). Then repeat the stepping movement and punch both fists in an uppercut (37. Cannon Through the Sky). Step onto your left foot and kick your right leg high and slightly left, so that it moves across your extended palms (38. Lotus Kick). Step to bring your feet into a "T" position and block up with your left hand. Pivot to face left, sink down on your left leg and punch and parry at chest level (40. Step Up to Form Seven Stars). Extend your right leg and arm back in a reverse lunge (41. Retreat to Ride the Tiger). Shift back onto your right leg and pivot to face forward, extending your right arm (42. Turn the Moon). Follow up with two short punches (43. Shoot Tiger With Bow). Form a mirror image of position 2, but with your forward foot flexed (44. Grasp Bird's Tail). Swing your hands up, crossing your palms at chest level, then lower your arms and turn so that you face forward in an erect posture (45. Conclusion).

Once this routine is mastered, it takes approximately 20 minutes to complete. Stretching exercises should be added to complete the T'ai Chi exercise routine.

Modifying a T'ai Chi Exercise Routine for the Frail Elderly

Although research has yet to be done on the modification of T'ai Chi exercises to accommodate increasingly frail patients, this author has had vast clinical experience in the modification of T'ai Chi routines. For instance, an individual who is unable to stand to do the T'ai Chi routine as recommended above can modify the exercise by sitting in a chair or on the edge of a mat and performing the upper trunk and extremity movements. These activities reflexively facilitate postural responses in the lower extremities, and ultimately result in the strengthening of the trunk and lower extremities. This therapist progresses the patient to less stable surfaces by placing a thick foam cushion or a SitFit cushion (Sissel Inc, Sumas, WA) on the chair or mat. A rocker board can also be used as a sitting surface to further facilitate balance responses and challenge the postural mechanisms.

As the patient gains agility and trunk strength, moving him or her onto a therapeutic ball, with the feet touching the ground, is a means of progressing towards the standing postures. Clinical experience lends credence to the fact that even the frailest patient can start T'ai Chi exercises in seated postures and progress to double stance exercise routines.

T'ai Chi's Preventive Qualities

Greater than 80% of all illness has been shown to have stress-related etiologies.[34] Medical and rehabilitation practices that seek only to "fix" the physical symptoms (body) without addressing the impact of emotional well-being on disease are missing the target. Although the origins of T'ai Chi exercise are based in ancient Eastern philosophy, it is a suitable form of exercise for tense Westerners. It has the advantage of regular exercise[1-18] combined with an emphasis on gracefulness and slowness of pace that Western society so conspicuously lacks. T'ai Chi can give those who live in a fast-paced environment a compensating factor in their lives.

From ancient Chinese medicine, it has long been recognized that there is mental as well as physical aspects of disease.[30-34] Traditionally, according to Eastern philosophies, the mental state of the individual was considered to be more important than the physical symptoms. Recently, a new basic science of Western medical research, called psychoneuroimmunology, has emerged.[1,2,11,12,34] This area of science is the study of the effect of emotions on disease. The new studies strongly indicate that virtually every illness, from a common cold to cancer and heart disease, can be influenced either positively or negatively by an individual's mental status. Today, Western health care professionals in both the physical and mental health professions are increasingly recognizing the role of the mind in the prevention and cure of illness. The health practitioner may encounter clients who do not seem to respond to traditional health care. Psychoneuroimmunology confronts these problems by employing the health traditions of other cultures and viewing the body and mind as a balanced whole.[1,2]

T'ai Chi is a specific technique for attaining peaceful mental states and therefore it can be extrapolated that it may help prevent or reverse disease processes. T'ai Chi integrates the body and mind through breathing and movement. The open and closed movements of T'ai Chi are coordinated with breathing. The benefits of this exercise form seem to be based in the fundamental combination of movements and breathing techniques in the basic T'ai Chi exercise routines. The entry level of the exercise has many similarities with medical treatments for respiratory illness (eg, deep breathing exercises, segmental expansion exercises, etc) and with walking exercise, the most recommended aerobic exercise for coronary artery disease.[4,6,9]

Current Research on the Effects of T'ai Chi

Recent research has investigated the physiological effects of T'ai Chi exercise and found that this exercise form has measurable effects on cardiorespiratory function, mental control, immune capacity, as well as the prevention of falls through the improvement in muscle strength, flexibility and balance parameters.[35,36] Circulatory status has also been found to improve in elderly individuals participating in T'ai Chi exercise routines.[37]

CARDIORESPIRATORY FUNCTION AND T'AI CHI

In a study by Lai et al,[6] it was determined that the elderly T'ai Chi exercisers showed a significant improvement in VO_2 uptake compared to an age-matched control group of sedentary elders. Lai and colleagues concluded that the data substantiated the practice of T'ai Chi as a means of delaying the decline in cardiorespiratory function commonly considered "normal" for aging individuals. In addition, T'ai Chi was shown to be a suitable aerobic exercise for older adults.[6] A subsequent study by Lai et al[9] further substantiated that T'ai Chi exercise is aerobic exercise of moderate intensity. In the past, it was believed, though never studied, that T'ai Chi exercise forms did not have a significant cardiorespiratory component and therefore were deemed non-aerobic. It has been clearly demonstrated in these studies that, despite the slow, steady, smooth pace of T'ai Chi exercise routines, there is a significant positive effect on the cardiorespiratory system.[3,6,9]

The low, slow intensity of the T'ai Chi exercise form has long been a point of therapeutic contention. It is argued that this type of movement is not intense enough to produce cardiovascular and respiratory effects. Lan and coworkers[38] obtained vital sign measures, recorded heart rate responses and VO_2 measurements during the practice of T'ai Chi, and obtained breath-by-breath measurement of cardiorespiratory function and sequential determination of blood lactate levels during T'ai Chi routines. The same measures were collected on an exercise group performing incremental aerobic exercise of leg cycling. The results of comparing the two exercise groups clearly demonstrated that T'ai Chi is an exercise with moderate intensity (despite it's appearance), and is aerobic in nature.[38] T'ai Chi exercise routines were found to be comparable to programs of moderate intensity aerobic exercise in reducing blood pressure in previously sedentary, hypertensive, elderly individuals.[39]

Fontana and colleagues[40] found that movements used to perform T'ai Chi require energy expenditure comparable with that for activities of daily living and for low level exercises currently recommended for persons with low exercise tolerance.[40]

A program of T'ai Chi Chih, a modified T'ai Chi exercise, was piloted in a study comprised of a small sample of individuals with heart failure.[41] Comparisons of pre- and post-measures of heart failure symptoms, general health, mental health, functional capacity, and energy perceptions support the potential of T'ai Chi Chih in managing heart failure symptoms and improving quality of life.[41] Lan and associates[42] studied the effects of T'ai Chi Ch'uan on patients following coronary artery bypass and demonstrated that this exercise form favorably enhances cardiorespiratory function and improved functional outcomes following surgery.[42] Danusantoso and Heijnen[43] established that T'ai Chi Ch'uan has a positive impact on the outcomes in patients with haemophillia.[43] Overall strength, flexibility, and functional measures improved in this population, and the number and severity of bleeding episodes decreased as a result of participation in T'ai Chi exercise routines.[43] Complementary therapies and healing practices have been found to reduce stress, anxiety, and lifestyle patterns known to contribute to cardiovascular disease.[44] T'ai Chi has been established as a primary component in cardiac rehabilitation programs.

BALANCE, FALLS, AND POSTURAL CONTROL AND T'AI CHI

The potential value of T'ai Chi exercise in promoting postural control, improving balance, and preventing falls has also been substantiated by several researchers.[3,5,7,8,10,18] Tse and Bailey[3] found that T'ai Chi practitioners had significantly better postural control than the sedentary non-practitioner. Province et al[5] found that treatments directed towards flexibility, balance, dynamic balance, and resistance, all components of T'ai Chi exercise, reduced the risk of falls for elderly adults. Wolfson et al[7] demonstrated that short-term exposure to "altered sensory input or desta-bilizing platform movement" during a treatment session—in addition to home-based T'ai Chi exercises—elicited significant improvements in sway control and inhibited inappropriate motor responses. The outcome measure of functional balance improved more substantially in the exercise group that combined the treatment sessions with the home program of T'ai Chi. Wolf et al[8] com-pared a balance training group, in which balance was stressed on a static to moving platform using biofeedback, to a group of T'ai Chi Quan exercisers. A third group served as a control for exercise intervention. This article did not provide information on the results of the effects of the two dif-ferent exercise approaches on balance and frailty measures, though it did provide a superb set of assessment tools for measuring balance. In a subsequent interview with Steven L. Wolf, PhD, PT, FAPTA by Jan P. Reynolds of the *PT Magazine of Physical Therapy*,[45] Wolf spoke positively about the therapeutic value of exercise forms such as T'ai Chi in delaying or possibly preventing the onset of frailty. The benefits of T'ai Chi in fall prevention has been also supported by a study by Judge et al[10] in which these researchers demonstrated improvements in single-stance postural sway in older women with T'ai Chi exercises. Wolf[13] in a summary of a series of investigations comparing computerized balance machines with T'ai Chi, ultimately found that T'ai Chi as an exercise form for older adults can have a substantially favorable effect in delaying the onset of fall events.

Yan[46] examined whether T'ai Chi practice could reduce the inconsistency of movement force and movement pattern output in older adults, a problem often associated with the increased incidence of falling. The findings suggest that T'ai Chi participants significantly reduce the vari-ability of movement patterns and the inconsistency of muscle force compared to participants in a traditional activity group after 8 weeks of practice. This study provides evidence that proposes that T'ai Chi practice may serve as a better real world exercise for reducing movement and muscle force variability in older adults.[46] Lan and associates[47] evaluated the effect of T'ai Chi Ch'uan on knee extensor strength and endurance in elderly individuals. As this muscle group weakness is directly associated with the increased risk of falling, the findings of this study are important. A significant improvement in muscular strength and endurance of knee extensors occurred following a 6-month program in T'ai Chi.[47]

The volume of research substantiating the use of T'ai Chi as a means of preventing falls has grown in the past few years. Regardless of the setting, evidence consistently supports the effective-ness of T'ai Chi exercise in improving balance and preventing falls.[18,48-54]

NEUROLOGICAL CONDITIONS AND T'AI CHI

Recently, research using T'ai Chi exercise as an exercise form has included neurological condi-tions of stroke, head trauma, and multiple sclerosis.[55,56] Rehabilitation after either stroke or severe head injury is a complex process that can be long and frustrating. New, more holistic methods for rehabilitation are constantly sought. The utilization of the slow, rhythmical movements in T'ai Chi have been found to significantly improve movement patterns, trunk stability, reduce tone, and improve balance in severely involved neurological patients.[55] Husted and colleagues[56] explored the psychosocial and physical benefits of an 8-week program of T'ai Chi in a group of patients with multiple sclerosis. The results demonstrated an increase in walking speed and greater flexibility, especially in the hamstrings. Patients experienced improvements in vitality, social functioning, mental health, and the ability to carry out physical and emotional roles.[56] This pilot study actu-ally led to the implementation of several similar programs for people with multiple sclerosis across the United States. T'ai Chi and other health promotion programs offer help toward achieving the goals of increasing access to a person's environment and services, maximizing independence, and improving quality of life for people with chronic disabling conditions.

Community-dwelling stroke survivers, on completion of 12 weeks on T'ai Chi Ch'uan showed improvement in social and general functioning skills including balance and speed of walking measures.[57]

MUSCULOSKELETAL CONDITIONS AND T'AI CHI

T'ai Chi has also been found to have beneficial effects for individuals with musculoskeletal problems. A comprehensive review of the research on complementary and alternative treatments on musculoskeletal disease was conducted at Stanford University.[58] The goals of the review were to establish a comprehensive literature review and provide a rationale for future research carrying the theme of "successful aging." Researchers found multiple studies showing that T'ai Chi was efficacious primarily as a complementary intervention for musculoskeletal disease and related disorders.[59] Hartman and associates[19] did a study to determine the effects of T'ai Chi training on arthritis self-efficacy, quality of life indicators, and lower extremity functional mobility in older adults with osteoarthritis. Their research indicated that moderate T'ai Chi intervention can enhance all of these parameters and is a safe and effective means of managing pain and improving lower extremity osteoarthritis.[19] Yocum, Castro, and Cornett[59] determined that programs using alternative therapies such as T'ai Chi and meditation in combination with traditional medications appear to be beneficial in managing the complex stress and pain mechanisms, which share many central nervous system pathways, in patients with rheumatoid arthritis. A long-term benefit was associated with quality of life measures. Rheumatoid arthritic patients who practiced T'ai Chi showed positive results in functional measures, social involvement, and long-term outcomes.[59] Strategies for the prevention and treatment of osteoporosis are directed at maximizing peak bone mass by optimizing physiologic intake of calcium and vitamin D and providing instruction in exercise that adds mechanical stress to bone.[60] Woo et al[60] determined that the combined stretching, strengthening, and balance components of exercise provided by T'ai Chi was the most effective in the prevention of bone loss and in decreasing falls. Prevention of bone loss is obviously preferable to any remedial measures, but, according to this study, T'ai Chi strategies provide a hopeful means of restoring deficient bone.[60,61]

One year of T'ai Chi training demonstrated the added musculoskeletal benefits of faster hamstring and gastrocnemius reflex reaction and improved knee joint position senses. These changes are not only associated with stronger and faster muscle contractions, but also improved dynamic standing and dynamic balance leading to significant balance improvements during exercise and sport activities and functional activities of daily living.[62] The influence of T'ai Chi training on reducing the risk of falling improved postural control by altering the center of pressure trajectory during gait initiation. T'ai Chi improved the mechanism by which forward momentum is generated and improved coordination during gait initiation, suggesting improvements in postural control.[63,64]

CANCER AND T'AI CHI

T'ai Chi is among the many complementary and alternative therapies that have been studied for management of pain, treatment side effects, and functional losses associated with the treatment of cancer.[65,66] T'ai Chi has been found to be an exercise technique that relieves stress and enhances well-being in the cancer patient. It has also been found to be effective in decreasing pain and improving functional outcomes, even in the frailest of patients with a cancer diagnosis.[65,66]

STRESS, EMOTIONAL, AND PSYCHOLOGICAL CONSIDERATIONS AND T'AI CHI

The stress reduction effects of T'ai Chi exercise, as measured by heart rate, blood pressure, urinary catecholamine, and salivary cortisol levels, were compared to a groups of brisk walkers, meditators, and quiet readers.[11] In general, it was found that the stress-reduction effect of T'ai Chi characterized those physiological changes produced by moderate exercise. Heart rate, blood pressure, and urinary catecholamine changes for the T'ai Chi exercise group were similar to those changes occurring in the walking group. Additionally, it was reported that the T'ai Chi group expressed the enhancement of "vigor" and a reduction in anxiety states. In a study by Brown et al,[12] unequivocal support is provided for the hypothesis that T'ai Chi exercise, which incorporates a cognitive strategy as part of the training program, is more effective than exercises lacking a structured cognitive component in promoting psychological benefits.

Self-rated health is a powerful and consistent predictor of self-care capability and health outcomes including mobility, morbidity, and mortality.[14] Additionally, exercise is important for maintaining health and improving functioning in older adults.[67] T'ai Chi has been found to not only improve an elder's perception of health, but also has been found to have a significant therapeutic value in improving overall quality of life measures.[14-17]

A very important component of quality of life measures is the measure of functional independence. Recent research has provided sound evidence that the practice of T'ai Chi leads to and improvement in functional and quality of life measures.[19-21] Li and associates[20,21] indicated that compared to a control group of inactive older adults, participants in the T'ai Chi group experienced significant improvements in all aspects of physical functioning over a 6-month intervention period. Overall, improvement occurred across all functional status measures from daily activities such as walking and lifting to moderate-vigorous activities such as running.[20,21] This strongly indicates that a self-paced and self-controlled activity such as T'ai Chi has the potential of being an effective, low-cost means of improving functional status in older persons.

As the above research indicates, there is clearly a positive effect on the sense of well-being of elders practicing T'ai Chi. A study by Chen, Synder, and Krichbaum[67] added a new dimension to the study of T'ai Chi by exploring the reasons (eg, facilitators and barriers) that elders seemingly practice T'ai Chi on a more consistent basis than other exercise forms. The results showed that encouragement from others was the most important factor for elders to regularly practice T'ai Chi, whereas positive health outcomes were the reason they continued to practice it beyond group settings.[62,63] Interesting, most of the initial non-T'ai Chi group participants felt that they were too weak to perform the T'ai Chi exercise. When this group was instructed in this exercise form following the comparative portion of the study, the significant and immediate improvements in health status and well-being measures prompted an even greater participation rate. This group was highly motivated and very enthusiastic about attending daily T'ai Chi sessions.[66] One of the reasons given by a member of this non-T'ai Chi-turned-T'ai Chi group was "T'ai Chi works better than regular exercise. It is not boring at all, in fact, it is rather enjoyable—like a dance."

A recent study looked at perceive, health status in frail older adults who participated in 1 year of T'ai Chi exercise.[68] These findings suggest that older women who are becoming frail benefited from T'ai Chi, demonstrated by an improved perceived health status and a sense that they were able to do more functional activities, including ambulation. These findings have significant implications for the potential of near-frail elderly individuals remaining in the community or being admitted to skilled nursing facilities or requiring higher levels of assisted living environments. Practicing T'ai Chi offers the potential to enhance the physical and mental health of older adults.[69] A short style T'ai Chi program found that older women practicing this form of exercise improved overall fitness levels, such as lower extremity strength, balance, and flexibility, and demonstrated significantly faster brisk walking speeds and reduction of risk of falling in community dwelling elders.[70]

▭ Case Example: Managed Care and T'ai Chi

Mr. K is an 84-year-old white male, admitted to the nursing home in a markedly reconditioned state, with diagnoses of coronary heart disease, tuberculosis, confusion, recent history of falls, depression, and malnutrition. He was referred to physical and occupational therapy for screening and recommendations. Screening by physical therapy resulted in an initial evaluation which revealed a significantly compromised cardiopulmonary response to any activity, flexed posturing in standing with occasional loss of balance during directional changes, ambulation with moderate assistance of one requiring verbal cueing, and a fluctuating cognitive status. He was quite congested and occasionally expectorated blood, especially with exertion. He had remarkable shortness of breath at rest and significant rubor of all extremities with 1+ pulses distally. He was withdrawn, minimally verbal, and obviously quite depressed. Based on our assessment his prognosis was deemed poor for functional recovery to his pre-morbid state and discharge unlikely.

Mr. K was placed on a fall prevention program that included trunk extensor strengthening, extremity strengthening, and flexibility exercises. Deep breathing exercises were initiated and a reconditioning walking program using a 12-minute test protocol was started. Buerger-Allen exercises were initiated for his circulation and to promote postural changes and mobility. He was also referred to a nutritionist and nursing was consulted regarding his skin and circulatory status. Patient gains were marginal in both physical and occupational therapy over a 3-week period. He continued to require minimal to moderate assist during ambulation, had a poor physiological response to activity of any sort, remained short of breath at rest, and was still withdrawn, now being virtually nonverbal and severely depressed.

Due to the restrictions placed on duration of intervention in a managed care delivery system driven by critical pathways, aggressive "skilled" intervention could no longer be justified. The insurer agreed to a 4-week trial of T'ai Chi exercises to be done 5 days per week in a group setting. The patient was initially instructed in breathing techniques and standing postures utilizing a set of T'ai Chi movements that did not significantly displace his center of gravity. Remarkable improvements were noted in respiratory status, that is, he was no longer short of breath at rest, and standing posture was distinctly improved by the end of the first week. It was noted that this elderly gentleman was much more alert and responsive to his surroundings and appeared to be less depressed. The T'ai Chi routine was expanded to encompass his increasing capabilities and weight shifting postures were started, though one-leg stance T'ai Chi activities were still omitted from his routine. By the end of the second week, this patient was ambulating to and from all activities with stand-by assistance and no verbal cueing. His extremity pulses had improved to 2+ with no extremity rubor. He still experienced shortness of breath on exertion, though was no longer short of breath at rest and not expectorating blood. He was noted to be spontaneously telling stories and joking with the staff and other residents. He reported amiably "where" his energy was going from time to time and stated that he was "eating everything on my plate."

Mr. K continued to progress in all areas of functional status. By the end of the third week he was ambulating to all activities independently and safely. He was alert and obviously happy. We were able to start one-legged stance postures in his T'ai Chi routine. He was independently taking a shower (which pleased him to no end). He was quite fondly acknowledged by his fellow residents due to his sense of humor, optimism, and compassion for their concerns.

By the end of the fourth week, Mr. K was happily discharged on a home program inclusive of T'ai Chi exercises. Since his discharge, he has enrolled in a T'ai Chi program at a local martial arts facility which he participates in for 2 hours, three times a week, and Mr. K comes back to the nursing home twice a week to assist as an instructor for our T'ai Chi classes.

Perhaps Mr. K's progress sounds too good to be true, but the reality of his improvement has been observed in many of our patients participating in the T'ai Chi classes. Beyond the physical aspects of this exercise form, the most notable improvement appears to be in the area of "outlook." Elderly individuals participating in the T'ai Chi classes express pure enjoyment in the slow, rhythmic movements and the group interaction. They report that they "feel stronger, more balanced" and that they feel as if they are "dancing not exercising." And, the insurers are overwhelmed with the functional successes that seem to be inherent in this mode of exercise. T'ai Chi is a low-cost, low-tech group activity.

Conclusion

The increasing body of research related to the use of T'ai Chi as a valuable therapeutic intervention substantiates our need as professionals, in a cost-containment arena, to evaluate the merits of this exercise form.[1-12] T'ai Chi is viewed as an "alternative" therapy and often perceived as "flaky," however, it has clinically been observed and now scientifically has been shown to enhance function in our elderly patients. This author cautions, however, that while individual complementary modalities, such as T'ai Chi, hold considerable merit, it is critical that the philosophy underlying these therapies be understood and honored.

Recently, the use of T'ai Chi has been identified by the National Institutes of Health as one of a list of "alternative therapies" that will be targeted for research funding as a legitimate area for investigation. We should seize the opportunity to provide leadership in this emerging area in rehabilitative medicine. T'ai Chi, though it is a "nontraditional" approach to therapeutic intervention, merits further traditional scientific analysis to quantify its apparent therapeutic validity.

References

1. Wanning T. Healing and the mind/body arts: massage, acupuncture, yoga, T'ai Chi, and Feldendrais. *AAOHN Journal.* 1993;41(7):349-351.
2. Lan C, Lai JS, Chen SY. T'ai Chi Chaun: an ancient wisdom on exercise and health promotion. *Sports Med.* 2002; 32(4):217-224.
3. Tse SK, Bailey DM. T'ai Chi and postural control in the well elderly. *Am J Occup Ther.* 1992;46(4):295-300.
4. Ng RK. Cardiopulmonary exercise: a recently discovered secret of T'ai Chi. *Hawaii Medical Journal.* 1992;51(8):216-217.
5. Province MA, Hadley EC, Hornbrook MC, et al. The effects of exercise on falls in elderly patients. A preplanned meta-analysis of the FICSIT trials. Frailty and injuries: cooperative studies of intervention techniques. *JAMA.* 1995;273(17):1341-1347.
6. Lai JS, Lan C, Wong MK, Teng SH. Two-year trends in cardiorespiratory function among older T'ai Chi Ch'uan practitioners and sedentary subjects. *J Am Geriatric Soc.* 1995;43(11):1222-1227.
7. Wolfson L, Whipple R, Judge J, Amerman P, Derby C, King M. Training balance and strength in the elderly to improve function. *J Am Geriatric Soc.* 1993;41(3):341-343.
8. Wolf SL, Kutner NG, Green RC, McNeely E. The Atlanta FICSIT study: two exercise interventions to reduce frailty in elders. *J Am Geriatric Soc.* 1993;41(3):329-332.
9. Lai JS, Wong MK, Lan C, Chong CK, Lien IN. Cardiorespiratory responses of T'ai Chi Chaun practitioners and sedentary subjects during cycle ergometer. *J Formosan Med Assoc.* 1993;92(10):894-899.
10. Judge JO, Lindsey C, Underwood M, Winsemius D. Balance improvements in older women: effects of exercise training. *Phys Ther.* 1993;73(4):254-265.
11. Jin P. Efficacy of T'ai Chi, brisk walking, meditation, and reading in reducing mental and emotional stress. *J Psychosom Res.* 1992;36(4):361-370.
12. Brown DR, Wang Y, Ward A, et al. Chronic effects of exercise and exercise plus cognitive strategies. *Med Sci Sports Exer.* 1995;27(5):765-775.
13. Wolf SL. From tibialis anterior to T'ai Chi: biofeedback and beyond. *Appl Psychophysiol Biofeedback.* 2001;26(2):155-174.
14. Taggart HM. Self-reported benefits of T'ai Chi practice by older women. *J Holist Nurs.* 2001;19(3):223-237.
15. Chen KM, Snyder M, Krichbaum K. Clinical use of T'ai Chi in elderly populations. *Geriatr Nurs.* 2001;22(4):198-200.
16. Yalden J, Chung L. T'ai Chi: towards an exercise program for the older person. *Aust J Holist Nurs.* 2001;8(1):4-13.
17. Ward J. T'ai Chi for older people. *Nurs Older People.* 2001;13(1):10-13.
18. Wolf SL, Sattin RW, O'Grady M, et al. A study design to investigate the effect of intense Tai Chi in reducing falls among older adults transitioning to frailty. *Control Clin Trials.* 2001;22(6):689-704.
19. Hartman CA, Manos TM, Winter C, Hartman DM, Li B, Smith JC. Effects of T'ai Chi training on function and quality of life indicators in older adults with osteoarthritis. *J Am Geriatr Soc.* 2000;48(12):1553-1559.
20. Li F, Harmer P, McAuley E, et al. An evaluation of the effects of T'ai Chi exercise on physical function among older persons: a randomized controlled trial. *Ann Behav Med.* 2001;23(2):139-146.
21. Li F, Harmer P, McAuley E, et al. T'ai Chi, self-efficacy, and physical function in the elderly. *Prev Sci.* 2001;2(4):229-239.

22. Liao W. *T'ai Chi Classics: New Translations of Three Essential texts of T'ai Chi Ch'uan*. Boston, MA: Shambhala Publications; 1990.

23. Lynoe N. Ethical and professional aspects of the practice of alternative medicine. *Scand J Soc Med*. 1992;20(4):217-225.

24. Wardwell WI. Alternative medicine in the United States. *Soc Sci Med*. 1994;38(8):1061-1068.

25. Kronenberg F, Mallory B, Downey JA. Rehabilitation medicine and alternative therapies: new words, old practices. *Arch Phys Med Rehab*. 1994;75(8):928-929.

26. Jou, TH, Shapiro S (trans, ed). *The Tao of T'ai Chi Ch'uan Way to Rejuvenation* Warwick, NY: T'ai Chi Foundation; 1988.

27. Blofeld J (trans, ed). *I Ching: The Book of Change*. New York, NY: E.P. Dutton & Co; 1965.

28. Da Liu. *T'ai Chi Ch'uan and I Ching*. New York, NY: Harper & Row Publishers; 1987.

29. Da Liu. *T'ai Chi Ch'uan & Meditation*. New York, NY: Schocken Books; 1991.

30. Huai CN. *Tao and Longevity*. New York, NY: Weiser Publications; 1984:8-12.

31. Legge J. *The Texts of Taoism*. Vol 1. New York, NY: Dover Publications; 1962:256-257.

32. Fung YL. *A History of Chinese Philosophy*. Vol 2. Princeton, NJ: Princeton University Press; 1953:436-444.

33. Sohn RC. *Tao and T'ai Chi*. Rochester, VT: Destiny Books; 1989.

34. Kirsta A. *The Book of Stress Survival: Identifying and Reducing Stress in Your Life*. New York, NY: Simon and Schuster; 1986.

35. Li JX, Hong Y, Chan KM. T'ai Chi: physiological characteristics and beneficial effects on health. *Br J Sports Med*. 2001;35(3):148-156.

36. Hong Y, Li JX, Robinson PD. Balance control, flexibility, and cardiorespiratory fitness among older T'ai Chi practitioners. *Br J Sports Med*. 2000;34(1):29-34.

37. Wang JS, Lan C, Wong MK. T'ai Chi Ch'uan training to enhance microcirculatory function in healthy elderly men. *Arch Phys Med Rehabil*. 2001;82(9):1176-1180.

38. Lan C, Chen SY, Lai JS, Wong MK. Heart rate responses and oxygen consumption during T'ai Chi Ch'uan practice. *Am J Chin Med*. 2001;29(3-4):403-410.

39. Young DR, Appel LJ, Jee S, Miller ER. The effects of aerobic exercise and T'ai Chi on blood pressure in older people: results of a randomized trail. *J Am Geriatr Soc*. 1999;47(3):277-284.

40. Fontana JA, Colella C, Wilson BR, Baas L. The energy costs of a modified form of T'ai Chi exercise. *Nurs Res*. 2000;49(2):91-96.

41. Fontana JA, Colella C, Baas LS, Ghazi F. T'ai Chi Chih as an intervention for heart failure. *Nurs Clin North Am*. 2000;35(4):1031-1046.

42. Lan C, Chen SY, Lai JS, Wong MK. The effect of T'ai Chi on cardiorespiratory function in patients with coronary artery bypass surgery. *Med Sci Sports Exerc*. 1999;31(5):634-638.

43. Danusantoso H, Heijnen L. T'ai Chi Ch'uan for people with haemophilia. *Haemophilia*. 2001;7(4):437-439.

44. Kreitzer MJ, Snyder M. Healing the heart: integrating complementary therapies and healing practices into the care of cardiovascular patient. *Prog Cardiovasc Nurs*. 2002;17(2):73-80.

45. Reynolds JP. Profiles in Alternatives: "East and West on the Information Superhighway": T'ai Chi. *PT: Magazine of Physical Therapy*. 1994;2(9):52-53.

46. Yan JH. T'ai Chi practice reduces movement force variability for seniors. *J Gerontol A Biol Sci Med Sci*. 1999;54(12):M629-M634.

47. Lan C, Lai JS, Chen SY, Wong MK. T'ai Chi Ch'uan to improve muscular strength and endurance in elderly individuals: a pilot study. *Arch Phys Med Rehab*. 2000;81(5):604-607.

48. Wu G. Evaluation of the effectiveness of T'ai Chi for improving balance and preventing falls in the older population—a review. *J Am Geriatr Soc*. 2002;50(4):746-754.

49. Kessenich CR. T'ai Chi as a method of fall prevention in the elderly. *Orthop Nurs*. 1998;17(4):27-29.

50. Choi JH, Moon JS, Song R. Effects of sun-style T'ai Chi exercise on physical fitness and fall prevention in fall prone older adults. *J Advanced Nurs*. 2005;51(2):150-157.

51. Tsan WW, Wong VS, Fu SN, Hui-Chan CW. T'ai Chi improves standing balance control under reduced or conflicting sensory conditions. *Arch Phys Med Rehab*. 2004;85:129-137.

52. Lin MR, Hwang HF, Wang Yw, Chang SH, Wolf SL. Community-based T'ai Chi and its effect on injurious falls, balance, gait, and fear of falling in older people. *Phys Ther*. 2006;86(9):1189-1201.

53. Li F, Harmer P, Fisher KJ, Mcauley E, Chaumeton N, Eckstrom E, Wilson NL. T'ai Chi and fall reductions in older adults: A randomized controlled trial. *J Gerontol Med Sci*. 2005;60A(2):187-194.

54. Zhang JB, Ishikawa-Takata K, Yamazaki H, Morita T, Ohta T. The effects of T'ai Chi Chaun on physiological function and fear of falling in the less robust elderly: An intervention study for preventing falls. *Arch Gerontol & Geriatrics*. 2006;42:107-116.

55. Shapira MY, Chelouche M, Yanai R, Kaner C, Szold A. T'ai Chi Ch'uan practice as a tool for rehabilitation of severe head trauma: 3 case reports. *Arch Phys Med Rehabil*. 2001;82(9):1283-1285.

56. Husted C, Pham L, Hekking A, Niederman R. Improving quality of life for people with chronic conditions: the example of T'ai Chi and multiple sclerosis. *Altern Ther Health Med*. 1999;5(5):70-74.

57. Hart J, Kanner H, Gilboa-Mayo R, Haroeh-Peer O, Rozenthul-Sorokin N, Eldar R. T'ai Chi Ch'uan practice in community-dwelling persons after stroke. *International J Rehabil Res.* 2004;27(4):303-304.
58. Brismee JM, Paige RL, Chyu MC, et al. Group and home-based T'ai Chi in elderly subjects with knee osteoarthritis: a randomized controlled trial. *Clin Rehabil.* 2007;21(2):99-111.
59. Yocum DE, Castro WL, Cornett M. Exercise, education, and behavioral modification as alternative therapy for pain and stress in rheumatic disease. *Rheum Dis Clin North Am.* 2000;26(1):145-159, x-xi.
60. Woo J, Hong A, Lau E, Lynn H. A randomized controlled trial of T'ai Chi and resistance exercise on bone health, muscle strength and balance in community-living elderly people. *Age Aging.* 2007;36(3):262-268.
61. Chan K, Qin L, Lau M, Woo J, Au S, Choy W, Lee K, Lee S. A randomized, prospective study of the effects of T'ai Chi Chun exercise on bone mineral density in postmenopausal women. *Arch Phys Med Rehabil.* 2004;85:717-722.
62. Fong SM, Ng GY. The effects on sensorimotor performance and balance with T'ai Chi training. *Arch Phys Med Rehabil.* 2006;87:82-87.
63. Hass CJ, Gregor RJ, Waddell DE, Oliver A, Smith DW, Fleming RP, Wolf SL. The influence of T'ai Chi training on the center of pressure trajectory during gait initiation in older adults. *Arch Phys Med Rehabil.* 2004;85:1593-1598.
64. Maciazek J, Osiski W, Szeklicki R, Stemplewski R. Effect of T'ai Chi on body balance: randomized controlled trial in men with osteopenia or osteoporosis. *Am J Chin Am.* 2007;35(1):1-9.
65. Cassileth BR. Evaluating complementary and alternative therapies for cancer patients. *CA Cancer J Clin.* 1999;49(6):362-375.
66. Cassileth BR. Complementary therapies: overview and state of the art. *Cancer Nurs.* 1999;22(1):85-90.
67. Chen KM, Synder M, Krichbaum K. Facilitators and barriers to elders' practice of T'ai Chi. A mind-body, low-intensity exercise. *J Holist Nurs.* 2001;19(3):238-255.
68. Greenspan AI, Wolf SL, Kelley ME, O'Grady M. T'ai Chi and perceived health status in older adults who are transitionally frail: a randomized controlled trial. *Phys Ther.* 2007;87(5):525-535.
69. Chen KM, Li CH, Lin JN, et al. A feasible method to enhance and maintain the health of elderly living in long-term care facilities through lon-term, simplified T'ai Chi exercises. *J Nurs Res.* 2007;15(2):156-164.
70. Audette JF, Jin YS, Newcomer R, et al. T'ai Chi versus brisk walking in elderly women. *Age Ageing.* 2006;35(4):388-393.

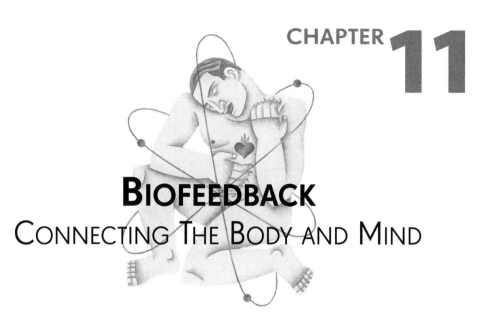

BIOFEEDBACK
CONNECTING THE BODY AND MIND

Jennifer M. Bottomley, PhD, MS, PT

T he suggestion that hemiplegia, migraine and tension headaches, asthma, hypertension, cardiac arrhythmias, visual acuity, torticollis spasms, pain, hyperkinesis, and functional and cognitive disorders of any of the body's systems may all be relieved by a single form of treatment sounds more like a 19th century pitch for snake oil than a true reflection of research. Yet biofeedback has been investigated extensively and has promising clinical applications in an astounding number of conditions.[1-124]

The last two decades have seen an increasing convergence of body and mind therapies. These new therapies are often labeled *psychosomatic* or *psychophysical* medicine.[1] As both names imply, these approaches to healing deal with the effect of the mind on the body. With them tremendous strides have been made in understanding mental influences on body systems ranging from the muscular to the immune system. This has led to treatment procedures that exploit this connection between mind and body. Biofeedback techniques for stress-related disorders and dysfunction and mental imaging using autogenic (a method of mind-over-body control based on a specific discipline for relaxing parts of the body by means of auto-suggestion) feedback to enhance the responsiveness of the autonomic nervous system and/or the immune system response are two good examples of this process. Biofeedback is one of the earliest and most accepted ways that rehabilitation professions have employed that integrates rather than separates the mind and body.[2]

Biofeedback, meaning "life-feedback," is a process of electronically utilizing information from the body to teach an individual to recognize what is going on inside of his or her own brain, nervous system, and muscles. Biofeedback refers to any technique that uses instrumentation to give a person immediate and continuing signals on changes in a bodily function that she or he is not usually conscious of, such as fluctuations in blood pressure, brainwave activity, or muscle tension. Theoretically and very often in practice, information input enables the individual to learn to control the "involuntary" function.[3,4]

Biofeedback acts as an output-input system whereby output is based in the motor unit and the input is via sensory pathways comprising proprioceptors, exteroceptors, and interoceptors.[2] Biofeedback provides a means of measurement of a physiological response using an electronic device. It aids the sensory side of a feedback mechanism assisting a compensated sensation, such as with a cerebral vascular accident or other brain injury, in responding appropriately (ie, motor unit training) by increasing conscious awareness of intact but usually unfelt sensation. Basically, biofeedback acts as a sixth sense by providing an artificial proprioception feedback. Via operant conditioning, a new association between a stimuli and a response is developed. The action the learner takes is voluntary and under their own control. The response is instrumental in producing a reward or removing a negative stimulus, and this reinforcement shapes behavior and function with successive stages.

Biofeedback transfers the responsibility for final success to the patient. Often, individuals seek medical help, hoping to place the responsibility of "curing" their problems on the clinician, while the patient takes an almost passive role in the treatment process. This is commonly known as an external locus of control. The patient should understand that he or she has the ability, with assistance from the appropriate medical professionals, to help him- or herself. Biofeedback provides a modality to accomplish this.

Principles of Biofeedback

The prefix *myo* is derived from the Greek word for muscle. In combination with the Greek word *graphos*, meaning to write, and the additional prefix *electro*, the word becomes electromyograph, an instrument for recording the electrical activity of the muscles. Electromyographic (EMG) biofeedback is a modality for measuring and displaying muscle activity, and is used primarily where any modification of muscular behavior is indicated. With its use, an individual can learn to become more aware of their own muscle activity, and thus, gain more complete control of functional activity. It also provides an ideal method for rehabilitation practitioners to record a patient's day-to-day progress.

The biofeedback device imparts objective information about the degree of activity occurring in a muscle, through surface electrodes, in audio and/or visual form, in much the same way that an electrocardiogram (EKG) provides information about cardiac activity or an electroencephalogram (EEG) displays brainwave activity. In an EMG biofeedback system, the electrical signal originating in the muscle under study is amplified and then translated into sound and visual reading which corresponds to increased and decreased muscle activity. EMG is the process of recording and interpreting the electrical activity of muscle. When a muscle contracts, it produces a characteristic spike (pulse) waveform that can be detected easily by placing an electrode on the skin over the muscle belly. For example, if you tightly grasp an object in your hand, the muscles in your arm will generate a specific electrical voltage, usually measured in millivolts (0.001 volt) or microvolts (0.000001 volt). As you squeeze the object tighter, the electrical voltage will increase as more motor units are recruited. As you relax your hand, the electrical voltage will decrease dramatically. EMG is, therefore, a direct physiological index of muscular activity and the state of relaxation.

The interior of a nerve cell is electrically negative with respect to the exterior during its resting phase. This negative potential, typically 50 to 100 millivolts, exists because of the "selective permeability" of the cell wall. On the outside of the cell membrane $Na+$ ions are more concentrated, and on the inside $K+$ ions are more concentrated along with $Cl-$ and other large, negative ions. The semipermeable membrane acts as a barrier to the free interchange of these ions, bringing about a condition like that of a charged battery. The membrane is, therefore, polarized, giving rise to a potential gradient across the cell membrane. This phenomenon is known as the resting potential of the cell.[2,5]

When a nerve cell is stimulated, its normal resting potential disappears. The permeability of the cell wall changes, permitting $K+$, $Na+$, and $Cl-$ ion migration through the wall. $Na+$ ions move from the interstitial tissue fluid surrounding the nerve cell into the nerve fiber. Eventually the sodium ion concentration inside the nerve fiber exceeds that in the interstitial fluid. Potassium ions move from within the nerve fiber to the interstitial fluid. The $Na+$ and $K+$ ion movements cause a reverse potential to build up (ie, the interior of the cell becomes more positive than the exterior) because the inside of the cell has been flooded with sodium ions. This reverse potential may reach a value of 30 to 50 millivolts. After a short time, the membrane regains its original permeability characteristics, and the normal ion distribution is re-established via the sodium-potassium pump. This changing potential produced when the nerve cell "fires" and then regains its resting voltage is known as the *action potential*.[2,5]

When a nerve cell fires, it influences adjacent cells and causes them to fire. These cells, in turn, cause firing of the nerve cells adjacent to them. In this manner, the action potential spreads rapidly from cell to cell. This traveling action potential is known as an impulse. Impulses move along nerve fibers to stimulate the associated muscle fibers, and along the muscle fibers to cause contraction. An impulse can travel in both directions away from the point of stimulation, but cannot reverse direction toward the starting point. Such reversal of direction is prevented because each nerve cell along the path of the impulse becomes momentarily refractory (ie, insensitive to stimulation for a short time after it has fired).[2,5]

The motor unit is a basic configuration of neuromuscular activity. It consists of a collection of muscle fibers controlled by a singe nerve fiber. When the nerve provides the "triggering" electrical impulse, the muscle fibers contract practically simultaneously. A motor unit may have only a few muscle fibers or thousands, and many motor units are needed to provide the mechanical force required to impart movement to the body.

The motor point is normally the most excitable point of a muscle and represents the area of the greatest concentration of nerve endings. It generally corresponds to the level at which the nerve enters the belly of the muscle.

The frequency spectrum is the range of frequencies present in a given electrical event, as measured in hertz. An example of such a frequency is the 60 cycle (hertz) waves given off from wall outlet voltage. The frequency spectrum of EMG signals covers the range from 20 to 5000 hertz.[5]

The raw, unprocessed EMG signal when amplified can be heard in a set of earphones or a speaker. These "muscle sounds" have been variously described as popping, crackling, hissing, freight train, airplane, and chugging sounds.[2] The raw EMG sound, however, is of little use as a feedback signal since the ear's ability to discern changes in signal amplitude is very limited. For this reason, the EMG signal is usually processed and converted to a variable frequency signal because the ear is much more sensitive to changes in tone.[2,5]

Both surface and needle electrodes have been used in EMG. Although the voltage from a single muscle fiber can be monitored by the use of a fine-tipped needle electrode, surface electrodes are commonly used for biofeedback in the rehabilitation setting. The voltage picked up by the surface electrodes is actually an average for the many muscle fibers below and near the electrodes. Although muscle action potentials as picked up by the electrodes could possibly be as high as 1000 microvolts, values between 100 and 500 microvolts are more representative.[5]

The principle advantage of needle electrodes is their high sensitivity to individual motor unit potentials, usually without interference from nearby muscles.[2] Therefore, they are usually used for diagnostic purposes. However, since physical therapists normally use EMG biofeedback for muscle re-education and relaxation purposes, surface electrodes have a number of advantages. For example, they eliminate the necessity of keeping all materials sterile and can be used easily on a home basis by the patient.

EMG biofeedback has been reported as being a successful procedure for assisting the rehabilitation of patients with a wide variety of neuromuscular problems,[2,6,7] providing muscle re-education and/or muscle relaxation in conditions which may include:

+ Relaxation in spasmodic torticollis[2]

+ Migraine headache pain[8-16]

+ Tension headache pain[8-14]

- Treatment of temporomandibular disorders[17-19]
- Improvement of functional deficits in paraplegia and quadriplegia[20,21]
- Improvement of postural instability, proprioception, and reduction of falls[21-25]
- Treatment of vestibular disorders[26]
- Treatment of cerebral palsied children for muscle re-education and relaxation[27,28]
- Cerebral vascular accident rehabilitation[25,29-36] for:
  - Foot drop and other gait problems
  - Posture and muscle tone improvement
  - Improved voluntary control of involved muscles
  - Muscle relaxation in associated reactions
  - Speech problems
- Gait training[37,38]
- Muscular training after nerve, muscle, ligament, or tendon injury, repair, or transfers[39-45]
  - Carpal tunnel syndrome
  - Hand dystonia
  - Rotator cuff and other shoulder pathologies
  - Lateral epicondylitis
  - Thorasic outlet syndrome
  - Patellofemoral pain
- Achilles tendon repairs
- Early joint mobilization after surgery[39-41,43,44]
  - Total joint replacements and other orthopedic surgeries
  - Re-education of affected muscle following radical mastectomy
- Measurement of endurance with sustained activity[46-48]
- Functional training and reduction of myoclonus following brain injury[49-52]
- Control of urinary incontinence and other pelvic floor disorders[53-65]
- Relaxation for intractable constipation symptoms and fecal incontinence[66-72]
- Respiratory control in asthma, emphysema, and chronic obstructive lung disease[73-78]
- Modification of hypertension[79-81]
- Treatment in diabetes, vascular disease, and symptoms of intermittent claudication[82-85]
- Parasympathetic control of cardiac arrhythmias[86]
- Stress management[87-94]
- Treatment of affective disorders; depression, anxiety, addiction[95-99]
- Intervention for dysphagia and other swallowing disorders[100-102]
- Muscle re-education following Bell's palsy[103,104]
- Pain management and reduction in chemotherapy related symptoms in cancer patients[105-115]
- Improvement of memory functioning[116]
- Wound healing[117]

Types of Biofeedback Interventions

Primarily, in the field of rehabilitation medicine, biofeedback techniques are used that focus on muscle re-education or voluntary inhibition (relaxation) of the muscle.[6,7] In these approaches, electrodes are place directly over the belly of the target muscle. Success is measured by appropriate muscle activation or relaxation. Techniques that are aimed at autonomic nervous system control include: placement of surface electrodes on the frontalis muscle and measurement of physiologic variables such as heart rate, blood pressure, breathing pattern and rate, and galvanic skin response. Another approach for biofeedback intervention is the use of a digital temperature monitor for measurement of physiologic response though body temperature.[32]

In addition to instrumentation for feedback purposes, treatment techniques often include guided imagery training or progressive muscle relaxation which are forms of autogenic relaxation techniques.[5,7] Deep breathing techniques have been shown to effectively regulate mental states,[88-90] and are often employed in combination with the above mentioned biofeedback techniques to enhance a state of relaxation. Guided imagery is frequently used as an adjunct to biofeedback to facilitate a state of excitation for athletic training. Blumenstein et al[88] found that significant tachypnea was observed during imagery of sprint running and in most cases studied, EMG biofeedback substantially augmented the physiological responses.

The mechanisms by which cognitive processes influence states of bodily arousal are important for understanding the pathogenesis and maintenance of stress-related morbidity. Critchley and associates[7] investigated cerebral activity related to cognitively driven modulation of sympathetic activity and found that biofeedback-assisted relaxation was associated with significant increases in left anterior cingulated, vermal, and globus pallidus activity.[7] These findings have potential implications for a mechanistic account of how therapeutic interventions, such as relaxation training in stress-related disorders, mediate their effects.

MUSCLE RE-EDUCATION

When using biofeedback for muscle re-education, it is important to place the muscle to be examined in the easiest position for the patient to elicit movement. For example, in testing the strength of the vastus medialis of the quadriceps muscle group, the patient might be positioned on his or her side, attempting to straighten his or her lower leg. Another useful position might be with the patient supine and the lower leg hanging off the edge of the table. For other patients, this movement might best be accomplished from a sitting position. It is generally easier to elicit motor unit firing when a muscle is in a fully-stretched condition and the patient is asked to move through a full range of motion. Visual observation by the patient of the motion to be performed can often be of great benefit.

At the initial treatment session, it is important for the therapist to familiarize the patient with the operation of the biofeedback unit. Placing electrodes on a normal muscle or on the corresponding muscle of the uninvolved extremity when possible, and going through the full range of motion or tensing and relaxing the muscle, will help prepare the patient to work with the affected muscle or muscle group. This approach will also give the patient practice in reading the meter and hearing the "muscle sounds."

To aid the patient in eliciting motor responses, all forms of exercise, proprioceptive neuromuscular facilitation (PNF) techniques, and body positioning may be employed. The objective is to discover any functional motor units in the muscle. If no active motor units are discovered at a particular therapy session, it does not necessarily mean that none are present. In a weakened muscle, there may be only a few active motor units, as compared to the thousands in a normal muscle. What we are searching for is "potential activity" of motor units in what appears to be a "paralyzed" muscle.

When active motor unit responses are found, the next step is to bring the responses under voluntary control. It should not be expected that when responses in an involved muscle are detected, they will remain at the same high level of activity at future therapy sessions. A great degree of variability can be expected initially, especially in the neurologically compromised muscle. Over an extended period of treatment, a muscle given regular, continued exercise is likely to show a continuing increase in strength and less tendency toward wide fluctuations in readings.

Motivation of the patient is the key. If the therapist approaches the patient optimistically with the attitude that EMG biofeedback can be of significant benefit in the rehabilitation process, and continually emphasizes reachable goals with good exercise programs, then real progress can be achieved and objectively measured. As the return of functional components for a desired task occurs, and the speed and accuracy of performance improve, biofeedback instrumentation may be gradually withdrawn.

It is important to remember that it is extremely easy for a person who has obtained some functional use of a muscle group to later let those muscles regress to a decreased level of function. This generally happens when muscles are not exercised for a period of time. It must be stressed to the patient that the natural sensory feedback mechanism of the muscles he or she is attempting to strengthen has been diminished, and that constant attention on a daily basis is required to increase muscle strength and function to an optimum level.

EMG biofeedback can also be used as a monitor for evaluation of progress with home exercise programs in subsequent follow-up sessions. A home unit is often helpful, and most EMG biofeedback units manufactured today have memory capabilities of 30+ treatment sessions, so that progress can be downloaded and compliance with the exercise program monitored. Since it is a natural tendency to decrease exercise as strength increases, patients should be re-evaluated on a periodic basis, and the therapist should reinforce the necessity of continuing their exercise programs. It is important to remember that if a total program of objective measurement of muscle activity is undertaken, clear, concise records must be kept to facilitate reimbursement by third party payors.[118]

MUSCLE RELAXATION

The procedure for training a patient in muscle relaxation techniques is much the same as for muscle re-education. The difference lies in the fact that instead of teaching the patient to increase motor unit firing, we are trying to inhibit or decrease the level of firing created by the tension or tone in the muscle. Again, electrodes should be attached over an unaffected muscle for demonstration of how muscle tension can be lowered after an initial muscle contraction. Only when the patient has thoroughly understood the relationship between muscle contraction and relaxation and the corresponding changes in auditory and visual displays should the electrodes be placed on the affected muscle.

The patient must understand that relaxing a muscle that has abnormal tone will not be as easy as relaxing a normal muscle, but that it can be done with practice and perseverance. Repeated orientation is necessary. The individual must understand that he or she controls the feedback and that the equipment does not control him or her. Among the best tools to assist a patient in decreasing muscle tension are deep breathing techniques focusing in on the abdominal region, music, relaxation tapes, and progressive relaxation exercises, such as those designed by Jacobsen.

To assist patients who have difficulty in decreasing muscle activity, the therapist should point out any strained posture, labored breathing, or noted lack of focus, etc interfering with the ability to relax. Ideally, for training practice sessions, the patient should be in a quiet, dimly lit room, free from outside distractions, and positioned for maximum comfort. It is sometimes helpful to begin training or practice sessions by having the individual imagine pleasant scenes or experiences. This allows the patient to clear his or her mind of any of the "built-in" tensions of everyday life. Clinical training sessions generally last 30 minutes on a two- to three-time per week basis. As the patient makes progress in decreasing the microvolts level in a structured situation, he or she should be encouraged to practice these relaxation techniques in the environment where the tension arises.

When working with patients who have muscle contraction or tension headaches, the electrodes are often placed on the skin over the frontalis muscle, about 2 inches apart and approximately 1 inch above the eyebrows. It should be explained to the individual that the electrodes are measuring the amount of muscle tension he or she is producing, and that this tension is a reflection of the tension throughout his or her whole body.

Some clinicians feel that the frontalis is not necessarily the best reflector of body tension for every patient, and with this author would agree. Another effective lead placement is suggested using a global technique. With this technique, the electrodes are attached to the flexor surface of each forearm. This electrode placement allows monitoring tension of all the muscles of the upper body, which comprise approximately 60% of the controlled muscles of the body.

In order to develop a complete program of muscle re-education or relaxation, it is important that the patient be instructed in the use of EMG biofeedback unit at home. This approach allows the patient to monitor and maintain the optimum level that he or she has achieved in the clinical environment.

Clinical Research in the Use of Biofeedback Techniques

IMMUNOLOGY

The role of the mind in healing the body is a fascinating subject that is steadily gaining in importance even within traditional medical practice. Mentally influencing the immune system, for example, is an exciting new field given the name *psychoneuroimmunology* (literally the effect of the mind through the nervous system on the immune system). This topic has been extensively covered in Chapter 1 of this book and is only mentioned here as it relates to the utilization of biofeedback techniques.

The effect of biofeedback-assisted relaxation on cell-mediated immunity, cortisol, and white blood cell count was investigated by McGrady et al[129] under low-stress conditions. Interestingly, the group of subjects trained in biofeedback-assisted relaxation techniques showed increased blastogenesis and a decreased white blood cell count, indicating a clear effect on the immune system.

The results of immunological responses of breast cancer patients to behavioral interventions is remarkable and promising.[130] Gruber et al[130] reports the results of an 18-month study of immune system and psychological changes in Stage 1 breast cancer patients provided with relaxation, guided imagery, and biofeedback training. Significant effects were found in natural killer cell activity, lymphocyte responsiveness, and the number of peripheral blood lymphocytes. This study clearly indicates that relaxation, guided imagery, and related biofeedback techniques have the potential for modifying the immune systems response in a positive manner.

MIGRAINE AND TENSION HEADACHE PAIN

Behavioral therapies such as biofeedback are commonly used to treat migraine and tension headache.[13-15] Controlling sympathetic activity is effective for controlling the pain in both disturbances[13] Grazzi and Bussone[13] confirmed the clinical efficacy of EMG biofeedback treatment for tension and common migraine headaches. In this study, the basal stress indices (plasma catecholamines and cortisol) were significantly different in the experiment group compared to no change in the controls, and the study group experienced a substantial decrease in frequency of headaches reported.

Functional activities of daily living are often restricted in the presence of tension headaches.[8-10] In a study by King,[8] EMG biofeedback was used to decrease upper trapezius activity related to tension headaches. It was this studies' belief that headaches were caused by general tension and anxiety and affected the individual's ability to adequately attend to activities of daily living, including child care, homemaking, and vocational activities. The program combined deep-breathing exercises, progressive muscular relaxation exercises, resisted shoulder elevation exercises, and EMG monitoring during upper extremity tasks, and a home exercise/relaxation program. EMG biofeedback was successful in assisting to eliminate tension headaches, and the patients reported an increased ability to attend to activities of daily living.[8]

Other studies[12,13] also strongly support the use of biofeedback-assisted relaxation techniques in the treatment of tension[12] and migraine[13,15] headaches.

Sarafino and Goehring[16] presented a review and archival analysis to assess age differences in acquiring biofeedback control and success in treating recurrent headache by using data from 56 studies with either adult or child subjects. All studies focused on treating headache with temperature biofeedback or electromyographic biofeedback. Results showed that both children and adults experienced substantial improvements in headache pain management with both forms of biofeedback. No age differences were found in the acquisition of biofeedback control indicating that regardless of age, biofeedback is a modality that can be applied for management of headache pain.[16]

TEMPOROMANDIBULAR DISORDERS

Often, individuals with temporomandibular (TMJ) disorders experience a great deal of jaw pain and can develop tension headaches. Mishra et al[17] studied the relative efficacy of different biopsychosocial treatment conditions on patients with chronic TMJ and found biofeedback intervention to be the most effective in decreasing pain scores. The results of this study demonstrated that, in terms of a self-reported pain score, individuals undergoing biofeedback compared to a no-treatment control group reported significantly decreased pain scores. Moreover, patients in the biofeedback group reported significantly improved involvement in overall daily activities and displayed significant improvements in mood states compared with the no-treatment subjects.[17]

Crider, Glaros and Gevirtz[18] reviewed and performed a meta-analysis of the available literature to determine the efficacy of biofeedback-based treatments in subjects with TMJ disorders. They determined that, although the effect of biofeedback interventions were limited in extent (ie, duration), the available data support the efficacy of EMG biofeedback treatment for TMJ disorders.[18]

An interesting comparison of muscular relaxation effects of transcutaneous electrical neuromuscular stimulation (TENS) and EMG-biofeedback in patients with bruxism during the night was studied by Foster.[19] Results showed tendencies of nocturnal bruxism decreased mean-EMG levels for individuals after biofeedback treatment sessions. The results indicated, not only that the individuals exhibited fewer bruxing episodes following treatment, but that gains from biofeedback were maintained 6 months following termination of treatment.[19]

This research has significant implications for rehabilitation professionals involved in the management of patients with TMJ.

IMPROVEMENT OF FUNCTIONAL DEFICITS IN PARAPLEGIA AND QUADRIPLEGIA

The efficacy of enhancing muscle function in spinal cord patients when administered in conjunction with physical rehabilitation therapy has been substantiated.[20] Evidence from the study by Klose et al[20] indicated that spinal cord injury patients in the study group using biofeedback and a conventional exercise program increased the amount of improvement seen compared to the control group who used a conventional exercise program alone to regain muscle strength and function.

POSTURAL INSTABILITY, PROPRIOCEPTION, AND FALLS

Postural instability, deficits in proprioception, and kinesthesia are associated with many neuromuscular pathologies and increase the potential of falling. Postural instability may be developmental, as in the case of the severely motorically impaired child with cerebral palsy or acquired later in life secondary to neural disease or trauma.[21] Beyond the pathological conditions creating postural instability, aging is also associated with trunk weakness, alterations in neuromuscular and musculoskeletal efficiency, and an increased incidence of falling.[22,23] In contrast to the use of biofeedback for neuromuscular re-education of muscles that are overactive or underactive, biofeedback for postural instability has been used to augment achievement of functional skills, such as head or trunk control, or symmetry of standing balance.[21] EMG biofeedback instrumentation is effective in detecting muscle activity and giving the patient objective information about the physiological functioning and movements not ordinarily perceived by the individual. In the case of postural instability, auditory and visual biofeedback signals provide the patient with information regarding head and trunk orientation and about symmetry of weight bearing through the lower extremities.[25,27-29]

The possibility of using learned physiological responses in control of progressive adolescent idiopathic scoliosis has also been investigated.[29] Wong and associates[29] found that a long-lasting active spinal control could be achieved through the patient's own spinal muscles facilitated by auditory biofeedback. Adolescent patients were able to decrease the use of, and in some cases eliminate the need for, bracing devices generally prescribed until skeletal maturity or cessation of curve progression.[29]

VESTIBULAR DISORDERS

It is well known that diseases of the vestibular system can be compensated by increased spontaneous activity of other systems engaged in maintaining equilibrium (eg, proprioceptive and visual systems). A complex approach using multisensory stimulation is the optimal way to achieve vestibular compensation. Hahn and associates[26] studied the effect of vestibular rehabilitative therapy using biofeedback techniques in patients suffering from vestibular disorders such as Meniere's disease, neuritis vestibularis, and vertebrobasilar insufficiency. All of these subjects showed improvement in equilibrium by visual and proprioceptive biofeedback mechanisms indicating a clear value and usefulness of biofeedback techniques in the treatment of vestibular disorders.[26]

CEREBRAL PALSY

In addition to the physical problems inherent in cerebral palsy, speech problems can often create a frustrating communication deficit in these individuals. In a study by Howard and Varley,[31] the use of electopalatography biofeedback was used to treat patients with severe speech production problems affecting articulation, phonation, and resonance. It was found that this form of instrumented biofeedback provided a valuable form of visual feedback for patients and revealed and clarified aspects of oral movements for speech and non-speech activity that had been difficult to capture via auditory perception.[31]

CEREBRAL VASCULAR ACCIDENT

Rehabilitation for individuals sustaining a cerebral vascular accident (CVA) has been shown to be enhanced by employing EMG biofeedback for neuromuscular re-education.[32] These authors found that problems such as foot drop and other gait problems, posture and muscle tone, voluntary control of involved muscles, and muscle relaxation in associated reactions were all improved with the use of biofeedback as an adjunct to physical and occupational therapy. A recent study investigated whether visual biofeedback/forceplate training could enhance the effects of other physical therapy interventions on balance and mobility following stroke.[36] Following intervention, higher scores were obtained in both the biofeedback and control groups on the balance measures. Research indicates no significant advantage to the use of visual biofeedback training combined with other physical therapy interventions. However, virtual reality training has been successfully used to rehabilitate functional balance and mobility.[36]

Sunderland et al[33] did a detailed study to determine the recovery of upper extremity function following an acute stroke, comparing orthodox physical therapy interventions with therapy regimes enhanced by the use of EMG biofeedback to encourage motor learning with behavioral methods. Six months following strokes, it was found that study subjects had a statistically significant advantage in recovery of strength, range and speed of movement. Moreland and Thomson[34] showed that a small but significant effect on muscle function was realized utilizing EMG biofeedback compared to conventional physical therapy for improving upper extremity function in patients following a stroke.

GAIT TRAINING

As discussed in relation to posture and balance, biofeedback techniques are often successfully employed to improve gait patterns. For example, residual limb recovery after a transtibial amputation depends largely on close monitoring of the weight-bearing activities during the early postoperative stage. Chow and Cheng[37] investigated the ability of individuals with transtibial amputations to replicate a prescribed amount of weight bearing using a bathroom scale versus using auditory biofeedback. Their weight-bearing characteristics with and without use of auditory biofeedback were continuously monitored and showed that the residual limb would be overloaded using the conventional bathroom scale method during early postoperative ambulatory training. It was demonstrated that audio biofeedback was useful in preventing the residual limb from being overloaded.[37] These findings could conceivably be employed in any condition where the amount of weightbearing during gait training was a consideration.

The use of EMG biofeedback to reduce Trendelenburg gait was evaluated by Petrofsky.[38] Physical therapy involved muscle strengthening and gait training in which biofeedback was used for a portion of each therapy session. A subset of patients were also given a EMG biofeedback training device for neuromuscular re-education outside the clinic. It was found that the strength of gluteus medius contraction was improved through auditory input. If too little gluteus medius activity occurred on the affected side or the step was too short in duration, an audio cue alerted the individual so that he or she could correct the deficit. Subjects undergoing clinical therapy showed approximately a 50% reduction in hip drop, whereas those participants that used the home training device showed almost normal gait after the 2-month treatment period.[38]

MUSCULAR RE-EDUCATION/RELAXATION FOLLOWING INJURY

The effects of biofeedback on carpal tunnel syndrome show promise in preventing this problem from reoccurring. In a study by Thomas et al[39] behavioral modification based on audible EMG biofeedback signals was used to discourage awkward hand postures and the exertion of excessive force with the fingers, which are suspected of causing carpal tunnel syndrome. They found a reduction in symptomatology and a learning affect related to proper ergonomic posturing.

Work-related upper extremity disorders present a significant challenge to health care providers, employers, and insurers.[40,41] Reynolds[41] describes a rehabilitation approach for keyboard operators following radial tunnel compression and release of the extensor origin of the right elbow.[41] An EMG biofeedback device was employed in this study to determine which work activities individuals should avoid or alter to reduce strain in the wrist musculature. It was found that reoccurrence of carpal tunnel symptoms was significantly reduced by re-educating workers through the use of biofeedback.[41]

Deepak and Behari[42] employed specific muscle EMG biofeedback with individuals with hand dystonia (writer's cramp). EMG biofeedback improved the clinical and EMG picture in those patients with hand dystonia who showed EMG overactivity of proximal limb muscles during writing.[42]

Rotator cuff and other shoulder pathologies are often accompanied by protective muscle guarding in the supraspinatus, infraspinatus, anterior and middle portions of the deltoid, and the descending part of the trapezius. By using biofeedback surface electrodes it has been found that subjects could reduce the EMG activity voluntarily in the trapezius.[28] This was not true for the other muscles investigated. When the trapezius activity was reduced there was a tendency towards an increase in EMG activity in the other shoulder muscle, particularly the infraspinatus. Palmerund et al[43] suggest that the findings may be related to relaxation from an initial overstabilization of the shoulder, or redistribution of load among synergists. It is suggested that the possibility of reducing trapezius activity may be of ergonomic significance.[43]

Voluntary posterior dislocation of the shoulder is a difficult condition to treat successfully. It has been shown that EMG biofeedback is a nonoperative treatment that has been successfully used to prevent recurrent dislocation.[44]

To determine the effects of EMG biofeedback in patients with patellofemoral pain syndrome, a recent study demonstrated that an effective treatment modality for improving quadriceps muscle strength after athroscopic meniscectomy surygery is biofeedback.[45]

MEASUREMENT OF ENDURANCE

The effect of psychological strategies upon cardiorespiratory and muscular activity during aerobic exercise has been widely employed in sports therapy. Kranitz and Lehrer[46] demonstrated that all cardiovascular parameters (eg, heart rate, respiratory rate, depth of ventilation, blood pressure) could be consciously altered using biofeedback monitoring.[46] Leisman et al[47] investigated the effects of fatigue and task repetition on the relationship between integrated electromyogram and force output of working muscles.[47] This study showed that with fatigue, integrated EMG activity increased strongly and functional force output of the muscle remained stable or decreased. Fatigue results in a less efficient muscle process. Through training using biofeedback, the efficiency of muscle contraction could be improved with volitional control and the level of fatigue reduced.[47]

In space program studies it was found that biofeedback techniques enabled astronauts to maintain specific levels of exercise or lower negative pressure within acceptable limits of cardiac function.[48] As it is difficult to produce conditions of aerobic training in microgravity environments, the use of biofeedback to facilitate aerobic cardiac responses may assist in maintaining endurance under these circumstances. Applicability of biofeedback-induced endurance training with bedridden and otherwise immobilized individuals could hold great potential and should be evaluated in future research.

BRAIN INJURY

Biofeedback has traditionally been used in the context of relaxation therapy along with stress management. Some recent studies have looked to extend the applicability of biofeedback by using it as a didactic tool for neuromotor rehabilitation. Duckett and Kramer[49] applied biofeedback with anoxic head injury patients unable to participate in transfers owing to severe myoclonicity. They trained the patients using autogenic relaxation along with EMG biofeedback to reduce the myoclonus and therefore participate actively with stand pivot transfers.

Guercio and colleagues[50] examined the effects of behavioral relaxation training and biofeedback on ataxic tremor of adults with acquired brain injury. Relaxation techniques were used as the foundation for biofeedback training. The results with specific skills (ie, use of a letter board for communication) when the participants were able to relax the appropriate musculature were positive. The research demonstrated that the individual was able to learn to significantly decrease the severity of tremor to accomplish a functional task. As a result, each participant became more proficient at communicating with a letter board. Collateral effects were increased attempts at communication and fewer episodes of anger.[50]

The mechanisms of feedback not controlled by our consciousness play an essential role in the functions of the central nervous system in the process of programming of activities, behavior, and control of these functions. In cases of deviations or errors of activities, imposed by brain injury and stroke, the possibility of their immediate correction exists.[51] Brain damage after trauma or caused by tumor disturbs normal feedback mechanisms producing varying symptom complexes. Kwolek and Pop[51] found that EMG biofeedback was advantageous in providing afferent information to the brain-damaged patient and enhanced the return of motor function more substantially than conventional physical therapy interventions.[52]

URINARY INCONTINENCE AND OTHER PELVIC FLOOR DISORDERS

Stress incontinence is a debilitating condition affecting a large proportion of the female population. Pelvic floor exercising with the aid of EMG biofeedback is well established as an effective treatment regime.[53-65] Current EMG monitoring devices are effective as they may also be employed in community-based home therapy.[53,54] Many of the units are both compact and accurate and suitable for ambulatory monitoring of vaginal pressure.

McIntosh et al[55] found that both urinary and fecal incontinence was improved through the use of EMG biofeedback-assisted pelvic floor exercise. These authors clearly demonstrated that a pelvic floor rehabilitation program was an effective alternative to surgical intervention in reducing the frequency of urinary and fecal leakage. Brubaker and Kotarinos[56] also demonstrated that pelvic floor muscle training utilizing EMG biofeedback was beneficial in the treatment of urinary incontinence. Numerous studies provide confirmation that urinary incontinence can conservatively be managed through physical therapy interventions utilizing biofeedback-assisted pelvic floor muscle training.[55-61] Postoperative complications following radical prostatectomy usually include urinary incontinence.[60] Milam and Franke[60] found that beyond surgical interventions, such as modified apical dissection and construction of a tubularized neourethra, EMG biofeedback provided a reliable alternative to management of urinary incontinence after prostatectomy.

The effective use of biofeedback for gynecological problems such as vulvar vestibulitis syndrome, marked by moderate to severe chronic introital dyspareunia and tenderness of the vulvar vestibule, has also been clearly demonstrated.[62] Women instructed in a home program employing biofeedback-assisted pelvic floor muscle rehabilitation exercises experienced an increase in pelvic floor muscle contraction strength, a decrease in resting tension levels of the pelvic floor muscle, a decrease in the muscle instability associated with this syndrome, and a remarkable decrease in pain.[62]

Recent systematic reviews on the conservative management of urinary incontinence in women have identified evidence for firm recommendations to include biofeedback in the conservative strategies for treating this condition.[63] A comparative study looking at the effectiveness of an intensive group physical therapy program with individual biofeedback training for female patients with stress incontinence showed improvement in both groups. Both the intensive therapy group and the biofeedback groups resulted in a significantly reduced nocturnal urinary frequency and improved subjective outcome. Only group therapy resulted in reduced daytime urinary frequency. Biofeedback resulted in a better subjective outcome and higher contraction pressures of the pelvic floor muscle.[64]

Floratos and associates[65] evaluated the comparative effectiveness of EMG biofeedback with verbal instructions as learning tools of pelvic muscle exercises in the early management of urinary incontinence after radical prostatectomy. It was determined that intensive verbal instructions and biofeedback were both very effective methods and learning tools, however, the biofeedback group responded favorably to the intervention in less time, significantly reducing the duration of treatment.[65]

INTRACTABLE CONSTIPATION AND FECAL INCONTINENCE

Some individuals have difficulty relaxing the striated muscles of the anal sphincters, sometimes referred to as animus. Fecal incontinence is often underreported by the older populaton. It is especially common in elderly persons residing in community or long-term settings. Physiological changes, including sphincter muscle and sensory abnormalities in the anorectal region, contribute to this problem and respond effectively to biofeedback techniques.[66,67] Once fecal incontinence is identified, management is important. Treatment with biofeedback is feasible in many older adults.

Although immediate results are good to excellent in a great majority of patients who undergo biofeedback treatment for chronic constipation and fecal incontinence, they tend to loose the benefit over time.[68] Therefore, it is important that patients be re-evaluated and biofeedback intervention be done on an ongoing basis. Although behavioral treatment (biofeedback) successfully treats the pelvic floor abnormalities in patients with idiopathic constipation, many patients also normalize their impaired bowel frequency. Emmanuel and Kamm[69] postulated that this response may be associated with altered cerebral outflow via extrinsic autonomic nerves to the gut. They found that a successful outcome after biofeedback treatment is associated with improved activity of the direct cerebral innervation to the gut and improved gut transit. This effect is gut specific, cardiovascular autonomic reflexes were not altered.[69] Most programs implemented to treat fecal incontinence result in improvements.[70-72] Biofeedback is a nonsurgical, less costly means of treatment that reportedly produces good results in 65% to 75% of fecally incontinent patients. In solid stool fecal incontinence, biofeedback training effects are robust and seem not to be explained by expectancy or nonspecific treatment effects.[70,71] Sensory retraining appears to be more relevant than strength training to the success of biofeedback.[72]

ASTHMA, EMPHYSEMA, AND CHRONIC OBSTRUCTIVE LUNG DISEASE

The use of biofeedback techniques has also been shown to have an impact on respiratory resistance in conditions of asthma and other resistive lung problems.[73-75] Hypothesis for the positive impact of both visual and auditory biofeedback effectiveness in these respiratory conditions is the activation of the parasympathetic nervous system providing more available oxygen and the influence of relaxation and deep breathing techniques in calming the system, thereby reducing respiratory resistance.[73,75] Blanc-Gras et al[74] provided substantial evidence for support of the learning effect facilitated by the use of visual feedback in control of respiratory pattern. This information indicates that EMG biofeedback could have a great deal of merit in the treatment of asthma and other stress-related breathing problems.

Laryngeal dyskinesis is a functional asthma-like disorder refractory to bronchodilator regimes. Age-related attenuation of biofeedback effects on cardiovascular variability does not diminish the usefulness of the metho for treating asthma among older adults.[75]

Lehrer and associates[76] demonstrated that biofeedback techniques were effective as a nonpharmacological psychophysiological treatment for improving pulmonary function in asthmatic children. Biofeedback training in these children resulted in an increase in the amplitude of respiratory sinus arrhythmia with significant improvements in forced expiratory maneuvers from maximum vital capacity.[76] Likewise, Kern-Buell et al[77] conducted a randomized controlled study examining the effects of biofeedback-assisted relaxation in individuals with asthma. Data were collected on asthma symptoms, pulmonary function, indicators of arousal, and cellular immune factors. The trained group evidenced a decrease in forehead muscle tension in comparison to the controls, though showed no changes in peripheral skin temperature. Decreases in asthma severity and bronchodilator medication usage for the experimental group were observed. Pulmonary function testing revealed a significant difference between groups in forced expiratory volume (FEV) and vital capacity (FVC) with the biofeedback group having a higher ratio of FEV1/FVC at posttest compared with the controls. The cellular immune data showed not significant group differences in total white blood cell or lymphocyte counts, but decreases over time were observed. Significant differences were observed in the numbers of neutrophils and basophils in the trained group compared to controls, which supports the concept of decreased inflammation.[77] These studies clearly support the use of biofeedback techniques in pulmonary diseases characterized by hyper-responsiveness of the airway, inflammation, and reversible obstruction. Respiratory tract infection, allergies, air pollution, and psychosocial factors impact the severity and frequency of asthma symptoms and biofeedback have the potential of being a major component in the management of asthma.[76,77]

MODIFICATION OF HYPERTENSION

The central mechanisms and possibilities of biofeedback of the systemic arterial pressure have been investigated extensively.[46,79,80] McGrady[79] studied a group of patients with essential hypertension for the effects of group relaxation training and thermal biofeedback on blood pressure and on other psychophysiologic measures: heart rate, frontalis muscle tension, finger temperature, depression, anxiety, plasma aldosterone, plasma renin activity, and plasma and urinary cortisol. A significant decline in blood pressure was observed in 49% of the experimental group. Of that group 51% maintained a lower blood pressure at a 10-month follow-up examination suggesting that relaxation training has beneficial effects for short-term and long-term adjunctive therapy of essential hypertension in selected individuals.

Yucha and associates,[81] in a study to determine the effectiveness of biofeedback in the treatment of stages 1 and 2 essential hypertension, found that both biofeedback and active control treatments (ie, medications) resulted in a reduction in systolic and diastolic blood pressure. However, only biofeedback, with related cognitive and relaxation training show a significantly greater reduction in both blood pressure measures. This research also found a significant latent effect of biofeedback interventions, whereas active treatment approaches lost their effectiveness soon after cessation of the drug.[81]

DIABETES, VASCULAR DISEASE, AND INTERMITTENT CLAUDICATION

Saunders et al[82] examined the therapeutic effects of thermal biofeedback-assisted autogenic training in a group of diabetic and vascular disease patients with symptoms of intermittent claudication. The individuals received thermal feedback from the hand for five sessions, then from the foot for 16 sessions, while hand and foot temperatures were monitored simultaneously. Within the session, foot temperatures rose specifically in response to foot temperature biofeedback, and starting foot temperature rose between sessions. Posttreatment blood pressure was reduced to a normal level. Attacks of intermittent claudication were reduced to zero after 12 sessions and walking distance increased by about a mile per day over the course of the treatment. It would appear that thermal biofeedback and autogenic training are potentially promising therapies for persons with diabetes and peripheral vascular disease.

Of interest is a study by Freedman et al[91] comparing the sympathetic activation using temperature feedback compared to autogenic training alone. Thirty-nine normal volunteers of both sexes were randomly assigned to receive eight sessions of temperature biofeedback or autogenic training to increase finger temperature. Temperature feedback subjects produced significant elevations in finger temperature during training, whereas those who received autogenic training did not. This study indicates that autogenic training alone may not produce vasodilatation.

Rice and Schindler[83] investigated the effect of relaxation training/thermal biofeedback on blood circulation in the lower extremities of diabetic subjects. A within-subject experimental design was used. During phase 1, all subjects used a self-selected relaxation method and recorded toe temperatures daily. During phase 2, subjects were taught a biofeedback-assisted relaxation technique designed to elicit sensations of warmth in the lower extremities and increase circulation and temperature. Subjects relaxed at home with the use of a designated relaxation tape. Each phase of the study lasted 4 weeks. Mean temperature change scores between phases 1 and 2 were 8.73% (phase 1) and 31.88% (phase 2). The greater increase in phase 2 was attributed to the biofeedback-assisted relaxation technique. These authors concluded that diabetic patients show significant increases in peripheral blood circulation with this technique. This noninvasive method could serve as an adjunct treatment for limited blood flow in some complications of diabetes, such as ulceration.

Of noted interest, stressful life events and negative mood have been associated with elevated blood glucose and poor self care in individuals with diabetes. McGinnis, McGrady, Cox and Grower-Dowling[84] studied the outcome of biofeedback assisted relaxation to determine its effect on mood state, specifically depression, anxiety, and means of dealing with daily hassles (ie, stress). Statistically significant correlations were found between high scores on stress, anxiety, and depression inventories and higher glucose levels. Biofeedback assisted relaxation interventions resulted in a overall improvement in the psychological measures and a reduction in blood glucose levels without other adjunct therapies.[84] These finding hold great clinical significance in the management of insulin dependent diabetics.

Phantom pain is a frequent consequence of the amputation of an extremity and causes considerable discomfort and disruption of daily activities. Harden et al[85] demonstrated complete elimination of phantom limb pain after biofeedback techniques were employed.[85]

CARDIAC ARRHYTHMIAS

Respiratory sinus arrhythmia, the peak-to-peak variations in heart rate caused by respiration, can be used as a noninvasive measure of parasympathetic cardiac control. In a study by Reyes del Paso et al,[86] they showed that subjects could actually alter their respiratory sinus arrhythmia (ie, decrease or increase the rate) by monitoring respiratory biofeedback apparatus in conjunction with consciously concentrating on their depth and rate of respiration. Vaschillo et al[87] also demonstrated that individuals were able to modify their heart rates volitionally when instructed in relaxation techniques using EKG biofeedback monitoring. Additionally, resonant frequency heart rate variability biofeedback increased baroreflex gain and peak expiratory flow. Biofeedback readily produces large oscillations in heart rate, blood pressure, vascular tone, and pulse amplitude via paced breathing.

STRESS MANAGEMENT

When we are truly relaxed, very definite and measurable changes take place in the body.[79,88-90] These changes distinguish relaxation from the opposite states of tension or arousal. Some of the most significant changes are triggered by the two branches of the autonomic nervous system. The sympathetic branch of the nervous system controls body temperature, digestion, heart rate, respiratory rate, blood flow and pressure, and muscular tension. The parasympathetic nervous system lowers oxygen consumption and reduces the following bodily functions: carbon dioxide elimination, heart and respiratory rates, blood pressure, blood lactate, and blood cortisol levels.[79,88-92] These bodily changes are collectively referred to as the "relaxation response."

Recent research also suggests that among the biochemical changes triggered by relaxation there is an increase in the body's manufacture of certain mood-altering neurotransmitters.[90,91] In particular, production of serotonin (the biochemical equivalent to Prozac [Lilly, Indianapolis, IN]) is increased. Seratonin is associated with feelings of calmness and contentment.

Lehrer et al[90] isolated the types of biofeedback techniques that worked most effectively in various conditions. Their study showed that instrumentation using biofeedback electrodes placed over the involved muscles was most effective in treating disorders with a predominant muscular component (eg, muscle strength and/or tone changes, tension headaches, carpal tunnel, etc). Disorders in which autonomic dysfunction predominates (eg, hypertension, migraine headaches) are more effectively treated by techniques with a strong autonomic component, such as lead placement on the frontalis muscle, or digital temperature monitoring, and progressive relaxation techniques.

AFFECTIVE DISORDERS

Biofeedback interventions have been proposed as a promising modality in the treatment of affective disorders.[95] It has been determined that brainwave activity can be altered using biofeedback techniques.[95,96] Moore[96] found that alpha, theta, and alpha-theta enhancements are effective treatments of the anxiety disorders. This research also demonstrated the alpha wave suppression is also effective, but less so. Perceived success in carrying out specific tasks seems to play a big role in clinical improvement and results in changes in alpha and theta rhythms.[96] Certain skin diseases and sensitivity have been associated with anxiety. Biofeedback employed with dermatologic problems associated with stress appears to provide favorable treatment outcomes.[97] Allen and colleagues demonstrated that individual differences in resting asymmetrical frontal brain activity can be used to predict subsequent emotional responses and is alterable utilizing biofeedback training.[98] Therefore, it is hypothesized that using biofeedback in the treatment of affective disorders can offer a non-drug approach to managing depression, anxiety, and other emotional disturbances. Trudeau[99] provides evidence that biofeedback is an effective treatment approach for addictive disorders. Employing brainwave biofeedback, addicts can alter their emotional response to external stimulus (the psychological components of addiction) and change their physiological need for the substance to which they are addicted.[99] The mind is clearly a powerful thing.

DYSPHAGIA

EMG and biofeedback techniques are well established in the disciplines of physical medicine for the retraining of muscle groups to approximate functional performance in swallowing.[100-102] Dysphagia is a swallowing disorder frequently encountered in the rehabilitation of stroke and head injury patients. Oral dysphagia refers to abnormalities in the oral phase of the swallowing mechanism[100,102] As this disorder is primarily based in muscle over- or underactivity, biofeedback devices rendering feedback of biomechanical parameters characterizing the oral phase of swallowing have been shown to be extremely effective in re-establishing swallowing patterns in neuromuscularly impaired individuals.[100] Leplow, Schluter, and Ferstl[30] demonstrated that the use of biofeedback was instrumental is assessment of muscle activity in facial and oral musculature. These authors demonstrated that proprioception of neuromuscularly involved patients was enhanced, especially in muscles richly supplied with muscle spindles and afferent fibers (ie, masseter muscle, zygomatus major muscle).

BELL'S PALSY

Neuromuscular rehabilitation can reduce the severity of chronic facial paralysis, but complete recovery is frequently impeded by synkinesis.[103,104] It has been determined that synkinesis could be minimized by preventing its possible reinforcement during rehabilitation by employing EMG biofeedback with the goal of eliciting smaller movements. Muscular re-education in Bell's palsy patients who have intact facial-motor innervation has clearly been found to be enhanced by the use of EMG biofeedback. Facial function typically improves with a more rapid recovery of symmetry and a decrease in synkinesis.[103,104]

PAIN MANAGEMENT IN CANCER PATIENTS

Pain is one of the most feared consequences of cancer. Control of pain from cancer has been shown to decrease discomfort and diminish the need for drugs that may induce other negative side effects.[105-107] Relaxation and related biofeedback techniques have been shown to be effective in the management of cancer pain.[107-109] Utilizing such interventions as progressive muscle relaxation, relaxation and systemic desensitization, hypnosis, and biofeedback and relaxation, researchers have determined that nonpharmaceutical interventions for pain management have a great deal of potential.[107-110] Filshie,[109] comparing many specific methods in the management of pain (including electrical nerve stimulation, acupuncture, sympathetic blockade, epidural and intrathecal blocks, and neurosurgical and psychological biofeedback techniques) showed that the noninvasive procedure of relaxation and biofeedback had the greatest overall effect on pain.

Chemotherapy protocols that induce severe protracted nausea and vomiting are stressful for cancer patients, and the fear that may be associated with chemotherapy often outweighs other negative aspects of the cancer experience. Stoudemire, Cotanch, and Laszlo[106] showed that many of the associated side effects of chemotherapy could be managed through pharmacologic approaches and maintenance of hydration, in addition to reducing stress levels through emotional support and the use of behavioral relaxation techniques supported by EMG biofeedback. Recent research provides evidence that sensory-behavioral pretreatments can ameliorate radiation therapy-induced nausea and vomiting[110-113] and significantly diminish and in some cases eliminate pain in the cancer patient.[112-115]

MEMORY FUNCTIONING

Remediation of memory deficits through the application of biofeedback techniques has been found to be effective.[116] Thornton[116] studied electrophysiological functioning involved in memory while applying biofeedback techniques (ie, the individuals ability to alter EEG wave patterns) and determined that memory could be improved in all subjects performing auditory memory tasks (prose passages and word lists). EEG biofeedback interventions were designed to increase the value of specific electrophysiological variables related to successful memory function. Improvements ranged from 68% to 181% in the study participants as a result of the interventions.[116]

WOUND HEALING

A new area of treatment usage for biofeedback has recently been evaluated. A prospective, randomized study was conducted to determine the effect of biofeedback-assisted relaxation training on foot ulcer healing.[117] For patients with chronic nonhealing foot ulcers, medical care was combined with a standardized biofeedback-assisted relaxation training program in the experimental group. The intervention was designed to increase peripheral perfusion, thereby promoting healing. There was a statistically significant improvement in healing rate in the experimental (87.%[5]) compared to the control (43.8%) group. These findings may greatly influence the noninvasive, conservative approaches employed in the treatment of chronic nonhealing wounds in the future.

COGNITIVE FUNCTION

Recent research shows that neurofeedback is an effective EEG biofeedback technique for training individuals with cognitive disorders via operant conditioning. It is of interest that biofeedback has been shown to have a positive effect on improving cognitive function in the elderly.[123]

VISUAL ACUITY

Visual acuity has also been shown to be affected by biofeedback, which could have tremendous implications for many individuals as we age. Persons with visual acuity problems caused by different ocular disorders, including macular degeneration, myopic macular degeneration, and presbyopia, underwent visual rehabilitation with an instrument for biofeedback. Visual acuity was found to improve.[124]

Summary

As a literate civilization, we are now more than 5000 years old. Physical needs have always kept the mind well occupied. Technologies have granted us a comfortable control over our environment. Yet, these technologies are costly. It is clear that medical problems can be caused by or aggravated by the mental status of the individual. Understanding this, it is an intriguing paradox that Western medicine has created in its concentrated efforts on developing extensive drugs and elaborate surgical techniques to deal with physical and mental compensations. With the evolution of Managed Care, the trend needs now to seek less costly alternative of care. This involves reaching inward and developing technologies which will allow us some insight into our inner world. It is time to equal the balance and attempt to solve some of the physical manifestations of pathologies from within.

Biofeedback has shown a remarkably positive benefit on the functional and treatment outcomes of numerous conditions.[121,122] Biofeedback instrumentation has been a growing part of physical therapy practice for over 20 years,[118] and physical therapists have contributed to researching its efficacy in treating varying conditions. Sophisticated contemporary equipment does much more in quantifying biofeedback techniques' worth than was originally envisioned. The importance of relating quantified movement-based data to functional measures has influenced the level of appropriate reimbursement for physical therapy services utilizing biofeedback. Physical therapy, as a integral member of the medical community, needs to continue to investigate self-awareness and self-control as a probable rehabilitative tool in the treatment of a multitude of conditions.

References

1. Ford CW. *Where Healing Waters Meet*. Barrytown, NY: Station Hill Press; 1989.
2. Peper E, ed. *Mind/Body Integration: Essential Readings in Biofeedback*. New York, NY: Plenum; 1979.
3. Chandler C, Bodenhamer-Davis E, Holden JM, Evenson T, Bratton S. Enhancing personal wellness in counselor trainees using biofeedback: an exploratory study. *Appl Psychophysiol Biofeedback*. 2001;26(1):1-7.
4. Duffy FH. The state of EEG biofeedback therapy (EEG operant conditioning) in 2000: an editor's opinion. *Clin Electroencepablogr*. 2000;31(1):v-vii.
5. Wirth DP, Barrett MJ. Complementary healing therapies. *International Journal of Psychosomatics*. 1994;41(1-4):61-67.
6. Wolf SL. From tibialis anterior to Tai Chi: biofeedback and beyond. *Appl Psycholphysiol Biofeedback*. 2001;26(2):155-74.
7. Critchley HD, Melmed RN, Featherstone E, Mathias CJ, Dolan RJ. Brain activity during biofeedback relaxation: a functional neuroimaging investigation. *Brain*. 2001;124(Pt 5):1003-1112.
8. Evetovich TK, Conley DS, Todd JB, Rogers DC, Stone TL. Effect of mechanomyography as biofeedback method in enhance muscle relaxation and performance. *J Strength Cond Res*. 2007;21(1):96-99.
9. Sheffied MM. Psychosocial interventions in the management of recurrent headache disorders: policy considerations for implementation. *Behavioral Medicine*. 1994;20(2):73-77.
10. Penzien DB, Holroyd KA. Psychosocial interventions in the management of recurrent headache disorders: description of treatment techniques. *Behavioral Medicine*. 1994;20(2):64-73.
11. Kaushik R, Kaushik RM, Mahajan SK, Rajesh V. Biofeedback assisted diaphragmatic breathing and systematic relaxation versus propranolol in long term prophylaxis of migraine. *Complement Ther Med*. 2005;13(3):165-174.
12. Arena JG, Bruno GM, Hannah SL, Meador KJ. A comparison of frontal electromyographic biofeedback training, trapezius electromyographyc biofeedback, and progressive muscle relaxation therapy in the treatment of tension headache. *Headache*. 1995;35(7):411-419.
13. Grazzi L, Bussone G. Italian experience of electromyographic-biofeedback treatment of episodic common migraine: preliminary results. *Headache*. 1993;33(8):439-441.
14. Blanchard EB. Psychological treatment of benign headache disorders. *Journal of Consulting & Clinical Psychology*. 1992;60(4):537-551.
15. Scharff L, Marcus DA, Masek BJ. A controlled study of minimal-contact thermal biofeedback treatment in children with migraine. *J Pediatric Psychol*. 2002;27(2):109-119.
16. Sarafino EP, Goehring P. Age comparisons in acquiring biofeedback control and success in reducing headache pain. *Ann Behav Med*. 2000;22(1):10-16.
17. Mishra KD, Gatchel RJ, Gardea MA. The relative efficacy of three cognitive-behavioral treatment approaches to temporomandibular disorders. *J Behav Med*. 2000;23(3):293-309.
18. Crider AB, Glaros AG, Gevirtz RN. Efficacy of biofeedback-based treatments for temporomandibular disorders. *J Appl Psychophysiol Biofeedback*. 2005;30(4):333-345.
19. Foster PS. Use of the Calmset 3 biofeedback/relaxation system in the assessment and treatment of chronic nocturnal bruxism. *J Appl Psychophysiol Biofeedback*. 2004;29(2):141-147.
20. Klose KJ, Needham BM, Schmidt D, Broton JG, Green BA. An assessment of the contribution of electromyographic biofeedback as an adjunct in the physical training of spinal cord injured persons. *Arch Phys Med Rehabil*. 1993;74(5):453-456.
21. Moore S, Woollacott MH. The use of biofeedback devices to improve postural stability. *Physical Therapy Practice*. 1993;2(20):1-19.
22. van Dijik H, Hermens HJ. Artificial feedback for remotely supervised training of motor skills. *J Telemed Telecare*. 2006;12 Suppl 1:50-52.
23. Allum JH, Carpenter MG. A speedy solution for balance and gait analysis: angular velocity measured at the centre of body mass. *Curr Opin Neurol*. 2005;18(1):15-21.

24. Wong MS, Mak AF, Luk KD, Evans JH, Brown B. Effectiveness of audio-biofeedback in postural training for adolescent idiopathic scoliosis patients. *Prosthet Orthot Int.* 2001;25(1):60-70.

25. Wolf SL, Binder-MacLeod SA. Electromyographic biofeedback applications to the hemiplegic patient. *Phys Ther.* 1983;63:1404-1413.

26. Hahn A, Sejna I, Stolbova K, Cocek A. Visuo-vestibular biofeedback in patients with peripheral vestibular disorders. *Acta Otolaryngol Suppl.* 2001;545:88-91.

27. Nashner LM, Shumway-Cook A, Marin O. Stance posture control in select groups of children with cerebral palsy—deficits in sensory organization and muscular coordination. *Exp Brain Res.* 1983;49:393-409.

28. Woolridge CP, Russell G. Head position training with the cerebral palsied child—an application of biofeedback techniques. *Arch Phys Med Rehabil.* 1976;57(4):407-414.

29. Shumway-Cook A, Anson D, Haller S. Postural sway biofeedback—its effect on reestablishing stance stability in hemiplegic patients. *Arch Phys Med Rehabil.* 1988;69(3);395-400.

30. Leplow B, Schluter V, Ferstl R. A new procedure for assessment of proprioception. *Perceptual & Motor Skills.* 1992;74(1):91-98.

31. Howard S, Varley R. Using electropalatography to treat severe apraxia of speech. *European Journal of Disorders of Communication.* 1995;30(2):246-255.

32. Heller F, Beuret-Blanquart F, Weber J. Postural biofeedback and locomotion reeducation in stroke patients. *Ann Readapt Med Phys.* 2005;48(4):187-195.

33. Sunderland A, Tinson DJ, Bradley EL, et al. Enhanced physical therapy improved recovery of arm function after stroke. A randomized controlled trial. *J Neurol Neurosurg Psychiatry.* 1992;55(7):530-535.

34. Moreland J, Thomson MA. Efficacy of electromyographic biofeedback compared with conventional physical therapy for upper-extremity function in patients following stroke: a research overview and meta-analysis. *Phys Ther.* 1994;74(6):534-547.

35. Edwards CL, Sudhakar S, Scales MT, et al. Electromyographic (EMG) biofeedback in the comprehensive treatment of central pain and ataxic tremor following thalamic stroke. *Appl Psychophysiol Biofeedback.* 2000;25(4):229-240.

36. Bisson E, Contant B, Sveistrup H, Lajoie Y. Functional balance and dual-task reaction times in older adults are improved by virtual reality and biofeedback training. *Cyberpsychol Behav.* 2007;10(1):16-23.

37. Chow CH, Cheng CT. Quantitative analysis of the effects of audio biofeedback on weight-bearing characteristics of persons with transtibial amputation during early prosthetic ambulation. *J Rehabil Res Dev.* 2000;37(3):255-260.

38. Petrofsky JS. The use of electromyograms biofeedback to reduce Trendenlenberg gait. *Eur J Appl Physiol.* 2001;85(5):491-495.

39. Thomas RE, Vaidya SC, Herrick RT, Congleton JJ. The effects of biofeedback on carpal tunnel syndrome. *Ergonomics.* 1993;36(4):353-361.

40. Nord S, Ettare D, Drew D, Hodge S. Muscle learning therapy—efficacy of biofeedback based protocol in treating work-related upper extremity disorders. *J Occup Rehabil.* 2001;11(1):23-31.

41. Reynolds C. Electromyographic biofeedback evaluation of a computer keyboard operator with cumulative trauma disorder. *J Hand Ther.* 1994;7(1):25-27.

42. Deepak KK, Behari M. Specific EMG biofeedback for hand dystonia. *J Appl Psychophysiol Biofeedback.* 1999;24(4):267-280.

43. Palmerund G, Kadefors R, Sporrong H, et al. Voluntary redistribution of muscle activity in human shoulder muscles. *Ergonomics.* 1995;38(4):806-815.

44. Young MS. Electromyographic biofeedback use in the treatment of voluntary posterior dislocation of the shoulder: a case study. *J Orthop Sports Phys Ther.* 1994;20(3):171-175.

45. Kirnap M, Calis M, Turgut AO, Halici M, Tuncel M. The efficacy of EMG-biofeedback training on quadriceps muscle strength in patients after arthroscopic menisectomy. http://www.nzma.org.nz/journal/118-1224/1704/. Accessed July 2, 2008.

46. Kranitz L, Lehrer P. Biofeedback applications in the treatment of cardiovascular diseases. *Cardiol Rev.* 2004;12(3):177-181.

47. Leisman G, Zenhausern R, Ferentz A, Tefera T, Zemcov A. Electromyographic effects of fatigue and task repetition on the validity of estimates of strong and weak muscles in applied kinesiological muscle-testing procedures. *Percept Mot Skills.* 1995;80(3 Pt 1):963-977.

48. Baranski S, Markiewicz L, Sarol Z. Physiological aspects of automatic physical training control by biofeedback in weightlessness. *Life Sci Space Res.* 1980;18(1):169-173.

49. Duckett S, Kramer T. Managing myoclonus secondary to anoxic encephalopathy through EMG biofeedback. *Brain Injury.* 1994;8(2):185-188.

50. Guercio JM, Ferguson KE, McMorrow MJ. Increasing functional communication through relaxation training and neuromuscular feedback. *Brain Injury.* 2001;15(12):1073-1082.

51. Kwolek A, Pop T. [Use of Biological Vicarious Biofeedback in the Rehabilitation of Patients with Brain Damage] [Polish]. *Neurologia I Neurochirurgia Polska.* 1992;Suppl 1:321-327.

52. Thatcher RW. EEG operant conditioning (biofeedback) and traumatic brain injury. *Clin Electroencephalogr.* 2000;31(1):38-44.

53. Jones KR. Ambulatory bio-feedback for stress incontinence exercise regimes: a novel development of the perineometer. *J Advanced Nursing.* 1994;19(3):509-512.

54. Teunissen TA, de Jong A, van Weel C, Lagro-Janssen AL. Treating urinary incontinence in the elderly—conservative therapies that work: a systematic review. *J Fam Pract.* 2004;53(1):25-30.

55. McIntosh LJ, Frahm JD, Mallett VT, Richardson DA. Pelvic floor rehabilitation in the treatment of incontinence. *J Reprod Med.* 1993;38(9):662-666.

56. Brubaker L, Kotarinos R. Kegel or cut? Variations on his theme. [Review] *J Reprod Med.* 1993; 38(9):672-678.

57. Stern RM, Vitellaro K, Thomas M, Higgins SC, Koch KL. Electrogastrographic biofeedback: a technique for enhancing normal gastric activity. *Neurogastroenterol. Motil.* 2004;16(6):753-757.

58. Bosshard W, Dreher R, Schnegg JF, Bula CJ. The treatment of chronic constipation in elderly people: an update. *Drugs Aging.* 2004;21(14):911-930.

59. Rayome RG, Johnson V, Gray M. Stress urinary incontinence after radical prostatectomy. *J Wound Ostomy Continence Nurs.* 1994;21(6):264-269.

60. Milam DF, Franke JJ. Prevention and treatment of incontinence after radical prostatectomy. [Review] *Seminars in Urologic Oncology.* 1995;13(3):224-237.

61. Smith DA, Newman DK. Basic elements of biofeedback therapy for pelvic muscle rehabilitation. *Urol Nurs.* 1994; 14(3):130-135.

62. Glazer HI, Rodke G, Sencionis C. Hertz R, Young AW. Treatment of vulvar vestibulitis syndrome with electromyographic biofeedback of pelvic floor musculature. *J Reprod Med.* 1995;40(4):283-290.

63. Weatherall M. Biofeedback in urinary incontinence: past, present, and future. *Clin Opin Obstet Gynecol.* 2000;12(5):411-413.

64. Pages IH, Jahr S, Schaufele MK, Conradi E. Comparative analysis of biofeedback and physical therapy for treatment of urinary stress incontinence in women. *Am J Phys Med Rehabil.* 2001;80(7):494-502.

65. Floratos DL, Sonke GS, Rapidou CA, et al. Biofeedback vs verbal feedback as learning tools for pelvic muscle exercises in the early management of urinary incontinence after radical prostatectomy. *BJU Int.* 2002;89(7):714-719.

66. Tariq SH, Morley JE, Prather CM. Fecal incontinence in the elderly patient. *Am J Med.* 2003;115(3):217-227.

67. Anonymous. Anismus and biofeedback. [editorial] *Lancet.* 1992;339(8787):217-218.

68. Ferrara A, De Jesus S, Gallagher JT, et al. Time-related decay of the benefits of biofeedback therapy. *Tech Coloproctol.* 2001;5(3):131-135.

69. Emmanuel AV, Kamm MA. Response to a behavioral treatment, biofeedback, inconstipated patients is associated with improved gut transit and autonomic innervation. *Gut.* 2001;49(2):214-219.

70. Norton C, Chelvanayagam S. Methodology of biofeedback for adults with fecal incontinence: a program of care. *J Wound Ostomy Continence Nurs.* 2001;28(3):156-168.

71. Heymen S, Jones KR, Ringel Y, Scarlett Y, Whitehead WE. Biofeedback treatment of fecal incontinence: a critical review. *Dis Colon Rectum.* 2001;44(5):728-736.

72. Chiarioni G, Bassotti G, Stanganini S, et al. Sensory retraining is key to biofeedback therapy for formed stool fecal incontinence. *Am J Gastroenterol.* 2002;97(1):109-117.

73. Lehrer PM, Vachillo E, Vaschillo B, et al. Biofeedback treatment for asthma. *Chest.* 2004;126(2):352-361.

74. Blanc-Gras N, Esteve F, Benchetrit G, Gallego J. Performance and learning during voluntary control of breath patterns. *Biol Psychol.* 1994;37(2):147-159.

75. Lehrer P, Vaschillo E, Lu SE, et al. Heart rate variability biofeedback: effects of age on heart rate variability, baroreflex gain, and asthma. *Chest.* 2006;129(2):278-284.

76. Lehrer PM, Smetankin A, Potapova T. Respiratory sinus arrhythmia biofeedback therapy for asthma: a report of 20 unmedicated pediatric cases using the Smetankin method. *J Appl Psychophysiol Biofeedback.* 2000;25(3):193-200.

77. Kern-Buell CL, McGrady AV, Conran PB, Nelson LA. Asthma severity, psychophysiological indicators of arousal, and immune function in asthma patients undergoing biofeedback-assisted relaxation. *J Appl Psychophysiol Biofeedback.* 2000;25(2):79-91.

78. Lehrer PM, Vaschillo E, Lu SE, et al. Heart rate variability biofeedback:effects of age on heart rate variability, baroreflex gain, and asthma. *Chest.* 2006;129(2):278-284.

79. McGrady AV. Effects of group relaxation training and thermal biofeedback on blood pressure and related physiological and psychological variables in essential hypertension. *Biofeedback & Self Regulation.* 1994;19(1):51-66.

80. Vasilevskii NN, Sidorov YA, Kiselev IM. Biofeedback control of systemic arterial pressure. *Neuroscience & Behavioral Physiology.* 1992;22(3):219-223.

81. Yucha CB, Tsai PS, Calderon KS, Tian L. Biofeedback-assisted relaxation training for essential hypertension: who is most likely to benefit? *J Cardiovasc Nurs.* 2005;20(3):198-205.

82. Saunders JT, Cox DJ, Teastes CD, Pohl SL. Thermal biofeedback in the treatment of intermittent claudication in diabetes: a case study. *Biofeedback & Self Regulation.* 1994;19(4):337-345.

83. Rice BI, Schindler JV. Effect of thermal biofeedback-assisted relaxation training on blood circulation in the lower extremities of a population with diabetes. *Diabetes Care.* 1992;15(7):853-858.

84. McGinnis RA, McGrady A, Cox SA, Grower-Dowling KA. Biofeedback-assisted relaxation therapy in type 2 diabetes. *Diabetes Care.* 2005;28(9):2145-2149.

85. Harden RN, Houle TT, Green S, et al. Biofeedback in the treatment of phantom limb pain: a time-series analysis. *J Appl Psychophysiol Biofeedback.* 2005;30(1):83-93.
86. Reyes del Paso GA, Godoy J, Vila J. Self-regulation of respiratory sinus arrhythmia. *Biofeedback & Self Regulation.* 1992; 17(4):261-275.
87. Vaschillo EG, Vaschillo B, Lehrer PM. Characteristics of resonance in heart rate variability stimulated by biofeedback. *Appl Psychophysiol Biofeedback.* 2006;31(2):129-142.
88. Blumenstein B, Breslav I, Bar-Eli M, Tenenbaum G, Weinstein Y. Regulation of mental states and biofeedback techniques: effects on breathing pattern. *Biofeedback & Self Regulation.* 1995;20(2):169-183.
89. Montgomery GT. Slowed respiration training. *Biofeedback & Self Regulation.* 1994;19(3):211-225.
90. Lehrer PM, Carr P, Sargunaraj D, Woolfolk RL. Stress management techniques: are they all equivalent, or do they have specific effects? *Biofeedback & Self Regulation.* 1994;19(4):353-401.
91. Freedman RR, Keegan D, Rodriguez J, Galloway MP. Plasma catecholamine levels during temperature biofeedback training in normal subjects. *Biofeedback & Self Regulation.* 1993;18(2):107-114.
92. Van Zak DB. Biofeedback treatments for premenstrual and prementrual affective syndromes. *International Journal of Psychosomatics.* 1994;41(1-4):53-60.
93. Ernst LS. Opening the door—biofeedback and meditation. *Beginnings.* 2002;22(1):11-15.
94. Uhlmann C, Froscher W. Biofeedback treatment in patients with refractory epilepsy: changes in depression and control orientation. *Seizure.* 2001;10(1):34-38.
95. Rosenfeld JP. An EEG biofeedback protocol for affective disorders. *Clin Electroencephalog.* 2000;31(1):7-12.
96. Moore NC. A review of EEG biofeedback treatment of anxiety disorders. *Clin Electroencephalogr.* 2000;31(1):1-6.
97. Sarti MG. Biofeedback in dermatology. *Clin Dermatol.* 1998;16(6):711-714.
98. Allen JJ, Harmon-Jones E, Cavender JH. Manipulation of frontal EEG asymmetry through biofeedback alters self-reported emotional responses. *Psychophysiology.* 2001;38(4):685-693.
99. Trudeau DL. The treatment of addictive disorders by brainwave biofeedback: a review and suggestions for future research. *Clin Electroencephalogr.* 2000;31(1):13-22.
100. Sukthankar SM, Reddy NP, Canilang EP, Stephenson L, Thomas R. Design and development of protable biofeedback systems for use in oral dysphagia rehabilitation. *Med Eng Phys.* 1994;16(5):430-435.
101. Bryant M: Biofeedback in the treatment of a selected dysphagic patient. *Dysphagia.* 1991; 6(3):140-144.
102. Reddy NP, Simcox DL, Gupta V, et al. Biofeedback therapy using accelerometry for treating dysphagic patients with poor laryngeal elevation: case studies. *J Rehabil Res Dev.* 2000;37(3):361-372.
103. Segal B, Hunter T, Danys I, Freedman C, Black M. Minimizing synkinesis during rehabilitation of the paralyzed face: preliminary assessment of a new small-movement therapy. *J Otolaryngology.* 1995;24(3):149-153.
104. Segal B, Zompa I, Danys I, et al. Symmetry and synkinesis during rehabilitatin of unilateral facial paralysis. *J Otolaryngology.* 1995;24(3):143-148.
105. Ferrell BR, Ferrell BA. Easing the pain. *Geriatr Nurs.* 1990;11(4):175-178.
106. Stoudemire A, Cotanch P, Laszlo J. Recent advances in the pharmacologic and behavioral management of chemotherapy-induced emesis [review]. *Arch Internal Medicine.* 1984;144(5):1029-1033.
107. Foley KM. The treatment of pain in the patient with cancer [review]. *CA: a Cancer Journal for Clinicians.* 1986; 36(4):194-215.
108. Contanch PH. Relaxation techniques as an independent nursing intervention for onocology patients. [Review] *Cancer Nursing.* 1987;10(Suppl 1):58-64.
109. Filshie J. The non-drug treatment of neuralgic and neuropathic pain of malignancy. [Review] *Cancer Surveys.* 1988; 7(1):161-193.
110. Blum RH. Hypothesis: a new basis for sensory-behavioral pretreatments to ameliorate radiation therapy-induced nausea and vomiting. [Review] *Cancer Treatment Reviews.* 1988;15(3):211-227.
111. Moher D, Arthur AZ, Pater JL. Anticipatory nausea and/or vomiting [review]. *Cancer Treatment Reviews.* 1984;11(3): 257-264.
112. Schafer DW. The management of pain in the cancer patient. *Comprehensive Therapy.* 1984;10(1):41-45.
113. Burish TG, Jenkins RA. Effectiveness of biofeedback and relaxation training in reducing the side effects of cancer chemotherapy. *Health Psychology.* 1992;11(1):17-23.
114. Steggles S, Fehr R, Aucoin P, Stam HJ. Relaxation, biofeedback training and cancer: an annotated bibliography, 1960-1985. *Hospice Journal.* 1987;3(4):1-10.
115. Ahles TA. Psychological approaches to the management of cancer-related pain. *Sem Onocol Nurs.* 1985;1(2):141-146.
116. Thornton K. Improvement/rehabilitation of memory functioning with neurotherapy/QEEG biofeedback. *J Head Trauma Rehabil.* 2000;15(6):1285-1296.
117. Rice B, Kalker AJ, Schindler JV, Dixon RM. Effect of biofeedback-assisted relaxation training on foot ulcer healing. *J Am Podiatr Med Assoc.* 2001;91(3):132-141.
118. Wolf SL. The relationship of technology assessment and utilization. Electromyographic feedback instrumentation as a model. *Int J Technol Assess Health Care.* 1992;8(1):102-108.
119. McGrady A, Conran P, Dickey D, et al. The effects of biofeedback-assisted relaxation on cell-mediated immunity, cortisol, and white blood cell count in healthy adult subjects. *J Behavioral Medicine.* 1992;15(4):343-354.

120. Gruber BL, Hersh SP, Hall NR, et al. Immunological responses of breast cancer patients to behavioral interventions. *Biofeedback & Self Regulation.* 1993;18(1):1-22.

121. Cassetta RA. Biofeedback can improve patient outcomes. *American Nurse.* 1993;25(9):25-27.

122. Montgomery DD. Change: detection and modification. *Appl Psychophysiol Biofeedback.* 2001;26(3):215-226.

123. Angelakis E, Stathopoulou S, Frymiare JL, et al. EEG neurofeedback: a brief overview and an example of peak alpha frequency training for cognitive enhancement in the elderly. *Clin Neuropsychol.* 2007;21(1):110-129.

124. Biorgi D, Contestabile MT, Pacella E, Barieli CB. An instrument for biofeedback applied to vision. *Appl Psychophysiol Biofeedback.* 2005;30(4):389-395.

CHAPTER 12

YOGA THERAPEUTICS
AN ANCIENT PRACTICE IN A 21ST CENTURY SETTING

Matthew J. Taylor, PT, PhD, RYT

> *Yoga is the control of the fluctuations of the mind.*
>
> Patanjali's Yoga Sutra 1.2; c. 150 C.E.

The recent popularity of hatha yoga appropriately presents a dichotomy of its own. The term *hatha* is composed of two Sanskrit words, *ha*, which means sun, and *tha*, which means moon. The polarized nature of these two terms is a metaphor for the spectrum of reality that life presents to the human being. On one hand, the popularity has exposed many Westerners to this ancient psychospiritual practice who may never have had an opportunity to experience it. There are presently more yoga teachers in California than in all of India. Yoga is practiced in studios, corporate settings, sports facilities, and major hospitals. The physical performance bias of our culture obviously suggests a direct application in physical rehabilitation as well. The opposite pole in the spectrum is that while yoga is incorporated within the framework of our physically based, consumptive culture, it is now used to sell everything from pharmaceuticals to brokerage services. Yesterday's step aerobics instructor is now certified in 2 days as a yoga teacher.

While the popularity and commercialization might appear to jeopardize the heart of yoga, the quantum impact of the transformative nature of the practice is bound to remain after the market frenzy recedes. The true power of yoga lies not in slick, lithe, and limber glossy images, but within the classic definition above. Feuerstein's[1] review of the term yoga further reveals that technically, yoga refers to that enormous body of precepts, attitudes, techniques and spiritual values that have been developed in India for more than 5000 years. In other words, the physical postures and motor performance outcomes that characterize so much of yoga within our culture is actually a byproduct of what is more accurately described as a technology for the evolution of the mind or consciousness. The essence of yoga is the experiential bridge it provides to the mind-body science, as described in Davis and Pert earlier in this book. The emerging awareness by Western science of the mind-body connection is actually a rediscovery of what has been the basis of the practice of yoga for thousands of years. A brief overview and history of yoga will set the stage for further discussion and potential application of yoga within the rehabilitation professions.

Table 12-1	PATANJALI'S EIGHT-FOLD PATH	
PATH	*DESCRIPTION*	
Yama	Moral precepts: nonharming, truthfulness, nonstealing, chastity, greedlessness	
Niyama	Qualities to nourish: purity, contentment, austerity (exercise), self-study, devotion	
Asana	Postures/movements: a calm, firm, steady stance in relation to life	
Pranayama	Breathing exercises: the ability to channel and direct breath and life energy	
Pratyahara	Decreased reactivity to sensation: focusing on senses inward, non-reactivity to stimuli	
Dharana	Concentration	
Dhyana	Meditation	
Samadhi	Ecstatic union, flow, "in the zone," spiritual support/connection	

Overview

The elements of yoga that directly address health concerns are known as yoga therapeutics and have been developed through the millennia. The Ayurvedic medical system of India and yoga therapeutics share many commonalties in their development to include a rich, allegorical language (ie, earth, ether, chakra, prana, etc) that is employed to this day. While these terms sound foreign to Western-trained medical professionals, closer examination reveals some striking similarity in their descriptions of disease and health.

The term yoga is derived from the Sanskrit verb yuj, meaning to yoke or unite, as in uniting the body, mind, and spirit. This union is achieved through various methods and technologies that include the familiar postures. A complete classic yoga practice (Table 12-1) has eight components that equate to moral restraints, personal behavioral observances, postures, regulation of breath, drawing the senses inward, concentration, and meditation.

Over time, this complete yoga practice results in increased strength, balance, stamina, flexibility, and relaxation.[2-5] These outcomes can be achieved without the occasional stereotypes that yoga requires bizarre body positions and occult religious practices. Simple body movements (*asanas*) done with mindfulness and attention achieve the outcomes without pain or extremes of range of motion (ROM). Yoga, as a life science philosophy, also makes no statement about any specific religious practice or spiritual belief and can be used to support all major faith traditions. The comprehensive approach of yoga (Table 12-1) can be likened to the widely embraced, present-day self-development theories that extol the virtues of the marketing theme "Body-Mind-Spirit."

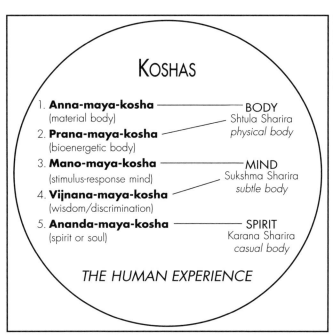

Figure 12-1. The Kosha and Sharira model. (Adapted with permission from Taylor MJ. What is health and illness? In: Taylor MJ, ed. *Integrating Yoga Therapy into Rehabilitation.* Embug, IL: Galena; 1999:15.)

The Yoga Therapy Health Model

Yoga therapy is a broad philosophical model of health based on the human experience; as such, it is a powerful tool in linking the historical "parts" paradigm to the quantum or integral model of human movement. This model was developed in an Eastern culture that used concrete images (bodies, sheaths, etc) to describe what was understood to actually be an interwoven, indivisible whole—or in Western terminology, quantum reality. The yoga model of health includes all dimensions of the patient's human experience and traces back c. 3000 to 4000 years to the Taittiriya-Upanishad, which hints at the Vedanta doctrine of the sheaths or koshas.[1] The koshas are illustrated in Figure 12-1, denoting layers or envelopes of reality within the realm of the patient's experience. Figure 12-1 illustrates how centuries later these sheaths were organized into three shariras (bodies) summarized as the body, mind, and spirit, or "physical, subtle, and causal bodies" in yogic terminology.[6] The modern-day clinical translations of the koshas are listed in Table 12-2.

These bodies, beginning with the physical level, by definition are progressively more subtle to perceive. Physical therapy training and practice focuses primarily on the first two levels, but addresses all five. Koshas may be better understood by the example of a patient with multiple sclerosis having an acute exacerbation of increased spasticity (first kosha) creating a bioenergetic hypertonicity (second kosha), triggering the pain cycle, functional self-consciousness, and varied emotional reactions (third kosha), making creativity, focus, and compassion challenging (fourth kosha) while generally sapping spirit, sense of support, and enthusiasm (fifth kosha). Clinically, this can also manifest as the opposite experience where the therapist senses that a physical impairment's etiology is the result of one or more other koshas such as fear, depression, or inappropriate stress/energy management.[7]

The yogic model of health describes health as balance and awareness within a free-flowing systemic interaction between all five of the allegorically porous, "thin" sheaths. Theoretically, imbalance or absence of awareness at any of the five levels results in dysfunction or disease, manifesting either directly or indirectly in one or more of the koshas. The holistic/quantum view also maintains that no rehabilitation condition exists, impacts, or results as a consequence of a single kosha level and, thus, thorough care must include consideration at each level.[6] A metatarsal

Table 12-2		
CLINICAL TRANSLATIONS OF THE KOSHAS		
SANSKRIT	*COMMON NAME*	*DESCRIPTION*
Anna-maya-kosha	Food sheath	Comprised of the physical solid aspect of the person (ie, cells, organs, bones, joints, etc)
Prana-maya-kosha	Life force sheath	The bioelectric forces and breath are a portion of the prana; similar to "Chi" or "Qi" concepts in Chinese medicine.
Mano-maya-kosha	Thought/primitive mind sheath	Includes emotions, reactive thinking reflexes or subcortical function; is largely shared with the rest of the animal kingdom.
Vijnana-maya-kosha	Wisdom/higher mind sheath	Includes the higher cortical functions of reflection, intuition, planning, and creativity; not as developed in animals.
Ananda-maya-kosha	Bliss sheath	Sometimes equated to the soul or spirit of the patient.

fracture would appear to be a purely physical condition. If the fracture resulted from an angry kick into a wall, the holistic view would state that the condition was not healed or "whole" until the individual worked at other kosha levels to determine the source and reaction to the anger, and developed appropriate strategies for the future. The right mix of higher kosha imbalances may trigger the sympathetic condition of reflex sympathetic dystrophy syndrome, which presently defies reductionistic explanation.

How Do Yoga Therapists Use the Model?

Yoga therapists (YTs) are trained to identify barriers to optimal function, create strategies or environments for enhanced proprioception and function, and retest outcomes. Their practice includes the assessment of structure and faulty motor sequencing/recruitment, and the prescription of remedial solutions. YTs also understand closed-chain kinematics, anatomical detail, fine motor sequencing, and the use of supports and manual facilitation techniques in managing their patients. On the surface, these roles share much in common with the traditional rehabilitation therapists. It is the frame of reference of this yogic health model that differentiates the two practices.

YTs recognize that stress-related illness is an increasing phenomenon with many conditions creating stress for the patient, are exacerbated by stress, or stress is a significant antecedent factor.[8] The yogic model defines stress as separation, or the sympathetic response, brought on by an imbalance or lack of integrity between koshas or within a particular kosha. The YT considers positive outcomes, or health, to occur as balance or homeostasis is achieved through a parasympathetic response and an integration of all five koshas. Benson's "remembered wellness," including accessing earlier motor strategies and the placebo effect, are additional outcomes present in this model focused on health optimization vs a crisis- or pathology-based system.[8]

Consider a YT working with a patient with hemiplegia post cerebrovascular accident (CVA). A CVA presents by definition as a physical (first kosha) disruption of circulation. However, in addition to the physical impairment, if the stroke was preceded by an episode or pattern of rage, anger, or depression, the holistic view would say the condition was not healed or "whole" until the individual worked at other kosha levels to determine the source and reaction to the emotion and developed appropriate strategies for the future. As such, the therapist will select interventions for both the current conditions and prophylactically since the subtler imbalances will also be addressed.

Clinically, the YT's assessment of the patient is composed of various stress or kosha-imbalanced factors, and the treatment goals generally include measurable relaxation phenomena. The YT assesses first and second kosha imbalances such as spasticity, low tone, guarding, decreased ROM and strength, splinting, thoracic/chest breathing, poor balance, and hypertension. The assessment also encompasses the remaining higher kosha presentations such as anger, depression, lethargy, anxiety, and fear. The goals, or intentions in the yoga vernacular, are to create an environment in which the student becomes aware of the present imbalances, is offered options for responding to those imbalances, and then experiences change toward balance or health. Those changes might present as decreased spasticity, balanced affect, full diaphragmatic breath, enhanced postural balance, decreased impairment, increased functional mobility, and a sense of efficacy.

The YT also directly addresses the fact that beyond the host of functional challenges that patients face, many often face a review of their life in the presence of the disease, disability, and in some circumstances, end-of-life concerns. They may ask such questions as: Who am I? Did or do I make a difference? What is next? Can I handle it? What will become of me? All are very "spirit" (fifth kosha) oriented questions that impact the role of the YT and the movement system of the lower koshas. This reflection of spiritual searching by the patient demands a complementary approach in assisting the patient to identify, understand, and achieve his or her goals. The broad depth of yoga addresses these concerns: changing roles and level of function, shifts between independence and dependence, fears and anxieties, end-of-life concerns and questions, and a strong support of faith or spiritual tradition. Yoga therapeutics supports this stage of rehabilitation by offering expanded tools beyond the mechanical (first and second kosha) movement of exercise.

The YT then selects from the eight paths (see Table 12-1), techniques, and methodologies that have been observed to create an environment for reconciling the imbalances of the koshas. The attractive simplicity of yoga therapeutics to the rehabilitation professional is that all of the koshas can be accessed through the therapeutic rehabilitation skills of positioning, movement, and breathing without having to directly address the more esoteric paths of yoga.

The Stress/Relaxation Response Model

Dr. Herbert Benson of the Harvard Mind-Body Institute first coined the term relaxation response in the early 1970s while studying transcendental meditators.[8] Benson documented the ability of the meditator to consciously elicit the relaxation response. The relaxation response's physiological mechanism is not fully understood. The relaxation response elicited by yoga has been associated with the psychophysiological responses that inhibit pituitary-adrenal activity by significantly decreasing blood levels of cortisol during and somewhat after practice.[9,10] Further, a decrease in blood pressure readings and anxiety scores has been demonstrated in several studies, one to include children and adolescents.[11-16] Harte, Eifert, and Smith[17] studied the effects of running and meditation on beta-endorphin, corticotropin-releasing hormone (CRH) and cortisol in plasma, and on mood. They found similar changes in mood and increased CRH immunoreactiv-

Table 12-3

THERAPEUTIC ASSESSMENT AND TREATMENT GOALS

STRESS ASSESSMENT	*TREATMENT GOAL/RELAXATION RESPONSE*
Increased muscle tone	Normalized tone
Cardiovascular stress	Cardiovascular ease
Anxiety/panic	Calm/relaxed
Elevated blood pressure	Normalized blood pressure
Fear/pessimism	Confidence/optimism
Dependent/passive	Independent/active
Distracted	Focused
Angry	Tolerant
Depressed	Balanced affect
Guarded, splinting	Fluid, graceful
Off balance	Balanced
Low energy	High energy
Thoracic/chest breathing	Diaphragmatic breathing

Adapted from Taylor MJ. *Integrating Yoga Therapy into Rehabilitation*. Galena, IL: Embug; 1999:24.

ity, indicating CRH release could be achieved with meditation without the physical exercise of running. Women practicing yoga produced improvement on scales of life satisfaction, mood, and coping with stress, while decreasing scores in excitability and aggressiveness.[18]

Clinically, the rehabilitation therapist's assessment is composed of various stress-related factors, and the treatment goals generally include measurable relaxation phenomena, achieved by traditional therapy treatments, as listed in Table 10-3. The previously mentioned studies suggest potential benefit from yoga in reducing the stress response. A deeper examination of the physiology of yoga breath regulation and postures (asana) will stimulate critical evaluation of the forthcoming literature review.

The Tools of Pranayama and Asana

One of the first physiologic responses produced under stress is an increase in respiration rate and decrease in tidal volume, accompanied by a shift from a diaphragmatic pattern to upper chest breathing. Miller[19] provides a thorough summary of the psychophysiological effects of both breathing patterns. There are more than 100 different combinations of yoga breath regulation patterns. These are used in yoga as energy management tools to affect either the high-energy, anxious response to stress or the opposite, low-energy, withdrawn, depressed pattern.[6] Raju et al[20] demonstrated that subjects who practiced pranayama could achieve higher work rates with reduced oxygen consumption per unit of work and without increased blood lactate, as well as significantly lower resting blood lactate levels. The full practice of pranayama is a complex one requiring careful instruction by an experienced YT. For the purposes of this introduction, the focus will be on the establishment of breath awareness and facilitating a full diaphragmatic breath, well within the competence and ethical realm of the rehabilitation professional. The yoga health model maintains that by having the patient direct the thinking mind (third kosha) to sensing and moving with the breath, there is little opportunity for that thinking mind to worry, despair, or become distracted. The focus of the mind on the sensation of breath and movement reduces stress, or the sympathetic response, which the model postulates allows the autonomic nervous system to move toward homeostasis with an inherent facilitation of sensorimotor integration (SMI). Instructing patients in diaphragmatic breathing with the intention of eliciting the treatment goals (see Table 12-3) is not only supported by research, but is a simple, cost-effective form of yoga therapy.

Asanas, or postures, are the other yoga therapeutic tools that share much in common with the rehabilitation counterpart, therapeutic exercise. There are literally thousands of asanas to choose from to create an environment of mindfulness and kosha awareness. One definition of asana is that of a postural pattern created by deviating the head and trunk from the center of gravity and having the pattern maintained purposefully for a length of time, then released in a smooth and effortless manner.[21] This postural pattern is initiated slowly and with attention to internal sensation and maintaining a full diaphragmatic breath. These patterns are prescribed and ideally performed using a minimum amount of voluntary effort and a minimum expenditure of energy for its maintenance and adjustment. True asana is classically described as having the qualities of stability (sthira), ease (sukha), and effortlessness or minimized effort (prayant shaithilya).[1,22] An asana is not, however, a braced or artificially sustained "posture" or a "pose." An experimental electromyogram (EMG) study revealed that in an asana performed isometrically there is a 30% increase in heart rate over the initial resting rate compared to only a 6% increase over resting rate when practiced the yoga way (ie, effortlessly and with full awareness).[23]

Another helpful description of asana is that the final stage of an asana (the "picture" in the book) is achieved through a natural sequence of ministages challenging the patient from midline stability to distal control, restoring stability and motor sequencing to address both primary and secondary impairments. The YT considers that each ministage may create a potential temporary disequilibrium by deviating the position of the center of gravity relative to midline or the base of support. Progressing slowly, through all key components of functional movement along a continuum from the core, proximal to distal, toward the full postural pattern with symmetry along the midline to ensure each ministage is mastered through integration of the koshas.

From the yoga therapeutic perspective, asana is also an attitude that is psychophysiological in nature in which state of mind or mindfulness is of the utmost importance, hence linking the physical position with the higher koshas. Every asana has the potential to have an effect on each of the five koshas. The YT utilizes this understanding to facilitate system balance based on the assessed imbalances. Since yoga is an experiential philosophy, the author directs his students and patients, "Do not believe what is written; experience it." Try the following: sit in a slumped forward head sitting posture for 10 breaths and sense the joy and enthusiasm of the asana. Now contrast that with upright, heart open, and arms spread wide overhead, face soft for 10 breaths. Feel the attitudinal difference? Every asana contains some of those subtle experiences as well as the physiological responses that are discussed below.

The YT's neurophysiological rationale of yoga therapeutics has been documented by Taylor and Majmundar.[21] Briefly, the rationale is that performance in the human movement system is impacted by not only structure and physiology but is also influenced by emotional, psychological, and spiritual conditions. The increased perception of proprioceptive information, awareness of thoughts and emotions, decreased cortical activity, and the development of nonreactivity to physical sensation result in the attainment of positive functional outcomes. Classically, the functional goal of the yogi was the elimination of postural sway, and from this practice it is believed comes the objective measures of increased flexibility, strength, and balance/postural stability.

To bridge the language of the two traditions, consider this yogic interpretation of the following Western motor concepts. Such an appreciation also resolves the dilemma of how one might document and record yoga therapeutic interventions. The above-stated postural efficiency depends on well-integrated and counteracting postural reflexes. There must be highly coordinated action between numerous muscles and joints, as well as an adequate foundation of muscle tone. All the while, proprioceptors, exteroceptors, and visceroceptors convey moment-to-moment information of head and body position in space to the lower brain structures of the midbrain, cerebellum, basal ganglia, and reticular activating system (pons and medulla).[24] This maintenance of a postural pattern and the equilibrium of the body during movement or stability in the asana is performed subcortically as an autonomic nervous system function. Muscles, ligaments, and joints are stretched statically in a passive response to gravity during the ministage or maintenance phase of asana. There is minimum muscular contraction and minimal voluntary effort as the decreased cortical activity and inward focus allows for the integration of the tonic system responsible for postural control and stability. There should be minimal energy expenditure to avoid cortical stimulation and subcortical compensatory motor patterns. Muscle tone is regulated as the feedback from the various muscle spindle fibers (types Ia and II), as well as the Golgi tendon organs, are allowed to integrate both peripherally and subcortically in a balanced or homeostatic autonomic nervous system.[25] The general rehabilitation goal of posture is stability and equilibrium of the body mass for safe interaction with the environment.

Asanas are often practiced as pairs, known as counterposes.[26] Biomechanically, this creates balance by soft tissue lengthening, hyaline cartilage compression and distraction, and reversing intervertebral disc pressures and dural stretch. These counterforces are also delivered to the internal organs, composed of smooth muscle, or the glands of the endocrine system. The patient experiences the more subtle effects of the higher koshas through this counterbalance, bringing about a balance in emotions and the subsequent biochemical signatures of that balance. This mechanical stimulation, coupled with the relaxation response, is cited as one potential source of many of the nonmusculoskeletal benefits of yoga.[27]

Weaving the principles of yoga with neurophysiological terminology not only facilitates communication within the medical community, but creates an internal subjective reconciliation for the therapist between the hemispheric dichotomies of linear and circular understanding. For a thorough review of the physiology of mindful movement, the reader is referred to Bottomley's coverage of the topic in this text. The tools of asana and pranayama precede meditation, or in medical parlance, psychosensorimotor integration. For a review of the neurophysiology of meditation, the reader is referred to King and Brownstone's review.[28]

Literature Review

Despite thousands of years of "clinical trials," there is a limited amount of objective, outcomes-based research on yoga as it applies directly to rehabilitation. There is also the design problem of creating a sham yoga intervention, since any movement done mindfully and with focus on the breath is technically yoga. A classic asana is not necessary to bring about the relaxation response.[8]

The psychophysiological literature on yoga documents some of the effects of practice to include improved ideal body weight, body density, cardiovascular endurance, and anaerobic power over a 1-year period of time.[29,30] The effect of long-term combined yoga practice has demonstrated a significant decrease in basal metabolic rate in healthy adults as a proposed result of reduced arousal.[31] A recent study of a group of 287 college students confirmed other research studies reporting the positive effect of yoga on the vital capacity of the lungs.[32] A short-term study of 6 weeks confirmed increased aerobic power but demonstrated decreased anaerobic power.[23] Contrary to the Western aerobic prescription of sustained moderate exercise for increasing energy metabolism, yoga has been demonstrated to create an increased thermic effect that persisted greater than 90 minutes after practice.[29] In the elderly, yoga has been shown to decrease resting heart rate, increase VO_2 max, and increase parasympathetic baroreflex sensitivity.[11] A study of women found yoga increased their maximum work output and decreased O_2 consumption per unit of work.[33] A 6-month trial with seniors resulted in improved sense of well-being, energy, timed one-legged standing, and forward flexibility.[34] Yoga also induces a state of blood hypocoagulability with decreased fibrinogen; increased fibrinolytic activity, hemoglobin, and hematocrit; and prolonged activated partial thromboplastin and platelet aggregation time.[35] Could this suggest that preventative medical management of patients at risk for thrombosis and emboli benefit from these effects of yoga?

Finally, appropriate since it is the final asana of every yoga class, the relaxation pose of Shivasana has been demonstrated to significantly facilitate recovery from induced physiological stress compared to two other postures (resting in chair and resting supine posture).[36]

Orthopedics

A summary review of yoga application in orthopedics is available in Taylor and Majmundar.[21] Yoga as rehabilitative intervention gained national attention with Garfinkel et al's study on yoga for carpal tunnel.[37] Utilizing a random, single-blind, controlled trial, the subjects received 11 yoga postures and a relaxation twice weekly for 8 weeks. Controls wore a wrist splint to supplement their treatment. The yoga group had significant changes in improved grip strength (from 162 to 187 mmHg, p=0.009) and pain reduction (decreased from 5.0 to 2.9 mmHg, p=0.02), with no significant changes in the control group. The yoga group had significantly more improvement in Phalen sign (12 subjects vs 2 in control, p=0.008). The yoga group tended to improve, but without significant differences in sleep disturbance, Tinel's sign, and median nerve motor and sensory conduction time. As a preliminary study, the sample size and generalizability were limited.

A study on yoga as treatment for osteoarthritis of the hands demonstrated significantly decreased pain during activity, tenderness, and increased finger ROM.[38] Emphasis was placed on attention to respiration and upper body alignment. There were favorable, though not statistically significant, differences in the treatment group's hand pain at rest and hand function. It was also noted there were no reported exacerbations while performing the asana. In both of Garfinkel's studies, a majority of the postures chosen either maintained the local tissue in a functional midrange position or in end-range without substantial overpressure for soft tissue deformation. There is considerable focus on proximal kinesthetic chain biomechanics, with special emphasis on core alignment and opening the chest. The yogic interpretation would describe both conditions as energetic imbalances and point to balancing the metaphoric heart as well as the musculoskeletal alignment.

An Iyengar yoga practice for reducing the symptoms of osteoarthritis of the knee as a pilot study with a very small sample utilized a 90-minute Iyengar yoga practice, once weekly for 8 weeks.[39] After the 8-week intervention, participants reported a significant reduction in pain, physical impairments, and negative emotions associated with their condition. Of note by the authors, 6 of the 7 participants were obese, and they suggested this study demonstrates the feasibility of using yoga as an intervention with obese individuals.

A designed yoga program on age-related changes in gait in a healthy senior population included 19 healthy adults (62 to 83 years old), all new to yoga, who participate in an 8-week Iyengar yoga program (two 90-minute yoga classes per week) specifically structured for seniors and designed to improve lower body strength and flexibility.[40] Participants were also asked to complete at least 20 minutes of home practice on alternate days. The study examined pre- and postintervention changes in peak hip extension, average anterior pelvic tilt, and stride length at comfortable walking speed. Peak hip extension and stride length significantly increased, and there was a marginally significant trend toward reduced average pelvic tilt. Participants who completed the home yoga practices were more likely to show this improvement Both the frequency and duration of yoga home practice predicted changes in hip extension and average pelvic tilt, leading the authors to conclude that home practice is an important part of yoga interventions.

Energetically, yoga also describes right nostril breathing as stimulating and left nostril breathing as relaxing. The pranayama technique of alternate nostril breathing is a powerful balancing technique to produce homeostasis.[19] Over a 10-day period, grip strength in children was shown to improve 4.1% to 6.5% after participating in single nostril or alternate nostril breath regulation (pranayama) without lateralization to one hand or the other. There were no changes in the other two groups that maintained breath awareness or practiced mudras (hand positions that direct prana).[41]

The yogic goal of drawing the senses inward to enhance focus and concentration, dharana, points to many interesting sport- and function-specific tasks requiring optimal performance levels. Yoga meditation combined with balance board training produced an enhanced balance index comprised of balance time and error for 5-minute duration trials.[42] The comparison group utilized amphetamine, which resulted in deterioration of task performance. There may also be an application in the patient with concomitant mental or neurological trouble attending to a task, or lack of dharana.

How does yoga compare to traditional therapeutic exercise intervention and what can the technique achieve in the presence of acute spasm? In "normals," yoga has been demonstrated to produce a 58% decrease in EMG muscle activity below basal rate for males and females.[43] One descriptive study of asana-based exercises for low back pain offers a series of test protocols and assignment of asanas based on the results.[44] Greater than 70% of the participants reported significant improvement. There are a number of major design flaws and some anatomical inaccuracies in the figures presented. There was a nonstatistical report of correlation between compliance and those that reported no improvement. Adding the simple variables of attention to and synchronization of movement with breath to the plethora of hamstring flexibility studies may yield new information.

While not described as a yoga intervention, the release of the anterior pelvis prior to forward bends or straight leg raises (SLR) is common yogic practice. Clark et al demonstrated increased passive unilateral straight-leg raise with ipsilateral anterior thigh soft tissue stretch.[45] Both the authors and the commentary by Sahrmann are unable to explain the results based on strict biomechanics (first kosha). The yoga explanation points to second and third kosha issues of security, fear, and anger, with those biomechanical areas said to be the psychoneuroimmunology storehouses of that emotional energy. Opening those areas biomechanically is thought to allow for balance and integration of that energy, manifested as enhanced hip flexion or forward bending. Do these emotions exist in patients with acute or chronic low back pain? In the yoga model, there is almost always some emotional stored energy, even in "normals," providing an Eastern interpretation of a documented Western orthopaedic outcome.

Back Pain

Yoga therapy for back pain gained national coverage with the publication of Sherman et al's studying comparing viniyoga-style yoga, physical therapy-led exercise and a self-care book for chronic low back pain.[46] The subjects included 101 adults (66% women, mean age of 44) with chronic low back pain, the majority of whom had experienced pain for longer than 1 year, and had experienced pain for more than 45 of the past 90 days prior to entering the study. After 12 weeks, patients in the yoga group had better back-related function than patients in the exercise or education groups. Reports of pain were similar in all three groups. At 26 weeks, patients in the yoga group reported better back-related function and less pain. They concluded over 3 to 6 months, yoga appeared to be more effective than traditional exercise or an educational book for improving function and pain in patients with chronic low back pain.

In another study, Galantino et al found trends in improvement of balance, flexibility, decreased disability, and depression in their modified hatha yoga pilot study.[47] Elsewhere a study examined the effect of Iyengar yoga for people experiencing back pain for an average of 11.2 years.[48]

Participants in the 16-week yoga group reported on a variety of outcomes at baseline, the end of the 16-week intervention, and at a 3-month follow-up. The yoga practice was associated with significant reductions in pain intensity, functional disability, and the use of pain medication, at both the 16-week point and the 3-month follow-up. In another study, researchers from the Duke University Medical Center examined the benefits of a traditional Buddhist loving-kindness meditation for chronic low back pain.[49] Participants were randomly assigned to either the loving-kindness intervention or to standard care. Researchers assessed patients' pain, anger, and psychological distress before and after the intervention. The loving-kindness group showed significant improvements in pain and psychological distress, but the standard care group did not. In addition, the more that an individual practiced loving-kindness meditation on a specific day, the less pain he or she experienced that day, and the less anger experienced the following day. Interesting results bearing in mind this included only meditation, no exercise or asana.

Poststroke Hemiparesis

A preliminary investigation of a yoga-based exercise program for people with chronic poststroke hemiparesis lent support for improvement in impairments and mobility in this patient population.[50] The primary outcome measures for the four subjects were the Berg Balance Scale and Timed Movement Battery. The 8-week intervention consisted of 1.5-hour yoga sessions, two times per week in the subject's home. The authors concluded further investigation is warranted to examine the effects of yoga in this population.

Sleep

The effects of yoga postures, self-regulated breathing, and relaxation techniques of yoga on sleep in a geriatric population were compared to Ayurveda and a wait-list control.[51] The yoga group of 40 showed a statistically significant decrease in time to fall asleep, and increase in total number of hours slept (average increase 60 minutes) and in the feeling of being rested in the morning after 6 months. In addition to improving the participants' quality of life, being able to decrease dependence on pharmaceuticals and fewer times up at night may decrease risks for fall in this population.

Mood

Given that depression and anxiety are key factors in treating pain, how yoga might impact both is of interest to physical therapists. Significant reductions were shown for depression, anger, anxiety, neurotic symptoms, and low frequency heart rate variability in the 17 completers of one study.[52] Eleven of the completers achieved remission levels post-intervention. Participants who remitted differed from the nonremitters at intake on several traits and on physiological measures indicative of a greater capacity for emotional regulation. Moods improved from before to after the yoga classes leading to the conclusion that yoga appears to be a promising intervention for depression as well as being cost effective and easy to implement.

In another study on yoga and fibromyalgia, the yoga group showed significant improvements in depression compared to the control group.[53] This randomized controlled trial examined effects on depressive symptoms in 91 women with fibromyalgia who were randomly assigned to treatment (n=51) or a waiting list control group (n=40). Somatic and cognitive symptoms of depression were assessed using the Beck Depression Inventory administered at baseline, immediately post-program, and at follow-up 2 months after the conclusion of the intervention.

Pain Management

The effects of chemical dependence and affective disorders, particularly depression, in pain management is well documented.[54,55] The perception and management of pain is closely linked to the mind-body connection. Yoga has been demonstrated to decrease somatic complaints in normal females.[18] Shivasana or corpse pose (lying supine) proved to be an effective technique for alleviating depression and significantly increasing positive change.[56]

Kabat-Zinn reported large and significant reductions in mood disturbance and psychiatric disorders (third and fourth koshas) using simple asana and meditation. He also reported producing a greater than 33% decrease in pain in 65% of the chronic pain subjects, and 505 patients reported greater than 50% relief on the pain index.[57] Kabat-Zinn's *Full Catastrophe Living*[58] provides a thorough description of the methodology of breath and movement.

What is the mood change following therapeutic exercise compared to asana, and could it impact compliance to home programs? Berger and Owen reported men performing yoga reported significantly decreased tension, anger, and fatigue over those who swam.[59] They also noted that greater mood changes correlated positively with compliance to the exercise.

Wound Healing

While not directly examining wound healing, these studies suggest exciting possibilities in wound management.

There was a significant reduction in hyperglycemia and indexed decreases in oral hypoglycemia and oral hypoglycemic drugs required for 104 of the 149 noninsulin-dependent diabetics after 40 days of yoga therapy.[5] Would this carry over to insulin-dependent diabetics and what would the long-term effects be in both groups?

Ornish's work in increasing coronary end-artery circulation utilizing diet, exercise, yoga, and group support shifted the paradigm of progressive coronary disease in cardiology.[60] Would such a program produce changes in end-artery compromise in distal extremities at risk or with wounds? What if this was accompanied with the type of guided imagery, mindful breathing meditation used in conjunction with ultraviolet (UV) therapy that produced a nearly four times faster healing rate for psoriasis than the control group that had UV therapy alone?[61] Might yoga, with its relative low expense and minimal side effects, offer most wound patients additional interventions as simple as listening to a taped guided yoga mediation on a daily basis?

Balance and Fall Prevention

A preliminary study was completed by Majmundar, Troy, and Sabelman on yoga for postural control and fall prevention in the elderly (Matra Majmundar, OTR, personal communication, August 2001). Citing falling as a major risk factor in the aging population, they compared a control group to a group that performed yoga asanas and breathing over a 12-week period. Utilizing a Wearable Accelerometric Motion Analysis System (WAMAS) developed at the Department of Veterans Affairs Health Care System Rehabilitation R&D Center in Palo Alto, Calif, they were able to gather three-dimensional upper body acceleration data through a variety of standard balance tests, measured pre- and postexperiment. They found decreased postural sway in tandem (toe-to-heel) standing with eyes closed in the yoga-trained group. Participants in the yoga group also reported subjective functional improvements, including relief of arthritis pain, enhanced stair climbing, increased ease in rising from and sitting down on the floor, and decreased frequency of urination through the night.

Respiratory Conditions

It is well documented that yoga has a positive impact on the pulmonary and autonomic function of asthma patients.[4,5,62-65] Tandon found that yoga, when compared to standard physical therapy treatment for chronic obstructive pulmonary disease, produced symptomatic improvement and significantly increased the mean maximum work by 60.55 kpm, whereas no change occurred with physical therapy.[66] The use of various hand mudras, bhandas, kriyas, pranayama patterns, and sustained restorative postures that mobilize the thoracic spine and chest wall have been valuable yoga therapeutic tools for the author. These techniques are performed by the patient, easy to perform as a home program, and very comfortable.

Case Example

The following intervention illustrates the clinical nuances of a yoga therapeutic approach to therapy for a chronic orthopedic diagnosis of mechanical low back pain.

HISTORY

A 38-year-old male with a 10-year history of progressively severe episodes of central low back pain with acute debilitating lateral shifts was seen weekly for eight 60-minute visits—an initial evaluation with seven 1-week follow-up visits. He had received many physical therapy interventions over the years to include spinal mobilization, craniosacral/myofascial release, and many of the approaches from existing schools of spine management. He reported a high level of compliance to therapeutic exercises, as well as utilizing various postural supports such as rolls, wedges, and ergonomically designed seating. His primary complaints were intolerance to sitting greater than 30 minutes and inability to garden vigorously without 3- to 4-day acute exacerbations. Activity level included running 30 minutes, 5 days per week with quality shoes, postexercise stretching, and twice per week strength training with good form and moderate resistance. Secondary complaints included an inability to comfortably play with his children on the floor, fear of participating in nonlinear sports, and chronic stiffness across the entire lumbosacral region (fourth, third, and first koshas). He related two different 1-week episodes that required complete bed rest. He utilized over-the-counter nonsteroidal anti-inflammatory drugs (NSAIDs) at prescription dosages as needed. He had a comprehensive knowledge base of postural care, ergonomics, and adaptive positioning because of a background in physical rehabilitation and fitness. He verbalized concern over continued symptom progression leading to a need for surgical intervention and/or chronic pain (third kosha). Socioeconomically, he related a busy social life but with few close friends (fourth kosha), and no acute financial concerns, yet a constant focus on the performance and balances of his financial accounts (first kosha). When questioned about past experience with yoga or breathing exercises, he related that he had no prior instruction in either but had been to several Feldenkrais workshops on back pain.

EXAMINATION

Static examination of posture revealed minimal forward head posture, well-developed musculature, and normal spinal curves; foot posture was symmetrical with slight pronation bilaterally but with a well-maintained longitudinal arch, and he reported greater weightbearing along the medial heels. There was no postural shift, and hips and shoulders were level. Functionally, he moved freely and without pain. Forward bending in standing was limited to midtibia with flattened lumbar spine; back bending was smooth and within normal limits. Hamstrings were tight with left at 45 degrees in 90/90 supine and 50 degrees right. Hips had 25 degrees internal rotation left; 35 degrees right; hip extension was 5 degrees bilaterally. He was nontender to palpation and no active trigger points were identified. His gait was WNL but with very little anterior/posterior scapular or pelvic movement. In standing, he exhibited no discernible movement associated with breath (second kosha). His respiration was shallow, originated in the chest, and at a rate of 17 breaths per minute. There was no observable spinal, shoulder, or abdominal movement associated with the breath. He was observed to maintain the left hand in a closed position relative to his open right hand (third kosha). During conversation, he was observed to lean forward, appearing to almost strain to hear or comprehend (first three koshas). When questioned, he related maintaining his tongue firmly against his lower teeth. Running gait was forward leaning, short strides, and a flat, immobile spine with bracing across the shoulders. On attempted long sitting forward bend, the knees were bent with shaking quadriceps, collapsed across the chest, little breath, and excessive upper cervical extension.

ASSESSMENT

The focus of the assessment was on the trunk stiffness, the secondary impairments of lower quarter dysfunction, inefficient gait (first kosha), and primarily directed at the restricted breath pattern (second kosha). A yoga therapeutic approach balances physical (first kosha) interventions by including asanas that not only address that level, but also address the more subtle koshas to include restricted breath pattern (second kosha), concerns/fears of surgery/chronic pain (third kosha), and the bracing or fearful attitude suggested by the noted apprehensive postural patterns (fourth and fifth koshas).

INTERVENTIONS

To that end, over the eight visits he was instructed in both a diaphragmatic and a full three-part yoga breath, prone and supine. Recruitment early on was inconsistent, ratcheted, and frequently out of sequence with upper chest accessory activity and regular queuing to release the tongue, hand, and hips. He verbalized frustration at his inability to overcome the clumsiness and awkwardness of many of the standing and seated poses, necessitating constant reminders to ease up, engage the full breath, and utilize props or supports for comfort. He was reassured this was an almost universal initial experience. Maintaining core awareness and the relaxation response through the diaphragmatic breath, he was then instructed in a supine back of the leg stretch with a strap. Emphasis was placed on waiting for the breath (fifth kosha) and initiating all movement as a radiation or wave from the belly. The next progression was a standing supported lunge with chairs and blocks. Mountain and Warrior II followed, with emphasis on symmetric and complete foot contact broadening the breath from pelvic floor to throat. Again, he verbalized frustration at sequencing, but with hand and verbal cues sequencing improved steadily. He was cautioned against excessive upper cervical extension and chin thrust on standing forward bends. To address the lack of pelvic mobility (first and second koshas), he was instructed in a supported pigeon pose to open both hip rotators and flexors. The right side was well tolerated, though on the left he noted a deep ache within the posterior hip as well as a strong sense of anger/fear when reclining forward over the left knee for more than 20 seconds. He cooperated but stated dislike for legs up the wall as a restorative pose, but was unable to articulate why he did not enjoy the pose. During final relaxation, he reported difficulty maintaining attention, with distracting thoughts either rehearsing or remembering numerous other parts of the day, causing him to have difficulty maintaining concentration. Modifying guided imageries to a more active, physically based reference helped, as did instruction in a pranayama technique of alternate nostril breathing, as both tend to provide a grounding task for the mind, making reflective ideation more difficult to pursue. He was instructed to attempt a gradual increase in endurance by extending the number of breaths he maintained in each posture, but without shaking or other signs of striving. He was given written instructions each time a new asana was assigned and told to perform the exercises daily. Follow-up weekly eventually led to a 40-minute session 5 to 7 days per week, including a 10-minute final relaxation.

OUTCOMES

Subjective

At 8 weeks, he noted an increased awareness of how "small" or restricted his breath had been most of the time (second kosha) and a strong correlation of the breath to the sensation of stiffness in his back. He noted that the breath was both comforting and relaxing (third through fifth koshas). He had experienced no acute pain or postural shifts during the treatment period. His compliance had been high with at least five times per week. He related significant improvement in sitting tolerance to where a recent 5-hour drive had been symptom free (first kosha). Morning stiffness and post-sitting stiffness were rare, and when they did occur, they were less than 25% of the previous level. He noted increased awareness of both physical tension (tongue, hand, and back) corresponded with perception of emotions such as frustration, anger, and fear (third and fifth koshas). His running gait felt more efficient (first kosha), but he also noted the insight as to how in the past he went to run to get away from stress or to experience the post-exercise relaxation. Lately, he had become more aware of running when he wanted to move, rather than "away from or because of something else" going on in his life. He incorporated the breath work at night, especially early morning when sleep was difficult, and found it both comforting and restorative (third and fifth koshas). He reported being able to comfortably play board games on the floor and wrestle with his children without discomfort or fear.

Objective

Static examination of posture was unchanged but related full foot contact weightbearing. Forward bending in standing was to midankle with reversed lumbar curve. Hamstrings were left at 65 degrees in 90/90 supine and 70 degrees right. Hips measured 40 degrees internal rotation left; 45 degrees right. Hip extension was 10 degrees bilaterally. His gait was WNL with both anterior/posterior scapular and pelvic movement. In standing, he had discernible movement associated with breath (second kosha) through the abdomen, flanks, shoulders, and chest. There was no observable spinal, shoulder, or abdominal movement associated with the breath. He demonstrated a fluid, full three-part sequenced breath at 9 breaths per minute (47% decrease in rate). He was observed to maintain an open hand position (third kosha). During conversation he sat comfortably erect, but with a casual ease, not leaning forward and with a softer facial expression (first three koshas). On questioning, he related still catching himself maintaining his tongue firmly against his lower teeth, but presently his tongue had been resting in the floor of his mouth. Running gait was an erect, natural stride length and a more supple spine with natural swing across the shoulders. On attempted long sitting forward bend, the knees were bent slightly but with no shaking, a neutral spine with open chest, full breath, and neutral upper cervical spine.

DISPOSITION

He was directed to continue with the series while gradually increasing the number of breaths, not to skip the final relaxation, and to monitor his physical comfort in relation to emotional stressors. He was discharged to his home program and planned to continue active participation in the local yoga class.

Practical Applications of Yoga

How can yoga therapeutics be incorporated in a rehabilitation practice? Some methods of incorporating yoga therapy techniques into a practice that is practical, seamless, and can be implemented in an acceptable, conservative manner are listed in Table 12-4. As with the other traditions, utilizing yoga techniques has the ethical considerations of knowing one's limits, receiving appropriate training for competency dependent on the skill level of the technique, and marketing in such

Table 12-4

PRACTICAL THERAPEUTIC YOGA APPLICATIONS

THERAPEUTIC TECHNIQUE	RATIONALE
Breath assessment instruction (*Pranayama*)	Optimize the autonomic nervous system through the relaxation response
Verbal cues (*Asana*)	More imagery for proximal-distal sequencing and greater recall
Guided imagery/restorative yoga (*Meditation and Samadhi*)	Capture Benson's "remembered wellness" for motor patterns
Pre-post body scan (*Asana*)	Embody proprioceptive baseline and intervention effects
ADL instruction (*Asana*)	Create conscious movement awareness
Journaling (*Niamyas—self study*)	Explore, analyze, and deal with psychoemotional-stress issues
Clinic environment (*Niamyas—purity*)	Facilitate a mindful, introspective, and stress-reduced environment
Home programs (*Ansana*)	Create movement sequences that are whole body, core initiated for subtle awareness and increased compliance
Group therapy (*Yamas and niyamas*)	Economical, socially, and emotionally rewarding to address chronic needs
Therapeutic exercise (*Asana*)	Synchronized with breath, whole body, core initiated

a manner as to preserve the integrity of yoga therapeutics. Networking with a local YT will create both business opportunities and professional development for each party. Because yoga therapy is provided literally across the entire lifespan from neonatal to end-of-life care, there is a wide variety of program development possibilities through such a relationship. The YT can share through the use of props, straps, bolsters, and restorative yoga (supported postures that are maintained for extended lengths of time). Yoga therapy is very accessible for all levels of movement capacity.

The primary principles in Table 12-4 involve bringing the patient's focus and attention internally. This requires the patient to be attentive to the feedback or proprioception he or she is experiencing from all koshas and within his or her capacity to communicate or manage this feedback responsibly. The only prerequisite for participating in yoga therapeutics is to be breathing, so please consider how you may already be or may begin to utilize these yoga techniques with all of your patients.

PROFESSIONAL QUALIFICATIONS FOR YOGA INSTRUCTION

The rehabilitation professions are the branches of medicine that specialize in the functional human movement system and related pathologies. As a profession, they seek new related knowledge and create clinical application with outcome-based research. The licensing process and knowledge base of anatomy, kinesiology, and physiology (to include respiration) justify academic, legal, and ethical use of the yoga techniques of postures with breath awareness. In the United States, there presently are no standards or legal restrictions as to who may instruct yoga or practice yoga therapy.

Deciding if and when a rehabilitation professional is "qualified" to use yoga therapeutic techniques is not clearly defined. Just as with the worldview paradigm, there is almost always a gray, rather than a black or white, standard. The question of who is qualified to teach yoga is no exception. Points of reflection and consideration are:

1. Yoga is far more than just asanas and breath regulation.
2. Limiting the instruction to just postures and breath misses an opportunity to address the deeper health model issues of the spirit being the causal body, and as such, can those issues be supported in a traditional clinical setting?
3. Because yoga instructors share an expertise in movement and balance, are they practicing physical therapy?
4. What could be gained from a collaborative effort?

There are no easy answers to these points, but if held in awareness by practitioners, a rich potential exists for better serving patients and clients. The author's experience is that physical and occupational therapists possess academic knowledge and scientific rigor that is sometimes lacking in the yoga community. The yoga community's intimate kinesthetic awareness and skill, coupled with being able to address higher kosha issues through breath and movement, could facilitate rehabilitation outcomes. What follows is intended to initiate that bridge building (yoking or yoga) between the two paradigms.

THE BRIDGES

Just as there are barriers or obstacles at all kosha levels in assisting a patient to achieve rehabilitation goals, so too do barriers exist when we expand professional paradigms. The largest barrier in the author's experience is the misconception about the word yoga, which may necessitate using descriptors such as movement therapy, mindful exercise, stretch and relax, integrative medicine, and mind-body science as more acceptable terminology. Yoga as a spiritual vehicle or life science philosophy can often be misunderstood to be a religion or in conflict with an individual's religious beliefs. Originating from the Hindu tradition, it makes no direct claims about a specific deity or dogma and can be adapted to conform to all of the world's major religions.[26]

Documentation is another barrier addressed earlier in the asana section. Initially, documentation appears daunting, such as envisioning a code for pranayama. In the allegorical language, the YT may prescribe bhujangasana (cobra) with hands-on correction for release of the particular chakra determined to be out of balance. Generically, describing the intervention in traditional therapeutic jargon solves the charting, coding, and outcomes dilemma. The yogic principles are used independently or in conjunction with standard therapeutic tools. The example above becomes performing prone press-ups with posterior-anterior glides while verbally directing attention to synchronizing movement with the breath, which can be coded as directed therapeutic exercise, neuromotor re-education, manual therapy, or some combination of codes dependent on time and emphasis. The outcomes might be documented as increased ROM for a task-specific activities of daily living (ADL), increased sitting tolerance, etc.

Breath Assessment/Instruction

The breath is both a mirror of the individual's autonomic nervous system and a tool for direct modulation. It is a tool to maintain internal focus by the patient with such techniques as incorporating all movement in synchrony with the breath (ie, opening the front of the body with inhale and closing the front of the body with exhale through the sagittal plane), or by counting breaths rather than repetitions, necessitating the patient to maintain internal focus. Diaphragmatic breathing is a cost-effective, simple form of yoga therapy. Remember, the patient will model or entrain with the therapist's breathing pattern as well.

Verbal Cues and Language

Monitoring the patient's vocabulary is a "safe," conservative method of addressing the higher, subtler aspects of the patient. Word selection is a window into the patient's relationship with his or her body, illness, and overall health responsibility. Does the patient claim ownership of his or her body and current complaint? Does he or she speak in the first or second person? Who is responsible for him or her getting better? Remember to also change your verbal cues to correlate with the way the mind works by using more visual imagery and active language vs Western measurable instruction (soften vs relax, telescope vs reach, lengthen/inflate vs stabilize, etc). These cue changes seem to augment proximal to distal sequencing more fluidly than linear, component directions.

Guided Imagery/Restorative Yoga

Use techniques of visualization, music, and guided imagery/relaxation, particularly during passive modalities. Provide enough of a period of time for sensorimotor integration (SMI) to occur during and after interventions versus "rushing the patient out the door." Anatomical, regional, or diagnosis-specific audiotapes can reinforce proprioceptive and kinesthetic awareness. A portable audio player and an audio file make this an easy intervention. Instruct the art of relaxation versus the patient's typical distraction/recreation scheme as a means of allowing the body to move into a full relaxation response and its consequent SMI. Judith Lasater, PhD, PT authored a book, *Relax and Renew*,[67] which is a rich introduction to this art.

Pre-Post Body Scans

Insist that the patient form both a preintervention baseline of internal awareness or proprioception, followed by a postintervention comparison, allowing SMI to reach a cognitive level of appreciation. Five minutes sensing the breath in and out is as complicated and expensive as this gets! An axiom of yoga of unknown origin is, "They can't heal what they don't feel."

Activities of Daily Living Instruction

Acknowledging that rehabilitation or yoga is far more than what is performed on the mat or in the clinic, how does the therapist create mindfulness throughout the day? The key is to create increased emphasis on self-awareness during ADL that might include asking the patient to note the direction of the breath (inhalation/exhalation) through activities, the sensations involved at various aspects of the body during an activity, or the altering of movements based on a focus at various areas of the body (ie, "Sense the sensation in your shoulder and how it changes if you breathe in or out as you reach, or as you press down more firmly with the big toe, etc").

Journaling

The use of a personal journal, to include reflections on the patient's impairment and all other experiences, can be an excellent tool for broadening the patient's awareness of more subtle issues and also expanding the therapist's understanding of the patient's situation. Whether this journal is kept privately or shared with the therapist is up to the patient's discretion. The act of journaling, if encouraged, can become a powerful tool for the patient to develop a deeper mind-body connection and sense of responsibility for his or her own health.

Passive Modalities/Clinic Environment

The holistic approach can be as simple as turning off the TV or radio; utilizing art, music, and color tastefully; providing positive waiting room material; and a quiet, warm environment. From the waiting room to departure, attention to breath can be tactfully encouraged. During passive modalities, breath awareness and listening to guided imagery relaxation tapes rather than reading the outdated news magazine can deepen the relaxation response. Anatomical, region-specific tapes can reinforce proprioceptive and kinesthetic awareness. Kabat-Zinn, using mindfulness meditation and asanas, demonstrated an uncoupling of the sensory dimension of the pain experience from the affective/evaluative alarm reaction so often found in patients experiencing pain.[57] This could provide a powerful interruption of the pain-spasm cycle at a higher kosha level.

Home Programs

Asanas tend, by definition, to be whole-body exercise and, as such, generally do not require as many different forms. They can also be sequenced in a pleasant, functional flowing manner of progression called vinyasas rather than linear, calisthenic-type sections. There is some evidence that exercise that improves mood is positively correlated with compliance.[59] While not yet studied, fewer, more relaxing, and flowing movements may enhance patient compliance.

Therapeutic Exercise

Many of the therapeutic exercises traditionally prescribed resemble asanas in form. McKenzie exercises in physical therapy look very much like crocodile (prone-lying), sphinx (prone-on-elbows), cobra (press-ups), and initiation of the triangle (lateral glides).[3] Focus on breath, movement synchronized with breath, decreased perceived exertion, and therapeutic intention differentiate asanas from therapeutic exercise. Therapeutic progression is similar within the parameters of intensity and gravity modification. Counting by breaths for duration rather than repetitions facilitates attention. Disruption of a smooth, full breath signals need for modification of intensity.

Asanas are identified with creating certain effects on all of the kosha levels. Similar biomechanical stretches may have very different "attitudes" or "spirits." The verbal and tactile cues utilized make use of the mind's ability to think in image, motion, and color by being more colorful and image-oriented to enhance kinesthetic learning ("drift" vs "reach"; "soften and release" rather than "relax"). Yoga asanas have been integrated into other movement therapies because of their effectiveness and complement to SMI. There is aquatic yoga, yogassage (soft tissue work in sustained asana), and Eleanor Criswell's somatic yoga, which blends the work of Moshe Feldenkrais and yoga.[68]

Group Rehabilitation

The group setting of yoga has anecdotally produced numerous improvements in a wide range of health conditions. Chronic spinal pain, fibromyalgia, multiple sclerosis, osteoarthritis, and joint replacement are just a few of the group classes being offered. While this contradicts our detailed, patient-specific evaluation and treatment prescription, what is this phenomenon and can it be utilized? Ornish contends group support may be the single most important factor in his studies.[69] Would delivering therapy to a group of similar diagnostic codes be cost effective in making services more affordable to those dependent on discretionary funds, yet maintain revenue rates? As direct access and increased financial responsibility fall to the individual, this may be a valuable model for delivery of services.

Professional Networking

Establishing a working relationship with the yoga community offers many personal, professional, and business opportunities. The therapist who develops a personal practice enjoys the health benefits of yoga, increased kinesthetic awareness, and expanded teaching tools of technique and vocabulary. As experts in movement science, this ongoing, mindful motor practice enhances both entry-level and continuing education for professionals while providing a psychomotor learning base not available from reflective academic study.

Offering workshops in both the rehabilitation and yoga community on common topics like back pain or women's health, off-hour space utilization, the introduction of cash-based programming, and increased market traffic can be bottom-line enhancements to practice management. Referrals between the professions will increase as familiarity with each other's capabilities expands. Cooperative program development in ergonomics, stress management, pain management, osteoporosis, and numerous other shared clientele areas can lead to additional revenue streams in niche markets with seminar presentations, books, and instructional audio- and videotapes. As the field of psychoneuroimmunology expands and delineates how the body, mind, and emotions interact to impact movement, the rehabilitation professional who understands how asanas express all of the koshas will be well positioned to incorporate the emerging science. Rather than turf wars and a scarcity mentality, the worldview paradigm embraces such collaboration and partnering.

Conclusion

The profession of yoga therapy is a broad and ancient practice still evolving as it gains acceptance in the West. Sufficient evidence exists to warrant further scientific investigation of the breadth of yoga therapeutic properties as they apply to motor performance. Five thousand years of fieldtesting held under the rigors of Western science promises to bring additional knowledge to the healing arts. The knowledge held with the expanded vision of integrative medicine will yield an invaluable rediscovery heralding attributes of the 21st century, integral rehabilitation therapist.

Acknowledgments

Special thanks to Dr. Kelly McGonigal, PhD, editor of the *International Journal of Yoga Therapy* of the International Association of Yoga Therapists (www.iayt.org) for her assistance in the literature review and evidence search.

References

1. Feuerstein G. *The Yoga Tradition*. Prescott, AZ: Hohm Press; 1998.
2. Horak FB. Clinical measurement of postural control in adults. *Phys Ther.* 1987;67:1881-1885.
3. Iyengar BKS. The Tree of Yoga. Boston, MA: Shambhala; 1989.
4. Jain SC, Rai L, Valecha A, Jha UK, Bhatnagar SO, Ram K. Effect of yoga training on exercise tolerance in adolescents with childhood asthma. *J Asthma.* 1991;28(6):437-442.
5. Jain SC, Uppal A, Bhatnagar SO, Talukdar BA. Study of response pattern of non-insulin dependent diabetics to yoga therapy. *Diabetes Res Clin Prac.* 1993;19(1):69-74.
6. LePage J. *Integrative Yoga Therapy Training Manual*. Aptos, CA: Printsmith; 1994.
7. Taylor MJ. Yoga therapeutics in neurologic physical therapy: application to a patient with Parkinson's disease. *Neurology Report.* 2001;25:56.
8. Benson H, Stark M. *Timeless Healing: The Power and Biology of Belief*. New York, NY: Fireside; 1997.
9. Blackwell B, Bloomfield S, Gartside P. Transcendental meditation in hypertension. Individual response patterns. *Lancet.* 1976;1(7953):223-226.
10. Jevning R, Wilson AF, Davidson JM. Adrenocortical activity during meditation. *Horm Behav.* 1978;10(1):54-60.
11. Bowman AJ, Clayton RH, Murray A, Reed JW, Subhan MM, Ford GA. Effects of aerobic exercise training and yoga on the baroreflex in healthy elderly persons. *Eur J Clin Invest.* 1997;27(5):443-9.
12. Platania-Solazzo A, Field TM, Blank. Relaxation therapy reduces anxiety in child and adolescent psychiatric patients. *Acta Paedopsychiatrica.* 1992;55(2):115-120.
13. Sahasi G, Mohan D, Kacker C. Effectiveness of yogic techniques in the management of anxiety. *J Pers.* 1989;5(1):51-55.

14. Miller JJ, Fletcher K, Kabat-Zinn J. Three-year follow-up and clinical implications of a mindfulness meditation-based stress reduction intervention in the treatment of anxiety disorders. *General Hospital Psychiatry.* 1995;17(3):192-200.

15. Murugesan R, Govindarajulu N, Bera TK. Effect of selected yogic practices on the management of hypertension. *Indian J Physiol Pharmacol.* 2000;44(2):207-210.

16. Grossman E, Grossman A, Schein MH, Zimlichman R, Gavish B. Breathing control lowers blood pressure. *J Hum Hypertens.* 2001;15(4):263-269.

17. Harte JL, Eifert GH, Smith R. The effects of running and meditation on beta-endorphin, corticotropin-releasing hormone and cortisol in plasma, and on mood. *Biol Psychol.* 1995;40(3):251-265.

18. Schell FJ, Allolio B, Schonecke OW. Physiological and psychological effects of hatha-yoga exercise in healthy women. *Int J Psychosom.* 1994;41(1-4):46-52.

19. Miller R. The psychophysiology of respiration: Eastern and Western perspectives. *Journal of the International Association of Yoga Therapists.* 1991;2(1):8-23.

20. Raju PS, Madhavi S, Prasad KV, et al. Comparison of effects of yoga & physical exercise in athletes. *Indian J Med Res.* 1994;100:81-86.

21. Taylor MJ, Majmundar M. Incorporating yoga therapeutics into orthopedic physical therapy. *Ortho Phys Ther Clinics N Amer.* 2000;9(3):341-360.

22. Iyengar BKS. *Light on Yoga.* New York, NY: Shocken; 1976.

23. Balasubramanian B, Pansare MS. Effect of yoga on aerobic and anaerobic power of muscles. *Indian J Physiol Pharmacol.* 1991;35(4):281-282.

24. Allum B, Hulliger M. Afferent control of posture and locomotion. *Progress in Brain Research.* New York: Elsevier; 1989.

25. Werner JK. *Neuroscience: A Clinical Perspective.* Philadelphia, PA: WB Saunders; 1980.

26. Desikachar TKV. *The Heart of Yoga.* Rochester, NY: Inner Traditions; 1995.

27. Monro R, Nagarathna R, Nagendra HR. *Yoga for Common Ailments.* New York: Simon & Schuster; 1990.

28. King R, Brownstone A. Neurophysiology of yoga meditation. *International Journal of Yoga Therapy.* 1999;9:9-17.

29. Agte V, Chiplonkter S. Thermic responses to vegetarian meals and yogic exercise. *Ann Nutr Metab.* 1992;36:3.

30. Malathi A, Damodaran A, Iyar N, Patel L. Effect of yogic training on body composition and physical fitness. *Physiotherapy: The Journal of the Indian Association of Physiotherapists.* 1999;1:19-23.

31. Chaya MS, Kurpad AV, Nagendra HR, Nagarathna R. The effect of long term combined yoga practice on the basal metabolic rate of healthy adults. *BMC Complementary and Alternative Medicine.* 2006:6:28.

32. Birkel DA, Edgren L. Hatha yoga: improved vital capacity of college students. *Altern Ther Health Med.* 2000;6(6):55-63.

33. Raju PS, Prasad KV, Venkata RY, Murthy KJ, Reddy MV. Influence of intensive yoga training on physiological changes in 6 adult women: a case report. *J Altern Complement Med.* 1997;3(3):291-295.

34. Oken BS, Zajdel D, Kishiyama S, et al. Randomized, controlled, six-month trial of yoga in healthy seniors: Effects on cognition and quality of life. *Altern Ther Health Med.* 2006:12:1:40-47.

35. Chohan IS, Nayar HS, Thomas P. Influence of yoga on blood coagulation. *Thromb Haemost.* 1984;51(2):196-197.

36. Bera TK, Gore MM, Oak JP. Recovery from stress in two different postures and in Shavasana—a yogic relaxation posture. *Indian J Physiol Pharmacol.* 1998;42(4):473-478.

37. Garfinkel MS, Singhal A, Katz WA. Yoga-based intervention for carpal tunnel syndrome. *JAMA.* 1998;280(18):1601-1603.

38. Garfinkel MS, Schumacher HR, Husain A. Evaluation of a yoga based regimen for treatment of osteoarthritis of the hands. *J Rheumatol.* 1994;21:12.

39. Kolasinski SL, Garfinkel M, Tsai AG, et al. Iyengar yoga for treating symptoms of osteoarthritis of the knees: a pilot study. *J Altern Complement Med.* 2005;11:689-693.

40. DiBenedetto M, Innes KE, Taylor AG, et al. Effect of a gentle Iyengar yoga program on gait in the elderly: an exploratory study. *Arch Phys Med Rehabil.* 2005;86(4):1830-1837.

41. Raghuraj P. Pranayama increases grip strength without lateralized effects. *Indian J Physiol Pharmacol.* 1997;41(2):129-133.

42. Dhume RR, Dhume RA. A comparative study of the driving effects of dextroamphetamine and yogic meditation on muscle control for the performance of balance on balance board. *Indian J Physiol Pharmacol.* 1991;35(3):191-194.

43. Narayan R, Kamat A, Khanolkar M. Quantitative evaluation of muscle relaxation induced by Kundalini yoga with the help of EMG integrator. *Indian J Physiol Pharmacol.* 1990;34(4):279-281.

44. Ananthanarayanan TV, Srinivasan TM. Asana-based exercises for the management of low back pain. *Journal of the International Association of Yoga Therapists.* 1994;4:6-15.

45. Clark S, Christiansen A, Hellman DF, Hugunin JW, Hurst KM. Effects of ipsilateral anterior thigh soft tissue stretching on passive unilateral straight-leg raise. *JOSPT.* 1999;29(1):4-11.

46. Sherman KJ, Cherkin DC, Erro J, Miglioretti DL, Deyo RA. Comparing yoga, exercise, and a self-care book for chronic low back pain: a randomized, controlled trial. *Ann Intern Med.* 2005;143;849-856.

47. Galantino ML, Bzdewka TM, Eissler-Russo JL, et al. The impact of modified hatha yoga on chronic low back pain: a pilot study. *Altern Ther.* 2004;10(2):56-59.

48. Williams KA, Petronis J, Smith D, et al. Effect of Iyengar yoga therapy for chronic low back pain. *Pain.* 2005;115(1-2):107-117.

49. Carson JW, Keefe FJ, Lynch TR, et al. Loving-kindness meditation for chronic low back pain: results from a pilot trial. *J Holist Nursing.* 2005;23(3):287-304.

50. Bastille JV, Gill-Body KM. A yoga-based exercise program for people with chronic poststroke hemiparesis. *Phys Ther.* 2004;84(1):33-48.

51. Manjunath, NK, Telles S. Influence of yoga and ayurveda on self-rated sleep in a geriatric population. *Indian J Med Res.* 2005;121(5):683-690.

52. Shapiro D, Cook IA, Davydov DM, et al. Yoga as a complementary treatment of depression: effects of traits and moods on treatment outcome. E-cam Feb, 2007. http://ecam.oxfordjournals.org/cgi/reprint/nel114v1.

53. Sephton SE, Salmon P, Weissbecker I, et al. Mindfulness meditation alleviates depressive symptoms in women with fibromyalgia: results of a randomized clinical trial. *Arthritis and Rheumatism.* 2007;57(1):77-85.

54. Nespor K. Psychosomatics of back pain and the use of yoga. *Int J Psychosom.* 1989;36(1-4):72-78.

55. Nespor K. Pain management and yoga. *Int J Psychosom.* 1991;38(1-4):76-81.

56. Khumar SS, Kaur P, Kaur S. Effectiveness of Shavasana on depression among university students. *Indian J Clin Psychol.* 1993;20(2):82-87.

57. Kabat-Zinn J. An outpatient program in behavioral medicine for chronic pain patients based on the practice of mindfulness meditation: theoretical considerations and preliminary results. *Gen Hosp Psychiatry.* 1982;4(1):33.

58. Kabat-Zinn J. *Full Catastrophe Living.* New York, NY: Delta; 1990.

59. Berger BG, Owen DR. Mood alteration with yoga and swimming: aerobic exercise may not be necessary. *Percept Mot Skills.* 1992;75(3 Pt 2):1331-1343.

60. Ornish D, Scherwitz L, Billings JH. Intensive lifestyle changes for reversal of coronary heart disease. *JAMA.* 1998;280:23.

61. Kabat-Zinn J, Wheeler E, Light T. Influence of mindfulness meditation-based stress reduction intervention on rates of skin clearing in patients with psoriasis. *Psychosom Med.* 1998;60(5):625-632.

62. Nagarathna R, Nagendra HR. Yoga for bronchial asthma: a controlled study. *Brit Med J Clin Res Ed.* 1985;291(6502):1077-1079.

63. Nagendra HR, Nagarathna R. An integrated approach of yoga therapy for bronchial asthma: a 3-54-month prospective study. *J Asthma.* 1986;23(3):123-137.

64. Vijayalakshmi S, Satyanarayana M, Krishna-Rao PV, Prakash V. Combined effect of yoga and psychotherapy on management of asthma: a preliminary study. *J Indian Psychol.* 1988;7(2):32-39.

65. Wilson AF, Honsberger R, Chiu JT, Novey HS. Transcendental meditation and asthma. *Respiration.* 1975;32(1):74-80.

66. Tandon MK. Adjunct treatment with yoga in chronic severe airways obstruction. *Thorax.* 1978;33(4):514-517.

67. Lasater J. *Relax and Renew: Restful Yoga for Stressful Times.* Berkeley, CA: Rodmell Press; 1995.

68. Criswell E. *How Yoga Works: An Introduction to Somatic Yoga.* Phoenix, AZ: Freeperson Press; 1989.

69. Ornish D. *Love & Survival.* New York, NY: HarperCollins; 1997.

Bibliography

Bhole MV. Some physiological considerations about asanas. *Yoga Mimamsa.* 1969;15:4:13-30.

Khanam AA, Sachdeva U, Guleril R. Study of pulmonary and autonomic functions of asthma patients after yoga training. *Indian J Physiol Pharmacol.* 1996;40(4):318-324.

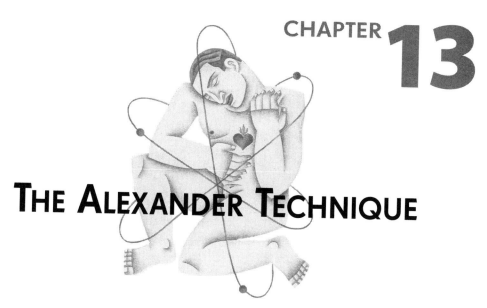

CHAPTER 13

THE ALEXANDER TECHNIQUE

Diane Zuck, MA, PT

Introduction

Frederick Matthias Alexander (1869-1955) developed the Alexander technique. On one level, his story is no different from yours or mine. On another, his search for personal healing and self-fulfillment led him down a path that changed his life and the lives of many others. Unlike most people, he possessed the capacity to observe himself and make systematic deductions about his movement and posture that he was then able to correlate with his symptoms.

At the age of 19, Alexander was already renowned as a Shakespearean elocutionist in the British theater. Recurrent hoarseness and loss of voice threatened his career. His physician recommended rest, which Alexander believed meant keeping his voice silent or not speaking above a whisper. The prescribed treatment worked and his voice returned for use in daily conversation. Then it was time for him to perform. Again and again, Alexander would experience hoarseness at the moment when his voice meant the most to him—during his delivery on stage.

As a result, his physician recommended surgery on the vocal cords. Unwilling and indeed unable to accept this drastic option, Alexander confronted his physician. He believed "...that it was something I was doing... in using my voice that was the cause of the trouble..."[1] Although the physician agreed with the theory, he was not able to help Alexander with the answer. Thus, Alexander was driven to help himself.

Over the next 3 years, Alexander devoted his time to the systematic observation of himself via mirrors with his most objective mind. He made thousands of observations of the same subject, himself, within the same controlled environment to prove or disprove his hypothesis that something he was doing was causing the trouble he was having with his voice.

Alexander observed himself in the act of speaking, or during his process of verbal behavior, under two conditions: when he intended to talk in an "everyday way," and when he intended to deliver a performance on-stage. The more revealing observation occurred when he intended to perform. As he took in a breath, even before he spoke, he heard himself gasp; he saw himself lift his chin and pull the head back and down, which then caused his stature to become short and narrow, to allow his upper chest to expand for air. As he sucked in the air, his larynx depressed. This action was not present when he spoke in conversation.

Later, Alexander would call the head-neck-back relationship the "primary control," and called the condition of the primary control "use."

He then focused on his actual speaking behavior when he intended to perform. Over and over, he saw himself lift his chin and pull his head back and down at the moment he intended to speak, but before a word was spoken. So then he waited, and before the word was said, he restored his head to a position that was not pulled down and back, and his stature to a place that was not short and narrow. This later became Alexander's "principle of inhibition."

As it turned out, the waiting gave Alexander a second chance—a chance to use himself, his body—in a different way. Regardless of his attempts to change his behavior, over and over he observed the same habit of his head pulling down and back.

In the next series of trials to change his behavior, he eliminated visual feedback. He felt himself breathe in with the intent to perform without speaking, he felt his pulled down and back habit, and then he waited. With internal feedback, he tried to undo his habit by moving his head to a position that was not pulled down and back. He intentionally moved his head forward and up. However, when he looked back to the mirror, nothing had changed. He found himself in his same habitual pattern of use, with or without visual feedback. This became Alexander's "principle of faulty appreciation."

He went back to his hypothesis that something he was doing was causing the trouble he had with his voice and began again. Not surprisingly, under the same conditions, the same results appeared. The more he tried not to repeat his habit, the more the habit appeared and reappeared. Later, this became the Alexander principle of "end-gaining" and a process called the "means whereby." But the story does not end here.

The result of his research, the 1918 publication of *The Use of Self*, included an introduction by the father of the description of the scientific method in America, Professor John Dewey. Alexander's discovery is described in his own words in the first chapter. The chapter, according to Dewey, is an "exemplar of all the major steps that are characteristic of a scientific inquiry."[2] Alexander's self-study parallels what we today describe as a single-case research design. In addition to proving his hypothesis, Alexander made a number of discoveries about himself that he later developed into the principles of the Alexander technique. Thus, John Dewey classified the descriptive research method employed by Alexander as exemplary of valid and reliable research.

Over time, Alexander became able to avoid pulling his head back and down which, he discovered, eliminated the sucking in of air and the depression of the larynx.

"The importance of this discovery cannot be overestimated, for through it I was led on to the further discovery of the primary control of the working of all the mechanisms of the human organism, and this marked the first important stage of my investigation."[1]

Alexander did not discover the universal primary control, for it turns out that we each use the structure of our head, neck, and back in unique ways. He did discover his own primary control and how it affected his use and function. This is the value of single-case research design. By discovering how his primary control affected his function, he could generalize the effect of one's primary control on one's function.

The Primary Control

The primary control is operationally defined as the organization of the head to the neck to the back. Anatomically, the head is defined as the skull with mandible and hyoid; the neck is defined as the top vertebrae of the spine; and the back is defined as the middle vertebrae of the spine, which supports the rib cage with the shoulder girdle and arms. The back also relates with the lower vertebrae of the spine, connecting with the pelvis and legs. The head is a center for receiving sensory input and houses the brain and midbrain until it exits the skull as the spinal cord. Muscles of the hyoid attach to the skull, the larynx, and the shoulder blade.

The head is delicately balanced on the neck, where cranial and peripheral nerves overlap, and, thus, the head on neck site is a major locus for reflex and voluntary and involuntary movement. The back supports the rib cage, housing many vital organs, supports the movement of the arms, and also supports the autonomic nervous system, which directs the function of our internal organs. The back extends into the lumbar and pelvic areas, where it supports other internal organs and the movement of the legs. The organization of the head-neck-back, the primary control, thus affects the functioning of each part of the organism.

"As the head moves, it imposes an attitude on the body [a dynamic influence] by redistributing muscular tonus."[2] The head houses the brain and is the center for our conscious and unconscious intentions and choices. Thus, the presence of consciousness is inseparable from the primary control. Therefore, each choice a person makes reflects the condition of the primary control and affects the dynamic state of the primary control, which in turn affects the entire organism and sets the conditions for the next choice. Conscious use of the organization of the head-neck-back (primary control) means consciously integrating the voluntary and involuntary experiences with constructive choice. This then results in the mutual development of the acts of inhibition and volition. This discovery of his own primary control led Alexander to discover the other principles of the Alexander technique.

Inhibition

Alexander's principle of inhibition expands the stimulus-response model to a stimulus-process-response model. At the moment Alexander intended to speak, he waited and observed his process. If he saw his habit emerge, he did not speak. He consciously inhibited the desire. During this pause, he reorganized his primary control and intended to speak again. If the habit reappeared, he continued to consciously inhibit it. In Professor Raymond Dart's mind, "the basic discovery Alexander made from 1888... was the practice of deliberate conscious inhibition."[3] Alexander accessed his primary control by conscious inhibition of pulling his head back and down through use of his intention to do just the opposite motion. He did not say to himself, do not pull the head back and down; instead he asked himself to move the head forward and up. In a sense, he gave his nervous system a positive direction, as the nervous system does not respond as well to what not to do. Alexander developed a series of directions, or orders, that he said to himself to sustain his level of inhibition and to maintain access to his primary control. He worked with these directions sequentially until they became a unity of intent, with each being a part and the whole in the same moment.

A stimulus-process-response model is supported by the work of Dr. Benjamin Libet, professor of physiology at the School of Medicine of the University of California, San Francisco. "Evidence indicates that there are 100 to 150 milliseconds within which a person may either prevent or allow an urge to move to become an action."[4] Frank Pierce Jones remarked "...I found that the paradigm of inhibition... could be applied equally well when the activity would be classed as mental or emotional."[2] Conscious inhibition brings to conscious awareness thought processes and intentions, leaving the individual able to choose a response. The habitual response is still available but now under the conditions of conscious control. Everyday events, previously thought to be not under our control, suddenly become available to our choice.

Conscious inhibition reveals that, given a stimulus, we are not bound to a habitual, learned response or reaction. Most of one's day is not dependent on life-threatening decisions which, if under true reflex control, we have no choice but to make. Instead, the nervous system has time between stimulus and response to process what's occurring before a response reaches the final common pathway. Three options of response are usually available. We can choose to act in our habitual way, to act in a brand new way, or not to act at all. To not act (to inhibit) is a valid, active response. To decide not to act is as equal a decision as to decide to act. In 1937, Sir Charles Sherrington wrote[5]:

*I may seem to stress the preoccupation of the brain with muscle. Can we stress too much that preoc-
cupation when any path we trace in the brain leads directly or indirectly to muscle? The brain seems a
thoroughfare for nerve action passing on its way to the motor animal. It has been remarked that life's aim
is an act not a thought. Today the dictum must be modified to admit that, often, to refrain from an act is
no less an act than to commit one, because inhibition is co-equally with excitation a nervous activity.*

Frank Pierce Jones also notes Sherrington's writings on inhibition: "There is no evidence that
inhibition is ever accompanied by the slightest damage to the tissue; on the contrary, it seems to
predispose the tissue to a greater functional activity thereafter."[2]

Professor Jones defines inhibition as[2]:

*In general, any suspension of activity or temporary withholding of a response. In Alexander's usage,
inhibition releases, rather than represses spontaneity by suspending habitual responses to stimuli long
enough so that intelligent guidance and reasoning can intervene. Alexander saw this ability to inhibit
automatic responses to stimuli, and to allow reason to intervene before making responses as "man's
supreme inheritance."*

In fact, Alexander's first book is entitled *Man's Supreme Inheritance.*[6]

Richard M. Gummere, Jr, past professor at Columbia University, wrote the prologue to the
1988 edition of Alexander's first book, describing it as "...a book of imperial scope."[6] In this book,
Alexander quotes Leonardo Da Vinci: "You can have neither a greater nor a less dominion than
that over yourself."

Faulty Sensory Appreciation

In the early stages, when he was working with his eyes closed, Alexander relied on his internal
sensory awareness for feedback. But even without visual feedback, his internal senses led to the
habitual outcome. Alexander concluded that his kinesthetic awareness, or appreciation, was wrong
and unreliable. He continued to work in front of the mirrors with his eyes open for the objective
view. He watched himself with the intent to deliver a speech using inhibition to access his primary
control until he could open his mouth without tilting his head back and down, could move his
head without moving his shoulders, and could take in a breath without shortening and narrow-
ing his stature. The directions became integral at this stage of his learning. With each direction,
he became more aware of new sensory information present with each conscious inhibition. Over
time, Alexander came to understand that he had retrained his nervous system to new ways of use
and function. The newer ways of use and function were available to him when he accepted his
sensory assessment as faulty, inhibited his response, gave direction, and chose to respond within
less familiar sensory surroundings.

Anatomically, our proprioceptive senses offer internal information about the body's position,
direction, and mass. Behaviorally, as we use our self in one way over time, we develop a response
that becomes habituated to the sensory information triggering that response.

In many habitual and much-practiced activities, such as those involved in balance and locomotion, sequences of "elementary motor acts" come to be assembled by the inclusion, in the gestalt
to trigger a specific element, of sensory messages that are parts of the kinesthetic reafference
occurring during the consummatory phase of other elementary motor acts performed earlier in
the sequence. Once a habitual motor sequence has been initiated, the successive stages follow one
another as in a chain reaction in which voluntary intervention can be effective. If this crucial stage
is omitted, the most assiduous practice serves merely to reinforce the undesired habit.[7]

Areas in our body also become contracted through use and habit. Habitual responses and contracted areas are deprived of sensory experiences, and new information may feel and be perceived
as wrong. For example, a person may habitually interlace his or her fingers with the left thumb
over the right thumb. It the same person performs the same act with the right thumb over the left,

it feels wrong or uncomfortable, so this new act may be excluded from the motor repertoire. This is a very simple experiment. But if that person chose to inhibit the usual response and to go with a new use, the person may find him- or herself open to receiving more information. If we are able to free our self from habit, areas open and new information brings a wider range of choices.

Alexander found that he could change his use by not relying on the familiar sensory information he knew to be wrong, by attending to conscious inhibition and direction, and by receiving new sensory feedback from his actions. Alexander was changing his habits by altering his kinesthetic re-afference. In the writings of JJ Gibson, "We can now suppose that the perceptual systems develop perceptual skills, with some analogy to the way in which behavioral systems develop performatory skills."[8]

End-Gaining and the Means Whereby

Alexander observed himself under two conditions: one, while intending to speak in an everyday way, and the other, while intending to deliver a performance. The latter was the act triggering the habit that caused his loss of voice. He discovered that if he could give up his desire to deliver a commanding performance, his use changed and he was able to speak his lines without any loss of affect or effect. He concluded that being solely attentive on the goal, or "end-gaining," took his awareness away from how he was going to get there, or the "means whereby." He discovered that his thought or intention alone was sufficient stimulus to elicit his undesired use. According to Professor Dart, in 1965, a decade after his death and three-quarters of a century after F. M. Alexander's self-analysis, an arresting neurological fact came to light through its having been recorded electronically in numerous encephalograms. Changes in electric potential take place in the nerve cells in the frontal lobes of human brains before, as well as during and after, voluntary muscular movements. Kornhuber and Deecke, two German neurologists, found that while an individual is thinking about carrying out an action, the action is being preceded by a slow negative wave occurring in the front region of his or her brain.[9]

Alexander used conscious inhibition to momentarily redirect his attention away from his goal and focus on his primary control and how he was using himself toward the goal. He brought his intentions to a level of consciousness that was accessible to a deeper desire to change his use. During this process, Alexander gave himself orders that later became the "directions."

Alexander's principle of end-gaining may seem obvious at first. We all strive for health, wealth, and happiness. We each have an understanding of what health, wealth, and happiness means, along with a plan of how to achieve them. Full understanding of the end-gaining principle is attained when it is applied to the simple, mundane activities of daily living. The everyday tasks of standing, walking, sitting down, standing up, drinking, eating, talking, etc, become actions integral with our goals. Everyday activities bring out typical patterns of use, or what is called postural set.[10] Even as you pick up a book and prepare to read, muscular tension increases and is enough to alter the relationship of the head, neck, and back. As you continue to read, you may literally be pulled in toward the goal of reading the words. In a short time, the head is pulled back and down as the shoulders become rounded and elevated with the effort of holding the book up against gravity. If you happen to be sitting against the back of a chair, you may easily fall into a slump and end up sitting on the sacrum. After years of this use, this may become the only postural set within which you are able to read a book. Such daily actions are not foremost in our consciousness because we have delegated them to the realm of automatic actions or habit. For example, locomotion can be accomplished on the spinal level and serves to move animals toward food and away from danger. Consciousness of the desire to walk toward a nonfood item, or approach a potentially dangerous item, is unique to human behavior. Humans have the ability to be aware of and to contemplate their actions.

"The means whereby" is the integration of awareness and attention. While studying the technique, Professor Jones commented, "It was only after I realized attention can be expanded as well as narrowed that I began to note progress."[2] And, "movement within an expanded field of attention is the means by which change is effected in the Alexander technique."[2]

In 1949, C. Judson Herrick wrote a biography of George Ellett Coghill, author of the document, "Appreciation: The Educational Methods of F. Matthias Alexander."[4] Coghill was a biologist and worked in comparative anatomy. While at Brown University, he was influenced by professors trained in the experimental psychology work of William James. Herrick reviewed Coghill's papers over varied topics but stated that all had a central theme "that was to correlate the development of behavior with the development of anatomical structure."[2-5] This is a more expanded view of the relationship between structure and function.

Professor Jones based this "extended field of consciousness" on the two ways that individuals gain knowledge from experience. One way is through the knowledge gained from within the individual, or introspection. The other way is through the knowledge gained from outside the individual, or what Herrick called extraspection. However, it is not one or the other focus of attention, but a unity of awareness.

"The attention is focused wherever it is wanted. But it is focused in such a way that when something in the environment is central, consciousness of the environment remains."[2] Thus, consciousness has a dual mechanism to gather information.

How is it possible for humans to be conscious of external and internal information in a coherent way that makes each avenue of information equally available? The intermediate relationship between structure, function, and environment is based on internal, interactive connections between the information received from within and without the organism.

A dual-mode sensory process model has been applied to the senses that serve behavior. In the visual system, the focal and ambient subsystems support visual input and perception.[11,12] The focal process provides for detail discrimination, and the ambient process provides for spatial orientation, movement detection, and balance. The functioning and use of each subsystem directly influences learning behavior. In the auditory system, Dr. Alfred Tomatis, developer of the Audio Psycho Therapy approach, describes the right ear focused on precise sound and the left ear on background sound.[13] A dual process of functioning within a sensory mode, like vision or hearing, is beyond a left-right brain model and goes deeper into the neural networks between the hemispheres, the cerebellum, and the midbrain. These sensory functions also subserve higher cortical functions which, if the whole is greater than the sum of its parts, may even be supra-cortical and literally out of the body within the realm of the mind. If the sensory systems subserve human consciousness, and if these subsystems work on a dual mode process, it is likely that the consciousness may also function in dual mode. Like the sensory systems, the consciousness can be accessed through educational and intentional efforts. For example, by utilizing the Alexander technique, a person accesses intention as he or she chooses how to respond to the sensory information at the moment. We are not bound to every response in our neural networks and can intercept the neural impulses through inhibition, choice, and a conscious change in direction.

Alexander did not cure his laryngitis. He did discover a way to integrate his mind and body to access a deeper desire to change his use, while moving toward a goal in such a way that prevented him from a hoarse voice at the time he most needed it. Aldous Huxley offers: "One has to make the discovery for oneself, starting from scratch, and to find what old F. M. Alexander called the means whereby, without which good intentions merely pave hell and the idealist remains an ineffectual, self-destructive and other-destructive end-gainer."[2]

This statement may mirror the essence of a controversy in physical therapy practice. Some practitioners are bound to science and use treatment procedures only if they have been firmly substantiated by rigorous, quantitative research. Other practitioners who are more open to the art in physical therapy can receive information that tells them something has worked to help a client and place validity on that information as it comes from a valued source.

Evidence of Efficacy

There is a growing body of evidence in the medical literature on the efficacy of the Alexander technique. The *Cochrane Database of Systematic Reviews* published a review of the efficacy of the Alexander technique in people with chronic , stable asthma in 2000.[14] Only randomized controlled trials were examined, but no trials were found that met the selection criteria of the search.

Ernst and Canter[15] published a systematic review of controlled clinical trials in a review article in the journal *Research in Complementary and Classical Medicine*. Of four clinical trials that met their criteria, two were found to be methodologically sound and clinically relevant. One of those was the following study.

Stallibrass, Sissons, and Chalmers[16] published "A randomized controlled trial of the Alexander technique for idiopathic Parkinson's disease" in *Clinical Rehabilitation* in 2002. This randomized controlled trial, with three groups of patients from London with idiopathic Parkinson's disease receiving "normal treatment," compared outcomes of one group receiving, additionally, 24 lessons in the Alexander technique (n=28, 2 lessons a week for 12 weeks), one group receiving 24 sessions of massage (n=29, 2 massages a week for 12 weeks) in addition to normal treatment, and one group with no additional intervention (n=27). The massage group was to control only for touch and personal attention, not to compare massage with the Alexander technique. The three groups were closely balanced using a special computer program for age, gender, duration of diagnosed illness, and severity of illness. Outcome measures included self-report on the Self-Assessment Parkinson's Disease Disability Scale (SPDDS) at best and worst times of day, and results from the Beck Depression Inventory and Attitudes to Self Scale. The Alexander group was comparatively less depressed at the conclusion of the study (p=0.03) on the Beck Depression Inventory, and at 6-month follow-up had improved on the Attitudes to Self Scale (p=0.04). The Alexander group improved significantly compared to the no additional intervention group pre-intervention to post-intervention both on the SPDDS at best and at worst. This improvement was maintained at 6 month follow up. The authors concluded that, despite the small sample size, the changes were statistically significant, and the reliability of the results was strengthened by the "consistently positive direction of results across a range of outcome measures."[16]

In a well-designed case report published in 2005 in *Physical Therapy*, Cacciatore, Horak, and Henry[17] describe the use of the Alexander technique with a 49-year-old woman neuroscientist with a 25-year history of left-sided idiopathic lumbosacral pain with observed changes in automatic postural responses. This patient could stand for no more than 30 minutes without exacerbating her pain. She took only an occasional ibuprofen for relief. She received 20 Alexander technique lessons from a certified teacher for 45 minutes each over a 6-month period. Outcome measures were posture coordination (automatic responses to surface translations using hydraulic platform, and one-legged balance) and pain (visual analog scale [VAS]). A 6-camera Motion Analysis system was used to measure kinematics. Also examined was the lateral curvature in the trunk during quiet stance. On being tested monthly for 4 months before the AT lessons and for 3 months after the lessons, results were quite positive. Before the lessons she consistently had laterally asymmetric automatic postural responses to translations. After the magnitude and symmetry of her responses and balance improved and her low back pain decreased (8.3 cm before to 1.9 cm after on the VAS) Her daily pain decreased to pain only 1 to 2 days a month and never again so severe that she had to lie down as previously. Balance ability improved for both legs.

In the *Journals of Gerontology*,[18] R. J. Dennis looked at the outcome of functional reach in normal older women following Alexander technique instruction. Women older than 65 (with the exception of one male control) were divided into three groups: a pilot group (group 1), an experimental group (group 2), and a control group (group 3). Groups 1 and 2 were given eight 1-hour, biweekly sessions of Alexander technique instruction with pre- and post-test of functional reach. Group 3 was simply given the pre- and post-test of functional reach. Groups 1 and 2 showed significant improvement in performance of functional reach. Group 2 was retested 1 month after post-test and showed a slight decrease in functional reach performance. Responses from members of groups 1 and 2 to a qualitative questionnaire indicated an overall positive response to the Alexander technique instruction. Dennis concluded that Alexander technique instruction may be effective in improving functional reach, thus perhaps improving balance and thereby reducing the tendency to fall in older.[18]

Austin and Ausubel from the Department of Radiology at Columbia University published an article in *Chest* in 1992 entitled, "Enhanced Respiratory Muscular Function in Normal Adults After Lessons in Proprioceptive Musculoskeletal Education Without Exercises."[19] The proprioceptive musculoskeletal education was instruction in the Alexander technique, which they described as "awareness and voluntary inhibition of personal habitual patterns of rigid musculoskeletal constriction." Ten healthy subjects (group 1) received 20 private Alexander technique lessons once a week. Spirometric tests including maximum static mouth pressures were assessed before and after each course of lessons. Ten healthy control subjects matched for age, gender, height, and weight (group 2) without instruction were tested over a similar interval. Using paired students' t-test, group 1 showed significant increases in peak expiratory flow (9%, $p<0.05$), maximal voluntary ventilation (6%, $p<0.05$), maximum inspiratory pressure (12%, $p<0.02$), and maximum expiratory pressure (9%, $p<0.005$). Group 2, the control, showed no significant changes. Austin and Ausubel suggest that, "possible mechanisms for the changes in the experimental group include an increased length and decreased resting tension of muscles of the torso, which in turn may increase their strength, increase thoracic compliance, and/or enhance coordination." They concluded that Alexander technique education may enhance respiratory function in normal adults.[19]

Why Learn the Alexander Technique?

A way to bring the mind and body into harmony seems desirous. Use of the consciousness and use of the body are equal and inseparable aspects of being human. The desire to meet a goal directs our bodily functions and vice-versa. Innate awareness of this mind-body/body-mind connection is present in each human at birth but is lost as we develop within environmental constrictions that limit learning about ourselves and about the choices we are free to make.

For example, young children exhibit innate use of the body. A child bends, squats, and sits on the ground with ease and poise. At some point, the child is required to sit in a chair and experiences an environmental constriction. Chair sitting is not innate. It is an acquired skill that is imposed upon the body-mind/mind-body process.

The Alexander technique offers a chance to regain mind-body harmony and has been called a method of psychophysical education. Professor Dewey "considered that the Alexander technique provided a demonstration of the unity of body and mind."[2]

Thompson[20] tells a revealing story of a 14-year-old boy who took lessons with him. The boy was strong and sturdy, played football, and would frequently beat up the kid next door. After the boy understood the principle of inhibition, Thompson worked with him through the postural set that accompanied his intent to "beat the kid up." The boy came to understand the kinesthetic difference he felt when he was or was not with his potentially harmful intent. He was sent home to perform an experiment. The next time he saw his target, the boy was asked to work with inhibiting his initial desire to fight and to decide if the circumstance was going to direct his response or if he could choose the extent to which the circumstance directed his response. The boy gave up fighting, gave up football, and took up music.

Focus on the outcome without attention to process requires being pulled toward that outcome in a way that strengthens habit and limits options. We become stuck in our own actions. The mind becomes stifled and the body eventually rebels. How individuals use their bodies then becomes a factor in many bodily ailments. Most musculoskeletal problems and some neurological problems have been greatly helped by giving the individual a way to control and manage his or her own body. Individuals striving for peak performance apply the technique with success. Musicians and athletes, for example, have taken Alexander lessons to improve physical and artistic performance. Even equestrians working with the technique experience a greater harmony between themselves and their mounts.

How the Alexander Technique Is Learned

Alexander thought his discovery was not that unique. It is possible for anyone to do what Alexander did—discover your own primary control. It also is possible to learn about the technique from books, journals, and articles and to apply what you have learned. Most people choose to find an Alexander teacher or are referred to one by a friend or medical professional.

Alexander used the directions to guide the student through the experience of discovering his or her own primary control and new use. The directions, or orders, can be an integral part of learning the technique but do not define the technique. At one point, Alexander stopped using verbal orders/directions while teaching others. He found he could use his hands on the student in a way that elicited the primary control and offered the student a different kinesthetic experience. The Alexander teacher will place his or her hands on the student for the purposes of bringing the student's awareness to areas of tension, assisting the student with inhibition of habitual use, and facilitating redistribution of postural tonus, thus providing the student with a different kinesthetic experience. Because the head, neck, and back area are central to the primary control, the teacher's hands will be in contact with these areas. The teacher's touch can be described as neutral, without effort or intent. The touch is a guide for support and trust. As the student becomes able to trust the support, the ability to let go and open up areas is experienced.

A teacher of the Alexander technique exemplifies the principles. As Jones stated, "You can't teach someone else an improved use of himself until your own manner of use has improved."[2] The teacher imparts his or her understanding of the principles through the use of voice and hands. Some Alexander teachers use their voice more than their hands or vice-versa, or use each in balance. Use of voice and hands also is variable within and across lessons. This is a matter of the teacher's teaching and the learner's learning styles. Sometimes it is good to work with several teachers before choosing one you want to work with over time. A teacher will have at least 1600 hours of teacher training over a period of 3 to 4 years.

Alexander lessons are not restricted to one location. For example, people receive lessons in their home, at their worksite, or their place of recreation. An Alexander teacher's studio has a few essentials like mirrors, chairs, and possibly a table/plinth. There is no need for the student or client to remove any clothes with the possible exception of shoes, which allow the feet to be more receptive to support from the floor. Chair work is very common. Alexander used sitting and standing from a chair as a typical example of an everyday activity that we are least likely to think about, and which is most likely to elicit our worst habits. Changes in habit are more likely to happen during a nonthreatening activity like standing up from a chair or walking across the room than during an activity of high tension like facing your boss. If you play the piano or ride a horse, the teacher may ask you to work with those intentions in mind and may later work with you sitting at your piano or on your horse. Table work and floor work can be used during lessons for the gravity-eliminated experience on the primary control (head, neck, back relationship).

An Alexander lesson is an experience of mutual respect. Each lesson is a recognition of the fine line between teacher and student. The aim of the lesson "...is to bring a pupil to the point of self-discovery that F. M. Alexander reached when he was able to translate what he saw in the mirrors into kinesthetic terms and to apply his new knowledge to the solution of his own problems and become in effect his own expert in the use of himself."[2]

Foundational Research and Documented Support

There is value in remembering that research cannot be limited to the controlled laboratory and must include the life experience.

Many people have found their way to the Alexander technique. Some are rather well-known figures in the world. Some have written about personal experience with the technique and others have reported rigorous research that has been conducted on the technique. This section summarizes the contributions of a few people. The reader is invited to follow along the path of these contributors and to identify his or her own personal interests.

Anatomist and anthropologist Raymond Dart was appointed chair of anatomy at the University of Witwatersrand, Johannesburg in 1922. In 1925, he published his findings of the Taung skull, later called *Australopithecus africanus*. Professor Dart showed the skull to be more man-like than ape-like. But because his conclusions did not support the prevailing theory, they were met with great speculation.[21] Eventually, after new fossils were uncovered, the Tuang skull was recognized for the traits resembling later forms of the genus *Homo*.[22] Significant to the Alexander technique, among those traits is the poise of the skull on the spine. In the evolutionary development of uprightness and bipedal locomotion, the downward weight of the cranium center of gravity and the upward support of the articulating cranial condyles became closer in space. The two forces are almost coincident in humans. Along with evolutionary changes in cranial shape and direction of muscle pull, the human uniqueness is the support of the cranium.[23] Professor Dart recognized that a critical feature of being human is the poise of the head on the neck.[24] In the same article, "The Attainment of Poise," Professor Dart states:[24]

> *Terminological failure to distinguish the static symbolism of posture from the dynamic plasticity of poise has thus been responsible for a great deal of confusion both in the nomenclature of, and medical thought concerning movement, ...a considerable number of intermediate positions are necessarily assumed...from the initial posture...to the terminal posture. These intermediate positions should always be positions of poise or equilibrium. Every phase of the movement...is in a state of mobile equipoise or balance.*

Professor Dart met Alexander in 1949, received lessons from him, and later from Miss Irene Tasker, and said:[3]

> *...Alexander was striving to explain... the body misuse and correction... Alexander's work is important because it is based on the fundamental biological fact that the relation of the head to the neck is the primary relationship to be established in all proper positioning and movement of the body.*

Alexander's only sibling, Alfred Redden Alexander, was probably his brother's strongest supporter and can be considered the "first teacher of the Technique." It is common within the Alexander community to refer to the brothers by their initials, F. M. and A. R. Both were born in Wynard, Tasmania. F. M. began taking students in 1894. In 1904, A. R. went to London with his brother to teach.

Ethel Webb was F. M. 's secretary and received lessons from him. She was also well read in the writings of John Dewey. Ms. Webb understood a connection between the Alexander technique and the work of Maria Montessori, and she went to Rome to study at the Montessori School. While she was there, she met Irene Tasker and Margaret Naumberg. Ms. Naumberg had studied with Professor Dewey at Columbia University and was instrumental in F. M. 's reasons for going to the United States and the eventual meeting with John Dewey. Ms. Naumberg later founded the Walden School. F. M. arrived in New York City in late 1914. Ms. Webb accompanied him and A. R. followed shortly after. In 1916, Ms. Tasker accepted an invitation to teach at Walden School and also enrolled at Columbia University to study with Professor Dewey. Ms. Tasker continued to take Alexander lessons and became F. M. 's assistant in 1918 and worked primarily with children. At this point in time, F. M. , A. R. , Ms. Webb, and Ms. Tasker were the only teachers of the Technique. As interest in the Technique grew, so did the need for a formal teacher training course. F. M. and A. R. had returned to London and the first teacher training course began in

1931 with 7 students. In 1935, A. R. returned to New York and traveled between there and Boston to start other training courses. A. R. died in 1946 after devoting his life to the teachings of his older brother. Ms Webb died shortly before F. M. (who died October 10, 1955), without naming a successor to his work. Ms. Tasker would have been the best claimant. A more thorough historical account of the Alexander technique can be found in Dr. Jones' book, *Body Awareness in Action.*[2]

American philosopher and educator John Dewey met Alexander around the year 1915, and was his first student in America. He took lessons throughout the 1920s and 1930s, the latter part of that time with Alexander's brother. In 1923, Professor Dewey wrote the Introduction to Alexander's book, *Constructive Conscious Control of the Individual.* He also described Alexander's discovery "as a new scientific principle with respect to the control of human behavior as important as any principle that has ever been discovered in the domain of external nature,"[2] and as "...comparable to the discoveries that were made in the Renaissance and that caused men to change their ideas..."[2] Dewey wrote several books during the time he was receiving lessons. It has been said that the reader's potential for learning from his books, *Art as Experience, The Quest for Certainty, How We Think, The Theory of Valuation,* and *Experience and Education,* is greater when understood in the light of the Alexander technique. In *Experience and Education,* Jones quotes Dewey stating, "The crucial educational problem is that of procuring the postponement of immediate action upon desire until observation and judgement have intervened."[2]

Dewey specifically referred to Alexander in *Human Nature and Conduct* and *Experience and Nature,* thus giving a written endorsement of the Technique. *Experience and Nature* is considered Dewey's best work and the one which most clearly and deeply exposes the Alexander principles.[2] Professor Dewey gave moral and intellectual support to Dr. Frank Pierce Jones to pursue research of the Technique. Unfortunately, Dewey died before Jones received sufficient financial support.

As a professor of classic Greek at Brown University, Dr. Jones first heard of the Alexander technique in 1930 from his colleagues in psychology. He was so drawn to the technique that he took a 3-year leave of absence to work with A. R. Alexander in the Boston training program. F. M. Alexander was at the training program during each of his visits to America. Dr. Jones qualified as an Alexander teacher in 1945. He met Professor Dewey in 1947, and both were greatly concerned by the lack of scientific foundation for the technique. He recognized the need to establish "...the physical equivalents of the great mental experience... to discover a mechanism that would account for the long-term effects on health and well-being."[2] Doctors in the Boston area were impressed by the physical improvements in their patients after Alexander lessons, but distressed because some form of nonscientific method was credited for the positive change. However, Jones knew "... a clinical study of the technique would be of little value until the principle it rested on had been demonstrated experimentally, and it could be shown that the clinical results followed from the means employed and could not be attributed to some other mechanism like suggestion."[2]

After a long search, and with encouragement from Professor Dewey, Dr. Jones gained a 7-year grant from the United States Public Health Service to find empirical support for the Alexander technique in the knowledge base of anatomy and physiology. Another long search gave Dr. Jones access to conduct his study at the Tufts University Institute for Applied Experimental Psychology.

Jones used the startle pattern as a model for postural malalignment demonstrating increased muscle tension and displacement of the head. He felt the same malposture was associated with lack of exercise, aging, or disease. In the research lab, he imposed a startle response stimulus to subjects and used photography and electromyography to record the pattern. The startle pattern is a primitive response that stays with the organism for its life span. The startle paradigm is "...appropriate for developmental and comparative studies," showing "...different types of plasticity such as habituation, sensitization, prepulse inhibition, and modification by prior associative learnings."[23]

Jones also studied subjects using multi-image photography (upon advice from Harold Edgerton at MIT), electromyography, x-ray photography, and force platform records during activities like rising from supine position, standing from a chair, and walking up and down stairs. He recorded the changes in a subject's habitual movement compared to guided movements facilitated by an Alexander teacher. Dr. Jones' research recorded that least muscle tension, least force, and least head displacement were achieved with guided movement.[24]

Jones also had subjects complete an adjective checklist to describe the kinesthetic effect of guided movement, and compared the subjective response with the objective measure. The descriptions of "lighter," "less familiar," "higher," and "smoother" were most consistent with measurable change. Jones concluded that his findings were consistent with the principles of physiology and psychology. Unfortunately, Jones died in 1975, just before completing the last chapter of his book, *Body Awareness in Action*, which was published the next year.

A lover of music and horse riding, Walter H. M. Carrington completed his training with Alexander in 1939. He continued on as Alexander's assistant and married a fellow teacher. Walter and his wife, Dilys, continued the teacher training program after Alexander's death in 1955. They continue to teach and are among the few living senior teachers of the Technique.

A London physician, Wilfred Barlow, met Alexander in 1938, and later married Alexander's niece, Marjory. Dr. Barlow's book, *The Alexander Principle*, summarizes 30 years of work and outlines the scientific basis of the technique. His articles on the Technique were published in many medical journals, and he wrote Alexander's obituary for *The Times* (London). Dr. Barlow died in 1991, and Marjory Barlow continues to teach in London.[25]

Renowned author Aldous Huxley was so crippled with pain he was bedridden, but continued to write with his typewriter on his chest. Huxley was one of F. M.'s students in America. His condition improved greatly with the lessons. In 1936, he wrote *Eyeless in Gaza*,[26] with a character based upon F. M. Alexander. In 1937, Huxley wrote *Ends and Means*,[27] which endorses the Alexander technique. In *The Alexander Principle*, Barlow[28] quotes a 1941 article by Huxley[28]:

> It is now possible to conceive of a totally new type of education, affecting the entire range of human activity, from the physiological, through the intellectual, moral and practical, to the spiritual... an education which, by teaching them proper Use, would preserve children and adults from most of the diseases and evil habits that now affect them: an education whose training would provide men and women with the psycho-physical means for behaving rationally.

Musician and film director Laura Archera Huxley addressed the Alexander community in 1991 and described the Technique as "...a window, opening on new and wider horizons...inviting us to apply its principles..." to our personal and professional lives.[29]

Physician and physiologist Nikolaas Tinbergen took lessons from several Alexander teachers. In 1973, Professor Tinbergen shared the Nobel Prize for Physiology and Medicine with Konrad Lorenz and Karl von Frisch. He devoted half his acceptance speech to the Alexander technique, and stated "...that many types of under-performance and even ailments, both mental and physical, can be alleviated, sometimes to a surprising extent, by teaching the body musculature to function differently..."[30]

A noted research scientist and university professor in physiology in the United Kingdom, Kathleen J. Ballard, PhD became certified as an Alexander teacher in 1984. She is a regular contributor to reference journals and presents her research at local and international meetings within the Alexander community. She is on the faculty at Walter Carrington's Alexander teacher training course in London. With her scientific background, Dr. Ballard helps to establish the validity of the Technique.[31]

Senior lecturer at the School of Physiology and Pharmacology, University of New South Wales, Australia, David George Garlick, MD, PhD has been a regular contributor to *Direction*, a journal on the the Alexander technique, and a presenter at international Alexander conferences. He edited *Proprioception, Posture and Emotion*,[32] a compilation of papers and posters at the Symposium on Proprioception, Posture and Emotion, sponsored by the Committee in Postgraduate Medical Education at the University of New South Wales in February of 1981. Dr. Garlick's support for the Technique included chairing the Fourth International Alexander Congress in Sydney, Australia in 1994.

A student of the Technique since 1969, Christopher Stevens now directs a teacher training program in Aalborg, Denmark. With his background in physics and physiology, he has conducted research on the Technique in the Department of Anatomy and Human Biology at Kings College, London, and in the Department of Anatomy, University of Copenhagen, Denmark. Stevens replicated Jones' study comparing habitual and guided sit to stand movements.[33] The findings of the two studies were consistent. Stevens did further study in postural stability between individuals who had taken Alexander lessons and individuals who had not taken lessons. He found the trained group had significantly less postural sway than the control group when standing with feet together and eyes closed.[33] He concluded that the Alexander-trained subjects had increased awareness of kinesthetic feedback to access for postural stability. Full details of Stevens' work can be found in his book *Toward a Physiology of the Alexander Technique*.[33-36]

While at Tufts University, Lester "Tommy" Thompson was a colleague of Frank Pierce Jones. Mr. Thompson studied the Technique with Dr. Jones for several years. Shortly before his death in 1975, Dr. Jones gave Thompson full approval and sanction to continue teaching the Technique. Since Dr. Jones' book was published after his death and there were many inquiries about his work and his records, Tufts University agreed to keep the records for a limited time unless further scholarly interest was evident. In 1982, the Frank Pierce Jones archives was established under the administration of Mr. Thompson, Dr. Richard Brown, and Mrs. Helen (Frank) Jones. In 1985, the Wessel Library at Tufts University agreed to keep the Jones Collection on a permanent basis. At the same time, a new collection of the F. M. Alexander papers was admitted. These collections include Dr. Jones' research papers and the correspondence he held with Alexander, Dewey, and others. Mr. Thompson directed the Archives until 1988. He continues to train Alexander teachers and is one of the 1993 founders and charter members of Alexander Technique International (ATI). The purpose of ATI is to promote and advance the F. M. Alexander technique and to disseminate information among its members and to the public.

This listing is by no means complete and only provides partial notes of a few people. Many individuals have contributed to the advancement of the Alexander technique through their practice, research, publications, and presentations.

Case Examples

Alexander did not approve of the use of case histories to substantiate his theories, believing this was a medical orientation toward research and he saw his work best applied in the field of education. "Case histories are important and do throw light on the mechanisms involved in the Technique. But they confuse by overstressing the medical aspect."[2] However, Alexander did cite "examples" of students who improved using the Technique. In fact, case examples can be found in Alexander's books[1,6] and in almost every other book written on the Alexander technique.

The first case example must be of Alexander himself. In discussing the authenticity of somatic pioneers, Don Hanlon Johnson states, "Alexander found that his laryngitis was not just a matter of germs infecting mucous membranes; it was also the result of the way in which he muscularly responded to expectant audiences."[37]

Dr. Barlow's book, *The Alexander Principle*, is illustrated with photographs of many subjects. Although photographs are limited, as they depict still moments in movement, the text clearly describes the dynamic aspects of misuse, especially the chapter on "Use and Disease."[28]

Tommy Thompson's presentation at The First International Congress of Teachers of the F.M. Alexander Technique at the State University of New York, Stony Brook in August 1986 cites two examples. The case briefly described earlier in this writing of the 14-year-old neighborhood bully demonstrates the moral implications of the Technique. The other tells of an National Football League player with neck and back pain interfering with his performance and demonstrates the influence of use on action. His body carried the actions of the game even though he was off the field. In other words, the somatic effects of previous games influenced his daily activities and the next game. The player never put his football down. Over the course of lessons, the player realized he could let go of the ball and receive the next play as a unique event. He was soon relieved of his pain and his performance on the field improved.[20]

An Alexander teacher and a physical therapist, Deborah Caplan has specialized her work to people with back problems. She frequently lectures to physical therapists and presents to the Alexander community. Case examples can be found in her writings.[38,39]

Students of F. M. Alexander and the Technique are a diverse group. Students of the technique include Henry Irving, Lily Langtry, Viola Tree, Oscar Asche, Matheson Lang, Paul Newman, Colin Davis, Roald Dahl, Edna O'Brien, Barry Tuckwell, John Cleese, Aldous Huxley, George Bernard Shaw, the Duchess of York, Sting, Sir Stafford Cripps, John Dewey, James Harvey Robinson, Sir Charles Sherrington, Professor G. E. Coghill, Archbishop William Temple, Frederick Perls, Moshe Feldenkrais, John Houseman, Paul McCartney, Mary Steenburgen, Irene Worth, Christopher Reeve, Joel Grey, Julie Andrews, Joanne Woodward, and Patrick Stewart.[2,23,33,40-44]

Some institutions that recommend or offer the Alexander technique in their curricula are the Julliard School, the Royal Shakespeare Company, the Israeli Air Force, the Los Angeles Philharmonic, the University of Wisconsin, the University of Washington, New York University, Boston University, Ohio State University, Southern Methodist University, and the American Conservatory Theatre.[43]

HOW AND WHY I CHOSE THE ALEXANDER TECHNIQUE

In 1982, my life fell into disharmony. I had been practicing physical therapy for 12 years and had just finished a master's degree. I was unhappy that my practice of physical therapy was draining me and I was unhappy with the way I felt. Over the next 5 years, I pursued every alternative approach that could possibly satisfy two basic needs: first, I looked for an approach that could help my aches and pains. Second, a taller order, I looked for an approach that I could believe in to the extent that I would learn it and be able to help others with it, even after I retired from physical therapy, and on until the day I died. Only in retrospect can I describe what my belief in an approach entailed. I wanted something I could do with my hands, one on one with another person, and something that had a scientific foundation I could accept. Essentially, "high touch and high tech." One evening in 1986, I went to an adult education center to hear an introductory lecture about "the" approach I had finally decided on, which was given by a teacher I had learned about in my search. An introduction to the Alexander technique was also on the agenda. I had never heard of this approach, nor of the person listed to present. Serendipity was with me that night because I found myself in the Alexander technique lecture given by my future teacher, Tommy Thompson. Within the first 5 minutes, I realized I had found what I was looking for—an approach that met my two criteria.

The Alexander technique was a hands-on approach based on sound, scientific reasoning and was amenable to research methods. It was also more educational and preventative than medical in orientation, and being more schooled in education than physical therapy, I was quite receptive. I scheduled a lesson but it was 6 months away. In the meantime, I read all of Alexander's books as well as those of Frank Pierce Jones and Edward Maisel. Reading F. M.'s books was like simultaneously stepping backward and forward in time. His style was difficult to read and not easy to comprehend. F.M. wrote about his work within a culture that was restrained. His insights were progressive and offered a solution to the human dilemma. I went to that first lesson with dread, because I'd read that F.M. Alexander would not accept therapists of any kind or teachers of physical education, who, he was sure, wanted merely to pick up a few new ideas to enliven their own teaching and be able to say that they were using the Alexander technique.[2]

My first degree was in physical education, the next in physical therapy, and the master's didn't matter. I had allowed myself into a situation with a two-strike score. If I failed this, I would be out. Tommy started my lesson with the usual hands-on approach. I literally took three steps back and said, "No! I'm just here to talk." We talked, and it was another 6 months before I had a real hands-on lesson.

I immediately understood the connection between the consciousness and body use. I also began to understand the reason for my aches and pains. I had several more lessons from Tommy and from a visiting teacher from Israel, and entered Tommy's training program in the fall of 1987. I continued my lessons and training. It took me 5 years, instead of the standard 3, to be certified. That was because of an "adjunct lesson" I took by breaking my leg. After two surgeries and 2 years to heal and process, I call my experience a sledgehammer lesson. I had not been paying attention to the moment-by-moment events affecting my life and I needed information I could not ignore. It took me 5 years to become certified as an Alexander teacher, but I did it the only way I could. I needed the extra time to learn my lessons my way. I often share my sledgehammer learning technique with my patients and there is immediate understanding.

Learning to be a teacher of the Alexander technique takes place within an apprentice model. I do not know why I was presented with the teacher I needed, or how I ended up in Tommy's lecture and training course. But over time, I came to understand and to value my teacher's lineage to Alexander himself. Tommy had studied with Frank Pierce Jones. Dr. Jones had studied with F. M. and A. R. Alexander. Thus, my training included the intuitive approach side by side with the anatomy and physiology foundation.

I have only had a handful of my own Alexander students, one of whom I have been seeing for several years. I had the opportunity to work with a 15-year-old boy with Wolfram syndrome, a rare, hereditary disorder causing diabetes mellitus, diabetes insipidus, optic atrophy, and deafness. I was told the lad has poor posture and poor awareness for the internal signs from his body. His mother had heard of the Alexander technique and connected with me through the grapevine. I have also worked with colleagues, family, and friends on an intermittent basis.

I was pleased to be able to help my father, a stoic person. As a child, he was plagued with allergies and asthma, which led to several serious bouts of bronchitis in adulthood. Several years ago, when Dad was about 76 years old, I learned he had been suffering from severe headaches almost daily. He was also quite curious about this approach, and eventually asked me to work with him. As I placed my hands on the "right upper quadrant," as physical therapists call it, I felt a subtle, yet powerful release. Although my hands were in contact with specific muscles overlying specific bones, I sensed the release was from deeper areas, closer to the core of his being. My father, who rarely shares his feelings, acknowledged that he too had sensed a change. Following this single session, he was headache-free for about 2 years, and now has an occasional, tolerable sinus-type headache. He also practices a home program I designed for him based on the principles to keep his spine, hips, and shoulders free from the daily build-up of tension.

COMBINING THE ALEXANDER TECHNIQUE WITH PHYSICAL THERAPY

Currently, I do not have a full Alexander practice, but I apply the principles of the Technique to my approach with patients while I am performing the standard tasks of physical therapy treatment. I work primarily in pediatrics with patients with vision and hearing deficits, head trauma sequelae, autism, and developmental delay, and also with adults in orthopedic sub-acute rehabilitation. I am impressed by two major changes in my work; how I use my hands to touch others and how my presence in treatment influences the well-being of each party. My touch is lighter and not directed toward a specific action. I also observe the words I use to reach the person. I talk less about the bones and muscles, and more about effort, grace, and poise. I accept that the individual has an understanding of what I say as I observe his or her use change. My presence in treatment is neutral, giving me room for acceptance of the individual's current position and needs. I no longer see total hip replacements or scoliosis or brain and birth traumas; I see individuals with unique life circumstances and life's imposed conditions. I am then able to work with individuals in a way that empowers them to change, and I do it without the need to carry their medical and emotional burdens on my shoulders. Physical therapy treatment, as with my Alexander lessons, then becomes an energizing experience. I am not drained or depleted of physical and emotional strength by what I should give to, or do for, the individual.

After I provide an Alexander lesson, I actually feel better than I did before the lesson. In an Alexander lesson, I have no intentions in mind (or inhibit my desire to plan a treatment) and allow the individual to lead me down the path he or she needs to explore. I act as a guide to suggest the means whereby the path may be taken. In physical therapy treatment, I have intentions because I have required functional goals and third parties to remind me, but I try to inhibit my desire to meet the needs of parties not present at the moment. Treatment outcome may be the same, and likely even more beneficial, because the individual has been given "unimposed upon space" to change his or her use, and thus to heal.

This is not to say the individual would have accomplished the same without me. I believe my presence, guided by the principles of the Alexander technique, facilitates a change in the whole person, directly affecting his or her condition in a positive fashion. And with the Alexander technique, I have a means to manage those moments that "push my buttons" or trigger my "internal tapes," and to be aware of other options available to direct my physical and emotional responses. I am reminded of Dr. Jones' first chapter in *Body Awareness in Action*,[2] entitled "Escape from the Monkey Trap." He opens this section with a quote from C.J. Herrick: "In an expanding system, such as a growing organism... freedom to change the pattern of performance is one of the intrinsic properties of the organism itself."[2]

F. M. Alexander, through his intense questions and motivation to find answers within himself, defined a new outlook and approach to human development, spanning the space between stimulus and response, therapy and education. Documented scientific studies explain quite clearly how this Technique facilitates the improvement of the whole person by teaching a method where conscious control and freedom of choice is used in preventing and healing habitual causes of pain and discomfort. Thus, the Alexander technique takes its rightful place, along with physical therapy and other healing approaches, as complementary to the modern search for health and well-being.

Resources

+ Alexander Technique International: www.ati-net.com
+ American Society for the Alexander Technique: www.alexandertech.org

Acknowledgments

I appreciate the help of the editor, Dr. Carol M. Davis, in searching the literature and adding the additional evidence for both the second and now the third edition of this text.

References

1. Alexander F. M. *The Use of Self*. Long Beach, CA: Centerline Press; 1984.
2. Jones FP. *Body Awareness in Action: a Study of the Alexander Technique*. New York, NY: Schocken Books; 1976.
3. Wheelhouse F. Dart and Alexander. *Direction*. 1988;3:100-105.
4. Sheppard D. Physiology and freedom: a report on Dr. Benjamin Libet's lecture to NASTAT's second annual meeting. *The Alexander Review*. 1989;4:5-17.
5. Alexander F. M. . *The Universal Constant in Living*. Long Beach, CA: Centerline Press; 1986.
6. Alexander F. M. . *Man's Supreme Inheritance*. Long Beach, CA: Centerline Press; 1988.
7. Roberts TDM. Balance and locomotion. In: Garlick D, ed. *Proprioception, Posture and Emotion*. Bankstown, Australia: Adept Printing Pty; 1982.
8. Mixon D, Burton P. Faulty sensory perception. *Direction*. 1989;4:128-134.

9. Dart RA. An anatomist's tribute to F. Matthias Alexander. Memorial lecture before the Society of Teachers of the Alexander Technique in London, England, March 20, 1970. In: *Skill, Poise, and The Alexander Technique*. Long Beach, CA: Centerline Press.

10. Jones FP. Method for changing stereotyped response patterns by the inhibition of certain postural sets. *Psych Rev.* 1965;3:196-214.

11. Schneider GE. Two visual systems: brain mechanisms for localization and discrimination are dissociated by tectal and cortical lesions. *Science.* 1969:163;895-902.

12. Trevarthen CB, Sperry R. Perceptual unity of the ambient visual field in human commissurotomy patients. *Brain.* 1973;96:547-570.

13. Joudry R. The use of the ear. *Direction.* 1995;3:23-25.

14. Dennis J. Alexander technique for chronic asthma. *Cochrane Database Systematic Review.* 2000;(2):CD000995

15. Ernst E, Canter PH. Alexander technique. *Research in Complementary and Classical Medicine* 2003;10:325-329.

16 Stallibrass C, Sissons P, Chalmers C. Randomized controlled trial of the Alexander Technique for idiopathic Parkinson's disease. *Clinical Rehabilitation* 2002;16:695-708.

17. Cacciatore TW, Horak FB, Henry SM. Improvement in automatic postural coordination following Alexander Technique lessons in a person with low back pain. *Phys Ther.* 2005;85(6):565-578.

18. Dennis RJ. Functional reach improvement in normal older women after Alexander technique instruction. *Biol Med Sci.* 1999;54(1):M8-11.

19. Austin JH, Ausubel P. Enhanced respiratory muscular function in normal adults after lessons in proprioceptive musculoskeletal education without exercises. *Chest.* 1992;102(2):486-90.

20. Thompson LW. Its practical application in pursuing the possibility of changes in moral and mental attitude and the extension of the range within which free choice and free will can operate. In: *The Scientific and Humanistic Contributions of Frank Pierce Jones on the F. Matthias Alexander Technique.* Long Beach, CA: Centerline Press; 1988.

21. Falk D. *Braindance.* New York: Henry Holt; 1992.

22. Tobias PV. Man, *The Tottering Biped: The Evolution of His Posture, Poise and Skill.* Bankstown, Australia: Adept Printing Pry; 1982.

23. Tobias PV. Man, the tottering biped: the evolution of his erect posture. In: Garlick D, ed. *Proprioception, Posture and Emotion.* Bankstown, Australia: Adept Printing Pty; 1982.

24. Dart RA. The attainment of poise. *So Afr Med J.* 1947;21:74-91.

25. Davis M. The mammalian startle response. In: Eaton RC. *Neural Mechanisms of Startle Behavior.* New York, NY: Plenum Press; 1984:287-351.

26. Huxley A. *Eyeless in Gaza.* New York: Harper & Row; 1936.

27. Huxley A. *Ends and Means.* New York: Harper & Row; 1937.

28. Barlow W. *The Alexander Principle.* London: Arrow Books; 1975.

29. Huxley L, Pappas C. Tribalistic thinking: enslavement or freedom? In: *The Third International Alexander Congress Papers, Engelberg, Switzerland.* Bondi, Australia: Direction; 1991.

30. Tinbergen N. Ethology and stress diseases. *Science.* 1974;185:20-27.

31. Ballard K. The Alexander technique and postural reflexes. In: *The Second International Alexander Congress Papers, Brighton, England.* Bondi, Australia: Direction; 1988:35-39.

32. Garlick D, ed. *Proprioception, Posture and Emotion.* Bankstown, Australia: Adept Printing Pty; 1982.

33. Stevens C. Experimental studies of the Alexander technique. In: *The Second International Alexander Congress Papers, Brighton, England.* Bondi, Australia: Direction; 1988:136-156.

34. Stevens C. *Alexander Technique.* London: Macdonald & Co; 1987.

35. Stevens C. Scientific research and its role in teaching the Alexander technique. *The Alexander Review.* 1989;4:171-194.

36. Stevens C. *Toward a Physiology of the Alexander Technique.* London: Stat Books; 1995.

37. Johnson DH. *Body: Recovering Our Sensual Wisdom.* Berkeley, CA: North Atlantic Books; 1992.

38. Caplan D. *Back Trouble: A New Approach to Prevention and Recovery.* Gainesville, FL: Triad Publishing; 1987.

39. Caplan D. The Alexander technique and its application to back problems. In: *The Second International Alexander Congress Papers, Brighton, England.* Bondi, Australia: Direction; 1988:73-77.

40. Barlow W. Posture, proprioception and the Alexander technique. In: Garlick D, ed. *Proprioception, Posture and Emotion.* Bankstown, Australia: Adept Printing Pty; 1982:228-245.

41. Brennan R. *The Alexander Technique: Natural Poise for Health.* Rockport, MA: Element; 1991.

42. Brennan R. *The Alexander Technique Workbook: Your Personal Programme for Health, Poise and Fitness.* Rockport, MA: Element; 1992.

43. Conable W. *How to Use the Alexander Technique.* Columbus, OH: Andover Road Press; 1995.

44. *Exchange: The Journal of Alexander Technique International.* 1996;4(2):20.

Suggested Reading

Alexander F M. *Constructive Conscious Control of the Individual*. Long Beach, CA: Centerline Press; 1984.

Austin JHM, Ausubel P. Enhanced respiratory muscular function in normal adults after lessons in proprioceptive muscu-loskeletal education without exercises. *Chest*. 1992;102:486-490.

Carrington W, Sontag J, eds. *Thinking Aloud: Talks on Teaching the Alexander Technique*. San Francisco, CA: Mornum Time Press; 1994.

Chance J, ed. The life and work of Raymond Dart. *Direction*. 1988;3:68-86,96-105.

Dewey J. *Experience and Nature*. New York: W. W. Norton & Co; 1929.

Dewey J. *Human Nature and Conduct*. New York: Modern Library; 1930.

Dewey J. *How We Think*. Boston, MA: D.C. Heath & Co; 1933.

Dewey J. *Art as Experience*. New York, NY: G.P. Putnam & Sons; 1934.

Dewey J. *Experience and Education*. New York: Macmillan; 1938.

Dewey J. *The Quest for Certainty*. New York: G.P. Putnam & Sons; 1939.

Dewey J. The theory of valuation. In: *International Encyclopedia of Unified Science*. Chicago, Ill; 1939.

Garlick D, ed. *Proprioception, Posture and Emotion*. Bankstown, Australia: Adept Printing Pty; 1982.

Huxley A. *Eyeless in Gaza*. New York: Harper & Row; 1936.

Huxley A. *Ends and Means*. New York: Harper & Brothers; 1937.

Huxley A. End-gaining and means-whereby. *The Saturday Review of Literature*. October 25, 1941.

Huxley A. *The Doors of Perception and Heaven and Hell*. New York, NY: Harper & Row; 1954.

Huxley LA. *You Are Not the Target*. New York: Farrar, Straus & Company; 1994.

Johnson DH, ed. *Bone, Breath & Gesture: Practices of Embodiment*. Berkeley, CA: North Atlantic Books; 1995.

Kodish SP, Kodish BI. *Drive Yourself Sane! Using the Uncommon Sense of General Semantics*. Englewood, NJ: Institute of General Semantics; 1993.

Maisel E. *The Alexander Technique: The Essential Writings of F. Matthias Alexander*. New York: Carol Communications; 1989.

Maisel E. *The Resurrection of the Body: The Essential Writings of F. Matthias Alexander*. Boston, MA: Shambhala Publications Inc; 1986.

Sanfilippo P. *The Reader's Guide to the Alexander Technique: A Selected Annotated Bibliography*. Long Beach, CA: Centerline Press; 1987.

Tobias PV. A Tribute to Emeritus Professor Raymond Dart. *Direction*. 1988;3:96-99.

Todd ME. *The Thinking Body*. Princeton, NJ: Princeton Book; 1988.

CHAPTER 14

FELDENKRAIS METHOD IN REHABILITATION

USING FUNCTIONAL INTEGRATION AND AWARENESS THROUGH MOVEMENT TO EXPLORE NEW POSSIBILITIES

James Stephens, PT, PhD, GCFP and Teresa M. Miller, PT, PhD, GCFP

Introduction

The authors have been impressed by the effectiveness that the use of the Feldenkrais Method has demonstrated in their clinical practice. Not only does the process usually allow the therapist and client to find an effective solution to the problems at hand, but it often subsequently empowers clients to more effectively solve problems in pursuit of their own health and function. The literature is beginning to describe this.

The goal of this chapter is to introduce the conceptual and practical processes of the Feldenkrais Method. The chapter will briefly introduce the man, Moshe Feldenkrais, who developed the method by presenting a picture of his creative process and thinking over time, which led to the development of his method of work. The chapter will then describe different aspects of working with a client using Functional Integration (FI) and Awareness Through Movement (ATM), presenting some of the related assessment processes and a case study for each approach. A review of the research literature will also be discussed. Finally, the chapter lists resources for people who are interested in pursuing further learning on their own.

Background

MOSHE FELDENKRAIS' LIFE AND WORK

From a base in physics, the work of Moshe Feldenkrais expanded into many other areas, including Gestalt psychology, progressive relaxation,[1] bioenergetics,[2] sensory awareness,[3] the hypnosis of Milton Erickson,[4] an ecological perspective on mind[5] and human perception,[6] and the physiological studies of Sherrington, Magnus, Pavlov, Fulton, and Schilder.[7]

Born in the Russia in 1904, Feldenkrais grew up in an educated, middle class family, the grandson of a revered Jewish holy man. At the age of 14, he trekked to Palestine. There he worked doing manual construction, surveying, and tutoring children who had difficulty learning.[8,9] During this time in Palestine, under the British mandate, there were attacks against the new Jewish settlers. Feldenkrais developed a form of hand-to-hand combat that was used by the settlers for self-defense, described in the book *Ju-Jitsu and Self-Defense*,[9] which he published in Paris in 1929.

Feldenkrais went to Paris in the late 1920s to continue his education at the University of Paris, where he studied mechanical and electrical engineering and later read for his doctorate in physics. While in Paris, he also studied the writings of Freud and Coue and in 1930 published a Hebrew translation with commentary of Coue's work, *Autosuggestion*.[9] In 1934, Feldenkrais met Jigaro Kano, the Japanese originator of Judo, who was doing demonstrations in Paris. Feldenkrais trained with Kano and became one of the first Europeans to receive a black belt and founded the Judo Club of France in 1936.[9] While playing soccer with a French club, he tore the meniscus of his left knee. He observed that there were times when he was able to move normally and other times, during which he seemed to be doing the same activities, he would become incapacitated by the pain in his knee. He took this as a challenge and over time learned to walk and move without pain.[7] This was his initial experience in using awareness to improve function.

During World War II, Feldenkrais fled to England and was assigned to the British Admiralty unit on antisubmarine warfare, and there found a group of people interested in studying Judo with him. These classes provided the opportunity for him to experiment with his own ideas that formed the beginning of his thinking on Awareness Through Movement.[8] During this time, he wrote and published several volumes on Judo.[10,11] In London, after World War II, Feldenkrais continued his study of psychology, anatomy, and neurophysiology and became familiar with the work of F. M. Alexander, who developed a system for changing postural habits through awareness and exercise. He also became familiar with the work of Elsa Gindler, who was teaching the importance of sensory awareness, and Gurdieff, who taught that personal development was a life-long process of improving self-awareness of the body and the spirit. In London, he also worked with D. G. Morgan, a psychiatrist who believed that the history of a person's experience was locked in the body and needed to be released by neuromuscular work. This wide-ranging study by Feldenkrais culminated in his publication of *Body and Mature Behavior* in 1949.[8] This book was the first comprehensive expression of the philosophy, science, and experience underlying his method of working.

In 1951, Feldenkrais returned to Israel to become head of armed forces research. In his spare time, he continued the development of his psychophysical methods by teaching small group classes on weekends and evenings. In 1968, Feldenkrais began his first training program with 14 clients in Tel Aviv.[12] This training lasted for 3 years. Later, some of these clients traveled with him to the first American training in San Francisco from 1975 to 1977. Sixty people were trained at that program. After the San Francisco training, the Feldenkrais Guild was established under Feldenkrais' guidance to support graduates of the training program and to plan and conduct future training programs. In July 1984, on the first day of one of the authors' (JS) training program in Toronto, Feldenkrais died. That program and subsequent training programs have been conducted by senior practitioners under the auspices of the Feldenkrais Guild. There are now many chapters of the Feldenkrais Guild throughout the world (see Resources).

PHILOSOPHICAL AND THEORETICAL BASIS

> *The human brain is such as to make... acquisition of new responses a normal and suitable activity... The active pattern of doing is therefore essentially personal. This great ability to form individual nervous paths and muscular patterns makes it possible for faulty patterns to be learned... The faulty behavior will appear in the executive motor mechanisms which will seem later... to be inherent in the person and unalterable. It will remain largely so unless the nervous paths producing the undesirable pattern of motility are undone and reshuffled into a better configuration.[13]*

The initial exposition of Feldenkrais' thinking is set out in *Body and Mature Behavior: A Study of Anxiety, Sex, Gravitation and Learning*.[13] The subtitle suggests the breadth of issues addressed.

Feldenkrais was interested in developing a method that would assist people to function at a higher level of maturity. In this state of maturity, a person would bring to bear on present circumstance only those past experiences that were appropriate and necessary.[13] This image was embodied for him by the Judo concept of Shizentai, balanced upright stance. This stance had two components: 1) posture from which a person could initiate movement in any direction with the same ease, without preliminary adjustments; and 2) performance of movements with the minimal amount of effort and maximum efficiency. Such a person would have the capacity to recover well from any kind of challenge or trauma. Basic to this ideal was a well-developed kinesthetic sense necessary for learning. He saw maturity as the state in which the capacity to learn had reached its highest level of development.

Physical learning is defined as an organic process in which the mental and physical aspects are fully integrated. It proceeds at its own pace; it is completely individualized and guided by the perception of an action feeling easier to do. It occurs most readily in short, focused intervals of attention and when the learner is in a good mood. The outcome of this process is the development of self-knowledge, the awareness of how we do an action. "Learning is the acquisition of the skill to inhibit parasitic action (components of the action which are unrelated to the intention of the action resulting from some secondary intention) and the ability to direct clear motivations as a result of self knowledge."[14] Initially when learning a new skill, many components of movement are done that interfere with the overall intention of the action. One by one, the parasitic movements are eliminated, leaving only the essential, differentiated action. This learning is different from training, practice, or exercise. In involves the discovery of new ways to do activities that one already knows how to do.[15] There is a broadening of the repertoire of behavior to give multiple options for doing any particular activity. Children develop this capacity naturally. For example, a 3-year-old girl will delight in demonstrating the many different ways to come down the stairs: sliding on her stomach head first, sliding on her stomach feet first, creeping backward, creeping forward, bumping on her butt while sitting, walking holding the rail, jumping two or three steps holding the rail, rolling, and finally walking and not holding the rail. Coming down the stairs is an exciting learning experience.

Each person learns to satisfy his or her basic needs in his or her own individual way. For an infant, dependent on adults for fulfillment of many of those needs and for safety, much of the learning process is interpersonal. The infant, thus, can develop what Feldenkrais called cross-motivation, in which gaining the approval of adults is more important than exploring and learning the task in an individualized way. Successful interpersonal learning occurs when adults support the exploration and satisfaction of needs in a positive and playful way while maintaining safety. However, adults may impose arbitrary and erroneous ideas of caution, prudence, and decent and indecent behavior on the child, and impose punishment or withdraw approval when the child does not perform to their expectations.[14]

Well-meaning adults may interfere with the process of organic learning, limiting the development of skill in acquiring multiple options for performing any activity. Imagine you, as a parent, have anxiety that your child will get hurt coming down the stairs any way but the conventional way of walking, and you withdraw approval from the child and even punish alternate ways of descending the stairs. Anxiety related to fear of falling might be produced in the child. Feldenkrais also believed that anxiety would be produced when our options were removed and we had no alternative ways of acting.[13] Imagine that you are faced with failing in your professional training and have no other idea of what you might do with your life! Or imagine the difference between walking on a 1-foot-wide beam that rests on the ground compared to a 1-foot-wide beam 20 feet in the air where stepping off is not an option.

Feldenkrais clearly conceived of the process of learning as producing new pathways, associations, and connections in the central nervous system. All the different patterns of innervation involved in the control of voluntary movement develop as the control of action is being learned. So the control of movement is integrated into what Feldenkrais called the vast background of vegetative and reflexive activity of the nervous system.[13] The imposition of anxiety, compulsion, or cross-motivation on this process of learning created what Feldenkrais called faulty learning. The child learned to produce the behavior that was expected, the posture that was approved of, or the expression that was acceptable, and did not learn to test behavior against present reality. The continual learning process that would go on throughout life in a mature person came to a standstill. How many 60- or 70-year-olds have nine different ways of coming down the stairs? In the adult, habitual patterns that were formed over the years have molded the body to produce, for example, flat feet or stiff shoulders and a neck that will not turn or a painful low back. The problem may not be with the feet, back, or neck. It may be with the parasitic neuromuscular patterns that have been formed and with the loss of the ability of the person to adapt to new situations by learning.[13]

Later in his career, Feldenkrais recognized that physical injury and malfunction of the nervous system interacted significantly with the process of neuromuscular habit formation. If the nervous system does not work properly in either its motor, sensory, or integrative/cognitive components, it becomes difficult or impossible to produce the normal functional control patterns used in everyday life. A musculoskeletal injury creates pain or alters the anatomy so as to interfere with normal function. Also, a person who has rigid and maladaptive neuromuscular habit patterns is more likely to be injured in an automobile accident and less likely to adapt and recover than a person who can learn and adapt quickly.[7]

What would it take for a 70-year-old to have a movement repertoire that included the nine ways of coming down the stairs mentioned earlier? Or to return the arm and hand of a concert flutist, damaged by a bullet, to its previous world-class level of function? Or for a child born with cerebral palsy to learn to walk? Feldenkrais believed that the key to these transformations was the education or re-education of the kinesthetic sense and resetting it to a normal course of self-adjusting improvement of all neuromuscular activity.[13] What is this process and how is it implemented?

Approaches to the Client

Feldenkrais Method is practiced in two forms: FI and ATM. These will be described below with examples of the process and case studies.

INTRODUCTION TO FUNCTIONAL INTEGRATION

An FI lesson is a one-on-one, hands-on approach to learning that occurs in a safe, supportive, and non-judgmental, environment. The practitioner uses passive movement and resistance to passive movement through the skeleton to explore the client's current state of functioning in the world. Lessons are aimed at increasing the client's awareness of how he or she moves, discovering alternative ways of functioning in the world beyond what is already familiar, and increasing the fluidity, ease, and efficiency of movement.

Environment and Context for Learning

The beginning of an FI lesson is generally performed with the client's body in a fully supported position so that the system is responding to a neutral, quiet environment in which learning can be optimized. Clients are guided to become more familiar with their current organization of body segments in relationship to each other and to the support surface. The way that the client most often organizes his or her body segments at rest and during functional activities is understood as a reflection of his or her orientation to the world and preparedness to move in different directions at any moment.

There is a minimal amount of verbal instruction. The practitioner utilizes gentle, noninvasive touch to stimulate awareness and curiosity, and an almost imperceptible level of force to explore willingness to move. The practitioner's hands are not used to push or manipulate, although there is intent to convey how the person functions easily and something new—some new possibility for movement—around that which is already easy.

When the body is relaxed and moved passively, there is a chain reaction of movement throughout the skeleton that is similar to the observed phenomenon of knocking over a set of dominos. If no muscles were present to constrain or influence passive movement through the skeleton, movement would travel through the skeleton unimpeded. During an FI lesson, the practitioner has no preconceived notion of how the person should move or what is normal, only what makes sense for that person based upon willingness to move in different directions and inherent structural constraints imposed by the skeleton for different movements.

Feldenkrais believed that use of effort and willpower to complete movements and maintain postures would tend to limit freedom of choice to more habitual ways of interacting with the world.[7] FI lessons are conducted passively to limit effort by the client. Lessons generally begin at slow speeds since faster motions often evoke a protective response and effort on the part of the client. As rapport and trust develop between client and practitioner, and as the client learns how to reduce effort, movements may become faster, larger, and more playful as the range of free, nonguarded movement increases.

Learning to reduce muscular effort is encouraged by passively supporting the client's body segments using rolls, pillows, bolsters, and/or the practitioner's hands to match and/or augment postures and movement patterns. Matching and/or augmenting postures and movement patterns that are easy sets the stage for a safe and familiar context for learning. Creating a sense of safety provides an opportunity for the client to explore novel combinations and alternative pathways of movement. This is analogous to the exploratory behavior of a toddler who runs back and forth between the safety of a parent and the curiosity of a new toy or person in the room. When the parent is not present, the child stops playing and becomes anxious. The presence of the parent provides a sense of security from which the child can explore. Likewise, matching rather than correcting or insisting upon change in posture or a movement pattern sets the stage for safe exploration and integration of alternative ways of using one's body.

Movement is repeated with the intent of learning to reduce effort on the part of the client and to have the client become more familiar with variations in the movement, making alternatives to the familiar way of moving feel less awkward. In addition, bringing a body segment in one direction and then returning toward the start position enhances the client's concept of movement ease in the reverse direction of what is familiar or easy. Repetitions of consistent stimuli can be used to determine if movement direction and amplitude have changed. Each repetition of a movement takes on a slightly different pathway, which expands upon the client's options for easy movement. Repetition of movement is used not for the sake of practice but to familiarize the person with what he or she has learned and to bring attention and awareness to a particular function. Frequent, brief rest periods are provided to allow the person to process comparisons of movement freedom in different directions.

In a hands-on lesson, the practitioner's ability to move freely and easily with the client can also affect the client's ability to learn. The lesson is similar to dancing with a partner, being free to listen to directional cues and move easily in all directions. The position of the practitioner relative to the client, the support surface, and the practitioner's own habit patterns play a role in the ability of the client to allow him- or herself to become completely receptive and engaged in the exploration. The practitioner's organization also influences the directions and magnitudes of movements that are possible. Practitioners spend a great deal of time during their formal training learning to organize themselves so that their own interactions in the world will be less likely to limit those of the clients with whom they work.

Lessons include playing with movement and movement combinations in different positions relative to gravity and as part of different functional activities to help generalize learning. There are no exercises to practice following a lesson, although the person may be asked to explore and compare movements to reinforce concepts learned during a lesson.

When pain, stiffness, and/or weakness are present, the practitioner generally begins working at a distant area of the body to minimize anxiety on the part of the client. In a situation where a person has suffered a neurological injury such as a stroke, the practitioner works with the stronger side of the body first, especially in a situation with sensory deficit. This process is less confrontational to the client and evokes less anxiety by focusing on movements that feel good and are successful for function. For example, if the client has a painful shoulder or neck, the practitioner may choose to start the lesson at the person's feet and build upon the ease of movement there. Small indirect movements may occur simultaneously at other segments.

Assessment and Reassessment

During an FI session, the practitioner observes the client's initial postural configuration (alignment of body segments relative to other segments and to the support surface) in sitting, standing, and/or lying. The arrangement and folds of the client's clothing and body contours can provide additional information about the way the individual organizes him- or herself in relationship to the world.

The practitioner then makes contact with the client's skeleton and using very gentle and slow passive movement, assesses the willingness of individual body segments and of the whole individual to move from the initial configuration. The practitioner feels for the first muscular response to limit the passive movement, while observing for dampening of the chain reaction through the skeleton. Constraints to the flow of movement between body segments are noted and brought to the client's attention, as are areas of the body that are used as pivots around which functional movements occur.

The practitioner assesses and reassesses the client's movement on a moment-to-moment basis throughout the course of a lesson.[16] The practitioner makes on-going judgments for how to proceed with the lesson that are based upon synthesis of observations, background information about the client, and/or movement findings. In addition the practitioner constantly considers positions and ways to support the client that will allow the client greater freedom and choices of movement.

Focus of Functional Integration Lessons

During a FI lesson, the practitioner has no preconceived notion of how the person should move or what is "normal." The practitioner takes into account the client's reports and requests, knowledge of the client's background, and the practitioner's knowledge and experience when designing a lesson for the client. Themes of a lesson include: 1) enhancing the client's orientation within the environment; 2) enhancing fluidity, ease, and efficiency of movement; and 3) enhancing the sense of differentiation or integration of body segments to the whole.[16]

Orientating the client to the environment includes working to enhance the client's sense of weight shift, awareness of orientation of the eyes at rest and during functional activities, sense of support of the skeleton in relationship to gravity and the support surface, self-image, and body image.

Lessons that are focused on enhancing fluidity, efficiency, and ease of movement include comparisons with effortful movement, resistance and/or constraint to movement, segments of the body where the client initiates movement from most often, and changes in the tonus of the muscles. Lessons focus on changing options for speed, direction, magnitude, and quality of movement.

Practitioners also structure lessons to enhance the client's perception of how movement translates between body segments and through the whole skeleton during function and during passive movement. Lessons of this nature include enhancing the client's perception of differentiation of movement of body segments from the whole and/or integrating movement of specific body segments to movements of the whole.

When the practitioner observes and/or palpates restrictions to movement through the skeleton from a particular vantage point, the practitioner may choose to change the point of contact of their hand(s) with the client's body segment, change the angle of or direction of movement, or switch to a different body segment to affect the flow of movement through the skeleton.

Three Case Examples

Case 1

A mature woman in her early 50s with cerebral palsy requested Feldenkrais lessons to improve the smoothness and safety of her walking. She also wanted to be able to stand on one foot. Her movement assessment showed that she had difficulty uncoupling the joints of her lower extremities in sitting, standing, lying down, and on all fours. Her lessons focused on supporting her initial configuration. When lying on her back, her pelvis was rotated to the right, her left lower extremities were both rolled toward the right, and there was little if any movement at her hip joints. As part of the lesson, her pelvis and lower extremities were rolled further toward the right and briefly compared to movement to the left. Her left lower extremity had greater availability of movement than the right so movement on that leg was explored first. Rolling her leg to the right automatically brought the pelvis to the right so the pelvic motion was augmented and then differentiated from the leg. The practitioner also worked on gently pushing from the sole of the foot through the leg to initiate movement of the leg in the socket of the hip. As the practitioner did this subtle movement, she varied the amount of roll of the leg slightly each time so that the client could begin to feel the movement of the leg in the joint. In amazement, the client said, "I didn't know I had a joint there." She asked to see an anatomy book to confirm that there was supposed to be a joint at her hip where she had never felt one. During that lesson, the practitioner was also able to bring the client's knee up toward her body by rolling her leg further out and bending the knee. They then explored movement at the hip joint within the tiny zone of comfort that was available with the hip and knee bent. When the client's muscles would grab, the practitioner would wait for the contraction to let up before they would explore another slight variation to the movement. The stiffness that had been so evident in her legs changed significantly. At the end of that lesson, they practiced lifting one leg in standing while holding onto the back of a chair. The client was able to march in place by raising her feet several inches off the floor without having to lean backward. She had learned to disassociate or uncouple her leg from her pelvis for the first time in her life.

Case 2

Often, the changes in postural configuration and functional abilities that occur are not linearly related to the lesson. For example, the practitioner had a client in her 90s who came for lessons to improve the way she was walking. She arrived for her first lesson with a walker and had a great deal of difficulty going up steps. She was very hunched over and complained of weakness and stiffness in her knees. When lying down, she was unable to fully straighten her hips or knees and needed two pillows under her head to accommodate her forward head position and rounded shoulders. Her FI lesson brought her further into her initial configuration of flexion of the trunk and lower extremities. Building upon her willingness to move into flexion and listening to her system for directions of ease versus resistance, eventually she was able to lie on her back curled in a ball and holding her knees. In this position, the practitioner was able to roll her side to side. Briefly, toward the end of the session with the woman still lying on her back, the practitioner helped her to explore pushing with one foot or the other into the table with bent knees. When she stood up, her posture was much more erect, and she reported that her legs felt stronger and less stiff. Several days later, the practitioner received a phone call from the client's daughter, who reported that her mother had taken a bath by herself for the first time in a year and had no problem getting out of the tub. The changes in function were nonlinear in the sense that the practitioner never worked on teaching her how to get in or out of the tub and never worked directly on improving her erect standing or walking.

Case 3

In addition to identifying ways that the initial configuration could be achieved more completely, the practitioner also helps to identify pathways of connections between body segments that are more consistent with the bony skeleton and with function. Take for example the 74-year-old woman who came for FI lessons complaining of pain in her right groin and knee that had been present for years. She had a history of several previous falls and had received physical therapy and acupuncture treatments with some short-term relief. Movement assessment revealed that she was organized with her pelvis rotated to the right and her upper body rotated to the left in sitting, standing, and lying down. In addition, her right shoulder was rolled forward and the right upper arm was held firmly at her side when lying down. When pressing down through her first rib to assess movement through her skeleton from the base of her neck toward her feet, the right side moved down easily, while the left did not. The body segment components of this configuration were augmented first. Then right and left side-bending of the trunk were compared. The right side bent easily in a direction of slight extension; however, when guiding the movement from the neck down, the motion traveled only down to the middle of the rib cage before moving off to the left. There was no connection to the feet. This was compared to the left side, which did not side-bend. The opposing configuration between the pelvis and the lower ribs was augmented and held to take over the work of habitual muscle contraction. Providing support into her initial configuration allowed her to relax and let her pelvis and lower ribs move more easily together to the left. Movement through the skeleton from the right side of the neck became more clear in the direction of the left pelvis and left leg but was still moving off to the left in the midrib area. As side-bend of the trunk at different levels was again compared, side-bend to the left became easier and movement down through the neck to the left foot was more consistent. From there, the lesson progressed to reversals of rolling to the left and onto the back, to sitting and eventually to standing. Reaching toward the left with the right arm in sitting and in standing was compared to its mirror image on the left. The client reported almost total relief of pain for several days following the lesson and reported being able to do heavy house cleaning that she was normally unable to do.

See References 7 and 17 through 20 for several general FI resources.

AWARENESS THROUGH MOVEMENT

ATM is a verbally directed movement process that can be done with one person or many people. Feldenkrais did public workshops with as many as 300 people participating. An ATM lesson can be presented on audiotape either commercially or by taping an individual lesson done with a client and letting him or her work with it at home. (Hundreds of lessons are available on CD or online. See the Additional Resources at the end of the chapter.) When a lesson is done with many people at the same time, people respond in very individualized ways using pieces of the action as they are able for mini-lessons at a level that they can manage.[21]

An ATM lesson is a structured movement exploration that makes use of common movement forms to explore how the individual organizes his or her control of movement. For the practitioner, it is rather like taking the client on a leisurely stroll along the edge of a canyon while feeling safe and in control, appreciating the view and knowing that there may be something different just over the edge. A lesson may be done in supine, side lying, prone, sitting, or standing, and involves small turns, bends, or weight shifts with the goal of being able to perceive the change that occurs while remaining in complete control of the movement process. The movement is used to generate changes in posture and movement pattern that can be perceived.

Slow, small, simple movements are done at first in order to reduce effort and optimize awareness. The Weber-Fechner principle[22] in sensory physiology shows us that excessive effort interferes with our ability to detect small changes. A lesson might begin with a very small movement involving external rotation of the hip with flexion of the knee in the supine position. This movement would be repeated in slightly different ways 10 to 20 times. During this process, awareness is directed to changes in other areas of the body related to this movement. There may be rotation of the spine so that the opposite hip lifts from the floor, a change in the pattern of breathing, maybe a stiffening of the opposite leg or foot, or pressing into the floor with the opposite leg. When this simple movement is optimally performed using the whole body, the opposite leg will be fully relaxed and the spine able to turn as weight is transferred laterally. Other parts of the body would be free to move in other directions: turning or nodding of the head, for example, should be easy. If a person discovers that he or she is holding the leg or foot stiffly, holding his or her breath, or not experiencing a weight shift through the skeleton, then it is possible to discover that he or she is making unnecessary, excessive, muscular effort to perform that movement. The effort spent on this habit interferes with the perception of action and control of movement.

These kinds of observations are the basis of the assessment performed in conjunction with ATM. We as practitioners look for how a person organizes his or her weight through the skeleton in relation to the base of support. Is the use of the skeleton optimal? How much effort does the person make to hold a position or do a transition from it? Are all the body segments organized to participate appropriately in the intention of the movement, or is one leg possibly anchoring a different intention, thus making the movement less efficient and potentially dangerous? Is the timing of control of one body segment contributing optimally to the movement of others? The more a person is able to reduce effort and discriminate small changes, the more finely he or she can control action.

ATM lessons commonly make use of novelty. Lessons can be structured in such a way that the outcome of the movement (rolling over, standing up) is not obvious during the process. This use of novelty allows the client to maintain better awareness of the details of the movement in progress without reverting back to habitual movement patterns for an action she already has a way of performing. In this way, new patterns of motor control can be developed.

Case Example

A 41-year-old clinical psychologist and professional singer was referred for her most recent episode in a 20-year history of recurring headaches and chronic pain in her upper back, neck, and lower back. Her diagnoses included left sacroiliac joint dysfunction, pelvic hypermobility, cervical and thoracic facet joint malalignment, and a mild (less than 20 degrees) scoliosis with apices at C5, T6, and L2. The precipitating event for this episode was trying to open a heavy door. The effort of opening the door caused a spasm of pain in her right low back, from which upper back and neck stiffness developed over the next day without resolution. Lifting or carrying even very light objects also set off her back pain, often incapacitating her for weeks. Because of this type of onset, she had severely limited her activities, leading to further loss of function and loss of independence in many daily activities. She had previously been treated in a variety of ways, including bed rest, heavy medication for pain, myofascial release, traditional strengthening and range of motion, and Pilates technique, all with limited success. Initial observations of her movement showed that she was unable to organize abdominal muscles well in supine transfers, depending more than usual on upper extremity assistance, and that she was unable to lift her head off the floor from supine. She also had a lot of fear about doing many movements because of the frequent disastrous consequences.

She had a general problem with effective motor control, not simply a problem of weakness. Lessons focused around how she could learn to use her abdominals again in a coordinated and powerful way. The ATM process outlined below was a part of her treatment plan. It unfolded slowly over the course of 6 weekly sessions. As she developed mastery of these movement problems, she ceased having headaches, had much less tension in her upper back and neck, and much reduced low back pain. She was able to bend, reach, lift, and carry light objects with much more ease and could lift her head up from supine and get up from the floor without any thought of difficulty. The process of learning abdominal control was organic, embedded in a variety of functional movement patterns.

A Set of Awareness Through Movement Lessons

Each bullet is a movement sequence that was explored in many repetitions and variations in the order presented. Her response is in italics:

+ From a long sit position on the floor leaning back on the hands, slowly bend the legs and posteriorly tilt the pelvis until the feet come off the floor. *Initially, she had difficulty with pain in her low back, upper back, and neck that eased as she found a way to take weight more symmetrically through her ischial bones and to bring her head forward closer to her base of support.*

+ Sitting on the floor with legs flexed and feet in the air, hands on the knees, slowly rock in different directions. A process of progressive approximation is used to develop a movement sequence. For example, begin with lifting one foot off the floor while shifting weight slightly toward the right ischium. Then lift both feet slightly off the floor while shifting weight to the right. Repeat similar movements to the left side. With both feet in the air, move one knee in small circles, then move the other knee in small circles. *She initially was able to move very little without losing her balance. Her range and control of motion increased considerably as she discovered how she could laterally flex and rotate her spine to bring her head closer over her base of support.*

+ While maintaining sitting balance on the floor, hands on knees, and feet in the air, slowly move and twist the legs side to side and turn the head in the same and opposite direction. *She developed skill in these movements as she discovered how to let her weight go further out to the side on her pelvis and turn her legs in a different direction at the same time.*

+ From sitting on the floor with hands on knees, slowly roll backward with a rounded back so as to roll the back to the floor with the pelvis coming up into the air and the weight shifting onto the shoulders, then roll back up to sitting. *Initially, she was very afraid to do this, and in her first attempts her back slapped flat against the floor. Slowly, she learned to curl her spine so that she could feel each vertebra as it met the floor. When she reached this stage of control, she was able to roll back to the floor and roll back up with minimal effort and use of momentum. At this point, she was able to stabilize her core and control its rotation effectively as she opened a heavy door in her home which she had been unable to do previously.*

Evidence of Efficacy: Review of the Research

There is growing literature in the field now called cognitive neuroscience that is expanding our understanding of brain plasticity in just the way that Feldenkrais imagined. This research has provided evidence that damage to the nervous system centrally or peripherally, engaging in novel or usual activities, and recovery from disease processes affecting the central nervous system stimulate change in central sensory and motor representations.[23-25] The question of whether this sort of plasticity occurs during the process of rehabilitation is only beginning to be addressed.[26-29] Functional magnetic resonance imagery (fMRI) has recently been used to demonstrate improved activation of the involved motor cortex paralleled by improved hand function following a Feldenkrais intervention in a patient 9 months post stroke.[30] This is the only evidence so far that Feldenkrais Method works at this level.

Much of the published work is in the form of single or multiple case studies. These reports contain detailed information about interventions that have been highly successful in producing functional gains. Examples of this type of literature include report of improved functional mobility in a group of people with spinal cord injury;[31] the reduction of stuttering in three people using FI;[32] dramatic functional improvements in two women who had traumatic brain injury;[33] resolution of back pain;[34,35] reduction of pain and improved mobility in four women with rheumatoid arthritis;[36] improved mobility and well-being in four women with multiple sclerosis;[21] improved balance and mobility in a woman with multiple sclerosis;[37] improved flexibility and mobility in a woman with hereditary spastic paraparesis;[38] and improved function in patients with Parkinson's disease.[39] In two separate papers,[40,41] Stephens has reported outcomes from clinical practice that demonstrate a greater than 80% rate of clients achieving 100% of initial goals, and a greater than 90% rate of clients achieving at least 75% of initial goals over a total of nearly 200 clients and more than 90 different ICD-9 diagnostic codes. The number of visits per episode of care fell well within the guidelines suggested by the *Guide to Physical Therapy Practice*.[42]

Ives and Shelly[43] reviewed the research published through 1996 and noted that in many of the studies reviewed well-controlled research designs were not used or there were other flaws in the experimental procedures. However, they concluded that further research was warranted due to the "sheer number of positive reports that fit within a sound theoretical framework." More recently, a number studies incorporating more effective methods, larger groups, and random assignment control group studies have been done. Four general areas of clinical outcomes will be presented: pain management, motor and postural control, functional mobility, and psychological and quality of life effects.

PAIN MANAGEMENT

More than 50% of clients seeking Feldenkrais intervention came with an initial complaint of pain interfering with function.[41] Fibromyalgia is an increasingly common diagnosis. In a study of five women with fibromyalgia using ATM twice weekly for 2 months, Dean et al[44] showed significant decrease in pain and improved posture, gait, sleep, and body awareness. In an attempt to replicate this work, Stephens et al,[45] using a repeated measures design with 16 people with fibromyalgia, observed changes in pain and mobility variables, but these were overshadowed by the high variability of repeated baseline measures. In another study of the fibromyalgia population, initial improvements found during the 15-week intervention were not maintained at the 6-month follow-up. Again methodological problems were cited in this study.[46]

Bearman and Shafarman[47] found large decreases in pain perception, improvements in functional status, reduction in use of pain medication, and a 40% reduction in the cost of medical care during a 1-year follow-up period for a group of seven chronic pain patients following an 8-week intensive Feldenkrais Method intervention. Working with 34 chronic pain patients in a retrospective study, Phipps et al[48] showed that the Feldenkrais Method helped to reduce the pain and improve function and that learned ATM methods were still used independently by patients 2 years post-discharge. In a study of 97 auto workers in Sweden, Lundblad, Elert, and Gerdle[49] found significant decreases in complaints of neck and shoulder pain and in disability during leisure activity in the Feldenkrais intervention group compared to randomly assigned physical therapy and no intervention control groups. The Lundblad study is the best experimental design done to date in the area of pain management.

DeRosa and Porterfield[50] included the Feldenkrais Method among a number of intervention methods that would most successfully address the motor control elements underlying much of the presenting back pain seen in physical therapy clinics. Since this work, it has been widely recognized that active exercise is a more effective intervention for back pain than other, more passive approaches. Maher[51] has recommended that Feldenkrais Method not be considered as an intervention for low back pain based on the idea that there is little high quality evidence supporting its efficacy. The same conclusion was reached with regard to mechanical neck pain.[52] Both of these reviews conclude that the lack of supporting evidence from large clinical trials is a reason to not use Feldenkrais Method. We suggest here that there is sufficient anecdotal, case and small study evidence to support further research in the form of larger clinical studies.

In other pain related work, Rogers[53] has provided evidence that people who have used Feldenkrais, ATM and other body awareness therapies have a greater awareness of the mechanisms of injury occurring during piano practice and therefore a better opportunity to develop preventative strategies. O'Connor[54] has reported that Feldenkrais Method can be used effectively as part of palliative care with people who are in chronic pain. In summary, Feldenkrais Method appears to be an approach that has great potential as an intervention for pain but that it is not well supported at this time with evidence from large randomized, controlled trials.

MOTOR AND POSTURAL CONTROL

In the area of motor control, three kinds of problems have been explored: changes in activity of a muscle group during a standard task, changes in postural control related to breathing, and postural control related to standing balance and mobility. In a study[55] involving 21 subjects, an ATM lesson exploring trunk flexion led to a decrease in abdominal electromyogram (EMG) activity and a perception of the standardized supine flexion task being easier. There was no similar change in a control group using imagery and suggestion along, but no movement, which suggests that the changes noted were a result of the exploratory movements alone. Another study[56] using 30 subjects reported an increase in supine neck flexion range of motion and a decrease in perceived effort in this movement compared to a control group. Several groups have been interested in studying effects on hamstring length. In studies looking at hamstring function, James et al[57] and Hopper, Kolt, and McConville[58] reported no change in hamstring length following a single ATM lesson designed to lengthen hamstrings compared to relaxation and normal activity control groups. These studies looked at effects of ATM following a single lesson. Stephens et al[59] studied effects of a set of hamstring lengthening ATM lessons used over a period of 3 weeks. There was a significant increase in hamstring length compared to a normal activity control group. This result suggests that a period of time longer than a single lesson may be required for adequate learning in most people.

Saraswati[60] showed changes in pattern of breathing involving increased movement of the abdomen, postural changes involving increased use of erector spinae muscles, and increased peak flow rates compared to a matched group of young, healthy controls following a series of ATM lessons. The use of ATM to improve breathing, mobility, and postural control has also been reported in a case study with a man with Parkinson's disease.[61]

In an initial study of four women with multiple sclerosis, Stephens et al[21] documented improvements in supine to stand transfers and a subjective report of generally improved control of balance and movement. In a follow-up study with a group of 12 people with multiple sclerosis, Stephens et al[62] found significant improvements in balance performance and balance confidence compared to a group meeting for educational purposes only, using a randomized control group design. Batson et al[63] have provided similar evidence of improved balance and mobility in a pilot study with stroke patients.

In a study with 59 well, elderly women randomly divided into three groups, Hall et al[64] found improvements in activities of daily living score, Timed Up and Go, Berg balance assessment, and three of eight scales on the SF-36 following a 10-week series of ATM lessons. Seegert and Shapiro[65] have also reported changes in static standing control in healthy, young subjects. In summary, in a series of studies, Feldenkrais Method has been shown to have a positive impact on postural and motor control in normal and impaired subjects. More research is needed in these areas.

FUNCTIONAL MOBILITY

Several studies have shown improvements in functional mobility using Timed Up and Go and other measures. These studies have been done with well elderly people,[66,67] people with multiple sclerosis[20] and CVA.[63]

PSYCHOLOGICAL AND QUALITY OF LIFE EFFECTS

As noted earlier, Feldenkrais thinking was driven by theory from psychology as well as physiology. An overriding interest was to find a method of improving the level of maturity with which people function in their lives. In a recent dissertation, Frank[68] has discussed the role of proprioception, what he refers to as "awareness through movement," in the development and regulation of self-perception throughout life. He came to the conclusion, in agreement with Feldenkrais, that a cohesive experience of the body is at the core of individual health and maturity. This suggests that changes in psychological variables such as body image, self-efficacy, anxiety, and life satisfaction should be studied. There is some research in these areas.

In a qualitative study of 10 people who had prolonged experience of FI, Steisel[69] found improvements in body awareness, motivation, self-esteem, and decreases in anxiety. In an interesting study using analysis of clay figure construction, Deig[70] described expansion in the detail and form of body image after a series of ATM lessons. This work was extended by Elgelid[71] who found improvements in body image resulting from a series of ATM lessons using the Jourard-Secord

Cathexis scale. Hutchinson[72] also used this scale and reported improvements in body image in a group of overweight women. The best-designed study in this area involved a matched, control group study of 30 young women with eating disorders. Laumer et al[73] used standardized psychological testing to measure outcomes. They concluded that a 9-hour course of ATM improved the level of acceptance of the body and self, decreased feelings of helplessness and dependence, increased self-confidence, and facilitated a general process of maturation of the whole personality in the experimental group. All these studies lend support to the idea that one of the fundamental impacts on Feldenkrais Method is on body image and awareness.

In 1977, Gutman et al[74] did the first research involving Feldenkrais Method in a well elderly population. Subjects were divided into three matched groups: 6 weeks ATM, 6 weeks standard exercise, and a no exercise control. Although they were unable to show additional benefits of Feldenkrais sessions in functional or physiological measures compared to exercise and no exercise control groups because of measurement and design problems, they did find a trend toward improvement in overall perception of health status in the Feldenkrais group. Also studying a well elderly population, Stephens et al[67] reported significant improvements in the vitality and mental health subscales of the SF-36 following a 2-day ATM workshop. This area of work has been extended by Malmgren-Olsson et al[75,76] to a group of 78 patients with a variety of musculoskeletal disorders, showing that Feldenkrais Method intervention was effective in reducing psychological distress as well as pain and in improving negative self-image. Lowe[77] has suggested that the same effect may occur in people who are engaged in a process of rehabilitation acutely after myocardial infarct.

More extensive study of effects of Feldenkrais Method on anxiety have been done by Kolt et al.[78,79] In several papers, they have found significant reduction of state anxiety across a single lesson increasing across 10 weeks of intervention. This conclusion was further supported by Netz[80], who compared effects on state anxiety, depressive mood, and subjective well-being and found ATM, swimming, and yoga all more effective than aerobic dance or a computer class control group in improving outcome measures in these areas.

Psychological and quality of life outcomes have been studied with patients in neurological rehabilitation as well. In the first study in this area in people with multiple sclerosis, Bost et al[81] demonstrated an improvement in well-being in a controlled study of 50 subjects over 30 days. In a small multiple case study involving four women, Stephens et al[21] found large increases in well being using the Index of Well-Being. In a follow-up study in which balance was also demonstrated to be improved, Stephens et al[82] have shown significant improvements in retrospective memory and positive social support in the ATM group compared to the control group with multiple sclerosis. And in a randomly assigned, crossover design, Johnson et al[83] found a significant decrease in perceived stress and anxiety following Feldenkrais sessions in a group of 20 people with multiple sclerosis. Research has begun in this area with the post-CVA population. Connors[84] described a patient with hemi-inattention who showed significant improvement on the Behavioral Inattention Scale after a 4-week intervention with Feldenkrais Method acutely following a right frontal hemorrhage. This improvement was not accompanied by motor improvement at this early stage of rehabilitation. Finally, in a recent study that is in preparation for publication, Batson et al[85] have found improvement in the ability to image movement, using the Movement Imagery Quotient, in a group of people more than a year post CVA. The most exciting aspect of this finding was the strong positive correlation found between improvement in motor imagery and improvement in balance and mobility measures.

Conclusion

The Feldenkrais Method begins with a great respect for the individuality and dignity of the client and proceeds with gentle exploratory processes, actively and passively, to engage the client in a process of learning. It has application to people with a wide range of disabilities and to people from very low to very high functional levels. The research supports efficacy in a variety of areas. Clearly, more research is needed to establish the range of useful application and to understand the processes by which this approach is effective.

Acknowledgments

We would like to thank all of the clients and patients with whom we have worked over the years for challenging our creativity and allowing us to challenge theirs.

References

1. Jacobson E. *Progressive Relaxation*. Chicago, IL: University of Chicago Press; 1938.
2. Lowen A. *Bioenergetics*. New York, NY: Coward, McCann and Geoghegan; 1975.
3. Brooks CVW. *Sensory Awareness: The Rediscovery of Experiencing*. Great Neck, NY: Felix Morrow Publishing; 1974.
4. Erickson M. *Hypnotic Realities*. New York, NY: Irvington; 1976.
5. Bateson G. *Mind and Nature*. New York, NY: EP Dutton; 1979.
6. Gibson JJ. *The Senses Considered as a Perceptual System*. Boston, MA: Houghton Mifflin; 1966.
7. Feldenkrais M. *The Elusive Obvious*. Cupertino, CA: Meta Publications; 1981.
8. Newell G. Moshe Feldenkrais: a biographical sketch of his early years. *Somatics*. 1992;7:33-38.
9. Hanna T. Moshe Feldenkrais: the silent heritage. *Somatics*. 1984;5(1):8-15.
10. Feldenkrais M. *Higher Judo*. Vol 3. London: Frederick Warne; 1942.
11. Feldenkrais M. *Judo*. London: Frederick Warne; 1942.
12. Talmi A. First encounters with Feldenkrais. *Somatics*. 1980;3(1):18-25.
13. Feldenkrais M. *Body and Mature Behavior: A Study of Anxiety, Sex, Gravitation and Learning*. New York, NY: International Universities Press; 1949.
14. Feldenkrais M. *The Potent Self. A Guide to Spontaneity*. San Francisco, CA: Harper & Row; 1985.
15. Shafarman S. *Awareness Heals: The Feldenkrais Method for Dynamic Health*. Reading, MA: Addison-Wesley Publishing; 1997.
16. Miller TM. Decision making processes of physical therapists and Feldenkrais practitioners. PhD dissertation. Temple University, Philadelphia, PA, May 2007.
17. Ginsburg C. The roots of Functional Integration: part I—biology and Feldenkrais. *Feldenkrais Journal*. 1988;3:13-24.
18. Ginsburg C. The roots of Functional Integration: part II—communication and learning. *Feldenkrais Journal*. 1989;4:13-19.
19. Ginsburg C. The roots of Functional Integration: part III—the shift in thinking. *Feldenkrais Journal*. 1992;7:34-47.
20. Kelso JA Scott. *Dynamic Patterns: The Self-Organization of Brain and Behavior*. Cambridge, MA: MIT Press; 1997.
21. Stephens JL, Call S, Evans K, Glass M, Gould C, Lowe J. Responses to ten Feldenkrais Awareness Through Movement lessons by four women with multiple sclerosis: improved quality of life. *Physical Therapy Case Reports*. 1999;2(2):58-69.
22. Kandel ER, Schwartz JH, Jessell TM. *The Principles of Neural Science*. 4th ed. Norwalk, CT: Appleton and Lange; 2000.
23. Kaas JH. Plasticity of sensory and motor maps in adult mammals. *Ann Rev Neuroscience*. 1991;14:137-167.
24. Nudo RJ, Milliken GW, Jenkins WM, Merzenich MM. Use-dependent alterations of movement representations in primary motor cortex of adult squirrel monkeys. *J Neurosci*. 1996;16(2):785-807.
25. Nudo RJ, Friel KM. Cortical plasticity after stroke: implications for rehabilitation. *Rev Neurol (Paris)*. 1999;155(9):713-717.
26. Kolb B, Gibb R, Gorny G. Cortical plasticity and the development of behavior after early frontal cortical injury. *Dev Neuropsychol*. 2000;18(3):423-444.
27. Friel KM, Heddings AA, Nudo RJ. Effects of postlesion experience on behavioral recovery and neurophysiologic reorganization after cortical injury in primates. *Neurorehabil Neural Repair*. 2000;14(3):187-198.
28. Florence SL, Boydston LA, Hackett TA, et al. Sensory enrichment after peripheral nerve injury restores cortical, but not thalamic, receptive field organization. *Eur J Neurosci*. 2001;13(9):1755-1766.
29. Liepert J, Uhde I, Graf S, et al. Motor cortex plasticity during forced-use therapy in stroke patients: a preliminary study. *J Neurol*. 2001;248(4):315-321.

30. Nair DG, Fuchs A, Burkart S, Steinberg FL, Kelso JAS. Assessing recovery in middle cerebral artery stroke using Feldenkrais Method. *Brain Inj.* 2005;19(13):1165-1176.

31. Ginsburg C. The Shake-a-Leg body awareness training program: dealing with spinal injury and recovery in a new setting. *Somatics.* 1986;Spring/Summer:31-42.

32. Gilman M, Yaruss JS. Stuttering and relaxation: applications for somatic education in stuttering treatment. *J Fluency Disorders.* 2000;25(1):59-76.

33. Ofir R. *A Heuristic Investigation of the Process of Motor Learning Using Feldenkrais Method in Physical Rehabilitation of Two Young Women With Traumatic Brain Injury* [unpublished doctoral dissertation]. New York, NY: Union Institute; 1993.

34. Lake B. Acute back pain: treatment by the application of Feldenkrais principles. *Australian Family Physician.* 1985; 14(11):53-77.

35. Panarello-Black D. PT's own back pain leads her to start Feldenkrais training. *PT Bulletin.* 1992;April 8:9-10.

36. Narula M, Jackson O, Kulig K. The effects of six-week Feldenkrais Method on selected functional parameters in a subject with rheumatoid arthritis [Abstract]. *Phys Ther.* 1992;72(Suppl):S86.

37. Stephens J. Feldenkrais Method: A case study of the application of Feldenkrais Method for a person with balance problems related to multiple sclerosis, evidence and practice. In: Deutsch J, Anderson E, eds. *Complementary Therapies for Physical Therapists: From Art to Practice,* Atlanta, GA: Elsevier; 2007 (in press).

38. Stephens J. Feldenkrais Method of somatic education. In: Umphred D, ed. *Neurological Rehabilitation.* 5th ed. Philadelphia, PA: Mosby; 2007.

39. Johnson M, Wendell LL. Some effects of the Feldenkrais Method on Parkinson's symptoms and function. Paper presented at: Annual Conference of the Feldenkrais Guild of North America; October 2001; San Francisco, CA.

40. Wildman F, Stephens J, Aum L. Feldenkrais Method. In: Novey DW, ed. *Clinician's Complete Reference to Complementary and Alternative Medicine.* St. Louis, MO: Mosby; 2000: 393-406.

41. Stephens J. Feldenkrais Method: background, research and orthopedic case studies. *Orthopedic Physical Therapy Clinics of North America.* 2000;9(3):375-394.

42. American Physical Therapy Association. Guide to physical therapist practice. 2nd ed. *Phys Ther.* 2001;81(1).

43. Ives JC, Shelley GA.The Feldenkrais Method in rehabilitation: a review. *Work.* 1998;11:75-90.

44. Dean JR, Yuen SA, Barrows SA. Effects of a Feldenkrais ATM sequence on fibromyalgia patients. Poster session presented at: Annual conference of the Feldenkrais Guild of North America; August 1997; Tamiment, PA.

45. Stephens JL, Herrera S, Lawless R, Masaitis C, Woodling P. Evaluating the results of using Awareness Through Movement with people with fibromyalgia: comments on research design and measurement. Paper presented at: Annual conference of the Feldenkrais Guild of North America; 1999; Evanston, IL.

46. Kendall SA, Ekselius L, Gerdle B, Soren B, Bengtsson A. Feldenkrais intervention in fibromyalgia patients: a pilot study. *J Musculoskel Pain.* 2001; 9(4):25-35.

47. Bearman D, Shafarman S. Feldenkrais Method in the treatment of chronic pain: a study of efficacy and cost effectiveness. *Am J Pain Manage.* 1999;9(1):22-27.

48. Phipps A, Lopez R, Powell R, Lundy-Ekman L, Maebori, D. *A Functional Outcome Study on the Use of Movement Re-Education in Chronic Pain Management* [unpublished master's thesis]. Forest Grove, Ore; Pacific University, School of Physical Therapy; 1997.

49. Lundblad I, Elert J, Gerdle B. Randomized controlled trial of physiotherapy and Feldenkrais interventions in female workers with neck-shoulder complaints. *J Occup Rehab.* 1999;9(3):179-194.

50. De Rosa C, Porterfield J. A physical therapy model for the treatment of low back pain. *Phys Ther.* 1992;72(4):261-272.

51. Maher CG. Effective physical treatment for chronic low back pain. *Ortho Clin North Amer.* 2004;35(1):57-64.

52. Kay TM, Gross A, Goldsmith C, Santaguida PL, Hoving J, Bronfort G. Exercises for mechanical neck disorders. *Cochrane Database of Systematic Reviews.* 2007;3.

53. Rogers SM. *Survey of Piano Instructors: Awareness and Intervention of Predisposing Factors to Piano-Related Injuries* [dissertation]. New York, NY: Columbia University Teachers College; 1999.

54. O'Connor M, Webb R. Learning to rest when in pain. *Euro J Palliat Care.* 2002;9(2):68-71.

55. Brown E, Kegerris S. Electromyographic activity of trunk musculature during a Feldenkrais awareness through movement lesson. *Isokinetics and Exercise Science.* 1991;1(4):216-221.

56. Ruth S, Kegerreis S. Facilitating cervical flexion using a Feldenkrais Method: Awareness Through Movement. *J Sports Phys Ther.* 1992;16(1):25-29.

57. James ML, Kolt GS, Hopper C, McConville JC, Bate P. The effects of a Feldenkrais program and relaxation procedures on hamstring length. *Australian J Physiother.* 1998;44:49-54.

58. Hopper C, Kolt GS, McConville JC. The effects of Feldenkrais Awareness Through Movement on hamstring length, flexibility and perceived exertion. *J Bodywork Movement Therapies.* 1999;3(4):238-247.

59. Stephens J, Davidson JA, DeRosa JT, Kriz ME, Saltzman NA. Lengthening the hamstring muscles without stretching using "awareness through movement. *Phys Ther.* 2006;86(12):1641-1650.

60. Saraswati S. *Investigation of Human Postural Muscles and Respiratory Movements* [unpublished master's thesis]. University of New South Wales; Australia; 1989.

61. Shenkman M, Donovan J, Tsubota J, Kluss M, Stebbins P, Butler R. Management of individuals with Parkinson's disease: rationale and case studies. *Phys Ther.* 1989;69:944-955.

62. Stephens J, DuShuttle D, Hatcher C, Shmunes J, Slaninka C. Use of Awareness Through Movement improves balance and balance confidence in people with multiple sclerosis: a randomized controlled study. *Neurology Report.* 2001;25(2):39-49.

63. Batson G, Deutsch JE. Effects of Feldenkrais awareness through movement on balance in adults with chronic neurological deficits following stroke: a preliminary study. *Complementary Health Practice Review.* 2005;10(3):203-210.

64. Hall SE, Criddle A, Ring A, Bladen C, Tapper J, Yin R. *Study of the Effects of Various Forms of Exercise on Balance in Older Women* [unpublished manuscript]. Nedlands, Western Australia: Healthway Starter Grant; 1999.

65. Seegert EM, Shapiro R. Effects of alternative exercise on posture. *Clinical Kinesiology.* 1999;53(2):41-47.

66. Bennett, JL, Brown BJ, Finney SA, Sarantakis CP. Effects of a Feldenkrais based mobility program on function of a healthy elderly sample. Poster session presented at: Combined Sections Meeting of the American Physical Therapy Association; February 1998; Boston, MA.

67. Stephens JL, Pendergast C, Roller BA, Weiskittel RS. Learning to improve mobility and quality of life in a well elderly population: the benefits of awareness through movement. http://www.iffresearchjournal.org/stephens2005.htm. Accessed June 9, 2008.

68. Frank R. Body awareness: the development of self-perception [dissertation abstract: 1997-95024-173]. *Dissertation Abstracts International: Section B: The Sciences and Engineering.* 1997;58(6-B):3315.

69. Steisel SG. The client's experience of the psychological elements in functional integration. *Dissertation Abstracts International, Massachusetts School of Professional Psychology.* Ann Arbor, MI: University Microfilms; 1993

70. Deig D. *Self Image in Relationship to Feldenkrais Awareness Through Movement Classes* [unpublished master's thesis]. Indianapolis, IN: University of Indianapolis; 1994.

71. Elgelid HS. *Feldenkrais and Body Image* [unpublished master's thesis]. Conway, AR; University of Central Arkansas; 1999.

72. Hutchinson MG. *Transforming Body Image. Learning to Love the Body You Have.* Freedom, CA: The Crossing Press; 1985.

73. Laumer U, Bauer M, Fichter M, Milz H. Therapeutic effects of Feldenkrais Method "Awareness Through Movement" in patients with eating disorders. *Psychother Psychosom Med Psychol.* 1997;47(5):170-180.

74. Gutman G, Herbert C, Brown S. Feldenkrais vs conventional exercise for the elderly. *J Gerontolog.* 1977;32(5):562-572.

75. Malmgren-Olsson EB, Branholm IB. A comparison between three physiotherapy approaches with regard to health-related factors in patients with non-specific musculoskeletal disorders. *Disabil Rehabil.* 2002;24(6):308-317.

76. Malmgren-Olsson E, Armelius B, Armelius K. A comparative outcome study of body awareness therapy (BAT), Feldenkrais, and conventional physiotherapy for patients with non-specific musculoskeletal disorders: changes in psychological symptoms, pain and self image. *Physiother Theory Pract.* 2001;17(2):77-95.

77. Lowe B, Breining K, Wilke S, Wellmann R, Zipfel S, Eich W. Quantitative and qualitative effects of Feldenkrais, progressive muscle relaxation, and standard medical treatment in patients after acute myocardial infarction. *Psychotherapy Research.* 2002;12(2):179-191.

78. Kolt GS. McConville JC. The effects of a Feldenkrais Awareness Through Movement program on state anxiety. *Journal of Bodywork and Movement Therapies.* 2000;4(3):216-220.

79. Kerr GA, Kotynia F, Kolt GS. Feldenkrais Awareness Through Movement and state anxiety. *Journal of Bodywork and Movement Therapies.* 2002;6(2):102-107.

80. Netz Y, Lidor R. Mood alterations in mindful versus aerobic exercise modes. *J Psychol.* 2003;137(5):405-419.

81. Bost H, Burges S, Russell R, Ruttinger H, Schlafke U. *Feldstudie zur wiiksamkeit der Feldenkrais-Methode bei MS-betroffenen.* Deutsche Multiple Sklerose Gesellschaft [unpublished manuscript]; 1994. .

82. Stephens JL, Cates P, Jentes E, et al. Awareness Through Movement improves quality of life in people with multiple sclerosis. Poster presentation at: APTA, Combined Sections Meeting; February 2004; Nashville, TN.

83. Johnson SK, Frederick J, KauFeldenkrais Methodan M, Mountjoy B. A controlled investigation of bodywork in multiple sclerosis. *J Altern Complement Med.* 1999;5(3):237-243.

84. Connors K, Grenough P. Redevelopment of sense of self following stroke, using the Feldenkrais Method. Poster Abstract from "Movement and Development of Sense of Self" Symposium, Annual Conference of Feldenkrais Guild of North America, Seattle, August, 2004.

85. Batson G. The effect of group delivery of Feldenkrais Awareness Through Movement on balance, functional mobility and quality of life in adults post-stroke [PhD Dissertation]. Rocky Mountain University, Provo, Utah, 2006.

Additional Resources

✦ **Feldenkrais Guild of North America (FGNA)**
   3611 SW Hood Avenue, Suite 100
   Portland, OR 97201 USA
   Phone: 800-775-2118
   Fax: 503-221-6616
   Email: guild@feldenkrais.com
   Web site: www.feldenkrais.com

Moshe Feldenkrais established the FGNA in 1977 as the professional organization of practitioners and teachers of the Feldenkrais Method. The guild provides training, certification, and continuing education for practitioners; protection of the quality of the Feldenkrais work; support for research; and is a source of information about the Feldenkrais Method for the public. The guild publishes *The Feldenkrais Journal* quarterly, containing case stories, practitioner reflections, historical information, and artwork. It also publishes *In Touch*, a quarterly newsletter about practice issues and Guild business.

The role of the FGNA has been to establish professional standards for training and practice, to support the continued learning and growth of practitioners, to authorize and conduct training programs, to deal with ethical issues, and to support research.

✦ **Feldenkrais Resources**
   830 Bancroft Way, Suite 12
   Berkeley, CA 94710 USA
   Phone: 800-765-1907
   Fax: 510-540-7683
   Email: feldenres@aol.com
   Web site: www.feldenkrais-resources.com

Feldenkrais Resources is a practitioner owned and run organization that is a resource for audiotape, videotape, and print instructional information and practice support materials. It is also responsible for making available documentary materials about the life and work of Moshe Feldenkrais.

✦ **International Feldenkrais Federation (IFF)**
   Web site: www.feldenkrais-method.org

The IFF is a virtual academy that publishes a regular newsletter and journal and maintains an information bureau. The mission of the IFF is to raise the level of competence of practitioners worldwide through continuous learning. To this end, they maintain a Web site that allows access to a video collection of Feldenkrais' work and more than 400 ATM lessons, sponsor conferences, training programs, and research promotion.

✦ **The Open ATM Project**
   Web site: http://iod.ucsd.edu/~falk/openatm

This is a site containing many prerecorded lessons by a number of different Feldenkrais practitioners. These can be downloaded as mp3 files. The Hamstring Lengthening lessons that were part of Jim Stephens' research, published in *PT Journal* in 2006, are available here.

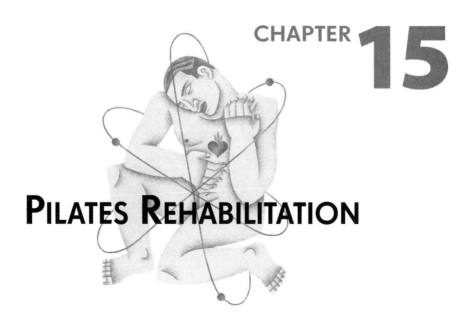

CHAPTER 15

PILATES REHABILITATION

Brent Anderson, PhD, PT, OCS

Origins of Pilates-Evolved Rehabilitation

As a child, German-born Joseph H. Pilates (Figure 15-1) suffered from a multitude of illnesses resulting in muscular weakness. Determined to overcome his frailties, he dedicated his life to becoming physically stronger. He studied yoga, martial arts, Zen meditation, and Greek and Roman exercises. He worked with medical professionals, including physicians and his wife Clara, a nurse. His experiences led to the development of his unique method of physical and mental conditioning, which he brought to the United States in 1923. In the early 1930s and 1940s, popular dance artists and choreographers such as Martha Graham, George Balanchine, and Jerome Robbins embraced Pilates' exercise method. As elite performers, dancers often suffered from injuries resulting in long recovery periods and inability to reach peak performance. Unique at the time, Pilates' method allowed and encouraged movement early in the rehabilitation process, by providing needed assistance. It was found that reintroducing movement with nondestructive forces early in the rehabilitation process hastened the healing. As a result, it was not long before the dance community at large adopted Pilates' work.

More than 70 years later, Pilates' techniques began to gain popularity in the rehabilitation setting. In the 1990s, many rehabilitation practitioners were using the method in multiple fields of rehabilitation, including general orthopedic, geriatric, chronic pain, neurological rehabilitation, and more. Within the rehabilitation setting, most Pilates exercises are performed on several types of apparatus (Figures 15-2 through 15-5). The apparatus work evolved from Pilates' original mat work, which proved difficult as a result of the effect of gravity on the body (Figure 15-6). On the apparatus, springs and gravity are used to assist an injured individual to successfully complete movements that otherwise would be restricted for multiple reasons, aiding in a safe recovery (see Figure 15-3). Ultimately, by altering the spring tension or increasing the challenge of gravity, an individual may be progressed toward achieving functional movement. The use of the Pilates principles with the variations of the traditional repertoire to meet the needs of patients is often referred to in the Pilates community as Pilates evolved. The Pilates environment consists of equipment used by Pilates practitioners, including the Reformer, Cadillac or trapeze table, chair, ladder barrel, and mat.

Figure 15-1. Joseph H. Pilates. (Photo courtesy of Polestar Education LLC.)

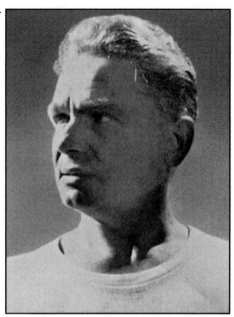

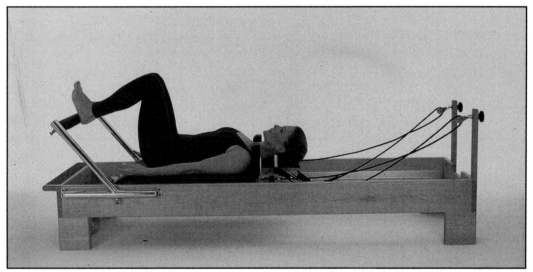

Figure 15-2. Footwork on clinical reformer. (Photo courtesy of Polestar Education LLC.)

Today, despite an increased number of health care practitioners using Pilates' principles for rehabilitation, there is still a lack of supportive literature examining the efficacy associated with Pilates-evolved techniques. Current scientific theories in motor learning and biomechanics are examined to help explain the principles of this old method of movement re-education.

Pilates' Principles

Joseph Pilates originally developed eight basic principles to guide his exercises, known as contrology. They consisted of concentration, control, precision and coordination, isolation and integration, centering, flowing movement, breathing, and routine.[1] However, Pilates was not a

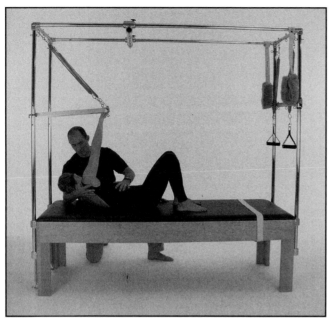

Figure 15-3. Neuromobilization with Tower Bar on the Cadillac. (Photo courtesy of Polestar Education LLC.)

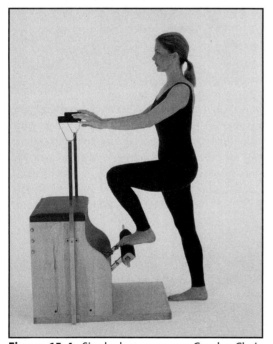

Figure 15-4. Single leg press on Combo-Chair. (Photo courtesy of Polestar Education LLC.)

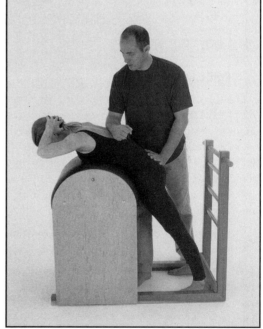

Figure 15-5. Limited thoracic spine extension over the Ladder Barrel. (Photo courtesy of Polestar Education LLC.)

prolific writer and, unfortunately, much of what is known about Pilates' principles has been passed down verbally from generation to generation. This has left much of his original work open to varying interpretations.

There are many avenues for Pilates certification around the world. Various Pilates education and treatment groups are known throughout the country and advertise widely.

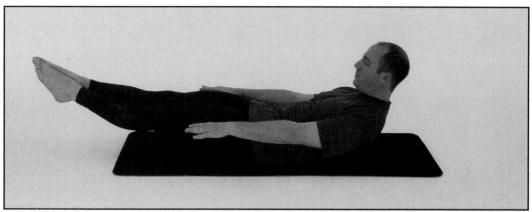

Figure 15-6. The hundred exercise on the mat. (Photo courtesy of Polestar Education LLC.)

The founders of Polestar Education (a Pilates education company specializing in rehabilitation, founded in 1992) studied with many of the first-generation Pilates enthusiasts and teachers. Though their repertoires were quite different from one another, they shared common principles. The therapists of Polestar took the opportunity to investigate the Pilates principles vs the original repertoire of Pilates and came up with the following six principles, supported with scientific foundations, to better explain the applications of Pilates for rehabilitation[2] (Table 15-1).

SIX BASIC PRINCIPLES

Principle I: Breathing

Breath, one of the key elements of Pilates training, is thought to be a facilitator for stabilization and mobilization of the spine and extremities. Faulty breath patterns are often associated with common complaints of pain and movement dysfunction. Pilates movements create an environment whereby breath is facilitated to increase the efficiency of air exchange, increase breath capacity, and facilitate thoracic postural changes. A rigid thoracic spine can be a causative factor in common cervical and lumbar pathology. The Pilates approach to breathing varies depending on which school of Pilates you graduated from, but one thing they all share in common is that breath is an integral part of each and every exercise.

Principle II: Axial Elongation/Core Control (Centering)

The principle of stabilization and axial elongation greatly relies on the research from Queensland, Australia. Such studies demonstrate that the transverse abdominus, multifidus, diaphragm, and abdominal oblique muscles are key organization muscles of movement in healthy individuals and are often lacking in individuals with chronic low back pain.[3-5] It is for this reason that many of Joseph Pilates' original teachings that refer to the powerhouse or the hollowing of the abdominal wall are becoming quite popular among rehabilitation specialists around the world. The principle of elongation is what has brought about the greatest interest in Pilates rehabilitation. Stabilization is not always the best descriptor of what Pilates can do for an individual. Motor control studies and theories of trunk organization and stabilization teach us that subthreshold contraction of global stabilization muscles provide safe movement throughout one's daily activities.[6] Dr. Shirley Sahrmann relates control of the trunk to a balance of stiffness between muscles in order to provide efficient control of dynamic posture.[7]

The principle of axial elongation is thought to organize the spine in its optimal orientation for efficient movement, thus avoiding working or resting at the end of range, which can place undue stresses on the inert and contractile structures of the trunk and extremities. This organization of

Table 15-1

CLINICAL APPLICATIONS OF THE PILATES PRINCIPLES

BREATHING

Breath can facilitate spine stability, spine articulation, core control, efficiency of movement, and movement can facilitate breath.

AXIAL ELONGATION/CORE CONTROL

Axial elongation should be present in every Pilates exercise, providing the optimal space, stiffness, and orientation of joints and supporting tissues to move throughout the day without the risk of injury.

ORGANIZATION OF THE HEAD, NECK, AND SHOULDERS

Providing the efficient expenditure of energy while moving will help maintain an optimal alignment of the head, neck, and shoulders on the trunk. This organization provides for safety, aesthetics, and energy conservation.

SPINE ARTICULATION

Knowing the properties of the spine and the groupings of the vertebrae (cervical, thoracic, and lumbar) allows for accurate imagery, verbal cueing, and tactile cueing to optimize movement.

ALIGNMENT AND POSTURE

Proper alignment and organization of the upper and lower extremities as they pertain to the trunk allows for safe, efficient movement of the body. Alignment often removes damaging stressors that prevent spontaneous healing.

MOVEMENT INTEGRATION

Movement integration not only consists of musculoskeletal movement integration but the integration of mind and body. Maximizing the mental involvement with the exercise creates almost a meditative state for the patient, enhancing body awareness and exploring new movement opportunities without pain. When the mind, body, and spirit are thought to be one, if one moves the body, one moves all systems.

---

spine and extremities also provides optimal potential for performance of sport and leisure activities. With an ever-growing population interested in feeling good and being able to perform daily activities and recreate without the risk of injury, axial elongation is a high priority and could account for many of the anecdotal spontaneous resolutions of low back pain that come with Pilates. Clinically, when a patient has the ability to reorganize his or her strategy of spine movement, spine stabilization, and movement of the extremities in conjunction with the spine, forces seem to be better distributed throughout the spine, and these are less likely to introduce harmful effects to the soft tissues surrounding the spine. It also appears that those who are diagnosed with spine pathology, even as grievous as disc pathologies, can often minimize the provoking forces at the site of the lesion, thus minimizing the pain response and accelerating healing. Pilates' exercises have an innate way of facilitating trunk organization at a subconscious level, allowing the individual to explore and assimilate a more efficient control of the trunk. These clinical observations warrant scientific investigation.

Figure 15-7. 90/90 on the Cadillac. (Photo courtesy of Polestar Education LLC.)

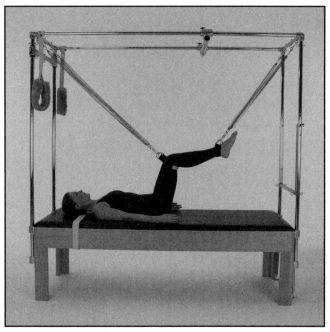

Pilates also provides an environment in which the difficulty of the exercise can be modified, thus facilitating successful execution of a desired movement outcome. The four basic tools referred to by Polestar Education in the Pilates environment are familiar to neurological rehabilitation: 1) modify the base of support, 2) decrease the center of gravity, 3) shorten the length of the levers, and 4) vary the assistance (spring tension). One of the basic exercises, 90/90, uses the springs for assistance. The tables allow the practitioner to lower the center of gravity and increase base of support, and the exercise can be modified by changing the length of the levers (Figure 15-7). This formula allows the therapist to facilitate motor changes of the trunk quickly, while giving ownership of the newly acquired movement to the patient or client.

Principle III: Efficient Organization of Head, Neck, and Shoulder Girdle (Flowing, Efficient Movement)

This principle focuses on the patient's ability to align the head, neck, and shoulder girdle. Efficiency of movement can be observed by the tone and posture of the head, face, neck, and shoulder girdle in relation to the thoracic spine and trunk. Many restrictions and unnecessary stresses can occur in this area. The benefits of this principle are increased range of motion, energy conservation, and minimized risk of lesions. Lesions usually occur at the end of a range of motion. Increasing the available range of motion and improving coordination of the scapula thoracic joints will decrease the likelihood of experiencing destructive forces to the shoulder and neck joints.

Principle IV: Spine Articulation (Isolation and Integration)

The distribution of segmental movement through the spine is a topic that researchers are anxious to measure. Does distributing the motion between spinal segments significantly reduce stressful forces from causing micro- and macrotraumas to the hypermobile segment? Currently, there are no instruments that can measure this accurately. A study carried out at Mount Saint Mary's University's physical therapy program used the Metrecom Skeletal Analysis System to measure the phenomena of distribution of motion following Pilates' exercises. Pilot studies showed that following one session of Pilates, healthy subjects had a significant increase in overall forward bending, an increase in motion of less mobile segments, and a decrease in motion of the previously measured hypermobile segments.[8] With limited research regarding this topic, it still can be hypothesized

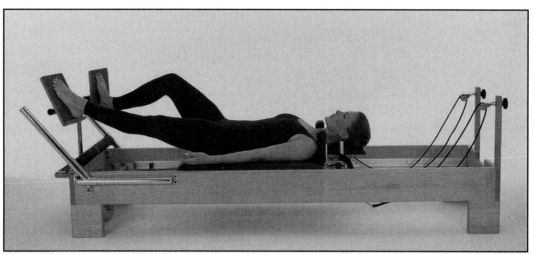

Figure 15-8. Footwork with proprioceptive T-Bar on Clinical Reformer. (Photo courtesy of Polestar Education LLC.)

that by increasing the motor awareness of spinal motion in all directions, one can extrapolate that distribution of movement is equivalent to a distribution of sheer force to the spine.

Principle V: Alignment and Posture (Centering, Precision, and Coordination)

Proper alignment and posture are foundational to efficient, coordinated movement. Postural organization can significantly decrease energy expenditure in daily activities. For example, if an individual allows the femurs to medially rotate while decelerating in gait, it will lead to a number of potential lesions (patella femoral pain, foot and ankle tendonitis, hip and pelvic pathologies). Faulty alignment in the extremities and spine can be the source of decreased range of motion, early fatigue of muscle groups, abnormal stresses on inert structures, and faulty movement patterns that can potentially be harmful.

Pilates pays attention to static alignment and posture but places greater emphasis on dynamic alignment and posture. With a device on the Clinical Reformer (one of the basic pieces of apparatus used by Joseph Pilates and modified for rehabilitation) known as the rotating T-Bar, a therapist can measure weightbearing asymmetries while squatting. Using the closed chain foot bar can assess asymmetries between hip rotators as they apply to alignment through a squatting range of motion (Figure 15-8). These diagnostic and treatment applications in the Pilates environment allow rehabilitation practitioners to better assess and treat alignment-related impairments not only in the lower extremity but also in the upper extremity and trunk.

Principle VI: Movement Integration (Concentration, Integration, Flowing, and Routine)

According to many Pilates rehabilitation specialists, this most important principle of rehabilitation could represent the unexplainable changes often experienced in the Pilates environment. The advanced mastery of movement requiring a connectedness between mind and body is thought by many Pilates rehabilitation practitioners to be one of the primary reasons for its success. Emphasizing holistic mind and body integration sometimes uncovers emotional causes for movement disorders. One anecdotal account of a therapist with a patient suffering from chronic low back pain for 5 years could be a good example of this principle. The patient's magnetic resonance imaging (MRI), myelogram, computerized tomography (CT) scan, tests were negative. She was referred to the therapist for an evaluation and Pilates intervention. After introducing the first few Pilates exercises, the hamstring arcs in particular (an exercise that supports the legs in straps while the patient lies supine, the legs are moved in circular motions) (Figure 15-9), the patient began to cry and express emotional releases. After being escorted to a private room, she proceeded to

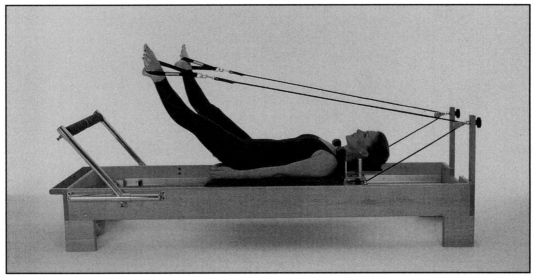

Figure 15-9. Leg circles on Clinical Reformer. (Photo courtesy of Polestar Education LLC.)

confide an experience in her childhood involving sexual molestation by a family member. She never shared this before, not even with her husband of 25 years. Within weeks, her symptoms significantly decreased and she was referred to the proper intervention.

According to experienced clinicians, this type of behavior is seen or expressed quite often. However, we usually do not talk about it because it does not fit within our current practice act. If movement integration is allowed to be expanded beyond just the musculoskeletal and allowed to incorporate the mind, emotions, subconscious, spirit, and physical body (including the digestive, circulatory, respiratory, and reproductive systems), this represents holistic movement integration of the entire person. Movement approaches that incorporate the movement of the whole person, such as Pilates, T'ai Chi, yoga, Feldenkrais, and gyrotonic expansion system, are going to continue to receive greater attention due to the increasing incidence of anecdotal improvements. The rehabilitation sciences will do well to look for ways of measuring outcomes as they pertain to movement of the whole person. Examples of possible movement-related research efforts might include self-efficacy studies pertaining to one's perception of self and one's ability to move, depression scales as they pertain to one's perception of ability to move or inability to move, and communication of disability through movement patterns.

🗁 Case Examples

An example of how perception influences motivation in movement was revealed in a man with a diagnosis of mechanical low back pain. He worked with the city street cleaning division and was looking forward to a long leave from work due to the back injury. His pain was local, aggravated with forward bending, twisting, and prolonged sitting. During his second visit, the physical therapist initiated Pilates exercises to teach him to minimize the unnecessary guarding and begin to increase awareness of his center and trunk control. During this session, the patient observed an elite dancer next to him doing an advanced move on the trapeze table. He made the comment, "I could never do that." He was told that he could do that exercise (hanging spine extension on the trapeze table) (Figure 15-10). On his next visit, the Pilates environment was manipulated such that he was able to perform the exercise safely and without discomfort whatsoever. As he sat on the edge of the table following his successful execution of what appeared to be an advanced exercise,

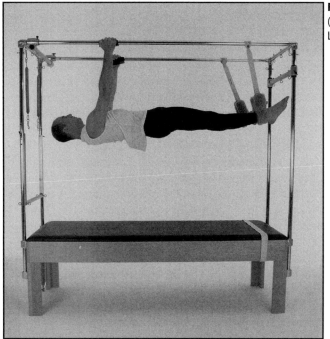

Figure 15-10. Hanging series on Cadilac. (Photo courtesy of Polestar Education LLC.)

he stated, "I can't believe I just did that exercise." The therapist waited a minute and then said to the patient, "That exercise is much harder than anything you would be required to do at work." There was silence and one could tell that the patient was reorganizing his neural network. What he thought was going to be a 6-month vacation now was reduced to 2 weeks. His previous motivation of the back injury was in conflict with his successful execution of an advanced movement on his third visit. He experienced a paradigm shift in his perception of what his mechanical low back pain meant to him.

In another example, a 76-year-old retired radiologist with a diagnosis of lumbar stenosis and Parkinson-like tremors was unable to walk greater than 100 yards without bilateral calf and lateral leg pain. He was taking medication for the tremor, pain, and inflammation. His previous activity included running, which he hadn't been able to do for more than 1 year. Objectively, his posture was very kyphotic with a significant forward head, with eye gaze on the feet. His gait was a slow shuffle and he often experienced a loss of balance. Active range of motion of his spine was limited to negative 15 degrees of extension, and he had no hip extension.

He did Pilates for approximately 1 year, one session per week accompanied by a walking program. The focus of his program was to facilitate his upright posture, axial elongation of the lumbar and thoracic spine, and to increase his ability to walk 1 to 3 miles per day. The Pilates environment (basic equipment and principles of Pilates) provided him with the ability to use assistance from the springs and varying orientations to gravity to learn how to safely walk upright in spite of his spine stenosis, increase his hip and thoracic extension, and bring his eye gaze into a parallel orientation to the floor while standing. Examples of two exercises used to help with balance, disassociation, and trunk extension are shown in Figures 15-4 and 15-5.

This patient now walks 1 to 3 miles per day with minimal complaints of lower leg pain. His medications have been reduced, and though he continues to battle the tremors, he has noted a significant decrease in loss of balance and near falls.

Evidence of Efficacy

Since the first edition of this text was published, there have been seven papers published pertaining to Pilates and health,[11-13] Pilates and aging,[14] and continued work on Pilates for low back care.[15-19] This number continues to grow as the interest and the awareness grows in the use of Pilates for rehabilitation and health practices. There are still a number of studies awaiting publication. These studies are looking at low back pain management, motor learning with spring-assisted movement training, and imagery facilitation.

One study awaiting publication[9] was designed to evaluate the effect of directed spring assistance and verbal guidance compared with verbal guidance alone on the skill acquisition of an abdominal curl-up. The subjects in the experimental group used a piece of Pilates equipment known as the Wall Unit. Subjects who were guided through movement with assistance from the springs demonstrated a 50% improvement in movement amplitude after intervention. An ANOVA analysis was performed and compared the difference between the control and experimental groups both pre- and post-test, and showed retention of benefit even higher than the original post-test results in the experimental group. These findings are important to the profession to demonstrate how assistance-guided movement potentially can affect the strategy of movement. If movement distributes throughout the spine, one could extrapolate that forces distribute as well.

In 1996, Mount Saint Mary's College in southern California conducted a pilot study that was presented at the California State Chapter Conference of the American Physical Therapy Association (APTA) as a poster presentation.[8] They concluded three very important findings. The research design consisted of a control and experimental group and pre- and post-test measures. The subjects consisted of a sample of all healthy students with no history of performing Pilates-based exercises. The pretest consisted of a standing flexion measured with a device to assess segmental motion of the spine in flexion. The average findings in this pilot study identified the strategy of forward flexion to take place primarily at the hip and L4-5 and L5-S1. The average angle of displacement in the lower two segments of the lumbar was 20 to 25 degrees. The angles significantly decreased from L4 upward, with the majority of the thoracic spine at 0 to 2 degrees maximum. The experimental group then proceeded with a 45-minute session of Pilates on the Reformer. Following the session, they returned to take their post-test. The control group took the pre-test with similar findings as the experimental group's pretest. They then rested for 45 minutes and returned to take the post-test with similar results as the pre-test. The interesting findings of the experimental post group were as follows: 1) overall flexion increased; 2) segmental motion increased by as much as 25% in the thoracic and upper lumbar segments; 3) and the most important finding was that at the levels L4-5 and L5-S1 there was a significant reduction in the angle of flexion by more than 50%, approximately 10 to 15 degrees per segment.

This pilot study could not be continued due to malfunction of the measurement instrument and withdrawal of the company's ability to validate its findings. However, the findings in the pilot study definitely laid the groundwork for further investigation regarding motor learning in the Pilates environment, which might explain how changing the strategy of movement can alleviate harmful forces that often continue the perturbation of lesions.

In January 2000, an article was published that discussed a case study using Pilates and the Gyrotonic Expansion System (Balanced Body Inc, Sacramento, CA) with favorable results.[10]

The most recent publications pertaining to low back care have shown a significant decrease in low back disability using Oswestry, Rolland Morris, and SF-36 scales.[15,17,19] A dissertation at the University of Miami demonstrated a significant improvement in back extension strength and the SF-36 Vitality measure when compared to massage alone. It is interesting that vitality, of all measures in the SF-36, demonstrated the strongest correlation with the Pilates intervention.[18] It could be that this positive movement experience without pain provides hope for a vital life. Rydeard et al study showed that Pilates-based approach was more efficacious than usual care in a population with chronic, unresolved lower back pain. This growing trend in the research continues to support Pilates as a legitimate intervention for physical therapy and health-related professions.

Two publications looked at Pilates training effects on flexibility and body composition. One showed a significant decrease in body fat composition and the other one did not. The difference between the two studies probably was due to the frequency of intervention and the duration. Jago et al had high school girls taking class 5 days a week for 4 weeks. Segal et al was not able to substantiate a significant decrease in body fat composition, but participants only participated in one class per week for 2 months, a significant decrease in actual contact hours compared to Jago et al. What Segal et al did show was a significant increase in flexibility. Anderson's dissertation also showed a trend of positive change in all of the physical measures for strength, flexibility, and coordination.

The Pilates Method Alliance—a nonprofit organization—and a few of its members including Polestar Pilates, continue to promote evidence-based research to substantiate the Pilates approach as a viable and valid intervention for rehabilitation and fitness. Polestar is currently conducting a number of studies and is supporting students from universities who are interested in conducting Pilates-based research.

Conclusion

In addition to the above principles, one of the greatest advantages that Pilates has to offer is its flexible environment to meet specific needs of the client. By manipulating gravity, base of support, length of levers, and center of gravity, the practitioner is much more capable of facilitating the patient's successful movement with less effort, less fatigue, and greater movement awareness retention. Pilates has been a tool for successful intervention with a large variety of patients of all ages with ranging diagnoses, from neurological to rheumatologic, pediatric to orthopaedic, and women's health to performance enhancement. Two basic assumptions we make in Pilates rehabilitation are 1) that movement exists within each person and 2) that the ability to heal lies within each individual. Ongoing studies will add to our understanding of the mechanisms of action that support these assumptions.

References

1. Pilates JH, Miller WJ. Result of contrology. In: *Return to Life Through Contrology*. New York, NY: JJ Augustin; 1945.
2. Anderson BD. *Polestar Education Instruction Manual: Polestar Approach to Movement Principles*. Coral Gables, FL: Polestar Pilates; 2001.
3. Richardson C, Jull G, Hodges P, et al. Local muscle dysfunction in low back pain. In: *Therapeutic Exercise for Spinal Segmental Stabilization in Low Back Pain*. London: Churchill Livingstone; 1999.
4. Richardson C, Jull G, Toppenberg R, et al. Techniques for active lumbar stabilization for spinal protection: a pilot study. *Australian Physiotherapy*. 1992;38(2):105-112
5. Richardson C, Jull G, Hodges P, et al. Overview of the principles of clinical management of the deep muscle system for segmental stabilization. In: *Therapeutic Exercise for Spinal Segmental Stabilization in Low Back Pain*. London: Churchill Livingstone; 1999.
6. Porterfield JA. Dynamic stabilization of the trunk. *J Orthop Sports Phys Ther*. 1985;6:271.
7. Sahrmann S. *Diagnosis and Treatment of Muscle Imbalances and Musculoskeletal Pain Syndromes* [workshop manual]; January 1996.
8. Daack M, Huntingdon J, Isaacson AF, Anderson B. The effects of Pilates based exercises on hypomobility of the spine in a healthy population. Poster presentation at: California APTA Conference; 1997.
9. Carr B, Day JA, Anderson BD. *Effect of directed spring assisted guidance on skill acquisition of thoracic spine*. [unpublished manuscript].
10. Duschatko DM. Certified Pilates and gyrotonic trainers. *Journal of Bodywork and Movement Therapies*. 2000:13-19.
11. Segal NA, Hein J, Basford JR. The effects of Pilates training on flexibility and body composition: an observational study. *Arch Phys Med Rehabil*. 2004;85:1977-1981.

12. Jago R, Jonker ML, Missaghian M, Baranowski T. Effect of 4 weeks of Pilates on the body composition of young girls. *Prev Med.* 2006;42:177-180.
13. Hutchinson MR, Tremain L, Christiansen J, Beitzel J. Improving leaping ability in elite rhythmic gymnasts. *Med Sci Sports Exerc.* 1998;30(10):1543-1547.
14. Smith K, Smith E. Integrating Pilates-based core strengthening into older adult fitness programs: implications for practice. *Topics in Geriatric Rehabilitation.* 2005;21(1):57-67.
15. Rydeard R, Leger A, Smith D. Pilates-based therapeutic exercise: Effect on subjects with nonspecific chronic low back pain and functional disability: a randomized controlled trial. *J Orthop Sports Phys Ther.* 2006;36(7):472-484.
16. Graves BS, Quinn JV, O'Kroy JA, Torok DJ. Influence of Pilates-based mat exercises on chronic low back pain. *Med Sci Sports Exerc.* 2005;37(5):S27.
17. Blum CL. Chiropractic and Pilates therapy for the treatment of adult scoliosis. *J Manipulative Physiol Ther.* 2002;25(4): e3.
18. Anderson BD. *Randomized Clinical Trial Comparing Active Versus Passive Approaches to the Treatment of Recurrent and Chronic Low Back Pain* [unpublished dissertation]. Miami, FL: University of Miami, Department of Physical Therapy; 2005.
19. Cowan T, Lackner J, Anderson BD, Polina J, Morigerato G, Hopkins L. *A Pilot Study of Pilates Exercise for Rehabilitation of Subacute Low Back Patients* [pending submission for publication]; 2003.

Additional Resources

+ Pilates Method Alliance
  Web site: http://www.pilatesmethodalliance.org

+ Polestar Centers for Physical Therapy and Pilates LLC
  Phone: 800-387-3651
  Web site: www.polestarpilates.com (site has extensive list of Pilates educators)

SECTION V

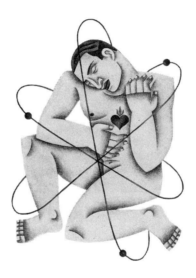

ENERGY WORK

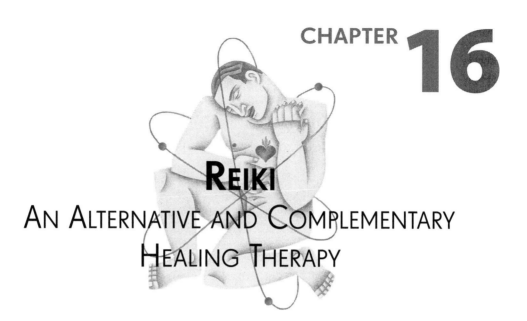

CHAPTER **16**

REIKI
AN ALTERNATIVE AND COMPLEMENTARY
HEALING THERAPY

Sangeeta Singg, PhD

Introduction

Although the notion that people suffering from mental or physical disorders can be healed by someone's touch is contemporary in the Western world, such practice has been in existence in the world since ancient times. With the advent of the Internet, it has become impossible for the Western medical establishment to prevent the invasion of ancient knowledge and practice of alternative medicine from looming as a new movement of healing with the help of so-called New Age modalities. It is ironic that the alternative healing modalities are being assigned to the New Age movement (some say a misnomer), which burgeoned in the West in the 1960s, whereas most alternative modalities are ancient. Modalities such as hands-on healing, T'ai Chi, hatha yoga, Ayurveda, prayer, acupuncture, Qi gong, Shiatsu, herbal remedies, and so on were the common practices in the ancient civilizations. All these systems view injury, dysfunction, and disease as manifestations of weak, unbalanced, or blocked vital energy. Energy in such a state is optimized with the help of alternative modalities, which leads to facilitated health and wellness.

For the most part, what caused the gap between ancient belief and modern medical practice is the rigorous adherence to the scientific method by the modern medical community and the rejection of ancient healing methods. Allopathic medicine is based on scientific inquiry, whereas alternative medicine is based on tradition and belief. The most important criterion for any drug or treatment to meet before the US Food and Drug Administration (FDA) will allow it to reach the American consumer is that it is able to withstand a double-blind controlled trial. Because many energy-based alternative modalities lack the stringent testing with double-blind controlled trials, they have been shunned as viable methods of treatment. In spite of the lack of controlled research, alternative healing methods are seeping into the treatment regimen of many patients either by their own undertaking or as a part of professional intervention. Many alternative modalities require involved training and internship; however, one modality called Reiki requires very little training and is the second most accessible modality (the first being the prayer).

Reiki (pronounced Ray-key) is a Japanese word, *Rei* meaning universal or omnipresent, and *Ki* meaning life force or energy. It is an all-knowing and all-encompassing universal life force that animates all living things.[1-4] It is the same as *ch'i* in Chinese, *prana* in Sanskrit, *mana* in Polynesian, *pneuma* in Greek, and *ruah* (breath of life) in Hebrew and in the Old Testament.[1,5]

There are as many words for the *universal life force* as there are the belief systems and languages. The author was interested in Reiki as a researcher and a psychologist for many years even though she did not know it by its Japanese name. As a result, she obtained training at all levels, from first degree to master level, and subsequently conducted and published a controlled Reiki study with graduate student Linda Dressen.[5,6]

Reiki practice has become quite well known all over the world. The Internet is replete with information on Reiki. There are several national and international Reiki organizations, and many Internet web sites, books, and anecdotal articles both in magazines and professional journals. However, there are very few controlled studies in the scientific literature supporting efficacy of Reiki healing. This chapter attempts to reconcile much anecdotal and limited empirical information, some of which is contradictory. Because the Reiki tradition is proudly referred to as "a rich oral tradition" by the practitioners (REF?), most of the theoretical and historical information about Reiki lacks written verification. Much of the information presented in this regard was obtained from interviewing several practitioners and reading a large number of informal and a few formal sources. Contradictory information from many of these sources is confusing. Thus, this chapter presents a coherent and widely accepted version of the Reiki story. Because of the vast amount of public domain information available on the Internet and via other sources, citing of all such sources is neither possible nor fair. As a result, only formal sources are cited here. Also, because of discrepancies among many sources, only that information is presented which appeared to be accepted by a majority of practitioners.

WHAT IS REIKI?

Reiki is a healing system that channels the universal life force through the practitioner's hands. The fundamental supposition of Reiki is that all living things are animated with the same infinite, monolithic, vital energy, and the source of this vital energy is spiritual. It is considered a holistic approach to health and well-being. The activation of Reiki is believed to promote energy balancing, healing, and a state of well-being in all living things. Therefore, Reiki may be called a form of *energy medicine*.[7] As such, it is practiced not only by professionals but also by laypersons to heal themselves and others in a variety of settings. The medical community is beginning to recognize the inevitable arrival of energy medicine in treatment. Gerber[8] has aptly stated, "Within certain subspecialties of conventional medicine... The permutation from conventional drug and surgical therapy to electromagnetic healing represents the beginnings of a revolution in consciousness for the medical profession."

As a noninvasive modality, Reiki is believed to flow via hands of a practitioner to a willing recipient. The practitioner serves as a conduit for the flow of this universal life force without using his or her own personal energy. This energy can be transmitted either by touching the recipient or intending its transmission from any distance. This universal life force is believed to be an intelligent energy that reaches the part of the body that needs it.[1,4,7] The practitioner does not need to know the ailment or diagnosis before administering a healing treatment. Although some alternatively believe that Reiki can be channeled to a specific place or problem in the body, most practitioners believe that this energy cannot be controlled or regulated in any way, and the energy will not work if one tries to direct it. This nondirective approach to healing is the major difference between Reiki and other hands-on healing methods.

Another difference from other manual therapies lies in the training procedure of the Reiki practitioner. Anyone can learn Reiki. However, unlike other hands-on healing methods, Reiki is not taught. Instead, it is transferred from the Reiki master to the student during the induction process called *attunement*.[5,7,9] Becoming attuned is a way of allowing oneself to open up to channel the universal life force. Once a person opens up to channel this energy, it is believed that he or she never loses it. However, a few believe that Reiki will "weaken and fade away when it is not exercised."[2] Also, some claim that you do not need to be attuned to practice Reiki, because the ability to tap into the universal life force is inborn in all of us. The author agrees with this contention. There are many ways to tap into this energy. Some are more tedious than the others; however, Reiki is considered one of the easiest and quickest ways to achieve this goal.

Intentionality is a crucial factor for the success of all natural healing modalities. Intentionality was the theme of two 1999 issues of *Bridges*,[10,11] the quarterly magazine of the International Society for the Study of Subtle Energies and Energy Medicine. Intentionality is described as the process of focusing attention of thought or concentration in a specific way so as to bring about a healing or balance by way of energy flow. Reiki practitioners are specifically taught to be cognizant of the recipient's voluntary intent to receive healing. Sending Reiki to an unwilling and unbelieving recipient is considered unethical. However, the situation is different when the recipients are children, animals, or seriously ill persons who cannot express their will in relation to receiving Reiki. It is believed that children, animals, and seriously ill persons lack barriers and are, therefore, very responsive to this life force.[4] If they do not want it, they will let the practitioner know by moving away from the practitioner's hands or simply by not accepting it.

THE EXPERIENCE OF RECEIVING REIKI TREATMENT

The experience of Reiki differs from recipient to recipient. Some commonly reported sensations are warmth, tingling, coolness, and subsequent general relaxation. Also, some feel a positive change in symptoms right away, and others report a positive change after a longer period of time. Reiki treatments are reported to produce no negative side effects. Respecting individual freedom is an important tenant of Reiki. The belief is that Reiki cannot be used against an individual's will or in a negative way. It can only be used with a willing recipient for the best possible outcome or the highest good because the intelligent life force knows what is best for the person.[1,2,4,7]

Because Reiki can be used along with allopathic treatment, patients in the hospital or under conventional medical care are very good candidates to benefit from Reiki. Reiki as a complementary modality can accelerate the healing process and reduce negative side effects of medicines and other procedures. It permeates all aspects of self from physical health to emotional well-being and spiritual awareness. Thus, it is believed to work simultaneously at the physical, mental, and spiritual levels. Because the universal life force is channeled through the practitioner, it benefits the practitioner as well.[1,2,4,7] As such, it is a double blessing; it blesses those who receive it and those who give it.

Historical Account

Different authors have presented different versions of the Reiki story.[1-7,12] All agree that Hawayo Takata (1900-1980), who lived in Hawaii, introduced Reiki to the West around 1937. While visiting her family in Japan, she became very ill and was admitted to a hospital to undergo an operation in 1935. In the operating room before the surgery, she strongly felt that there was another way to get better. Upon her inquiring, she was directed to a clinic run by Dr. Chujiro Hayashi (1878-1940), who learned Reiki from Dr. Mikao Usui (1865-1926), the founder of the Usui System of Reiki. In 1925, Hayashi, a retired Naval officer, became impressed with Usui's commitment and dedication and joined him in his cause of helping people with Reiki. Following Usui tradition, he established the first Reiki clinic after Usui's death in 1926. This is where Takata was treated. After her recovery, she received Reiki training from Hayashi and returned to Hawaii in 1937. A few weeks later and just before World War II, Hayashi came to Hawaii and trained Takata to teach Reiki to others. In February 1938, she was named a Reiki master. It is believed that Hayashi trained about 17 masters. Takata returned to Japan at Hayashi's request, and Hayashi passed the Reiki torch to her as his successor. Soon after this, he died in 1940.[1-7,12]

Takata practiced Reiki in Hawaii and later moved to California. She continued using and teaching Reiki until her death on December 11, 1980. She trained 22 Reiki masters, including her granddaughter, Phyllis Furomoto, to carry out the Reiki tradition.[1-4] After her death, two leaders emerged, creating two different branches of the Usui system of Reiki. Furomoto founded The Reiki Alliance in 1981. In 1982, another student of Takata, Dr. Barbara Weber Ray, founded the American International Reiki Association, Inc.[1,2] Currently, there are several organizations and versions of Reiki claiming their authenticity. They can be located on the Internet.

THE ORIGINS OF REIKI

How did the originator, Usui, learn Reiki? The legend is that Usui, a Christian minister, was heading a Christian boys' school in Kyoto, Japan. (Some believe he was a Buddhist monk. Yet, others say that he was neither a Christian minister nor a Buddhist monk, but was simply a spiritual healer.[1-7,12] He may have been both because many Buddhist spiritualists are not bound by strict religious beliefs or boundaries.) While working at the boys' school, he became interested in researching the miracles performed by Jesus. To learn the healing methods that Jesus might have used, he traveled to the United States but did not find the information he sought in Christian schools. He was then directed to study Buddhist writings seeking knowledge of what Buddha had taught about healing.

There are conflicting statements about Usui's visit to America. Some say that he never came to America, while others contend that he received his doctorate in theology from the University of Chicago. In any event, many practitioners in old Eastern societies in the late 1800s were labeled doctors without a medical degree if they learned the medical practice while assisting a doctor, many opening up an independent practice of their own after several years of training under a medical doctor.

In Japan, Usui searched for an answer in many temples and finally found Sanskrit writings in the form of Sutras, which explained how the healing was done. However, although he had found the information that explained the mechanisms of healing, he did not feel empowered to heal others. He then turned to another ancient Indian method of achieving enlightenment, one Buddha had used. He performed tapasya (penance) by fasting and meditating on Mount Koriyama, some 17 miles from Kyoto. At the end of the 21st day, he was enlightened with the knowledge of healing.

Usui used this knowledge to give healing to many people in Japan. He believed that in order to free humanity from illness and suffering, this healing method should be made available to the public. Therefore, he trained 18 or 19 Reiki masters before his death. Although most of the formal and informal information about Reiki practice pertains to healing others, the most important aspect of Reiki is self-healing. He also gave five spiritual precepts to his students to practice in daily life—for today only: do not anger, do not worry, be humble, be honest in your work, and be compassionate to yourself and others.[1-7,12]

It has been said that Usui rediscovered Reiki in the late 1800s, however the author disagrees. Rediscovery denotes that some lost thing has been found again. Reiki is an ontological reality that always existed regardless of our knowledge of it. It was in existence before Usui and before Buddha. What might be a more accurate statement is that Usui practiced Reiki based on an ancient Buddhist practice, which was introduced to the Western world in late 1930s by Takata. However, after Takata's death in 1980, Reiki practice became more structured and formalized than the original oral intuitive method. The goal, however, remains the same as Usui envisioned it: personal and global healing.

Some believe that both Usui and Hayashi did not leave any written instructions about Reiki, yet there are others who claim that they both had written some sort of manuals. During her training sessions, Takata maintained the oral tradition and did not allow her students to take notes.

However, this changed after her death.[1-7,12] At present, it appears that there are as many manuals as there are Reiki masters, and several Reiki masters claim to have unique Reiki systems (with different names). However, they all claim their lineage to Usui.

Because Reiki is not associated with any religion, both the practitioner and the recipient do not have to accept any religious beliefs as prerequisites to Reiki healing.[1-7,12] Although it comes from an ancient Tibetan Buddhist practice, it is not connected to Buddhism as such. It surpasses professional, cultural, and religious boundaries. Reiki practitioners include a variety of professionals and laypersons from many religions and cultures. For example, the International Association of Reiki Professionals[13] claims a global membership of Reiki practitioners and master teachers from 47 countries. There are several directories available via Internet that list Reiki practitioners from all over the world. *The National Directory of Reiki Healers and Masters*[14] lists American practitioners and masters. Of course, not all persons attuned to be Reiki practitioners are listed in these directories.

Reiki Training

Reiki training is provided by the Reiki masters at three to four levels presented in 3 to 10 stages depending on the master's training and association. However, traditionally, Reiki training was divided into three levels, *Shoden* (first teachings), *Okuden* (inner teachings), and *Shinpiden* (mystery teachings). They are now called first, second, and third (Reiki master) degrees, respectively.[4] Usui, Hayashi, and Takata have been considered the Grand Masters among Reiki practitioners; however, Takata did not appoint a successor. In fact, some have tried to claim this title.[1-4] Since Takata's death, several modifications of the traditional Reiki system have come into existence. Proponents of different variations have altered the classification and training system according to their preferences.

Even though the training methods may differ slightly, the ultimate goal at every level is a series of *attunements*. Attunement is a form of initiation that prepares one's body for channeling the universal life force. Attunement is believed to prime one to receive the flow of energy and empower to be able to channel this energy from the top of one's head through the palms. These cannot be explained in the text, however, because secrecy is maintained and disclosed only during master degree. Completion of the training is not heralded by any formal examination, because the major component of the training is the experience of attunement. Keeping in line with Takata's tradition, the beginner's level, or first degree training, begins with masters relating the Reiki story and sharing of anecdotal cases. The use of the word master is equivalent to teacher/mentor here. In the East, the title master or guru is bestowed on those who have achieved the highest levels of knowledge and enlightenment in a certain area and who are capable of imparting knowledge and mentoring others in that area. Some masters may also provide the information on research supporting the efficacy of Reiki. Students are then given attunements. They are also given a manual that shows different hand positions, which they then practice on themselves or others in class. Considerable time is spent on supervised practice. The number or sequence of laying hands on a recipient's body may differ from master to master. The number of hand positions may range from 5 to 15 depending on the master.

The advanced level, or second degree training, is available to all those who have completed the first degree. In second degree training, additional attunements are given and a series of special symbols are revealed. This allows for a deeper Reiki experience involving work on a mental/emotional level and added ability to send Reiki to a distant source. It is also called distant or absentee healing. The master level, or third degree training, is for those who are experienced Reiki practitioners both at the first and second degree levels. Some divide this level into third degree and master's level depending on a student's preparation and interest. During their attunement, participants learn a final symbol for attuning others and experiencing Reiki at the deepest level possible.

This training empowers the participants to become Reiki masters who are capable of providing all three levels of Reiki training to others.

Each Reiki training workshop may last from a half day to several days. Certificates of completion are provided at the end of each workshop for each level of Reiki training. Many masters have developed their own manuals in an attempt to personalize their training, and students receive these manuals during their training.

Reiki Treatment

The process of attunement allows one to channel Reiki immediately. Practitioners usually place their palms (some specify to cup them) in a sequential pattern on or just above the body of a recipient who is fully clothed. The hand positions are designed to cover the head, front, back, and feet, providing Reiki to the body's major organs and endocrine and lymphatic systems. The complete process may take from 60 to 90 minutes.[1-7] However, the time spent in a Reiki session can vary from situation to situation and place to place. Sometimes, the Reiki touch may last for only a few moments.[6] Such flexibility has made Reiki very useful for those professionals who have a very limited amount of time for each patient and a large number of patients to care for. That is a major reason why Reiki is popular with nurses and Reiki training is acceptable as part of their continuing education.[15] Sometimes the recipients may not wish to be touched or they may be in such condition that their skin cannot be touched (eg, burn victims). Reiki can be administered by holding hands 3 to 4 inches over the recipient's body, functioning as a distant healing.[1,7]

Evidence of Efficacy for Reiki Practice

Although the literature is full of anecdotes by Reiki practitioners and clients claiming healing at all levels, only a handful of scientific studies are found in support of such claims. Also, most of the studies have small samples and major methodological flaws.[5] Findings of these studies are summarized below.

Wetzel[9] compared two groups of participants on the basis of their blood hemoglobin and hematocrit values. The experimental group consisted of 48 adults who were in a Reiki training program in California in 1988, and the control group consisted of 10 medical professionals not involved in Reiki training. The participants in the two groups were not assigned randomly. Two blood samples, 24 hours apart, were obtained from each participant. The experimental group had the first degree Reiki training in these 24 hours. The results showed a significant change in hemoglobin and hematocrit values between two blood samples of the group that received Reiki training, however, the directionality of the change in these parameters was not defined. No significant change in these blood values was found in the two blood samples of the group that had no Reiki training. Later, in a case-by-case analysis, increase in the blood values was found in over half (28) of the experimental group participants. Because of the obvious methodological problems, the findings of this study did not contribute much to the scientific support of the subjective claims by those who practice Reiki.

Several studies were conducted by Wirth and colleagues,[17-19] who used Reiki in conjunction with LeShan or Therapeutic Touch (TT), intercessory prayer, and Qi gong at the Healing Sciences Research International at Orinda, CA. Although these healing modalities differ in their methods of application, they all tap into the same divine source of healing. Reiki and LeShan are nondirective approaches, whereas TT and Qi gong are directive approaches to healing. A brief discussion of the four healing modalities used by Wirth and colleagues is presented in the following text.

LeShan, developed by a clinical psychologist Lawrence LeShan, is a consciousness-based healing system in which the practitioner experiences universal oneness and interconnectedness. The practitioner does not focus on healing, but on being with the patient in a loving and caring way. Healing process is believed to be a natural human ability that can be enhanced by meditative techniques. TT, by Dora Kunz, a healer, and Dolores Krieger, a nursing professor, is based on the ancient practice of the laying-on of hands for healing. The TT practitioner scans the body of the patient by holding his or her hands 2 to 6 inches away from the body. If energy depletions are detected, then the practitioner conveys energy; and if excesses of energy are found, then the practitioner draws energy. Intercessory prayer is a most ancient and common method of healing used in all cultures and religions by invoking Divine intervention through prayer. The manner in which prayer is done differs from person to person, culture to culture, and religion to religion. However, a belief in existence of a higher power is a crucial factor in intercessory prayer. Intercessors can work from any distance. Qi gong is a Chinese method of self-healing (internal Qi gong) and healing of others (external Qi gong). External Qi gong was used in research by Wirth and colleagues. A Qi gong master can transmit his or her internal Qi (energy) to the acupuncture points of the patient's body.[16-18]

The first study by Wirth, Brelan, Levine, and Rodriguez[19] used a randomized, double-blind, within-subject, crossover design using 21 patients experiencing iatrogenic pain after extraction of asymptomatic, impacted lower third molar teeth. These patients went through two separate operations. They were randomly assigned to the treatment or control condition before operating the first time and then crossed over to the opposite condition for the second operation. Contrary to the control condition, the treatment condition was followed by Reiki and LeShan healing after the operations. The results showed that the participants experienced significantly less postoperative pain after the healing treatment.

In another study, Wirth, Chang, Eidelman, and Paxton[17] examined the effect of TT, Reiki, LeShan, and Qi gong in combination on blood assays using a point-of-care i-STAT clinical analyzer (East Windsor, NJ). They used a randomized within-subject, double-blind, crossover design, and randomly assigned 14 (21 to 41 years of age) healthy participants to treatment and control conditions for two 1-hour evaluation sessions separated by a 24-hour period. The treatment intervention consisted of Reiki and LeShan practitioners working conjunctively from a distance and Qi gong and TT practitioners working independently through a one-way mirror. The results showed significant treatment effects on urea nitrogen and glucose values (decrease). However, the majority of subjects who experienced a reduction in blood-glucose levels had a baseline measure higher than normal. After receiving the combination therapy, the glucose readings decreased to normoglycemic range. Also, the participants were Qi gong students and patients who had previous exposure to a complementary healing study. Because Reiki was combined with other modalities, any positive effects could not be attributed to Reiki alone. Findings of this study were considered preliminary due to several methodological limitations.

Later, a series of five experiments were designed by Wirth, Richardson, and Eidelman[18] to examine the efficacy of TT either in isolation or in conjunction with Reiki, LeShan, and intercessory prayer on the re-epithelialization rate of full-thickness human dermal wounds. Wound size varied from 4 to 8 mm. The experiments were well controlled using randomized and double-blind design. The sample sizes for five experiments ranged from 15 to 44. The results of the two experiments yielded statistically significant accelerated rate of re-epithelialization for the treatment groups as compared to the control groups. However, researchers found the overall results of the five experiments to be inconclusive, because a consistent reproducible treatment effect was not derived. Also, because Reiki was used in conjunction with several other complementary therapies, the results were not too helpful with regard to establishing validity of Reiki.

Neklason[20] examined the effects of Reiki on telepathic communication and the Taylor-Johnson Temperament Analysis (T-JTA) variables. The T-JTA is a measure of nine personality traits (nervous/composed, depressive/light-hearted, active-social/quiet, expressive-responsive/inhibited, sympathetic/indifferent, subjective/objective, dominant/submissive, hostile/tolerant, and self-disciplined/impulsive) and may serve as an indicator of emotional disturbances. The results showed that Reiki influenced telepathy trial scores. However, the data were considered insufficient for statistical analysis of T-JTA scores because there were only two participants in the treatment group and three in the control group. In another study of five patients who either had multiple sclerosis, lupus, fibromyalgia, or thyroid goiter, Brewitt, Vittetoe, and Hartwell[21] used the Life Information System Ten (LISTEN) device (Busywork Inc, Orem, UT) to measure the electrical skin conductance at 40 acupuncture points. The electrical skin conductance measures were taken after the first, third, and last treatment sessions. A total of 11 Reiki sessions were given. Three skin points, referred to as neuroendocrine-immune points, showed significant changes. An abnormally low mean conductance was recorded before treatment, which improved to normal range after the third Reiki session. Low conductance was considered to indicate depleted energy and illness. All patients reported increase in relaxation and mobility, decrease in pain, and a sense of "centeredness" after Reiki sessions. Obvious methodological problems limited the findings of this study.

In a pain management study of 20 participants who experienced pain due to several conditions, Olson and Hanson[22] combined Reiki and opioid therapies. This study at the Cross Cancer Institute at Edmonton, Alberta, Canada was designed to explore the effectiveness of Reiki as an adjuvant to opioid therapy. A visual analogue scale and a Likert scale were used to measure pain. Pain was shown to be significantly reduced on these instruments following the Reiki treatment. In absence of a control group, the results of this study remained inconclusive.

A study by two nursing professors, Wardell and Engebretson[23] at the University of Texas Houston Health Science Center, examined the effect of Reiki on anxiety, blood pressure, skin conductance, muscle tension, skin temperature, and biological measures of salivary IgA and cortisol. A single group repeated measure design was used with a nonrandom sample of 23 participants. Data were collected before, during, and immediately after a single 30-minute Reiki session. The results comparing before and after measures showed a significant reduction in anxiety, a significant rise in IgA levels, and a significant drop in systolic blood pressure. These findings suggested that even a single Reiki session was successful in reducing anxiety, increasing relaxation, and increasing humoral immunological functioning. The authors suggested further research in the area of immune response.

In an effort to control some extraneous variables, two experiments used nonhuman subjects to measure effects of Reiki. Baldwin and Schwartz[24] divided 16 male Sprague Dawley rats into four groups housed in four separate but similar rooms. The rats in three of the four groups were subjected to 15 minutes of 90 dB white noise for 3 weeks and rats in the fourth room were the quiet control group. Because loud noise stress can damage the mesenteric microvasculature causing leakage of plasma into the surrounding tissue, the rat groups were varied in four conditions to determine whether Reiki as a healing energy can reduce microvascular leakage. The four groups were No Noise group, Noise group, Noise and Sham Reiki group, and Noise and Reiki group. The Noise and Reiki group received a daily 15-minute Reiki treatment prior to the noise. The experiment was performed three times and in all three experiments, Reiki significantly reduced the average number and area of microvascular leaks compared to the other noise groups. However, authors questioned whether the effects were caused by Reiki itself or the relaxing effect of the Reiki practitioner and recommend using distant Reiki in the future experiments.

A second study by Rubik, Brooks, and Schwartz[25] examined effects of Reiki, a "universal life energy," on growth of heat-shocked *Escherichia coli* cultures. Growth was considered a measure of vitality and well-being in bacteria. Researchers also examined whether or not practitioner well-being influenced the effects of Reiki on bacterial culture growth. Fourteen Reiki practitioners provided 15 minutes Reiki to boxes of bacterial cultures and completed pre- and post-test measures of well-being. Each practitioner completed three runs in which bacteria were treated called "non-healing context," and two runs for "healing context" in which they first treated a pain patient for 30 minutes. In the "healing context," Reiki significantly improved the growth of treated bacterial cultures as compared to controls. Also, initial level of well-being of the practitioners correlated with the bacterial culture growth. The Reiki-treated bacterial counts were higher than controls for practitioners starting with a higher level of well-being, whereas for a practitioner starting with a diminished level of well-being control, counts were higher. It was concluded that Reiki might be modulated by the human biofield influenced by the practitioner's psychophysiological state which challenged two of Usui lineage beliefs: 1) the Reiki practitioner is a passive conduit and 2) Reiki can be practiced in "any state of practitioner consciousness." The researchers warned that due to the small number of practitioners in the study, no definitive conclusion could be made and further studies were needed to confirm and extend the findings of this study.

Personal Research Experience With Reiki

Hailing from India, I grew up knowing about many alternative healing modalities such as yoga, Ayurvedic medicine, homeopathy, healing through touch and prayer, herbal remedies, etc. Consequently, when I first learned about Reiki at the 1997 Annual Conference of the International Society for the Study of Subtle Energies and Energy Medicine (ISSSEEM), I was not surprised. I assumed that Reiki was similar to some healing practices that have been in existence for centuries in India. If you have ever seen the pictures of Hindu gods and goddesses, you would notice that they have their right hands up facing you with energy bursting out of them. This energy repre-sents the divine energy that heals and blesses. Also in India, when younger persons touch the feet of elders as a form of greeting, the elders place their palms on the younger persons' heads and shoulders giving them ashirwad, which means blessings.

At any rate, having earned three graduate degrees in America and being involved in research for over two decades, I learned to put my subjective feelings about what constitutes effective healing practice aside and profess only that which was verified via scientific method. But my exposure to Reiki at the ISSSEEM awakened the memories of my experiences with alternative healing methods of India. Also, I met doctors, bioengineers, nurses, psychologists, professional counselors, social workers, and laypersons at the ISSSEEM meeting who practiced Reiki and other forms of alterna-tive and complementary therapies. Inspired by their testimonies, I sought the training and earned my first degree in Reiki on July 20, 1997.

I was very excited about being initiated into this art of healing called Reiki and could not wait to share my experiences with my psychology students. Besides telling them about this hands-on heal-ing modality, I shared my frustration about the lack of scientific evidence demonstrating the effi-cacy of Reiki practice. I had decided to conduct research in this area to satisfy my own curiosity. One day after an undergraduate counseling psychology class, my student Linda Dressen stopped me and said, "I was looking for a mentor, and I think I have found her." She then shared with me her enthusiasm about Reiki and commented that she was a Reiki master. I shared my research ideas and hypotheses with Linda and asked her if she would like to get involved in the project. She agreed immediately and enrolled in an independent research class with me and later participated in the Reiki study. I designed and directed the study in which five Reiki masters and four layper-sons helped in collecting data from chronically ill patients in the West Texas area. The impressive results prompted me to submit the study for presentation at the Ninth Annual Conference of the ISSSEEM in Boulder, CO. Our paper[6] was one of the four technical papers accepted from over 110 submissions worldwide for the 1999 ISSSEEM conference. Later, our study was published in *Subtle Energies & Energy Medicine*.[5] Following is a summary of the study.

This was the first experimental study that compared Reiki with progressive muscle relaxation, control, and placebo conditions to examine the efficacy of Reiki for emotional, personality, and spiritual changes in chronically ill patients. Sex and type of treatment were the independent vari-ables of the study. Treatment groups were Reiki group (R), progressive muscle relaxation group (PMR), wait-list control group (C), and placebo group (P). The dependent variables included present pain intensity; total pain rating index-R (PRI-R); PRI-R: sensory quality of pain; PRI-R: affective quality of pain; PRI-R: evaluative quality of pain, depression, state anxiety, trait anxiety, self-esteem, locus of control, realistic sense of personal control, and belief in God's (higher power)

Table 16-1

MAIN EFFECTS OF TREATMENT AND ONLY SIGNIFICANT TREATMENT X SEX ANOVA AND OMEGA SQUARED RESULTS USING PRETEST/POST-TEST CHANGE SCORES FOR 12 DEPENDENT VARIABLES

DEPENDENT VARIABLE	F	P	ω^2
Global pain intensity	9.67	0.0001	0.18*
Pain Rating Index-R: Sensory	2.87	0.03	0.05
Pain Rating Index-R: Affective	0.17	0.91	ns
Pain Rating Index-R: Evaluative	5.43	0.001	0.13
Pain Rating Index-R: Total scale	2.24	0.09	ns
Depression	23.57	0.0001	0.34*
Depression x sex	2.98	0.03	0.03
State anxiety	18.56	0.0001	0.28*
Trait anxiety	17.29	0.0001	0.29*
Self-esteem	3.29	0.02	0.05
Locus of control	5.18	0.002	0.10
Unrealistic sense of control	3.79	0.01	0.07
Faith in God	2.80	0.04	0.04
Faith in God x sex	2.68	0.05	0.02

*Large effect size

assistance. These variables were measured by the following instruments: General Information Questionnaire (GIQ), Social Readjustment Rating Scale, McGill Pain Questionnaire, Beck Depression II Inventory, State-Trait Anxiety Inventory, Rotter I-E Scale, Rosenberg Self-Esteem Scale, and Belief in Personal Control Scale.[5]

The study included 48 men and 72 women (N=120) who were chronically ill with headaches (45%), heart disease (10%), cancer (8%), arthritis (7%), peptic ulcer (6%), asthma (7%), hypertension (12%), or human immunodeficiency virus (HIV) infection (5%). They were predominantly Caucasian (92%) with average age of 41.34 years (SD=11.32). These participants had no prior experience with Reiki, PMR, or any type of hands-on healing therapy, and they all experienced some type of pain. These volunteers were randomly assigned to one of the four treatment groups resulting in eight (treatment x sex) subgroups (ns=30). All participants received 10 30-minute sessions twice a week. The R group received Reiki sessions and the PMR group received sessions of PMR and deep breathing exercises. The participants in group C read any material of their choice for 10 30-minute sessions and did not receive Reiki treatment. The group P received false Reiki treatments by four lay assistants who did not receive Reiki attunement, but learned the hand positions used on group R participants. The group R participants were contacted after 3 months for follow-up testing to assess the change in dependent measures from post-test to follow-up.[5]

The results using the 4 x 2 factorial ANOVA and Omega Squared (ω^2) for pretest/post-test change for all dependent variables are presented in Table 16-1. Although the ANOVA results for 10 independent variables were significant, only three main effects showed medium and four main effects showed large effect sizes. Large treatment effects (Omega squared of 0.15 or larger is considered large treatment effect 0.24) were found on present pain intensity, depression, and state

Table 16-2

ILLUSTRATION OF THE TUKEY/KRAMER PROCEDURE RESULTS FOR POST HOC PAIRWISE COMPARISONS

VARIABLE	TUKEY/KRAMER PROCEDURE RESULTS PATTERN
Present pain intensity (A)	Group R > PMR ∫C ∫P
Pain Rating Index-R: Sensory (A)	Group R > PMR ∫P
Pain Rating Index-R: Evaluative (A)	Group R > PMR ∫C ∫P
Depression (A)	Group R > PMR ∫C ∫P
A x B	R ♂ > R ♀
State anxiety	Group R > PMR ∫C ∫P
Trait anxiety	Group R > PMR ∫C ∫P
Self-esteem	Group R > PMR ∫C ∫P
Locus of control	Group R > PMR ∫C ∫P
Unrealistic personal control	Group R > PMR ∫C
Faith in God (A)	Group R > PMR ∫C
A x B	R ♀ > PMR ♀∫C ♀♂∫P ♀
	P ♂ > PMR ♂♀∫C ♂♀∫P ♀

Key: A=Treatment; A x B=Treatment x sex interaction; R=Reiki group; PMR=progressive muscle relaxation group; C=control group; P=placebo group; >=significantly greater change; ∫=no significant difference in change; ♂=men; ♀=women

and trait anxiety. Medium treatment effects were noted on PRI-R: evaluative, locus of control, and unrealistic sense of control; while treatment effects were small on PRI-R: sensory, self-esteem, and faith in God. Significant interaction effects of treatment x sex were found only on depression and faith in God. Tukey/Kramer procedure was used for all post hoc pairwise comparisons. The direction of significant Tukey/Kramer procedure results are documented in Table 16-2.

The post-test and follow-up comparison results of group R showed significant reduction in sensory and affective qualities of pain along with the overall pain measure. All other comparisons did not yield significant results.

This was the first study of Reiki that randomly assigned men and women experiencing similar levels of life-event stress to experimental conditions and compared Reiki with PMR therapy, no therapy, and false Reiki. One of the major contributions of this study was to demonstrate how a placebo group can be used in Reiki studies. To my knowledge, no study prior to this study used a placebo group (false Reiki). After our study, studies are now designing experiments and quasi-experiments including a placebo or "sham Reiki" group.

Cooperation from patients and their health care providers was an important factor for the success of this study. Also, the patients were highly motivated to participate, perhaps due to their need to experience reduction in chronic pain resulting from their medical conditions. Some limitations of the study were that the sample was self-selected and some uncontrolled variables might have influenced the results, for example, "seriousness of the illness, multiple experimenters, multiple sites, religiosity, and social support available to the patient."[5] However, the random assignment of the participants and other controls used in the study provided some safeguards. Six major conclusions of the study are presented in the following section:

1. Reiki is an effective modality for reducing pain, depression, and state anxiety. Of those receiving Reiki, men tend to show greater reduction in depression than women after receiving Reiki.

2. Reiki is effective in enhancing desirable changes in personality. Persons tend to show decreased trait anxiety, self-esteem enhancement, and greater sense of internal locus of control. Further, their belief in their personal control tends to become more realistic.

3. Reiki enhances one's faith that God is a powerful agent whose help can be enlisted. Women tend to experience this enhancement in faith more than men.

4. Attunement is necessary for practice of Reiki. A false Reiki practice would not be effective in enhancing desirable changes in pain, affective states, personality traits, and spirituality.

5. The gains made by Reiki tend to persist over longer periods of time. After a 3-month period, significant reduction tends to occur in sensory and affective qualities of pain and the Total Pain Rating Index.

6. Chronically ill patients experiencing high stress and pain would be receptive to Reiki practice.[5]

Current Application and Future Directions

Reiki is currently being used by many doctors and nurses as an adjunct to conventional medical practice in America. The major application of Reiki is in the areas of stress reduction and pain management of chronically ill patients.[4,7,15] Other areas in which Reiki is being used are physical healing, emotional healing, attitudinal changes, and facilitation of the dying process.[1,7,15,27,28] Some are using it as a psychotherapy tool. Barnett and Chambers[7] state, "Reiki accelerates the process of psychotherapy by eliciting additional insights regarding the client's situation as well as by allowing the emotional residue to gently release from the body's cells. The result is a sense of well-being and empowerment."

Because of medical and psychological applications, Reiki training has become acceptable as part of continuing education for many types of helping professionals. For example, see the following excerpt from the American Psychological Association (APA)[29] Web site:

> **19-20C>Second Degree Reiki For Mental Health Professionals=/ Boston, MA/$190/10 CE credits**: Consists of the transmission of two attunements, lecture, discussion, guided meditations and practice time. Attention will be given to the integration of Reiki into the psychotherapy practice. Richard Curtin, PsyD, MA, School of Professional Psychology.

The APA has rigorous guidelines for approving continuing education workshops, and a workshop presenter has to submit a proposal that has to be approved by a continuing education committee. The APA's acceptance of the Reiki training for as many as 10 continuing education units is a strong sign that the mental health establishment of America recognizes the psychotherapeutic promise of Reiki.

In last few years, Reiki practice has also entered the hospital setting. In 1997, all but one physician at the Columbia/HCA Portsmouth Regional Hospital in Portsmouth, NH agreed to allow an option to receive a 15-minute Reiki treatment for preregistered surgery patients.[30] Sawyer[31] and Wing and Wolf[32] also took Reiki practice into the Dartmouth-Hitchcock Medical Center in Lebanon, NH and Department of Oncology at Women and Infants Hospital in Province, RI, respectively. Their articles provide information that can be helpful to professionals in making similar attempts.

Rand[33] has an online article on the Web site of the International Center for Reiki Training that discusses the efforts of several doctors, nurses, and Reiki practitioners who succeeded in having hospitals include Reiki as an adjunct therapy among their patient services. Some of the hospitals are the Columbia Presbyterian Medical Center, New York, NY; the Tucson Medical Center, AZ; the Manhattan Eye, Ear and Throat Hospital, New York, NY; the Memorial Sloane Kettering Hospital, New York, NY; the Marin General Hospital, Greenbrae, CA; the California Pacific Medical Center, San Francisco; the University of Michigan Hospital, Ann Arbor; and the Foote Hospital, Jackson, MI. Many benefits have been reported as a result of using Reiki as an adjunct therapy in hospitals, such as reduction in pain, reduction in anxiety, faster recovery, lessened blood loss during surgery, fewer side effects of chemotherapy, and less use of medications.

Ethics and Insurance

The International Association of Reiki Professionals (IARP) has been trying to regulate the practice of Reiki by creating a membership registration, a code of ethics, and a liability insurance program. The IARP has two slightly differing versions of the code of ethics, one for practitioners and another for master teachers. Of the 10 principles, principle 2 is the only one that differs in wording from the practitioner's version to the teacher's version. Therefore, the two wordings of principle 2 are presented in Table 16-3, along with the common wordings of the other nine principles.[34]

A professional liability insurance program is also available through IARP,[13] which covers Reiki practitioners as well as teachers in the United States and Canada. The insurance policy protects against malpractice suits resulting from services provided by practitioners and teachers. Besides providing the protection and support for its members, this program is believed to be useful because hospitals and other health care settings often require Reiki practitioners to have liability insurance to practice in these settings.

GUIDELINES FOR FUTURE RESEARCH

All research on Reiki to date is preliminary, because most findings have not been replicated under controlled conditions and lack extended follow-ups. However, findings of all types of studies serve as guidelines for future research. Science builds itself on all types of empirical studies, ranging from observational studies to rigorously controlled studies.

Nield-Anderson and Ameling[35] discuss several methodological and philosophical reasons for difficulty in conducting scientific research on the efficacy of Reiki. Although the author of this chapter agrees with their general contention that it is difficult to conduct Reiki studies using traditional scientific method, she does not think that it is an impossible task. For example, they say, "This healing method cannot be masked, per se, so that double-blind studies involving random assignment of subjects to standardized treatment protocols and control groups are not possible."[35] Several Reiki studies[5,17-19,36] have shown that random assignment of participants, standardized treatment protocols, and placebo and control groups are possible. Another difficulty stated by Nield-Anderson and Ameling is that randomization and group assignment render participants without choice in treatment, which may be a threat to a practitioner-client relationship.[35] This problem can be handled by using crossover experimental design and wait-list control group, as done in several studies.[5,17-19,36] Yet, another problem with Reiki studies mentioned in the article by Nield-Anderson and Ameling is that the studies of efficacy of Reiki "deal almost exclusively with well populations." There are several studies[5,17,22] that used patient samples.

Even though some researchers are making efforts to investigate the efficacy of Reiki, there are still many research questions demanding answers. For example, do we need multiple hand positions? If it is to be believed that Reiki is a self-directing and intelligent force that goes where it is needed, why not use only one hand position? Research needs to be designed comparing the single hand position, such as shoulders, to multiple hand positions.

Table 16-3

Code of Ethics for Registered Practitioners (RP) and Registered Teachers (RMT)

THE REGISTERED REIKI PRACTITIONER (RP)/REGISTERED REIKI MASTER PRACTITIONER AND TEACHER (RMT) AGREES TO:

1. Abide by a vow of confidentiality. Any information that is discussed within the context of a Reiki session is confidential between the client and practitioner.

2. Provide a safe and comfortable area for sessions or classes and work to provide an empowering and supportive environment for clients and students.

3. Always treat clients and students with the utmost respect and honor.

4. Have a pure and clear intention to offer your services for the highest healing good of the client and highest potential of the student.

5. Provide a brief oral or written description of what happens during a session and what to expect before a client's initial session. Provide a clear written description of subjects to be taught during each level of Reiki prior to class and list what the student will be able to do after taking the class.

6. Be respectful of all others' Reiki views and paths.

7. Educate clients/students on the value of Reiki and explain that sessions do not guarantee a cure, nor are they a substitute for qualified medical or professional care. Reiki is one part of an integrative healing or wellness program.

8. Suggest a consultation or referral for clients to qualified licensed professionals (medical doctor, licensed therapist, etc.) when appropriate.

9. Never diagnose or prescribe. Never suggest that the client/student change prescribed treatment or interfere with the treatment of a licensed health care provider.

10. Be sensitive to the boundary needs of individual clients and students.

11. Never ask clients to disrobe (unless in the context of a licensed massage therapy session at the client's option). Do not touch the genital area or breasts. Practice hands-off healing of these areas if treatment is needed.

Reproduced with permission from IARP.

Another question arises. Do practitioners need to pay attention during the session or could they be talking, watching television etc? It is believed that no focus or attention is required by the practitioner during the Reiki session. All one needs is to place the hands on another, and the Reiki will go where it is needed. Future studies need to examine this axiom, for example, by comparing a group receiving Reiki while watching TV to a group receiving Reiki in a quiet, private setting without any distractions for the practitioner as well as the recipient. This condition could be further varied by testing a session that is distracting for the practitioner (eg, use of head phones) but not for the recipient, and vice-versa. Several other questions are listed below.

How long do Reiki sessions need to be? Do longer sessions produce better results than the shorter sessions? How long should each hand position be held? Which hand positions are better for which disorders? Is the relaxed position in which the recipient is lying down better than a sitting or standing position? Could the attunements be removed if a person wished to have this done?

Reiki has a long way to go to be fully integrated into practice of medical professionals, because these unanswered questions might lead to their reluctance. Our scientific world rests on results of controlled studies, and that is what is needed to further the standing of Reiki in the medical field.

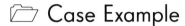 # Case Example

Jim is a 66-year-old retired military officer whose wife passed away after experiencing complications following surgery. He has two grown sons who are married and live in other states. Jim chose to retire in a small town with a military base. After his wife's death, he began experiencing shortness of breath and insomnia. Also, his knee pain got worse. Some days he had trouble walking. He sought medical help and was diagnosed with arthritis and anxiety. Doctors did not find anything wrong with his heart or lungs. Jim was given medications to manage his knee pain and anxiety. However, he did not take them regularly and said, "they did not help that much." He also complained that the anti-anxiety medication made him too tired during the day. He inquired about Reiki because he had learned about my interest in Reiki from one of my students. I told him about the Reiki protocol and suggested that he should consult his doctor and keep him informed about his condition while we worked with Reiki.

Before his first session, I asked him to rate his knee pain on a scale from 0 (no pain) to 10 (excruciating pain). He rated his pain to be 8. I gave him a 1-hour session three times a week for 2 weeks, and then once a week for 2 more weeks. After his first session, Jim reported some reduction in his knee pain (rated it 7). After the second session, he rated his pain to be 6. At the end of the first week (third session), Jim reported that he had not experienced the shortness of breath and his knee pain was less. After the second week (sixth session), his rating of pain had come down to 3. He said that the shortness of breath had not returned and he could walk most of the time without hurting. He also reported sleeping better. At that time, he was initiated into the first degree Reiki, which allowed him to do Reiki on himself. After a month of self-healing, Jim reported that his pain level fluctuated from 0 to 3, and after consulting his doctor, he had stopped taking anti-anxiety medication. He said he used Reiki to manage his pain and anxiety. I suggested that he should continue practicing self-healing with Reiki every morning as he had been doing. After 2 more weeks, Jim reported that his pain continued fluctuating between 0 and 3 and that he decided not to take any medication. He further reported that he was eating more balanced food and walking 30 to 45 minutes most every day. At the 3-month follow-up, Jim said that he was enjoying fishing again and had become active in his church, where he met a special female friend. He also said that he continued practicing self-healing with Reiki.

Conclusion

Reiki represents an ancient art of self-healing and healing others. It is a simple modality that can be learned by anyone regardless of their nationality, creed, culture, sex, age, and wellness level. One does not need to go beyond the first degree, because it provides all that one needs to facilitate healing oneself or others. However, all three Reiki degrees can be achieved by anyone who has a continued desire of experiencing Reiki at deeper levels. Reiki is believed to facilitate relaxation, manage pain, reduce stress, and promote healing. Although there are many anecdotal stories of positive physical, mental, and spiritual changes in people after receiving Reiki healing, the scientific evidence to support these claims is scant. More well-designed and controlled studies on efficacy of Reiki are needed for it to be accepted within the mainstream health care system. Because Reiki is so easy to learn, a time may come when health care professionals may advise it to be included in the preventive care program in addition to balanced diet and exercise. However, there is some evidence of overcommercialization of Reiki, which seems to give ammunition to those who are critical of this modality. In his recent book on spiritual healing research, Benor[16] listed three limitations of Reiki. Besides inadequate preparation of later generations of masters and lack of formal structure for supervision/certification, he assessed high fees (up to several thousand dollars) for master level training as a limitation. Therefore, it bears great responsibility on those who are committed to preserving the integrity of Reiki practice that they work toward keeping the practice free of internal bickering, competition, outrageous profit schemes, power struggle, gimmicky commercialization, and other such evils of modern materialism.

References

1. Baginski BJ, Sharamon S. *Reiki: Universal Life Energy*. Mendocino, CA: Life Rhythm; 1988.
2. Haberly HJ. *Reiki: Hawayo Takata's Story*. Garrett Park, MD: Archedigm Publications; 1990.
3. Jarrell DG. *Reiki Plus Natural Healing*. Celina, TN: Hibernia West; 1991.
4. Rand WL. *Reiki, The Healing Touch: First & Second Degree Manual*. 3rd ed. Southfield, MI: Vision Publications; 2000.
5. Dressen LJ, Singg S. Effects of Reiki on pain and selected affective and personality variables of chronically ill patients. *Subtle Energies & Energy Medicine*. 1998;9:51-82.
6. Singg S, Dressen LJ. Desirable self-perceived psychophysiological changes in chronically ill patients: an experimental study of Reiki. Presented at: Ninth Annual Conference of the International Society for the Study of Subtle Energies and Energy Medicine; June 1999; Boulder, Colo.
7. Barnett L, Chambers M. *Reiki Energy Medicine: Bringing Healing Touch into Home, Hospital, and Hospice*. Rochester, VT: Healing Arts Press; 1996.
8. Gerber R. *Vibrational Medicine: New Choices for Healing Ourselves*. Santa Fe, NM: Bear & Company; 1988.
9. Wetzel WS. Reiki healing: a physiologic perspective. *J Holist Nurs*. 1989;7(1):47-54.
10. International Society for Study of Subtle Energies and Energy Medicine. Intentionality and consciousness. *Bridges*. 1999;10(3).
11. International Society for the Study of Subtle Energies and Energy Medicine. Intentionality and consciousness: expanding horizons in energy medicine. *Bridges*. 1999;10(4).
12. Horan P. *Empowerment Through Reiki: The Path to Personal and Global Transformation*. Wilmot, WI: Lotus Light Publications; 1989.
13. The International Association of Reiki Professionals (IARP). Available at http://www.iarp.org. Accessed November 3, 2003.
14. Reiki Healers Association. *The National Directory of Reiki Healers and Masters*. Frederick, MD: Author; 1997.
15. Van Sell SL. Reiki: an ancient touch therapy. *RN*. 1999;59(2):57-59.
16. Benor DJ. *Spiritual Healing: Scientific Validation of a Healing Revolution* (Healing Research Vol I). Southfield, MI: Vision Publications; 2001.
17. Wirth DP, Chang RJ, Eidelman WS, Paxton JB. Hematological indicators of complementary healing intervention. *Complement Ther Med*. 1996;4:4-20.
18. Wirth DP, Richardson JT, Eidelman WS. Wound healing an complementary therapies: a review. *J Altern Complement Med*. 1996;2(4):493-502.
19. Wirth DP, Brelan DR, Levine RJ, Rodriguez CM. The effect of complementary healing therapy on postoperative pain after surgical removal of impacted third molar teeth. *Complement Ther Med*. 1993;1(3):133-138.
20. Neklason ZT. *The Effects of Reiki Treatment on Telepathy and Personality Traits* [unpublished master's thesis]. California State University, Hayward; 1987.
21. Brewitt B, Vittetoe T, Hartwell B. The efficacy of Reiki hands-on healing: improvements in spleen and nervous system function as qualified by electrodermal screening. *Altern Ther*. 1997;3:89.
22. Olson K, Hanson J. Using Reiki to manage pain: a preliminary report. *Cancer Prev Control*. 1997;1(2):108-113.
23. Wardell DW, Engebretson J. Biological correlates of Reiki Touch healing. *J Adv Nurs*. 2001;3(4):439-445.
24. Baldwin AL, Schwartz GE. Personal interaction with a Reiki practitioner decreases noise-induced microvascular damage in an animal model. *J Altern Comp Med*. 2006;12(1):15-22.
25. Rubik B, Brooks AJ, Schwartz GE. In vitro effect of Reiki treatment on bacterial cultures: role of experimental context and practitioner well-being. *J Altern Comp Med*. 2006;12(1):7-1.
26. Keppel G. *Design and Analysis: A Researcher's Handbook*. Engelwood Cliffs, NJ: Prentice Hall; 1991.
27. Ray B. *The Reiki Factor*. St. Petersburg, FL: Radiance Associates; 1985.
28. Bullock M. Reiki: a complementary therapy for life. *Am J Hosp Palliat Care*. 1997;14(1):31-33.
29. American Psychological Association. APA Education Information: CE June 1998 Calendar of Events. Available at http://www.apa.org/ce/cecal.html. Accessed November 3, 2003.
30. Alandydy P, Alandydy K. Using Reiki to support surgical patients. *J Nurs Care Qual*. 1999;13(4):89-91.
31. Sawyer J. The first Reiki practitioner in our OR. *Association of Operating Room Nurses Journal*. 1998;67(3):674-677.

32. Wing J, Wolf A. How we got Reiki into the hospital. *Reiki News*. 2000;Sept:28-29.

33. Rand WL. Reiki News Articles: The International Center for Reiki Training. Reiki in Hospitals. Available at http://www.reiki.org/reikinews/reiki_in_hospitals.html. Accessed November 3, 2003.

34. International Association of Reiki Professionals. IARP Code of Ethics. Available at http://www.iarp.org/ethicscode.html. Accessed July 10, 2008.

35. Nield-Anderson L, Ameling A. The empowering nature of Reiki as a complementary therapy. *Holist Nurs Pract*. 2000;14(3):21-29.

36. Mansour AA, Beuche M, Laing G, Leis A, Nurse J. A study to test the effectiveness of placebo Reiki standardization procedure developed for a planned Reiki efficacy study. *J Altern Complement Med*. 1999;5(2):153-164.

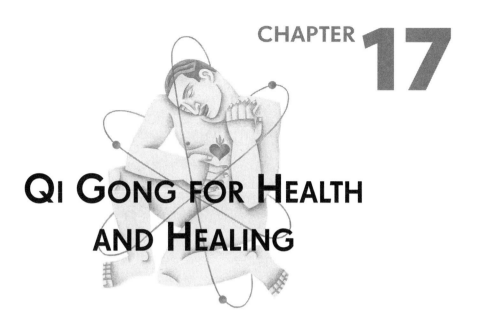

Qi Gong for Health and Healing

Jennifer M. Bottomley, PhD, MS, PT

Introduction

Qi gong is a therapeutic Chinese practice that has been used for thousands of years to optimize and restore energy (Qi) to the body, mind, and spirit. Elements of Taoist and Buddhist philosophies form the foundation of Qi gong, which promotes health and vitality through gentle exercises for the breath, body, mind, and voice.[1] Qi gong is an alternative therapy that recognizes the strong connection between the body and the mind. Qi gong is an ancient traditional form of a group of techniques considered energy medicine.[2] Energy medicine techniques derive from traditional Chinese medicine and are based upon the concept that health and healing are dependent upon a balance of vital energy, a still mind, and controlled emotions. Physical dysfunctions result from disordered patterns of energy of long standing. Reversal of the physical problems, according to Qi gong theories, requires a return to balance and ordered energy.[3] Qi gong is a system that teaches an individual to live in a state of energy equilibrium. Hypothetically, Qi gong relies on no external physical interventions, but rather, relies on mind control to prevent illness, heal existing physical and emotional problems, and promote health and happiness. This chapter will describe the use of these techniques with people who have long-term physical disabilities and other pathologies.

Qi gong is an exercise form, similar to T'ai Chi, that is particularly helpful in an elderly population because of its slow, controlled, non-impact-type movements and postures, which displace and thereby stimulate the cognizant control of the center of gravity. In fact, T'ai Chi was derived from Qi gong and has the same philosophical origins. Qi gong exercise form incorporates all of the motions that often become restricted with inactivity and aging. A distinguishing element of Qi gong is the use of static postures which, from a therapeutic perspective, are particularly helpful in individuals with movement limitations and those who are frail. Qi gong integrates deep breathing and meditation as well as self-massage, movements, and postures. Qi gong improves respiration, stresses trunk control, expands the base of support, improves rotation of the trunk and coordination of isolated extremity motions, and helps to facilitate awareness of movement and position.

Self-massage techniques stimulate circulation and affect nutritional absorption, flexibility, and sensory awareness. The meditative component of Qi gong serves to make an individual more aware of his or her body; enhance his or her ability to control muscle tension, posturing, and movement; and facilitates a peacefulness of mind that leads to a overall sense of well-being.[4,5]

Defining Qi Gong

Qi gong (pronounced chee-gong) translates as *breathing exercise* or *energy skill* and has a long history in China.[6,7] It has been recorded in medical literature since ancient times and is an important component of traditional Chinese medicine. It has been practiced by the Chinese people for thousands of years, both to improve and maintain health and to develop greater power for the martial arts. *Qi* is the energy that circulates within the body, and *Gong* means work or exercise, so Qi gong means the cultivation of the body's energy to increase and control its work capacity through the increase of circulation and energy flow.[1-7]

Qi gong exercise includes different methods of practice, breathing, self massage, movement, postures and meditation. In theory, by adopting various postures of the body and regulating breathing and mind, a person can cultivate vital energy to cure illness and maintain health.

In order to understand Qi gong, there are several concepts to be understood. The following is a brief description of each of the principles of Chinese Qi gong.

Vital Energy (Ch'i or Qi): Concept of Ch'i and Energy Flow

The first concept is that of *Qi*. Qi is the foundation of all Chinese medical theory as well as Qi gong.[3] It corresponds to the Greek "pneuma" and the Sanskrit "prana," and is considered to be the vital force and energy flow in all living things. Qi can be best explained as a type of energy very much like electricity, which flows through the human or animal body. It is a theory of traditional Chinese medicine that "vital energy" or Qi has profound effects on health and that breathing exercise can increase vital energy thereby preventing illness. Vital energy is the material foundation of the movement of life, the essence of life. It activates the physiological functions of the internal organs. Qi, prana, pneuma, life force, or internal energy (also: steam, vapor, air) describes the enhancement of energy flow though breathing exercise. When life stops, the circulation of vital energy disappears. A strong vital energy gives good health and a weak one poor health.[1,3]

Qi can also be explained as a medium of sensing or feeling. For example, if an individual injures an extremity, the Qi flow in the nerves of the extremity is disturbed and stimulated to a higher energy state. This higher energy state causes a sensational feeling that is interpreted as pain by the brain. The difference in energy potential causes an increased flow of Qi and blood to that area to begin repairing the damage. Complete healing occurs when the energy is once again balanced. If the damage is not completely repaired the energy remains unbalanced and pain will persist.

Yin and Yang Energy = Ch'i

Qi gong is also based upon the principle of *Yin* and *Yang*, which describes the relationship of complementary qualities such as soft and hard, female and male, dark and light, or slow and fast. Yin and Yang are often described as the unity of opposites (sympathetic and parasympathetic; north and south; positive and negative; heavy and light; life and death; day and night). One can not exist without the other. They are two opposing but complementary forces exerting universal influence. Yin is heavy and tends to sink downward. Yang is light and tends to float upward. Yin is the black or negative, while Yang is the white or positive. Yin is passive and tang is active. Yin represents quiet and rest, whereas Yang represents movement.

Figure 10-1, in the chapter on T'ai Chi, represents the universally accepted concept of Yin and Yang energy pictorially. Yin (greater) always contains some Yang (lesser), Yang (greater) always contains some Yin (lesser). The purpose of Qi gong exercises is to achieve a balance of Yin and Yang. Refer to Chapter 8 for a more comprehensive discussion of the concept of Yin and Yang.

Meridians and Channels

Qi channels or meridians refer to the pathways that create the relationship between vital energy and nature.[1-4] A channel or meridian is a major connector of each internal organ with the rest of the body. Imbalance in the energy levels of any organ will affect all of the other organs of the body. These channels frequently follow the major nerves and arteries.[3-7]

Another concept of Qi gong is the acupuncture points. Along each channel are the "cavities," points where electrical conductivity is higher than the surrounding area, commonly known as acupuncture points, which are used to stimulate the entire Qi system. Figures 17-1A to F display the commonly accepted energy channels as represented in acupuncture points. Energy channels throughout the body regulate Ch'i (Qi) flow. The body is hypothetically composed of eight energy channels (thought of as Qi reservoirs) and has 12 meridians (thought of as Qi rivers) that run throughout the body. The meridians and channels systematically include all parts of the trunk and extremities. When Qi is stagnant in one channel, the corresponding organ will be affected.[1,3]

The Five Elements

Another principle in Qi gong is that of the five elements. The five elements are understood better as forces, energy, and agents rather than as material elements. The emphasis is on principles and laws of nature, the outlook is dynamic and not static. The emphasis of this philosophy is placed on harmony and balance of these elements. The concept is one of unity in multiplicity. Table 17-1 provides a summary of how each of the five elements is associated with particular organs, colors, flavors, emotions, and the like.

No element is superior to the others. Each interacts with the other four differently and yet a balance is maintained in nature. For instance, we might say that water can dowse a fire, but fire can boil water and change it to steam. It is hypothesized that the circulation of Qi is governed by the time of day and the season of the year. Qi circulates within the body from conception to death, but the part of the body where the Qi is strongest changes around the clock.

Qi gong is interwoven with the five element theory and the movements are connected to different organs, sounds, emotions, etc. For instance, the *bear posture* in Qi gong is felt to be useful when there is an imbalance of energy flow in the area of the kidneys. The *bird posture* stimulates the heart channel and allows for opening the chest and reduction of pressure in the back and chest area. Yawning, scratching, rubbing, stretching, groaning, even crying are activities that are considered to bring the body into a more comfortable state. The practice of Qi gong recognizes that the internal and external are connected. Energy flowing through the internal organs, for instance, will express itself through an external posture or movement or emotion. Movements such as neck stretching, face rubbing, laughing, in fact all movements that we often practice involuntarily, can be said to have behind them a Qi gong theory based on the flow of energy through the channels and meridians. Every spontaneous posture or movement is thought to be a natural attempt to bring about balance and systemic homeostasis.

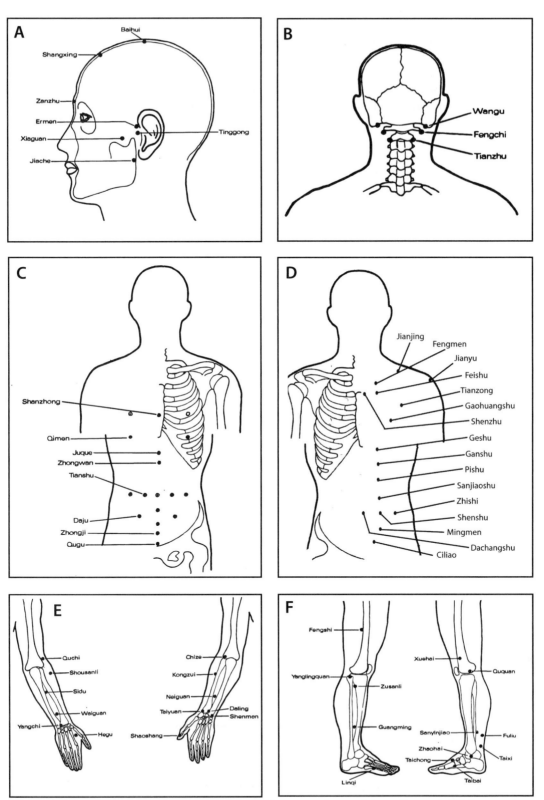

Figure 17-1. (A) Acupuncture points on the head. (B) Acupuncture points on the neck. (C) Acupuncture points on the front of the trunk. (D) Acupuncture points on the back of the trunk. (E) Acupuncture points on the arms. (F) Acupuncture points on the legs.

Table 17-1	THE FIVE ELEMENTS				
	WATER	*WOOD*	*FIRE*	*EARTH*	*METAL*
Organs	Kidneys	Liver	Heart	Spleen	Lungs
Animal	Bear	Deer	Bird	Monkey	Tiger
Color	Blue/black	Green	Red	Yellow	White
Sound	Groaning	Shouting	Laughing	Singing	Weeping
Smell	Putrid	Rancid	Scorched	Fragrant	Rotten
Taste	Salty	Sour	Bitter	Sweet	Pungent
Emotion	Fear	Anger	Joy	Sympathy	Grief
Season	Winter	Spring	Summer	Late Summer	Autumn
Time of Day	3 to 7 PM	11 PM to 1 AM	11 AM to 3 PM 1 to 11 PM	7 to 11 AM	3 to 7 AM

HYPOTHETICAL RELATIONSHIP OF MIND-BODY EXERCISE TO HEALTH

Current research indicates that the practice of mind-body forms of exercise, such as Qi gong and T'ai Chi, can improve balance, reduce falls, and increase strength and flexibility. In addition, these exercise forms enhance cardiovascular, respiratory, and immune system function[8] and promote emotional and spiritual well-being. Qi gong, and its derivative T'ai Chi, has been found to lower blood pressure and the stress hormone cortisol levels. Hypothetically, Qi gong maintains the balance and homeostasis of the entire system. Practice of Qi gong helps generate, channel, conserve, and direct energy.[9]

Evidence of Efficacy

ELECTRICAL ACTIVITY AND ENERGY FLOW

Although a number of studies on traditional Chinese medicine, such as Qi gong, have explored physiologic changes associated with this intervention, few studies have evaluated human cerebral evoked potentials in relation to Qi gong. Xu and associates[10] examined the changes in evoked potentials and electroencephalogram during Qi gong stimulation. These researchers found significant changes in evoked potential components originating from the cortex suggesting both facilitating and inhibitory effects on the cortex during Qi gong. No significant changes occurred in these measures in the subcortex. Qi gong stimulation had an effect by increasing electrical activity of the somatosensory, visual, and auditory pathways up to the cortex suggesting that this postural/exercise modality has the potential of stimulating and balancing the energy flow in the neurological tracts.[10]

NEUROENDOCRINE AND HORMONE LEVELS

Omura and coworkers[11,12] evaluated hormone and neuroendocrine activity associated with Qi gong stimulation and found enhanced neurotransmission in organs related to the meridians involved during the posture or movement of the exercise. These studies found that within the boundary of most acupuncture points and meridian lines were high concentrations of neurotransmitters and hormones, including acetylcholine, methionine-enkephalin, beta-endorphin, adrenocorticotropic Hormone (ACTH), secretin, cholecystokinin, norepinephrine, serotonin, and gamma-aminobutyric acid (GABA); and the hormones dopamine, dynorphin,[1-13] prostaglandin E1, estrogen (especially estriol and estradiol), testosterone, and progesterone. No significant amounts of these neurotransmitters and hormones were found at the surrounding area outside of meridian and acupuncture points.[11]

Stress hormones (as measured by salivary cortisol levels) have been found to significantly drop during and after exercise practice.[13,14] This is not only important in managing stress and tension related pathologies, but also in improving the overall immune system's ability to maintain homeostasis. Sun and co-workers found a significant immune response as measured by a marked increase in blood T-cells during and after practice.[15]

Stress hormones (as measured by salivary cortisol levels) have been found to significantly drop during and after exercise practice.[16,] This is not only important in managing stress and tension related pathologies, but also in improving the overall immune system's ability to maintain homeostasis. Sun and co-workers found a significant immune response as measured by a marked increase in blood T-cells during and after practice.[15]

Lee and colleagues[16] observed the response of plasma growth hormone, insulin-like growth factor-I, and testosterone to a period of Qi-training with Qi gong exercise and relaxation techniques. They found that plasma growth hormone increased greater than seven-fold in elderly trainees compared with close to two-fold in younger subjects. Insulin-like growth factor-I showed a significant increase in young subjects, but no response in the elderly.[16] Conversely, testosterone showed a significant increase in elderly subjects and no response in the young. These results suggest that Qi gong is a potential method for modulating the secretion of growth hormone in the young and elderly and possibly effect disorders such as growth hormone deficiency in children and osteoporosis in the elderly.[16] In another endocrine study by Lee and associates[17] the effects of Qi gong training on the secretion of thyroid and parathyroid hormones in elderly subjects was investigated. Qi gong induced a slight increase in thyroid stimulating hormone. Triiodothyronine (T3) and throxine (T4) were shown to significantly increase and closely correlated. An increase in the plasma level of T3 was associated with the secretion of T4.[17] The plasma concentrations of calciton and parathyroid hormone were increased, however, there was a slight decrease in ionized calcium. These results suggest that Qi gong training modulates the secretion of thyroid hormones, calcium metabolism, and parathyroid hormones in the elderly.[17]

CANCER

Though definitive studies demonstrating significant changes in outcomes with cancer interventions and Qi gong specifically have not been undertaken, alternative exercise forms have been shown to enhance the immune system, provide pain relief, and result in relief of symptoms often accompanying radiation, chemotherapy, and surgery.[18] Qi gong exercise, postures, meditation, self-massage, and breathing has been found to positively affect mood, outlook, and quality of life measure; enhance overall strength, flexibility, and functional capabilities; and result in greater relaxation and pain management.[19,20]

With the practice of Qi gong therapy, breast cancer patients demonstrated an improvement of the side effects of chemotherapy. The white blood cell count also decreased during the first course of chemotherapy in breast cancer patients.[21] Clearly further research is warranted in determining if there is a relationship between cancer prevention and treatment and Qi gong.

IMMUNOLOGICAL FUNCTION

Qi gong is a type of psychosomatic exercise that integrates meditation, slow physical movement, and breath, to which numerous physical as well as mental benefits have been classically ascribed. Research indicates that Qi gong also has a beneficial effect immunological function. One month of practicing Qi gong resulted in significant immunological changes that enhanced leukocyte, immunoglobulin, and other immune system components in older individuals whose immune system function had been deemed to be suppressed.[22] These findings are important in frailer older individuals who succumb to simple infection due to an unresponsive or sluggish immune system function.

CARDIOVASCULAR AND CARDIOPULMONARY MEASURES

Cardiovascular endurance improves with Qi gong and T'ai Chi exercises. These movement therapies have been found to increase the resistance to cardiovascular diseases and may actually delay the decline of cardiorespiratory function in older adults.[23] Qi gong improves the ability to maintain activity levels and allows for a high energy return for daily activities. Though the observation of Qi gong exercise would not lend to the thought that it was an aerobic activity, research has found that it is in fact a low-to-moderate-intensity exercise with a significant aerobic effect.[24,25] It has also be found to be a safe exercise for individuals at high risk for cardiovascular disease.[26]

Qi gong may be prescribed as a suitable aerobic exercise for older adults[27] and is the most recommended aerobic exercise for coronary artery disease. An additional benefit to Qi gong and T'ai Chi exercise has been realized by a significant reduction in both systolic and diastolic blood pressure.[28]

To investigate the physiologic effects of Qi gong training, Lee and associates[29] investigated changes in blood pressure, heart rate, and respiratory rate before, during, and after Qi training (meditative/relaxation postures in Qi gong training). Heart rate, respiratory rate, systolic blood pressure and rate-pressure product were significantly decreased during Qi gong postures suggesting that Qi gong training has physiological effects that indicate stabilization of cardiovascular system.[30] Progressive relaxation and Qi gong exercise improved the quality of life for cardiac patients with reference to physiologic and psychological measures in a recent study.[31] The calming effect of Qi gong is one very notable consequence of routine participation in this exercise mode in cardiac patients.[32,33]

Respiratory function has also been shown to improve with enhanced ventilatory capacity without cardiovascular stress.[34] Research indicates that one of the primary benefits is the efficient use of ventilatory volume and extremely efficient breathing patterns.

DIABETES

Tsujiuchi and associates[35] studied the effect of Qi gong relaxation exercise on the control of type II diabetes mellitus. They found a reduction in daily insulin needs as a result of daily practice of Qi gong meditation and postures.[35] Further studies are indicated to determine if Qi gong exercise have a long-term effect on the progression of diabetes.

FLEXIBILITY AND MUSCLE STRENGTH

Flexibility is improved through the stretching and eccentric/concentric contraction of the muscles. Qi gong provides increased resistance to muscle and joint injury and prevents mild muscle soreness if done before and after vigorous activity.

Muscle strength has been shown to improve through daily Qi gong activities. Movement patterns become less strenuous as muscles become stronger. Strong abdominal and lower back muscles prevent lower back problems. Stronger postural muscles improve posture. The appearance of muscle fitness improves as muscles become firmer. Generally, Qi gong practitioners have a higher level of endurance because of the improvement in muscle strength and flexibility.[36]

Omura, in the process of evaluating the external effects of Qi gong, showed that Qi gong energy has a polarity which influences the strength of muscles.[37] A positive polarity enhanced muscle strength and velocity measures, whereas a negative polarity resulted in a decrease in muscle force production and a slowing of contraction velocity. Depending on how Qi gong exercises are done (eccentric/concentric contractions or relaxation phases) and from which part of the body movement and energy emanate, the polarity changes. In general, it was found that when a positive polarity is facilitated during active contraction and movement involving painful areas, spastic muscles, or extremities with arteries in vasoconstriction it results in a subsequent reversal of polarity (negative) and relief of symptoms associated with these disturbances. It was found that Qi gong not only improved the microcirculatory disturbance and relaxed spastic muscles and vasoconstrictive arteries, but also reduced or eliminated the pain and selectively enhanced drug uptake in these areas.[37]

BALANCE AND POSTURE

Balance is substantially better in individuals practicing Qi gong and T'ai Chi exercises. Tse's studies demonstrated improvement in strength, mobility, balance, and endurance,[38] and Wolfson and coworkers[39] showed a significant improvement in balance capabilities through gentle movement exercises. As a result, there have been studies that indicate a significant reduction in falls. Wolf and associates[40] found that daily practice of T'ai Chi exercises reduced falls by 47%. Significantly, there was a concomitant reduction in the fear of falling.

BONE MASS AND JOINT INTEGRITY

As Qi gong is an inherently weight-bearing exercise that improves muscle strength, intuitively it can be stated that it would also increase bone mass. This could be a future research study in relation to the use of Qi gong or T'ai Chi in the presence of osteoporosis. Kirsteins and colleagues[41] found that these exercise forms were very effective in individuals with inflammatory joint diseases. No exacerbation in joint symptoms of individuals with rheumatoid arthritis were experienced by exercise participants.[41]

PAIN

Wu and associates[42] studied the effects of Qi gong on treatment-resistant patients with late-stage complex regional pain syndromes. The experimental group received instructions in directing Qi energy flow and instructions in Qi gong exercise (including home exercise) by a Qi gong master. The control group received similar instructions by a sham master. Exercises were performed in six 40-minute Qi gong sessions over a 3-week period with daily home exercises. Outcome measures included thermography, swelling, discoloration, muscle wasting, range of motion, pain intensity rating, medication usage, behavior assessment (activity level and domestic disability), frequency of pain awakening, mood assessment, and anxiety assessment. The authors reported that the genuine Qi gong group report 82% less pain by the end of the first training session compared to 45% of the control group. By the sixth session, 91% of the experimental group reported pain relief compared to 36% of the control group. The researchers concluded that Qi gong training results in pain reduction and long-term reduction of anxiety.

In elderly individuals with chronic pain syndromes, recent research indicates that Qi gong is a non-medication approach to managing pain without the significant side effects often experienced by older adults.[43] Older individuals with fibromyalgia, an otherwise functionally debilitating condition, have also been found to experience substantial pain relief after short term Qi gong therapy.[44] This has significant ramifications for treatment of pain and the quality of life in frailer older individuals.

PARKINSON'S DISEASE

Irrespective of limited evidence, not only traditional physical therapy but also an array of complementary methods have been applied in the treatment of patients with Parkinson's disease. A recent investigation found immediate and sustained effects of Qi gong on motor and non-motor symptoms of Parkinson's disease. Immediate outcomes were a decrease in rigidity, improved initiation of movement, control and coordination, and greater endurance. These motor symptoms were sustained as long as Qi gong exercise continued. Additionally, depression scores decreased in Parkinson's patients participating in regular Qi gong exercise over a 6-month period.[45]

PSYCHOPHYSIOLOGICAL REACTIONS AND MOOD

Based on Qi gong exercisers' self-reports, there is a significant effect on mood states. The improved sense of well-being has been documented by reported reduction in tension, anxiety, fatigue, depression, and confusion.[13-15] Additional benefits were improved mental attitude toward work, self, and life in general; a greater ability to cope with stress; better regular, restful sleep patterns; healthier eating habits; a greater ability to avoid or control mild depression; and a sense of harmony reported by a better communication pathway among body, mind, and spirit (eg, a sense of well-being).

The physiologic effects of Qi gong linked with psychophysiological reactions include changes in electroencephalogram (EEG), electromyography (EMG), respiratory movement, heart rate, skin potential, skin temperature, sympathetic nerve function, function in stomach and intestine, metabolism, and endocrine and immunity systems.[46] Psychological effects are motor phenomena and perceptual changes: a sensation of warmness, chilliness, itching sensation in the skin, numbness, soreness, bloating, relaxation, tenseness, floating, dropping, a sensation of floating, circulation of the intrinsic Qi, electric shock, and other reported sensations during Qi gong exercise. These phenomena appear to be transient and associated with the actual exercise period or latent effects for brief periods following the termination of exercise.[46]

Psychological effects of Qi gong therapy have also been demonstrated in the treatment of depression. One study showed that regular Qi gong practice could relieve depression and improve self-efficacy and personal well-being among elderly persons with chronic physical illness and depression.[47]

Identifying alternative exercise modalities in an effort to stimulate and promote participation in physical activity, especially among older adults, is a critical health consideration and challenge. Medical Qi gong has been shown to be a moderate-intensity physical activity that demonstrates both physiological and psychological benefits for older individuals. Additionally, it is a form of exercise that results in greater compliance than more traditional exercise forms.[48] In other words, older individuals are much more likely to enjoy Qi gong exercise and be motivated to participate in this alternative exercise modality on a regular and ongoing basis.

ADDICTION

Li, Chen, and Mo[49] explored the effectiveness of Qi gong therapy on detoxification of heroin addicts compared to medical and non-medical treatment. The interventions were as follows: a Qi gong group practiced Qi gong exercise and received Qi adjustments from a Qi gong master daily. A medication group received a detoxification drug by a 10-day gradual reduction method. A control group received only basic care and medications to treat severe withdrawal symptoms. Reduction of withdrawal symptoms in the Qi gong group occurred more rapidly than in the other groups. From the first day of intervention, the Qi gong group had significantly lower mean symptom scores than did the other groups. The Qi gong and medication groups both had significantly lower anxiety scores compared to the control group, however the Qi gong group had significantly lower scores on this measure than did the medication group. By the fifth day of treatment, all subjects in the Qi gong group had negative urinalysis results. It took the medication group 9 days and the non-medical group 11 days to clear the heroin from urine tests. These results suggest that Qi gong may be an effective alternative for heroin detoxification without side effects.[49] Though research in other areas of addiction has not included the use of Qi gong, the results of Li and co-workers study surely warrants evaluation in other addictive groups.

OVERALL MIND-BODY FITNESS AND WELL-BEING

Mind-body fitness therefore is associated with integration and balance in muscular strength, flexibility, balance, coordination, and perhaps most importantly from a *health promotion* viewpoint, improved mental development and self-efficacy. Qi gong combines mindfulness with physical activity and generates a temporary self-state or inwardly focused contemplative state: *mindful exercise.* It incorporates a focus on the present moment, in contrast to conventional exercise performance that emphasizes fat burning, body sculpting, or heart rate elevation.

In addition, research has found a significant participant recidivism.[50] In other words, because an individual enjoys the exercise form, he or she is more likely to stick with it. Qi gong teaches the patient/participant to be mindful of the intrinsic energy from which he or she may ultimately perceive greater self-control and empowerment by becoming intentionally aware of breathing and specific proprioceptive sensations while performing gentle, fluid movements. It is an *authentic mastery experience*—self-mastery is the hallmark of mind-body fitness conditioning.

Thoughts, perceptions, attitudes, and proprioceptive awareness affect bodily functions. Body-mind functions and kinesthetic sensations evoke changes in perception, attitude, or behavior. There is a strong basis in neuroscience for this. Neurons, neurotransmitters, and associated receptor proteins are activated. Some 80+ billion neurons exist in the adult human brain. Each receives input from 5 to 40,000 other neuronal axons. The perception of self or an environmental event (eg, exercise, anger, joy) is directly related to the number of neurons, neurotransmitters, and associated receptor proteins that are activated.

This slow controlled movement involves the limbic system (thalamus, hypothalamus, hippocampus). The electrochemical information from active neuronal circuits is ultimately transduced by the various structures of the limbic system into the hormones of behavior.[51-53] Much of this transduction is accomplished by the putative hypothalamic-pituitary-adrenal (HPA) axis. There is a reduction in catecholamine and glucocorticoid production. This axis can be viewed as one neuroendocrine pathway for mind-body interventions that focuses on reducing stress-related catecholamine and glucocorticoid production. One principle in molecular biology is that the synthesis and function of neuro-active substances are dictated by a range of genetic and environmental influences. Mind-body therapies such as hypnosis, T'ai Chi, Qi gong, and meditation alter the neurophysiology of this process by increasing parasympathetic tone.

The theoretical difference in mechanisms responsible for exercise-associated affective states comparing conventional vs mindful exercise:

+ The "endorphin high" is a consequence of aerobic exercise: endorphins are a class of endogenous neuro-active substances with morphine-like actions

+ Considerable evidence shows that to elicit an endorphin-mediated response, one must stress the musculoskeletal system to some critical duration of exercise intensity threshold

+ Alternatively, evidence shows that much of the reduction in tension with aerobic exercise is somatic (eg, muscular) whereas meditative activity instills more of a central relaxation response

Meditative states have long been associated with changes in EEG activity.[54-56] Analysis of the EEG activity indicates that the meditative state is a unique state of consciousness and separate from wakefulness, drowsiness, or sleep.[54] There appears to be a significant difference between EEG activity during meditative states of Qi gong compared with rest states with eyes closed. Zhang and associates[54] found a clear difference in EEG waves during the Qi gong state compared to the resting state. The EEG alpha activity during the Qi gong state occurs predominantly in the anterior regions. The peak frequency of EEG alpha rhythm is slower than the resting state during Qi gong and the change of EEG during Qi gong between anterior and posterior half is negatively correlated.[55,56] Changes of EEGs of Qi gong masters during the Qi gong state were different from those recorded during the resting state with closed eyes.[56]

Table 17-2

COMPARATIVE PHYSIOLOGIC RESPONSES TO ACUTE MEDITATIVE ACTIVITY AND AEROBIC EXERCISE

	MEDITATION	MUSCULAR EXERCISE (70% TO 80% VO$_2$MAX)
Neurobiological	Increased alpha EEG activity Right hemisphere activation Decreased SNS arousal Decreased HPA activation	Decreased alpha EEG activity Left hemisphere activation Increased SNS arousal Increased HPA activation
Cardiorespiratory	Decreased heart rate and BP Increased HRV Decreased VO$_2$	Increased heart rate, BP, and Q Decreased HRV Increased VO$_2$
Metabolic	Neutral RQ (eg, 0.85) Decreased blood lactate	Increased RQ (CHO) Increased blood lactate
Musculoskeletal	Relaxation Decreased EMG activity	Contraction Increased EMG activity
Endocrine	Decreased EPI, cortisol Decreased serum GH, TSH Decreased serum prolactin Decreased ACTH Decreased beta-endorphin	Increased EPI, cortisol Increased serum GH, TSH Increased serum prolactin Increased ACTH Increased beta-endorphin
Cognitive	Decreased arousal	Increased arousal

SNS=sympathetic nervous system; HPA=hypothalamic-pituitary-adrenal; BP=blood pressure; Q=cardiac output; HRV=heart rate variability; VO$_2$=oxygen consumption; RQ=respiratory quotient, ratio of carbohydrate (CHO) to fat oxidation; EMG=electromyographic activity, muscular tension EPI=epinephrine; GH=growth hormone; TSH=thyroid stimulating hormone; ACTH=adrenocorticotrophic hormone

Liu and colleagues[52,53] found that Qi gong training caused an enhancement of brainstem auditory evoked response with a concomitant depression of cortical (stress) responses. These observations may be related to healing and other health benefits of Qi gong.

In order to generate the greatest potential for affective beneficence, some combination of muscular exercise and mindful activity should be incorporated into the individual's exercise program. The response to mind-body exercise hypothetically falls in a range between meditation and vigorous aerobic exercise. Activity with a meditative component is less prone to activating the HPA axis and associated increases in tension and anxiety.

Table 17-2 presents a summary of the comparative physiological responses to acute meditative activity and aerobic exercise assimilated through this author's study of mind-body exercise.

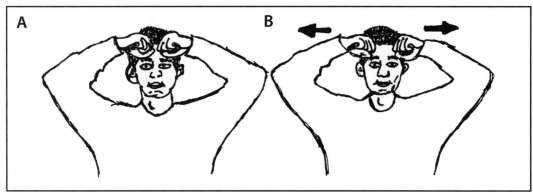

Figure 17-2. Rubbing the forehead. Place both fists in the center of your forehead with the knuckles together (A), then gently side the fist across the forehead towards the temple in a smoothing action (B).

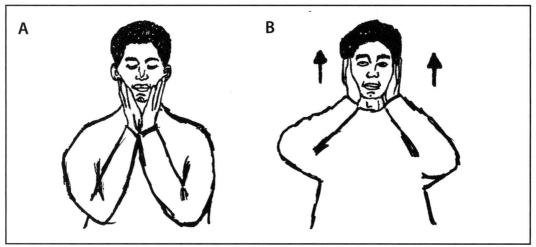

Figure 17-3. Stroking the sides of the face upward. Place the hands on the side of the face, palms inward, with the finger tips just below the ear (A). Stroke the face with the hands in an upward motion (B).

Techniques Used in Qi Gong

SELF-MASSAGE

This method of exercise is said to calm the mind and stimulate the internal organs. Self-massage is a "wake-up" exercise practiced before Qi gong postures, movement, and meditation. People have always instinctively rubbed or massaged sore muscles and other painful areas to ease their pain and to help the sore muscles recover more quickly. The therapeutic effects of massage are known worldwide. The Japanese have used acupressure-based massage, which is derived from Chinese massage, for centuries. The Greek have used a form of massage—slapping the skin—to treat various disorders. The Qi gong system of self-massage fully systemizes massage to harmonize with the theory of Qi circulation. Primarily, self-massage in Qi gong follows the pathways of the channels and meridians.

Figures 17-2 through 17-12 demonstrate the methods of self-massage use to calm the mind and stimulate the internal organs. Self-massage has been said to benefit many chronic problems including insomnia, anxiety, stomach and intestinal problems, cardiac diseases, pulmonary disorders, and high blood pressure.

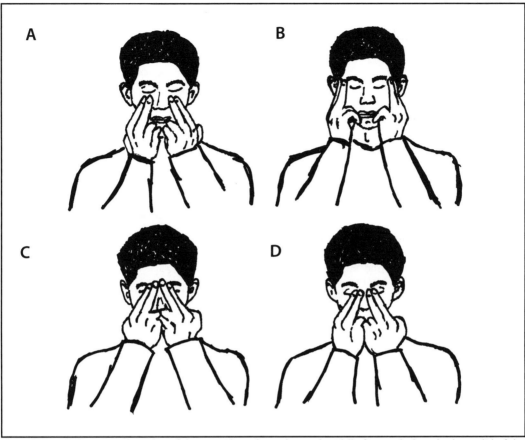

Figure 17-4. Massaging the orbit of the eye. Place the index and middle fingers below the lower lid of the eye, starting in the inner corner (A). Gently rub the eyes in a circular direction moving to the outside (B), over the eyes, under the eyebrows (C), down on the inside of the orbit completing the circle (D). Repeat three times.

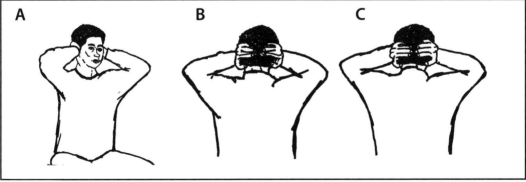

Figure 17-5. Sounding the drum. Place the palm of the hands over the ears, covering the area just over the most forward area of the ears (laogong point) with the fingers behind the head (A). Place the index finger across the middle finger (B), then slide the index finger off and back alongside into its natural position (C). Repeat six times.

Figure 17-6. Opening the sinus. Make a fist, then using both hands, place the first joint of the thumb on the bridge of the nose (A), then gently draw both fists away in a smooth action across each check (B).

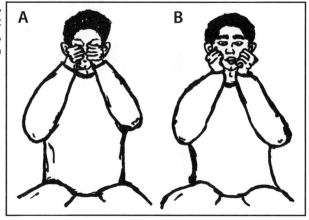

Figure 17-7. Washing the mouth with Qi. Purse the lips and draw in air. Hold the air at the back of the mouth (A) and then push to the front of the mouth, without exhaling (B). Swallow the saliva and exhale. Repeat 10 times.

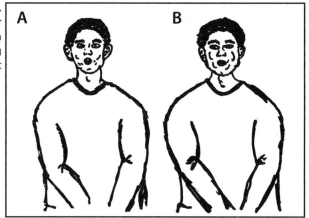

MOVEMENT AND POSTURES

Movement and postures are major components of Qi gong exercise. The theory of combining postures and movement is based on the principle of Yin and Yang. Passive and active. Still and moving. In the postures, specific muscle groups are stressed, but they are not tensed. For example, in one posture the arms are extended in front of the body as if they were hugging a tree (see Figure 17-15). This position is held and what is experienced is that the nerves, muscles, and circulation in the areas of the shoulder and arm become "excited." The muscles holding the posture might fatigue and fasciculate, and there may be a sense of warmth or tingling in the areas of the arms, shoulders, and trunk that are being challenged. This is considered to be the generation of Qi or energy. When the arms are relaxed and dropped, the kinetic Qi seems to flow into the areas of lower potential much like an electric battery circulates electricity when a circuit is made. These postures not only improve strength and flexibility, but have been shown to significantly improve endurance and aerobic capacity. Figures 17-13 through 17-16 are examples of static meditative Qi gong postures.

With practice of the individual standing postures, there is typically a progression to sequencing of mixed standing postures. These are invigorating and more physically demanding. Due to the length of this chapter, these postures will not be dealt with here. The reader is referred to the list of additional reading materials for instructional materials on these postures. Mixing standing postures is a means of focusing the energy in each of the 12 channels (meridians).

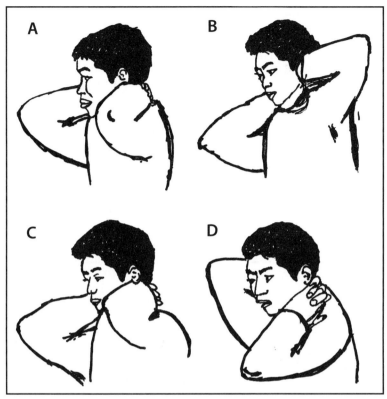

Figure 17-8. Rolling the arms while stroking the neck. Place the hands on the back of the neck, interlocking the fingers (A). Slide the hands from side (B), back to the center (C) and to the opposite side (8C). Repeat 10 times.

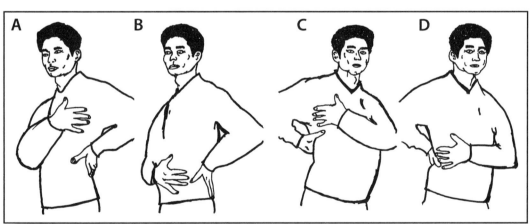

Figure 17-9. Releasing chest pressure. Place the right hand on the left side of the chest, at the same time taking the left hand behind and placing it on the back (A). Move the hands in a downward stroke finishing at the waist (B). Breathe out slowly when the hands reach the finishing point. Repeat this on the right (C & D). Do this three times alternating sides.

In moving, the mind concentrates on the breath and at the same time imagines guiding energy to a specific area. With concentration on the movement, the control of Qi is more efficient and the muscles can exert maximal power. Emphasis during movement is placed on a calm, relaxed, and natural movement pattern. Strongly tensed muscles are felt to narrow the Qi channels. Repeated movements away from the center of the body and then back in a slow and controlled fashion have been shown to build strength and flexibility. More importantly, because movement always challenges the center of gravity, awareness of kinesthetic and proprioceptive stimuli become acute.

Figure 17-10. Stroking the dantien in a circular motion. Place the right hand under the left hand, placing them on the dantien, 2 inches below the navel. Rotate the hands in small circles going from right to left, gradually making the circles larger, before decreasing to small again. Repeat 10 times.

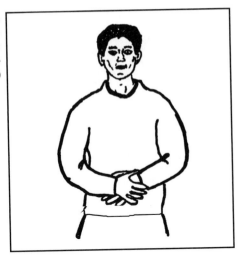

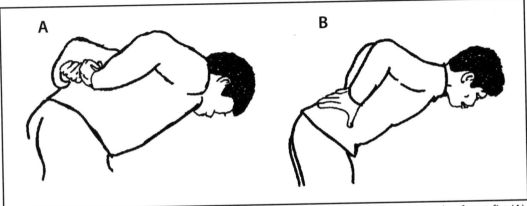

Figure 17-11. Kidney rub. Standing up, lean forward and rub the low back with the inside of your fist (A). Alternate this with a downward stroking motion (B). Repeat 10 times.

Figure 17-12. Circling the knees. Standing up, lean forward with your hands on your knees, and the knees bent slightly (A). Open and close the knees in an outward circling motion, then an inward circling motion (B). Repeat 10 times in each direction.

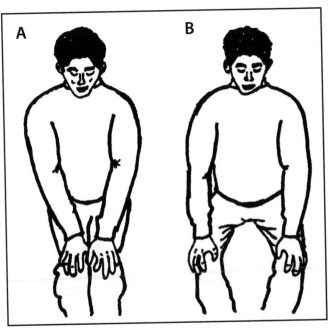

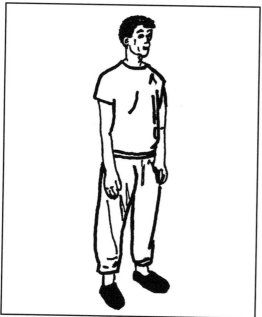

Figure 17-13. Simple standing posture. Stand upright naturally, raising the crown of the head. Close the mouth, relax the shoulders, concentrate on the dantien (2 inches below the navel), half close your eyes to avoid visual distractions.

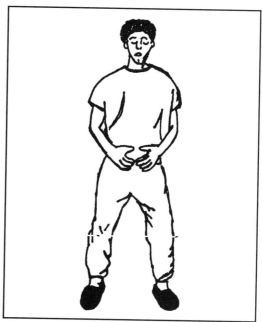

Figure 17-14. Holding the Qi in the dantien. Stand, slightly bending the legs, hold both hands as shown in front of the dantien. Keep the mind on the dantien and while keeping the shoulders and chest relaxed let your stomach move out when you breathe.

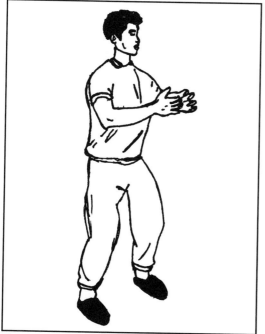

Figure 17-15. Hugging the tree. Stand erect, with shoulders relaxed and legs slightly bent, creating a circle in front of the body with your arms. This posture is one of the oldest Qi gong methods of practice handed down known for strengthening all systems.

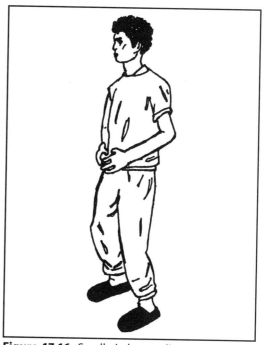

Figure 17-16. Small circle standing position. Half closing the eyes without focusing, bend your knees and concentrate on the dantien. Relax the shoulders and the back and hold the hands over the dantien region without touching the abdominal area.

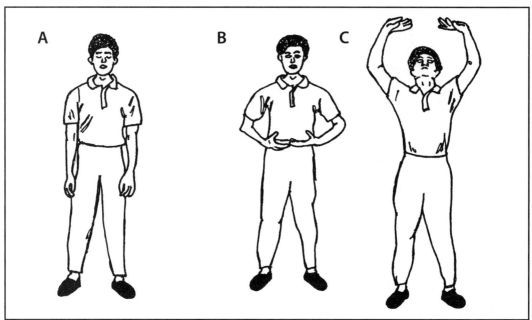

Figure 17-17. Supporting the sky with two hands. Stand in a relaxed position with feet under hips (A). Look straight ahead and breath through nose. Relax all joints and meditate for a few moments to gain concentration. Slowly raise arms in a circle in front of your body while inhaling (B), turn palms over and stretch up as though holding up the sky. At the same time lift heels off ground (C). Exhale while lowering arms and heels returning to the starting position. Health benefits: relaxes the muscles and stretches the arms, legs, and torso. Accompanied by deep breathing, it affects the chest, abdomen, and pelvis. It helps correct poor posture.

There are many exercise routines practiced by Qi gong practitioners. A popular routine is called the *Eight Pieces of Brocade* (or *Silk*). There are several varieties and distinct styles of this exercise form, all of them effective. The name comes from brocade or silk cloth which was originally used when doing the exercises. Today, the exercises are typically done without pieces of silk. Figures 17-17 through 17-24 depict a commonly used exercise routine.

BREATHING

Breathing techniques are employed with postures and movement. During postures it is believed that Qi can be accumulated with breathing and concentration (meditation), and that it is possible to guide the flow or circulation of Qi by directing the breath. Movement patterns also lend well to facilitating breathing techniques and directing the flow of energy. When the movement opens up an area, such as in the arm movement away from the chest, inspiration accompanies the motion. Deep breathing can be directed toward the fingertips and the breath held momentarily at the completion of the movement. Upon return to the resting posture, exhalation relaxes the individual back to the starting position. Self-massage also utilizes breathing during massage techniques. Meditatively, awareness of the areas being massaged and directing the Qi (the breath) to that area further enhances the beneficial effects on circulation, oxygenation, and the flow of energy.

MEDITATION

The key to successful practice of Qi gong exercises is concentration on the area being moved or postured and concentration on the breath as described above. This is meditation. Meditation is defined as close or continued thought, serious contemplation, or mental reflection. The concen-

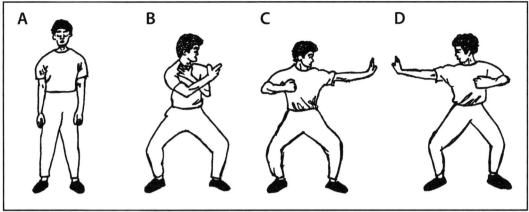

Figure 17-18. Drawing the bow to the left and right. (A) Stand in a relaxed position. (B) Step to left and bend knees to assume a horse-riding position. Cross arms in front of chest, right arm outside, left arm inside. Then with thumb and forefinger of left hand extended and other three fingers curled, stretch left arm out to left, eyes following, breathing in. (C) At the same time clench right hand and stretch to right as though pulling a bow. Return to preparation position while exhaling. (D) Repeat to opposite direction. Health benefits: movement concentrates on the chest, shoulder and arm muscles; provides weight shifting; helps circulation.

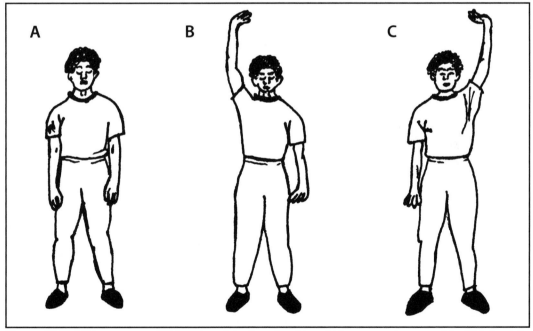

Figure 17-19. Lifting one arm. (A) Stand straight, feet shoulder width apart and arms at side. (B) Raise right arm over head, palm up, fingers together and pointing to left; at the same time press left hand down, palm down, fingers together and pointing straight ahead. Breath in while doing this. Return to preparation position while exhaling. (C) Repeat to opposite side. Health benefits: stretches arms and trunk; affects liver, gall bladder, spleen and stomach; strengthens the digestive system.

tration on movements and sensations of the Qi gong movements focuses the mind on movement patterns and postures. This moving meditation is of great importance in gaining the full benefits of this exercise form.

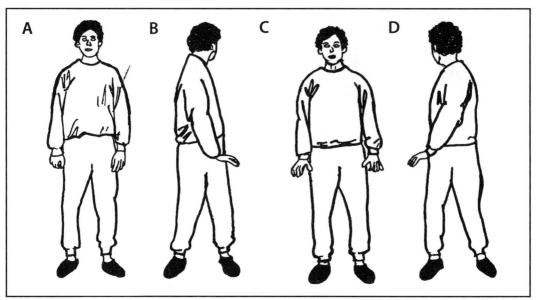

Figure 17-20. Looking backward. (A) Stand straight with palms lightly touching thighs, extend wrist with palms down and fingers forward. (B) Turn head to left slowly while inhaling and looking over your shoulder (keeping pelvis forward). (C) Return to starting position while exhaling. (D) Turn head to right slowly while inhaling and leading movement with eyes looking backward. Return to preparation position while exhaling. Health benefits: involves turning the head, rolling the eyeballs, challenging balance, and stretching trunk; strengthens neck and trunk muscles; revitalizes the nervous system.

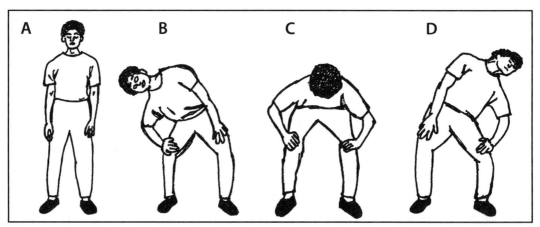

Figure 17-21. Killing heart fire by rotating head and body. (A) Stand straight with arms at side, bend knees to assume a horse-riding position with legs wide apart, placing hands on thighs with thumbs pointing outward. (B) Bend forward from waist and rotate body toward left while inhaling; at the same time sway buttocks toward right. (C) Return to start position while exhaling. (D) Repeat in opposite direction. Health benefits: this movement involves using the whole body and is excellent for relaxation.

THREE PRIMARY METHODS OF QI GONG

Of interest are the different forms and applications of the techniques described above. There are three primary philosophies in the practice of Qi gong. The Taoist philosophy strives for the balance between Yin and Yang, and so Qi gong methods include postures and movements in addition to breathing and meditation. The Buddhist philosophy of Qi gong is primarily one on Yin. They seek calm through maintaining postures and incorporating the components of respira-

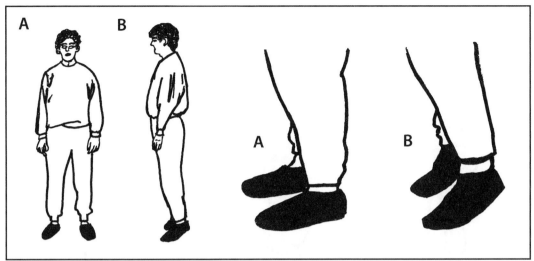

Figure 17-22. Raising the heels seven times. (A) Stand naturally with your feet shoulder width apart. (B) Keeping both legs straight, raise heels off the floor while inhaling. While exhaling let go and lower heels to the ground. Do this seven times in succession in time with your breathing. Health benefits: beneficial for the spine, posture, circulation, and the internal organs.

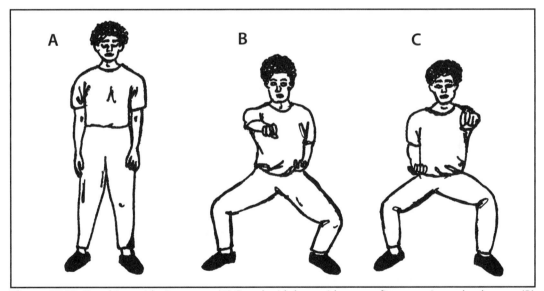

Figure 17-23. Punching with tiger eyes. (A) Stand with legs wide apart, fists at waist and palms up. (B) Bend knees to assume a horse-riding position. Inhale. With palms turning down and glaring eyes following movement, stretch right fist slowly forward as in a punching movement while exhaling. Return to starting position while inhaling. (C) Repeat on left. Health benefits: the emphasis here is on glaring eyes; exercise with eyes following thrusting fist helps concentration; movement builds up energy and strength.

tion and meditation. Moving meditation is primarily the philosophy used in medical or martial arts. This philosophy incorporates Yang and directed toward dynamic movement such as that experienced in T'ai Chi. Though this latter philosophy is more commonly practiced by health practitioners, this author is finding that the combination of movement and postures is substantially more efficacious from a clinical perspective when working with an older adult population. This is certainly an area that should lead to some significant research projects in the future.

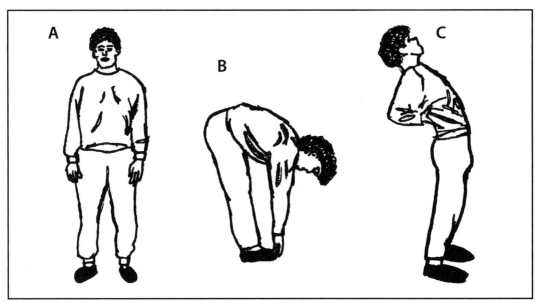

Figure 17-24. Holding the feet with two hands. (A) Stand in a relaxed position. (B) Keeping knees straight and head slightly raised, bend forward slowly and hold toes or ankles while exhaling. (C) Return to starting position and with hands holding back at waist level bend slowing backwards while inhaling. Repeat. Health benefits: good for kidneys and other internal organs; challenges balance and vestibular system; stretches and strengthens trunk muscles which in turn affects internal organs.

Conclusion

There is so much to Qi gong that it is impossible to cover all of the theory and training in a short chapter. It is recommended that if the clinician is interested in studying and acquiring skills in Qi gong that one seeks out a Qi gong master. A Qi gong teacher will instruct you in the form, however, serious study of this movement form requires the understanding of the philosophy behind the movements and principles underlying the application of each movement, posture, breathing technique, self-massaging technique, and the very important component of meditation. There are also numerous videotapes that are available to guide you in this exercise form for the therapeutic use of this movement modality with your older patients.

It is well known that Qi gong practice is beneficial to human health,[57] but it is less know that Qi gong may also be effective therapy to treat many otherwise "untreatable" conditions. The use of Qi gong has been identified by the National Institutes of Health as one of a list of alternative therapies that has been targeted for research funding. The increasing body of research related to the use of Qi gong as a valuable therapeutic intervention substantiates our need as professionals to evaluate the merits of this exercise form.

References

1. McCaffrey R, Fowler NL. Qi gong practice: a pathway to health and healing. *Holist Nurs Pract.* 2003;17(2):110-116.
2. Hankey A, McCrum S. Qi gong: life energy and a new science of life. *J Altern Complement Med.* 2006;12(9):841-842.
3. Sancier KM, Holman D. Commentary: multifaceted health benefits of medical Qi gong. *J Altern Complement Med.* 2004;10(1):163-165.
4. Witt C, Becker M, Bandelin K, Soellner R, Willich SN. Qi gong for school children: a pilot study. *J Altern Complement Med.* 2005;11(1):41-47.

5. Wagner B. Chinese meditation pattern. Qi gong: to learn from tigers and bears. Series: relaxation techniques 1. Centers of vital energy. *Forschr Med.* 1999;117(8):55-57.

6. Jouper J, Hassmen P, Johansson M. Qi gong exercise with concentration predicts increased health. *Am J Chin Med.* 2006;34(6):949-957.

7. Tang KC. Qi gong therapy—its effectiveness and regulation. *Am J Chin Med.* 1994;22(3-4):235-242.

8. Fukushima M, Kataoka T, Hamada C, Matsumoto M. Evidence of Qi-gong energy and its biological effect on the enhancement of the phagocytic activity of human polymorphonuclear leukocytes. *Am J Chin Med.* 2001;29(1):1-16.

9. Lee MS, Kim MK, Ryu H. Qi-training (Qi gong) enhanced immune functions: what is the underlying mechanism? *Int J Neurosci.* 2005;115(8):1099-1104.

10. Xu M, Tomotake M, Ikuta T, Ishimoto Y, Okura M. The effect of Qi-gong and acupuncture on human cerebral evoked potentials and electroencephalogram. *J Med Invest.* 1998;44(3-4):163-171.

11. Omura Y, Lin TL, Debreceni L, et al. Unique changes found on the Qi gong (Chi Gong) master's and patient's body during Qi gong treatment; their relationships to certain meridians and acupuncture points and the re-creation of therapeutic Qi gong states by children and adults. *Acupunct Electrother Res.* 1989;14(1):61-89.

12. Omura Y. Connections found between each meridian & organ area of corresponding internal organs in each side of the cerebral cortex; release of common neurotransmitters and hormones unique to each meridian and correspond-ing acupuncture point and internal organ after acupuncture, electrical stimulation, mechanical stimulation (includ-ing shiatsu), soft laser stimulation or Qi gong. *Acupunct Electrother Res.* 1989;14(2):155-186.

13. Jin P. Efficacy of T'ai Chi, brisk walking, meditation, and reading in reducing mental and emotional stress. *J Psychosom Res.* 1992;36(4):361-370.

14. Jin P. Changes in heart rate, noradrenaline, cortisol and mood during T'ai Chi. *J Psychosom Res.* 1989;33:197-206.

15. Sun XS, Xu Y, Xia YJ. Determination of E-rosette-forming lymphocytes in aged subjects with Tai Chiquan exercise. *Int J Sports Med.* **1989;10:217-219.**

16. Lee MS, Kang CW, Ryu H, Kim JD, Chung HT. Effects of ChunDoSunBup Qi-training on growth hormone, insu-lin-like growth factor-I, and testosterone in young and elderly subjects. *Am J Chin Med.* 1999;27(2):167-175.

17. Lee MS, Kang CW Shin YS, et al. Acute effects of chundosunbup Qi gong Qi-training on blood concentrations of TSH, calcitonin, PTH and thyroid hormones in elderly subjects. *Am J Chin Med.* 1998;26(3-4):275-281.

18. Lee MS, Yang SH, Lee KK, Moon SR. Qi gong's therapeutic effects in managing pain in cancer patients. *Eur J Cancer Care.* 2005;14(5):457-462.

19. Quah TC. Alternative and complementary cancer treatments. *Oncologist.* 1996;1(5):324-325.

20. Yan X, Shen H, Jiang H, et al. External Qi of Yan Xin Qi gong differentially regulates the AKT and extracellular signal-regulated kinase pathways and is cyotoxic to cancer cells but not to normal celss. *Int J Biochem Cell Biol.* 2006; 38(12):2102-2113.

21. Yeh ML, Lee TI, Chen HH, Chao TY. The influence of Chan-Chuang Qi-Gong therapy on complete blood cell counts in breast cancer patients treated with chemotherapy. *Cancer Nurs.* 2006;29(2):149-157.

22. Manzaneque JM, Vera FM, Maldonado EF, et al. Assessment of immunological parameters following a Qi gong training program. *Med Sci Monit.* 2004;10(6):CR264-270.

23. Lai JS, Lan C, Wong MK, Teng SH. Two-year trends in cardiorespiratory function among older T'ai Chi Chuan practitioners and sedentary subjects. *J Am Geriatr Soc.* 1995;43(11):1222-1227.

24. Lee MS, Kim MK, Lee YH. Effects of Qi-therapy (external Qi gong) on cardiac autonomic tone: a randomized placebo controlled study. *Int J Neurosci.* 2005;115(9):1345-1350.

25. Zhuo D, Shephard RJ, Plyley MJ, Davis GM. Cardiorespiratory and metabolic responses during T'ai Chi Chuan exercise. *Can J Appl Sport Sci.* 1984;9(1):7-10.

26. Schneider D, Leung R. Metabolic and cardiorespiratory responses to the performance of Wing Chun and T'ai Chi Chuan exercise. *Int J Sports Med.* 1991;12(3):319-313.

27. Lai JS, Wong MK, Lan C, Chong CK, Lien IN. Cardiorespiratory responses of T'ai Chi Chaun practitioners and sedentary subjects during cycle ergometer. *Journal of the Formosan Medical Association.* 1993;92(10):894-899.

28. Ng RK. Cardiopulmonary exercise: a recently discovered secret of T'ai Chi. *Hawaii Medical Journal.* 1992;51(8): 216-217.

29. Lee MS, Lim HJ, Lee MS. Impact of Qi gong exercise on self-efficacy and other cognitive perceptual variables in patients with essential hypertension. *J Altern Complement Med.* 2004;10(4):675-680.

30. Lee MS, Kim BG, Huh HJ, Ryu H, Lee HS, Chung HT. Effect of Qi-training on blood pressure, heart rate and respiration rate. *Clin Physiol.* 2000;20(3):173-176.

31. Hui PN, Wan M, Chan WK, Yung PM. An evaluation of tow behavioral rehabilitation programs, qiqong versus progression relaxation, in improving the quality of life in cardiac patients. *J Altern Complement Med.* 2006;12(4):373-378.

32. Nui PN, Wan M, Chan WK, Yung PMB. An evaluation of two behavioral rehabilitation programs, Qi gong versus progressive relaxation, in improving the quality of life in cardiac patients. *J Altern Complemtary Med.* 2006;12(4):373-378.

33. Stenlund T, Lindstrom B, Granlund, Burell G. Cardiac rehabilitation for the elderly: Qi gong and group discussions. *Europeon Soc Cardiology.* 2005;12(1):5-11.

34. Cheung BM, Lo JL, Fong DY, et al. Randomised controlled trial of Qi gong in the treatment of mild essential hypertension. *J Hum Hypertens.* 2005;19(9):697-704.

35. Tsujiuchi T, Kumano H, Yoshiuchi K, et al. The effect of Qi-gong relaxation exercise on the control of type 2 diabetes mellitus: a randomized controlled trial. *Diabetes Care.* 2002;25(1):241-242.

36. Bottomley JM: The use of T'ai Chi as a movement modality in orthopedics. *Orthop Phys Ther Clin N Am.* 2000; 9(3):361-373.

37. Omura Y. Storing of Qi gong energy in various materials and drugs (Qi gongnization): its clinical application for treatment of pain, circulatory disturbance, bacterial or viral infections, heavy metal deposits, and related intractable medical problems by selectively enhancing circulation and drug uptake. *Acupunct Electrother Res.* 1990;15(2):137-157.

38. Tse SK, Bailey DM. T'ai Chi and postural control in the well elderly. *Am J Occup Ther.* 1992;46(4):295-300.

39. Wolfson L, Whipple R, Derby C, et al. Balance and strength training in older adults: intervention gains and T'ai Chi maintenance. *J Am Geriatric Soc.* 1996;44:498-506.

40. Wolf SL, Barnhart HX, Kutner NG, et al. Reducing frailty and falls in older persons: an investigation of T'ai Chi and computerized balance training. *J Am Geriatric Soc.* 1996;44:599-600.

41. Kirsteins AE, Dietz F, Hwang SM. Evaluating the safety and potential use of a weight-bearing exercise, Tai-Chi Chuan, for rheumatoid arthritis patients. *Am J Phys Med Rehabil.* 1991;70(3):136-141.

42. Wu WH, Bandilla E, Ciccone DS, et al. Effects of Qi gong on late-stage complex regional pain syndrome. *Altern Ther Health Med.* 1999;5(1):45-54.

43. Yang KH, Kim YH, Lee MS. Efficacy of Qi-therapy (external Qi gong) for elderly people with chronic pain. *Int J Neurosci.* 2005;115(7):949-963.

44. Astin JA, Berman BM, Bausell B, Lee WL, Hochberg M, Forys KL. The efficacy of mindfulness meditation plus Qi gong movement therapy in the treatment of fibromyalgia. *J Rheumatol.* 2003;30(10):2257-2262.

45. Schmitz-Hubsch T, Pyfer D, Kielwein K, et al. Qi gong exercise for the symptoms of Parkinson's disease: a randomized, controlled pilot study. *Mov Disord.* 2006;21(4):543-548.

46. Xu SH. Psychophysiological reactions associated with Qi gong therapy. *Chin Med J.* 1994;107(3):230-233.

47. Tsung HW, Fung KM, Chan AS, Lee G, Chan F. Effect of a Qi gong exercise programme on elderly with depression. *Int J Geriatr Psychiatry.* 2006;21(9):890-897.

48. Kjos V, Etnier JL. Pilot study comparing physical and psychological responses in medical Qi gong and walking. *J Aging Phys Act.* 2006;14(3):241-251.

49. Li M, Chen K, Mo Z. Use of Qi gong in the detoxification of heroin addicts. *Altern Ther Health Med.* 2002;8(1):50-54, 56-59.

50. Levine DM. Behavioral and psychosocial factors, processes, and strategies. In: Pearson T, Criqui MH, Luepker RV, Overman A, Winston M, eds. *Primer in Preventive Cardiology.* Dallas, TX: American Heart Association; 1994.

51. Bloom FE, Lazerson A. *Brain, Mind, and Behavior.* 2nd ed. New York, NY: WH Freeman & Co; 1988.

52. Liu GL. Changes in brainstem and cortical auditory potentials during Qi-Gong meditation. *Am J Chin Med.* 1990; 18(1):5-11.

53. Liu GL, Cui RQ, Li GZ, Huang CM. Changes in brainstem and cortical auditory potentials during Qi gong meditation. *Am J Chin Med.* 1990;18(3-4):95-103.

54. Zhang JZ, Zhoa J, He QN. EEG findings during special physical state (Qi gong state) by means of compressed spectral array and topographic mapping. *Comput Biol Med.* 1988; 18(6):455-463.

55. He QN, Zhang JZ, Li JZ. The effects of long-term Qi gong exercise on brain function as manifested by computer analysis. *J Tradit Chin Med.* 1988;8(3):177-182.

56. Zhang JZ, Li JZ, He QN. Statistical brain topographic mapping analysis for EEGs recorded during Qi gong states. *Int J Neurosci.* 1988;38(3-4):415-425.

57. Chen KW, Turner FD. A case study of simultaneous recovery from multiple physical symptoms with medical Qi gong therapy. *J Altern Complement Med.* 2004;10(1):159-162.

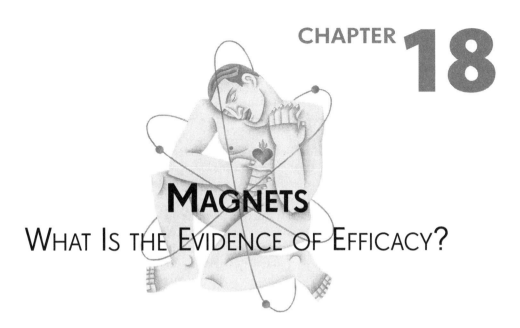

CHAPTER 18

MAGNETS
WHAT IS THE EVIDENCE OF EFFICACY?

Neil I. Spielholz, PT, PhD, FAPTA

Introduction

I am a skeptic. The reason for being so can be summed up in one word: experience. In the 47 years since I graduated from physical therapy school at Columbia University, and the 30 years since obtaining my PhD from the Department of Physiology and Biophysics at New York University Medical Center, I have witnessed the comings and goings of so many fads—the hopping on and off of so many bandwagons—that I view with a jaundiced eye reports of "cases that got better" with such-and-such a treatment.

Indeed, I even had such an experience shortly after graduating from physical therapy school. I was working at the Veterans Affairs Hospital in Manhattan and was assigned a patient who had a stroke 3 to 4 months prior to being transferred. When I first saw him, he was still fairly flaccid on the right side of his body. As part of a muscle re-education protocol, the referring physiatrist requested electrical stimulation of the patient's involved wrist extensors and ankle dorsiflexors. During the first week, I tetanized the target muscles, and the patient was delighted to see the "paralyzed" muscles contracting so strongly. I instructed him to try to contract the muscles himself as I applied the stimulation. By the end of the first week, he had regained all use of his right side. You could not tell he ever had a problem. He walked out of the hospital, blessing all of us (and me in particular) for working "miracles." After all, his first doctor had told him he would be paralyzed for the rest of his life!

For the next 2 years, every patient with hemiplegia who was treated by us had electrical stimulation as part of their treatment program. Guess what? None ever made a similar recovery. We could have written up our successful case and attempted to make a big deal out of it, but our further experience prohibited that. (This reminds me of the research warning, "If the experiment succeeds the first time, don't repeat it.") Why the patient made that remarkable recovery is unknown, but the "treatment" was certainly not generalizable.

This was when my skepticism began. I do not want to hear only about the patients who got better, also tell me about those who did not. Do not just tell me "they got better," tell me what

305

the outcome measures were. Do not just tell me *that* you "treated" them, tell me *how* you treated them. Tell me also about your controls, and how you reduced the chance of bias. In other words, convince me that your results are meaningful and can probably be attributed to your unique treatment. By the way, these are good questions to ask anyone who is trying to convince you that a particular treatment is effective. Maybe they are correct, but only time (and appropriate research) will tell the story. Do not be taken in by glitz and hype masquerading behind pseudoscience (some examples will be given later). On the other hand, be prepared to accept a change if it can be shown effective. There is a fine line between being gullible (and falling for anything) and being pig-headed (by refusing to accept anything that is "new"). Keep an open, but critical, mind.

This chapter attempts to compare and contrast unsubstantiated claims of efficacy with studies that have either supported or denied such claims. It attempts to point out when a report simply makes a claim, and when a report satisfies the criteria necessary to being considered credible. As the reader will see, however, the final chapter on whether static magnetic fields are beneficial or not is yet to be written (it is surely not this one!), so let's begin.

The idea that magnetic fields may influence certain functions of the body is neither surprising nor new. However, whether these "influences" have any beneficial (or detrimental) effects is another issue. This chapter reviews first how magnetic fields (both changing and static) may interact with physiology, then reviews claims for benefit of exposure to static (or unchanging) fields.

Electricity and Magnetism

Although it is now recognized that electrical phenomena and magnetism are intimately associated, this realization was not always the case. In fact, the two were considered distinctly different "forces" until a public demonstration in 1820 by the Danish physics professor Hans Christian Oersted. Professor Oersted found that a compass needle placed parallel to a wire shifted its north-south orientation somewhat when a direct current (DC) flowed through the wire. Reversing the flow of current caused the compass needle to deflect in the opposite direction. This simple observation indicated that the current flowing in the wire generated a magnetic field around itself and set the stage for other investigations (especially by Andre-Marie Ampere and Michael Faraday), ultimately leading to the recognition of *electromagnetism*. For an in-depth account of the events and people involved in this area over the centuries, Gerrit L. Verschuur's book, *Hidden Attraction: The Mystery and History of Magnetism,*[1] is recommended.

Basically, electromagnetism describes the reciprocal relationship between flow of current (electricity) and a surrounding magnetic field. Current flowing in a conductor generates a circular magnetic field around the conductor, and the direction of the field depends upon the direction of current flow (the so-called "right hand rule"). Conversely, if a conductor in which no current is flowing is exposed to a magnetic field that is *changing* in intensity (ie, one whose strength is time-varying), current is induced to flow in the conductor. Recall that in electricity, current is the flow of electrons (or charge) in one direction or the other.

The physiological implications of the above for are obvious. Since many biological functions are based on bioelectrical phenomena (such as demonstrated by the electroencephalogram [EEG], electrocardiogram [EKG], electromyogram [EMG], and others), the flow of these currents in the body must generate magnetic fields; conversely, subjecting the body to a *fluctuating* magnetic field must induce currents to flow within the body. But even static magnetic fields (ie, those that are not changing in intensity) can have effects by either attracting, repelling, or rotating molecules and/or atoms that are "polarized."

From this, it is certainly logical to anticipate that the application of electromagnetic fields to the body should be associated with some type of effects. Indeed, such is the case. Just a few examples include:

1. *Diathermy* (long wave, short wave, and microwave) for heating of deep tissues (very popular when the author was a student) and for electrocautery. The devices used for these purposes deliver electromagnetic radiation at frequencies greater than 1 million times a second (ie, >1 MHz) by means of high-frequency tuned circuitry. This radiation penetrates the body and induces currents to flow in conductors (tissues containing large amounts of electrolytes). This current flow, in turn, is converted into heat, as described by Joule's Law:

   J=I²Rt, where J=joules measured in calories, I=the current flowing in the conductor (note that this value is squared), R=the resistance of the conductor in Ohms, and t=time the current is flowing, in seconds.

2. *Magnetic resonance imaging* (MRI) for the visualization of tissues and structures within the body. The devices used for these purposes employ so-called superconducting magnets that deliver electromagnetic radiation in the radio frequency range. The magnetic field strengths delivered are of 1.5 Teslas (T) (terminology for measuring field strengths will be described later). MRI is based on the absorption and emission of energy by hydrogen atoms that are exposed to these high-frequency magnetic fields.

3. *Transcranial magnetic stimulation* (TMS) of the brain, an essentially painless way for stimulating the motor cortex (for certain electrodiagnostic procedures), which is now being investigated as a possible treatment for depression. The devices used for these purposes deliver magnetic field strengths that depend on the size of the coil used for delivering the stimulation and can range from 1.5 to 5 T. When positioned close to the skull over the motor cortex, the currents that are induced to flow by the application of these localized fields are sufficient to depolarize neurons to threshold and thereby produce responses from appropriate muscles.[2]

These techniques utilize sophisticated equipment that deliver pulsed magnetic fields. By contrast, the therapeutic use of magnets discussed in this chapter relies on simple, permanent magnets that deliver stationary (or static) fields of some particular strength. It is important to remember that stationary, or nonchanging, magnetic fields do not induce current to flow in conductors that may be in their spheres of influence. In this way, the magnets discussed here are quite different from those having the known effects previously mentioned. In other words, it is improper to try to draw a similarity between the known abilities of changing magnetic fields to exert physiological influences, and the yet-to-be proven abilities of static magnetic fields to relieve pain, decrease edema, facilitate wound healing, or improve strength. The reader should not lose sight of this distinction. Do not be taken in by those who play loose and easy with the literature, and who erroneously mention studies with these technologies and use them to "prove" the benefits of magnet therapy.

Some Definitions

MAGNETS AND MAGNETISM

Magnets exert their "effects at a distance" due to the presence of a magnetic field emanating from them. The effects of these fields include the well-known attraction of iron, or if two magnets are present, the attraction (or repulsion) of unlike (or like) poles. Magnetic fields can be visualized by placing a bar magnet under a sheet of paper, and then sprinkling iron filings on top of the paper. Figure 18-1 is a diagrammatic representation of how the lines of magnetic force arc between the north and south poles of the magnet in the surrounding space.[1] Also by convention, these lines of force (or the direction of the field) are considered to flow from the north pole to the south pole outside the magnet.[1] Another way to look at this convention (and seen in Figure 18-1) is that the direction of the field is the direction a "north pole" would be urged to move, which is, of course,

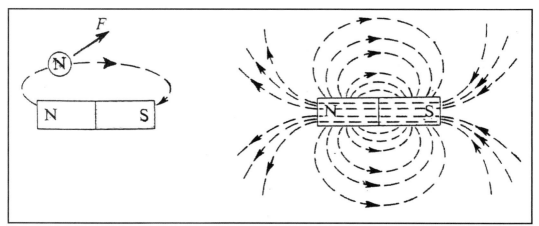

Figure 18-1. Simplified representation of magnetic field surrounding a bar magnet. On the right, the arrows represent the convention that the lines of force flow from the north to the south poles in the field outside of the magnet. On the left, a hypothetical north pole is "urged" to move in the external field away from the magnet's north pole toward its south pole. (Adapted from Verwiebe FL, Van Hooft GE, Saxon BW. *Physics: A Basic Science.* 5th ed. New York, NY: American Book Company; 1970.)

away from the magnet's north pole, toward its south pole. But this is only a convention. It would be just as true to define the direction of the field as along the path a "south pole" would be urged to move, which would then be from the south pole toward the north pole. This concept of convention will be discussed again later.

The reader also needs to keep in mind certain other conventions about the naming of magnetic "poles." In a compass (which is simply a lightweight elongated magnet free to pivot about its center), the pole that is labeled "N" is the pole that points somewhere in the direction of the Earth's geographic north pole, that is, the magnetic north pole does not coincide exactly with the geographic north pole. Since unlike poles attract, if we consider the northward-pointing pole of the magnet to be a north pole, then it must be pointing toward a south magnetic pole that is situated in the northern hemisphere of the earth. Conversely, if the pole labeled N in the compass is really a north-seeking pole, then it is in reality a south pole being attracted to a north magnetic pole situated in the earth's northern hemisphere. Either way, the pole marked "N" is pointing north. Furthermore, most regular bar magnets, such as those included in educational kits for teaching children (and adults) about magnetism, have their ends marked "N" and "S" similar to a compass. In other words, in these magnets, the "N" means it is a north pole and is pointing north toward a magnetic south pole. In fact, a magnet (or compass) labeled in this way is sometimes referred to as a "navigator's compass," for obvious reasons.

Now here comes a switch. In *therapeutic* magnets (sometimes also referred to as biomagnets), the pole marked "north" is *behaving as the earth's north pole* and will attract the north-seeking pole of a compass if the two are brought close to each other. In the therapeutic magnet, the "N" does mean north pole; that is, it will attract the north-seeking pole of a compass. Just to add to this confusion of terms, in therapeutic magnets the "N" also stands for "negative." Later, this chapter will discuss how this other term came about and a simple way to determine whether "N" on any magnet means north-seeking pole (ie, it is a navigator's magnet), or if it means the north and negative pole of a therapeutic magnet.

Getting back to magnets in general, the lines of force that surround it are called the *magnetic flux*, and are measured in terms of *Webers*. Flux density, which describes the number of lines of force per square meter perpendicular to the field at a point, would be Webers/m^2. In turn, 1 Weber/m^2 is a Tesla, while 1 T equals 10,000 gauss (or, 10^4 gauss=1 T). A gauss represents 1 line of force per centimeter squared perpendicular to the field.

There are two ways that a magnet's strength is reported. One is in milli Teslas (mT), and the other is in gauss. Just keep in mind that 10 gauss=1 mT, and you'll have no trouble going from one to the other.

It is also worth noting at this point that the three technologies mentioned above that are known to have biological effects, emit changing magnetic fields that have peak values in the Tesla range. Conversely, the static magnets we will be discussing in this chapter are usually rated in the hundreds or few thousand gauss. Therefore, these magnets are considerably weaker than the technologies mentioned. For further comparison, the Earth's magnetic field, although it varies depending upon position, has an average strength of 5 x 10^{-5} T, or 0.5 gauss. Therefore, the magnets we will be discussing are considerably stronger than the Earth's magnetic field.

Another point to keep in mind, however, is that magnets are rated at their surface. In reality, the strength of the magnetic field at any point in the field depends upon the medium that the field is projecting through (eg, a vacuum, air, water, or some other material), and it depends also upon the distance from the magnet to the point of interest. With respect to the latter, the field strength follows an inverse square relationship. In other words, if field strength at a certain distance from the magnet is known, doubling that distance leads to a field strength that is one-fourth of the original. Therefore, knowing that a magnet is rated as having 500 gauss (or 50 mT) does not tell you how many gauss are actually present at some depth within the body.

The permanent magnets used today for their presumed therapeutic purposes are usually one of two types. The first is a "ceramic" or "ferrite" magnet, in which the ingredients are either barium ferrite or strontium ferrite combined with iron oxide. The second is a "neodymium" magnet, in which the ingredients are neodymium (one of the so-called rare earth metals), iron, and boron. These are sometimes referred to as NdFeB magnets, for their chemical symbols. The latter magnets are somewhat more expensive and can achieve higher gauss ratings than the former, but both types hold their magnetism well. A research paper should indicate the type of magnet used in its Methods section.

OTHER MAGNET TERMINOLOGY

Manufacturers frequently advertise their magnets as being either *monopolar* or *bipolar*. This terminology is at first counterintuitive since a magnet has to have two poles, but the designations simply mean how many poles (one or two) are facing the skin. For example, a monopolar magnet is more like a "conventional" magnet, in which one end (or side) is the north pole and the other end (or side) is the south pole. Usually, the north pole (sometimes times referred to as the "negative pole" and imprinted with the letter "N" on it) is the side in contact with the skin. A bipolar magnet is fabricated from many small individual magnets lying either side by side or concentrically, with adjacent magnets alternating their polarity. In other words, in a bipolar magnet the north pole of one magnet, is next to the south pole of an adjacent magnet, and so on. In this situation, the side of the magnet in contact with the skin contains both poles and is therefore called *bipolar*.

Each manufacturer, of course, touts why their configuration is "better" than the others. For example, Magnetherapy Inc, the manufacturer of Tectonic Magnets (Leicester, United Kingdom), claims that their unipolar configuration permits one to "better exploit the basic laws of physics and assure a greater depth of penetration... generally four to eight times larger than bipolar magnets." This is because, they claim, the adjacent pole configuration of certain competitors results in some cancellation of field strength due to having alternating north and south poles near one another. Therefore, their argument goes just because a unipolar and a bipolar magnet may have similar gauss ratings (which are taken from the surface of the magnet), the unipolar magnet will produce a greater field strength some distance away.

On the other side of this debate (no pun intended), manufacturers of bipolar magnets claim other advantages of their arrangements, as will be described shortly. Now though, let's revisit the "convention" of equating north and south poles of therapeutic magnets to the terms *negative* and *positive*, which are used in electronics, and also to the origin of the term monopolar magnet.

In 1974, Davis and Rawls[3] published a book in which they described the effects on certain conditions using a monopolar magnet. Davis and Rawls claimed, based on previous work by Davis, that the conventional wisdom concerning magnets and magnetism was wrong. They claimed that magnetism was not a single "force," whose external field arcs in unbroken lines between the north and south poles (as seen in Figure 18-1), but two separate and distinct forces (which they named negative and positive), with "cables of force" (not lines of force) that emanate from one pole and re-enter the magnet at its middle. In other words, in the Davis and Rawls model, the poles are not connected in the field outside the magnet, but "are separate and distinct." Now, because these outside fields are separate, Davis and Rawls went on to claim that (using an elongated bar or rod magnet, so that the poles are relatively far apart), one can "treat" an area with either the north (which they named negative) or south (which they named positive) pole and, thus, gave rise to the concept of a monopolar or unipolar magnet. Therapeutic magnets today that are classified as monopolar are simply flattened versions of the ones used by Davis and Rawls.

To say the least, this concept that magnetism is made up of two distinct "energies" never gained acceptance in the scientific community. Why? Because Davis and Rawls have never presented unambiguous evidence substantiating their claim. In fact, and this is indeed unfortunate, in everything I have read by Davis and Rawls,[3,4] there is no true experimental evidence of any claim they make, and they have claimed to having made some astounding changes in organisms by exposing them to one pole or the other. However, not one piece of documentation accompanies their claims.

It is beyond the scope of this chapter to go into details concerning this lack of documentation by Davis and Rawls, but I refer the reader to their book *The Magnetic Blueprint of Life*.[4] In one chapter, Davis and Rawls amazingly publish a review of their work by a consultant of the American Cancer Society (Davis and Rawls claim to arrest, if not cure, cancer). In commenting upon their claims, the reviewer writes[4]:

> *These assertions by the authors are not supported by any described experiments... The reviewer sees no basis for crediting the assertions of the authors in the absence of experimental evidence... The observations are made repeatedly but the experiments are not adequately described... The design of the experiments, including the handling of controls, as well as analysis of results with error analysis, is not given. In the absence of such important details, this reviewer does not see any basis for the conclusions by the authors.*

The litany of identified problems goes on. Is it any wonder that nothing written by Davis and Rawls can be found in the peer-reviewed scientific literature?

In this same book, Davis and Rawls not only declare that the scientific community has been successful in squelching their work because their revolutionary findings go against the "establishment," they even suggest that Dr. Davis should be awarded the Noble Prize in cancer research for his contributions to the field![10] Readers may draw their own conclusions.

However, since Davis and Rawls are behind much of what is said concerning magnetic therapy, we must continue with how they determined that the north pole of a magnet is negative, and the south pole positive, regardless of what they say about magnetism being two separate energies. First, it turns out that their terminology has nothing to do with an excess or deficiency of electrons, or the presence of negative or positive ions, as in electrical circuits. Instead, the Davis and Rawls designations have to do with what they claim are physiological effects of the north and south poles, and whether these effects cause a decrease (negative effect) or an increase (positive effect) of some phenomena. An illustration of this is shown in Table 18-1.

A similar table can be found on page 30 in a book by Philpott and Kalita.[5] Like the books by Davis and Rawls,[3,4] the one by Philpott and Kalita[5] contains many claims based on anecdotes, but no scientific (ie, experimental) evidence.

Furthermore, readers familiar with classical electrotherapy will also note certain similarities between the effects of the negative and positive magnetic poles described by Davis and Rawls with those known to occur under the negative and positive poles of a DC circuit. For example, Table 18-2 is from the electrotherapy book by Watkins.[6]

Table 18-1

HEALTH EFFECTS OF DIFFERENT POLES

Research conducted by Albert Roy Davis and Walter C. Rawls Jr. concludes that the north and south poles of a magnet have different effects. Specifically, north pole energies rotate in a counter-clockwise direction and cause mass to contract. South pole energies rotate clockwise and cause mass to expand and dissipate. North pole energy is referred to as negative because it reduces or attracts and has alkaline properties. South pole energy is referred to as positive and has acidic properties. The following effects for each pole are as follows:

NORTH (NEGATIVE) POLE	SOUTH (POSITIVE) POLE
Promotes tissue alkalinization	Promotes tissue acidity
Increases tissue oxygenation	Decreases tissue oxygenation
Reduces swelling	Increases swelling
Relieves pain	Accelerates growth indiscriminately
Calms the nervous system	Promotes anxiety
Promotes sound, restful sleep	Makes sleep less sound and restful

Clearly, unless there is a specific reason for using the south pole of a magnet, it should be avoided. Use of the north pole is recommended in nearly all cases. This means that the north pole of the magnet should be facing, or in contact with, the area to be treated.

Table 18-2

EFFECTS OF THE DIRECT CURRENT

	PHYSIOCHEMICAL	*PHYSIOLOGICAL*
Positive pole (anode)	Acid reaction; repels metals and alkaloids	Hardening of tissue; decrease of nerve irritability
Negative pole (cathode)	Alkaline reaction; repels acids and acid radicals	Softening of tissues; increase of nerve irritability

Reprinted with permission from Watkins AL. *A Manual of Electrotherapy.* 3rd ed. Philadelphia, PA: Lea & Febiger; 1968. Copyright ©2003 Lippincott Williams & Wilkins.

In addition, the negative electrode has been reported to have an edema-reducing effect, presumably due to repulsion of negatively charged proteins in edema fluid, thereby osmotically drawing water away from the area. Watkins refers to this as *electro-osmosis.*[6] The electrical phenomena described by Watkins are based on experimental evidence. But where are the data showing this also occurs under the static magnetic poles, as claimed by Davis and Rawls? No such "proof" could be found in their writings, only the claims. A claim is not data.

There is yet another problem introduced into the literature by the Davis and Rawls[3,4] classification, and agreed to by Philpott and Kalita.[5] In the Philpott and Kalita book we read, "All magnets have two poles; one is called a north pole (negative) and the other a south pole (positive)... This use of *positive* and *negative* as applied to magnetism is recommended rather than the geographic definitions, which may cause confusion in regard to human physiology."[5] Here is the problem: in another popular book on magnets, namely that by Lawrence and Rosch,[7] we read, "Positive and negative are also misleading and inaccurate terms that originated with the British Admiralty's efforts to improve the compass... The end of the needle that pointed north was called the north or positive pole of the magnet. Actually, it should have been called the "north-seeking" pole, which would have meant that it was actually negative rather than positive."[7] So this means that since the north-seeking pole of a compass is in reality the south pole of a magnet (which we already stated), then the south pole is negative rather than positive (according to Lawrence and Rosch's definition).

Indeed, when a manufacturer of magnetometers and gaussmeters (eg, AlphaLab Scientific Instruments, www.trifield.com), was contacted in regard to how they equated north and south poles with negative and positive, their response was: "The north pole of a magnet emits an out-ward-pointing field, which is usually described as positive; the south pole emits an inward-pointing field, which is usually described as negative." So it does indeed appear that the Davis and Rawls classification is contrary to the tests and measurement classification. However, for our purposes, the point to keep in mind is that Davis and Rawls gave the designations negative and positive based on what they claimed were physiological effects, and many manufacturers of "therapeutic" magnets appear to follow that convention.

What then is a therapist to do if uncertain whether the "N" inscribed on a magnet stands for north pole that would be equivalent to the Davis and Rawls negative, or does it stand for negative, equivalent to the tests and measurements south pole (which is the north-seeking pole of a compass)? It is very simple. If you wish to double-check the polarity of a monopolar magnet, obtain a compass and approach it slowly with the magnet. The north-seeking pole of the compass will turn toward the north pole of the magnet (ie, the one mimicking the north pole of the Earth), and that pole will be the negative pole of Davis and Rawls.[3,4] So, if the magnet has an "N" on one side, and the compass needle rotates toward that side, then the "N" stands for the negative pole. Simple.

Even if Davis and Rawls,[3,4] Philpott and Kalita,[5] and Lawrence and Rosch,[7] have not supplied us with rigorous evidence that magnets exert the benefits they claim, it might still be the case that they are correct. Indeed, even if the theory "explaining" these benefits is wrong (or at least highly questionable), we would be equally wrong if we simply dismissed all of this as meaningless. Let us now put the hype aside and turn our attention to the issues that really confront us in the realm of clinical and experimental data.

Data vs Anecdote

Like many others in physical therapy, the first I heard about the "healing powers" of magnets was from a manufacturer. The literature to support the claim consisted primarily of well-known athletes, mostly professional golfers, attesting to how the manufacturer's magnets not only relieved their neck, back, or shoulder pain, but made them better golfers. Interesting, but certainly not proof of efficacy. Then, and adding to the mix, other manufacturers came along with different types of magnets, each extolling why theirs was better than the others, again offering anecdotal evidence, usually from professional athletes. But what about scientific studies?

Early Experiments

Prior to these recent claims of reducing pain, edema, and inflammation in humans, the potential effects of static magnetic fields on peripheral nerve function had been studied. Review of these papers, however, shows that the species examined were the frog[8-10] and the lobster,[11] and the nerves were studied in vitro (ie, out of the body). These different studies employed magnetic fields ranging from 1850 gauss to 2 T, with exposure times up to 4 hours. Findings were controversial. Some found no effects on parameters such as conduction velocity or amplitude of the compound nerve action potential, whereas others found that these measures increased.

One might conclude that the contradictory findings may be related to the different field strengths and exposure durations employed (a reasonable suggestion), but it seems the more important issue is whether these findings (either positive or negative) on isolated nerves of frogs and lobsters have anything to do with the intact physiology of humans? And how might the increases in conduction velocity and amplitudes of the nerve action potentials (if these indeed occur in humans) result in reducing pain, edema, and inflammation (as made by the claims)?

More recently, however, there have been an interesting series of in vitro studies using a form of bipolar magnet named MagnaBloc (Quixtar Inc, Grand Rapids, MI). This magnet incorporates four magnets of alternating polarity (the manufacturer has named this a "quadrapolar" configuration), embedded side-by-side in a 3.5-cm diameter disc. Field-intensity measurements have shown that due to the proximity of the poles to one another, a very steep positive-negative gradient exists in the field. This gradient, in turn, has been reported to block the generation of nerve action potentials in what were presumably mechanoreceptor and nociceptor neurons.[12-14] In these studies, which also compared different magnet configurations including monopolar, the field strength appeared not to be as important as the field gradient. It was also suggested, from the nature of the data, that the blockade of action potentials was due to altering the configuration of sodium channels that are necessary for depolarization to occur. Of course, whether these effects in vitro, where the magnets and target tissues were quite close to one another (estimated in the papers to be within 5 mm), translate to human situations has yet to be seen. This will be brought up again later, but if this arrangement indeed blocks action potentials in nociceptive fibers, then a possible mechanism for pain reduction has been demonstrated. Note that this would be despite the claims of those who believe that only the negative pole is beneficial. Now let's turn our attention to human nerves in situ.

Hong[15] studied motor conduction velocity and the excitability index of the median, ulnar, and peroneal nerves of 10 normal subjects (age 17 to 39 years) whose nerves were exposed to a 1-T static field for 15 seconds. All we are told about the magnet (besides its strength) was that it was "a 6-inch round electromagnet connected to a rectifier/controller" and was placed perpendicular to the nerves of interest. This is presumably a monopolar magnet, but there is nothing said about which pole was closest to the skin, nor the distance from the skin (inadequate description of methods). The excitability index was defined as the ratio of the amplitude of the compound muscle action potential evoked by a submaximal stimulus during or after magnetic exposure compared to that elicited before exposure, using the same intensity of stimulation. In other words, an increase in this ratio would indicate that the nerves are more excitable than before exposure, and vice-versa. Hong reported no significant change in the conduction velocity, although the excitability index significantly increased. The increased excitability was observed as early as 5 seconds after exposure started, and disappeared by 3 minutes after exposure stopped.[15]

Again, the clinical significance of this is unclear. First, we know nothing about the type of magnet used, nor the polarity employed. Second, the 1-T field is much stronger than the magnets for which claims are made, and the exposure time was only for 15 seconds, far shorter than the hours (sometimes days) that magnets are usually worn. Third, why should an increase in nerve excitability lead to a reduction in pain (as usually claimed)? So, although this was a study in humans, its findings are of questionable clinical significance for our purposes.

Studies on Pain in Humans

Hong et al[16] attempted to replicate a study by Nakagawa in Japan, who had reported that a magnetic necklace was effective in treating "magnetic deficiency syndrome, which includes stiffness of the shoulders, back, and scruff of neck," as well as a host of other complaints. Hong et al employed 101 volunteers (46 males and 55 females). Fifty-one of these volunteers had chronic neck and shoulder pain (either periodically or consistently) for more than 1 year. These 101 subjects were divided into two major groups, one who had chronic pain and one who had no pain. These major groups were then subdivided into two each, one of which was assigned to wear a necklace that had a true magnet incorporated into it, and the other had a placebo magnet incorporated into it. The true and placebo magnets were supplied by TDK Magnet Corporation (Garden City, NY). The necklace consisted of 11 drum-shaped elements (8 mm in length, 2.2 mm in diameter) spaced periodically along its length. The magnetized elements had "a surface density of approximately 1300 gauss that decreases rapidly away from the surface."[16]

Outcome measures were of two types: objective and subjective. The objective measures consisted of the excitation threshold of the suprascapular nerve, with recordings from the supraspinatus muscle; and the proximal conduction time of the ulnar nerve, as determined by the axillary F-loop latency. The subjective measures required the volunteers to rate, on scales ranging from 0 to 4, the intensity and frequency of pain and stiffness before and after 3 weeks of continuously wearing the necklace.[16]

Following the initial outcome measures, subjects with and without pain were randomly assigned to either the true or placebo magnet groups (see paper for details of assignments and the statistical analyses performed). At the end of the 3 weeks, it was found that patients with pain who had received either the true or placebo magnets both reported significantly less pain and less frequency of pain, but that there was no significant differences between these groups. The authors concluded, "Thus, there is evidence of a placebo effect."[16]

Concerning the objective measures, there were no significant changes in excitation threshold with either true or placebo magnets. However, there was a significant decrease in the ulnar nerve conduction time with the magnet, but this occurred only in the group that had no pain to begin with. Remember, though, that a decrease in conduction time means a faster conduction velocity, so the clinical significance of this finding, if it indeed means anything, is unclear. For our purposes, this study did not show a benefit, other than placebo, of wearing a magnetic necklace for subjectively reducing neck and shoulder pain. It also did not confirm the findings of Nakagawa.[16]

TRIGGER POINTS IN POST-POLIO SYNDROME

Vallbona et al[17] reported a double-blind placebo-controlled study of 50 patients with post-polio syndrome who also had "muscular or arthritic pain." These patients had trigger points or a circumscribed region that was painful to palpation. If a patient had more than one trigger point, only one was examined and treated. Two outcome measures were employed: in one, patients subjectively graded (on a scale of 1 to 10) the pain experienced when "firm application of a blunt object approximately 1 cm in diameter" was applied to the trigger point. The authors also noted that such application to a nonpainful area was experienced as pressure, but not pain. The second outcome measure was the completion of a McGill Pain Questionnaire to provide a subjective evaluation of their general pain experience.[17]

Following the above pretreatment determinations, patients were randomly assigned to receive either a true (500 gauss or 300 gauss, depending upon the magnet's size) or placebo magnet. These were Bioflex magnets (Bioflex Medical Magnets Inc, Oakland Park, FL), which contained concentric circles of alternating polarity (ie, a bipolar configuration). Devices were applied to the skin overlying the trigger point for 45 minutes. The outcome measures were then repeated. It was only after the post-treatment measures were taken that the "code" was broken and it was determined which patients received the true magnet and which received the placebo.[17]

Analysis showed that while pretreatment scores were essentially identical between the two groups, post-treatment scores were significantly different. The visual analog scores (VAS) decreased in the treated group a mean of 5.2 ± 3.2 (SD), while the placebo group decreased only 1.1 ± 1.6. It is noted, though, that while the authors stated that the second outcome measure was the McGill Pain Questionnaire, nothing appears in the paper about those results. No adverse side effects were reported. There were also no data concerning whether there were any longer-lasting benefits of the treatment.[17]

Therefore, all that can be said about this study is that in this group of patients, there does appear to be an "immediate" reduction of pain when a trigger point has pressure applied to it. More importantly, we do not know whether this pain reduction was maintained, nor do we know whether this pain reduction had any effects on the "everyday" pain experienced by these patients (ie, the pain they may have been experiencing without pressure being applied to the trigger points). Therefore, the clinical significance of these interesting findings is unknown. Were these patients really helped or not? Is it proper to tout this research as one "justifying" the use of magnets?

HEEL PAIN

Caselli et al[18] randomly assigned 40 patients with heel pain into two groups. The treatment group wore an insole (PPT/Rx Firm Molded Insoles from Langer Biomechanics) containing a Nikken 500 (Irvine, CA) gauss magnetic foil placed in the heel. The sham-treatment group wore the same insole but without the magnetic foil. Subjects used the insoles for 4 weeks and refrained from taking any medications. The outcome measure was the "foot function index" prior to and after the 4 weeks. The foot function index measures "the impact of foot pathology on function in terms of pain, disability, and activity restrictions." The three subscales (pain, disability, and activity restrictions) consisted of 20 items (items six, nine, and five, respectively) that patients grade on VAS. A total score was obtained, with higher values representing more impairment.[18]

Nineteen patients in the treated group and 15 patients in the sham group completed the treatment. Caselli et al reported that 11/19 (58%) patients treated with the magnetic foil added to the insole "reported an improvement in foot function," while 9/15 (60%) of patients treated with just the insole also "reported improvement." This difference in patients reporting improvement (58% vs 60%) was not significantly different. Also, there was "no significant difference in the improvement made by the magnetic foil group versus the molded insole group as measured by the percentage difference in the mean scores on the foot function index." Caselli et al concluded, "The magnetic foil offered no advantage over the insole."[18]

From the research standpoint, however, this paper has two serious problems. First, the authors did not specify what difference in the overall score between the pretreatment and post-treatment measures constituted an "improvement." A reader has no way of knowing, therefore, how the authors determined that 11/19 and 9/15 patients reported improvements. Second, this problem is exacerbated by this confusing description: "The score before the foot function index was 34 for the magnetic foil and 29 for the PPT insole. The score after the foot function index was 31 for the magnetic foil and 28 for the PPT insole." How can there be a "score" before and after the foot function index, when the foot function index was the score? Or did the authors mean "before treatment, the index scores were... while after treatment, the scores were..."? It should not be up to readers to try to interpret what an author was trying to say.

Even more damaging to the entire paper is the fact that in these two sentences we learn that the treated group went from a foot function index of 34 (presumably the mean value for the group, although this is not specified) to 31 after treatment, while the sham group went from 29 to 28. How these apparently minimal group changes allowed the authors to claim that "Approximately 60% of patients in both groups reported improvement" is quite unclear.

So, although this paper reports "negative" results for the effects of magnetic insoles in treating heel pain, it is difficult to deduce how one comes to any conclusion, either for or against, these benefits.

DELAYED ONSET MUSCLE SORENESS

Borsa and Liggett[19] performed a randomized, single-blind, placebo study investigating the effects of static magnets on delayed onset muscle soreness (DOMS). DOMS was induced in the biceps brachialis muscle of the nondominant arm in 45 volunteers. Outcome measures (the dependent variables) were pain perception (determined by the standard 10-cm VAS), range of motion of elbow flexion and extension, upper arm girth (as a composite score of three sites), and static force production of elbow flexion with the forearm in neutral and elbow flexed 90 degrees. These measurements were taken before the DOMS-producing protocol and then 24 hours later. Following this second measurement, subjects were randomly assigned to one of three groups (n=15 in each): an experimental group, a placebo group, and a true control group. The experimental group had a Nikken 700 gauss bipolar flexible magnet taped over the exercised muscle, which was worn continually except when bathing. The placebo group had identical-looking magnets, but which had no field strength (sham magnet), and the control group had no "treatment" at all. Subjects were asked to refrain from any analgesic, anti-inflammatory, or physical therapy treatments. Repeated measurements were then made after another 24, 48, and 72 hours.[19]

Repeated measures ANOVA showed no significant differences in any of the outcome measures between the three groups at any of the time intervals. If anything, the experimental group reported (on average) more pain than the other two groups 24 and 48 hours after the first post-exercise measurements, but this difference was not statistically significant.[19] Therefore, this study revealed no particular benefit of the magnetic therapy for reducing pain, increasing range of motion, or hastening return of static force production compared to either sham magnets or no magnets at all. With respect to this experimental production of DOMS, 700 gauss bipolar magnets did nothing to hasten the natural recovery process.

Another study on DOMS was reported by Reeser et al.[20] This was a double-blind, randomized control trial, in which 23 healthy subjects served as their own controls (contrast this design with the one by Borsa and Liggett just described). Elbow flexors on both sides underwent exhaustive eccentric exercises known to produce DOMS. Sides were then randomly chosen to receive either true or placebo treatments, using the same magnet types as reported by Vallbona et al (reviewed earlier). Treatments were carried out for 5 days at 45 minutes per treatment. Outcome variables included a 100-mm VAS for describing pain, maximum elbow flexion torque, elbow flexion angles both at rest and on maximum flexion, and arm circumference. These were all determined before eccentric exercise and then after each treatment, bilaterally. Subjects were required to refrain from taking any analgesics during this time.

Analysis showed that there were no statistically significant differences in any of the outcome measures between the true and placebo magnet sides at any of the time intervals. The authors conclude, "Our study offers no evidence to support a therapeutic role for magnets in treating DOMS resulting from exhaustive eccentric exercise."

Similarly, Mikesky and Hayden[21] reported a double-blind, placebo-controlled trial in which 20 subjects exercised both arms and then one arm or the other received either the true or placebo magnet. Magnets and placebos were contained in armbands worn continually for the next 7 days except when bathing. Again, there were no significant differences at any time in any of the outcome measures.

Note that of the three studies just described, only the one by Borsa and Liggett[19] employed a three-arm research design (true treatment, placebo treatment, and true control, or a natural history group). The other two studies were two-arm designs where the true treatment group was compared to a placebo treatment group. We will come back to this later.

PAINFUL NEUROPATHY

Weintraub[22] reported on 19 patients (out of an initial 24) with painful neuropathy due to either diabetes (n=10) or some other causes (n=9). These 19 completed a double-placebo crossover trial that lasted 4 months. Treatment consisted of magnetic insoles (475 gauss) or placebo insoles, one for each foot, for the first 30 days (phase I). These were then switched for another 30 days (phase II). In phase III, all subjects received two active insoles for the next 2 months. Unfortunately, nothing is said about who made the magnets, nor whether they were monopolar or bipolar. We are told, though, that no new pharmacological interventions were allowed during these 4 months. Subjects rated their complaints of burning, numbness, and tingling pain for each foot using a 5-point (0 to

4) VAS twice a day. Patients also underwent neurological and electrodiagnostic testing before and after these interventions.[21]

In the abstract, Weintraub reported[22]:

> *Improvement was significantly more pronounced in the diabetic cohort, 90% versus 33%, at the end of the 4 months (p<0.02). During the first month, the placebo response was noted to be the same in both groups (22%) for symptoms of burning and numbness and tingling, whereas in the second month, the placebo effect was greater in the diabetic peripheral polyneuropathy cohort than in the nondiabetic peripheral polyneuropathy cohort (38% versus 22%, respectively). This was felt to represent an overshoot phenomenon. At the end of 4 months, improvement was significantly more pronounced in the diabetic cohort for burning (p<0.05) and numbness and tingling reduction (p<0.05).*

A placebo response was defined as "a significant reduction in baseline pain scores (>25%) for burning and numbness and tingling when sham magnets (controls) were utilized."[22] It is apparent from this that a placebo effect can be expected in some patients (not surprisingly). Perhaps more importantly for our purposes, while there appeared to be a benefit greater than the placebo in the diabetic polyneuropathy (DPN) cohort (9/10 responding favorably), the nondiabetic polyneuropathy (N-DPN) cohort did not show such a benefit (only 3/9 responding favorably, which was not much different than the sham responses). In other words, 67% of subjects with nondiabetic painful peripheral polyneuropathy did not obtain particular benefit from the "treatments."

This study, of course, suffers from the obvious deficiency of small sample sizes (10 vs 9). Too much, either in favor or not in favor of magnets, cannot be read into its findings. However, the paper contains a number of other flaws and inconsistencies that detract from its overall credibility. For example:

1. The paper states that at the beginning of the study, "The mean spontaneous pain intensity (VAS scores) for burning was slightly higher in the N-DPN group (2.5 vs 2.1), whereas numbness and tingling scores were similar (2.1)." However, inspection of Figures 1 and 2 of the paper does not show this. Instead, for the "Burning" scores, the nondiabetic patients appear to be starting between 1.5 and 1.6, whereas the diabetic patients had initial "Burning" scores of about 0.9. And for "Numbness and Tingling," the initial values are between 2.1 and 2.4 for the nondiabetics, and 1.2 and 1.9 for those with diabetes. Therefore, what is said in the body of the paper is different from the data shown in the figures.

2. There are other inconsistencies between values given in the paper compared to what can be seen from simple inspection of the figures (this should have been picked up by the journal's reviewers to begin with). Table 18-3 shows the changes in VAS scores between the initial values prior to instituting magnet therapy, and the values obtained after completing the 4-month period. For both groups of patients, the scores are given depending upon whether the foot received sham treatment first or active treatment first during phase I of the trial.

   The negative sign before each value shows that the subjective rating decreased (on average) over the course of the 4 months. It is also apparent that, as described in the paper, patients with DPN showed larger decreases in VAS scores over the 4-month period than did patients with N-DPN. However, the values determined from Figures 1 and 2 in the paper do not agree with the much larger mean decreases described in the body of the paper, which range as high as 2.10. It is not at all clear where those values come from, although the trend described in the paper, namely that patients with DPN obtained more relief than those with N-DPN, is still seen.

3. Another shortcoming of this paper, and acknowledged by Weintraub,[22] is the fact that neither the patients nor the examiner were blinded to which foot had the placebo and which foot had the active magnet during phases I and II of the study. During the final 2 months (phases III and IV), both feet had active magnets. While this nonblinding could theoretically "bias" how patients rated their sensations, inspection of the data graphed in

Table 18-3

CHANGE SCORES DETERMINED FROM FIGURES 1 AND 2 IN WEINTRAUB

	DPN	N-DPN
Burning		
Sham first	−0.88	−0.20
Active first	−0.88	−0.18
Numbness/tingling		
Sham first	−1.06	−0.29
Active first	−0.7	−0.02

Adapted from Weintraub MI. Magnetic biostimulation in painful diabetic peripheral neuropathy: a novel intervention—a randomized, double-placebo crossover study. *AJPM*. 1999;9:8-17.

Figures 1 and 2 show that both active and sham magnets produced some decreases in VAS scores. Therefore, the nonblinded aspect of this study did not seem to have an impact on the results.

4. Although the author tells us that 90% of the patients with DPN showed statistically significant improvements in VAS scores, we are not told what change in these 9 out of 10 subjects qualified for being considered "statistically significant." Perhaps it was the change of >25% as indicated earlier for the placebo response, but this fact is not stated specifically in the paper, so we are left guessing as to what is meant.

5. Nothing is said about whether these changes in VAS scores were accompanied by improvements in the quality of life of these patients. Did they sleep better? Did they walk better? Were medications decreased? All we know is that VAS scores decreased, which while good to know, is really only a beginning. Clearly more properly designed research is needed.

BACK PAIN

Collacott et al[23] compared 300 gauss bipolar magnets and sham magnets worn across the backs of 20 subjects with chronic low back pain. The study was a randomized, double-blind, placebo-controlled, crossover design. Subjects wore either the active or sham devices for 6 hours, 3 days a week (Monday, Wednesday, and Friday) for 1 week. This was followed by a 1-week wash-out period, and then the next week switched to the other device, which was again worn for 6 hours a day for the same 3 days. These patients, therefore, were exposed to 18 hours each of both active and sham devices.

Outcome measures were VAS scores, the pain rating index (PRI) of the McGill Pain Questionnaire, and measurement of range of motion (ROM) of the lumbosacral spine using the 2-inclinometer method. Before the study began, the authors performed a power analysis for the VAS scores, assuming that a 2-point difference with a standard deviation of 1.5 would represent a significant reduction in pain. The analysis showed that to achieve a power of 0.8, 20 subjects would be needed. Twenty-four subjects originally met the study criteria, but for different reasons only 20 completed the full protocol. Subjects were asked to avoid any new treatments during the study period and not to change their use of medications (if any).

Subjects rated their pain before and after each treatment, and up to 3 days after all treatments ended. ROM was determined weekly. At the beginning of the study, the average VAS score for the active magnet group was 4.7±2.9, while for the sham group it was 5.0±2.4. Three days after treatments ended, the average change scores were −0.49±1.6 and −0.40±1.8, respectively. These values fell far short of the drop of 2 points that would have been considered significant changes and were not significantly different from each other (p=0.87). Similar nonsignificant changes or differences were found for the PRI scores and ROM.[23]

Collacott et al discussed possible reasons for their negative findings.[23] The most obvious, of course, is that magnets have no effect on low back pain. However, other possibilities that have to be considered include:

+ The magnets used in the study were not strong enough (300 gauss) to influence the regions generating the sensation of pain.

+ Treatment times were not long enough (perhaps the magnets should be worn all day, not just 6 hours a day, 3 days a week).

+ Perhaps a different magnet configuration should be employed (monopolar as opposed to bipolar).

To the credit of these authors, they caution why these negative findings cannot be generalized to the population at large with chronic low back pain. Issues mentioned included small sample size, subjects were only those who could travel to and attend the treatment sessions, and the fact that there was only one female in the study (subjects had been recruited from a Veterans Affairs clinic).

Holcomb et al[24] described two adolescents with "debilitating, medication-resistant, chronic pain in the low back and abdomen." Both had undergone multiple evaluations and treatments by various specialists, including appendectomies, but with no relief. Finally, MRIs revealed L5-S1 disc impingement in one patient, and T12-L1 disc protrusion in the other (see paper for other details). Both patients were then offered treatment with the quadrapolar MagnaBloc magnet described earlier. The paper reports rapid (ie, within minutes) reduction of pain, with long-lasting benefits with continued use.[24]

KNEE PAIN

Segal et al[25] studied the effects of the MagnaBloc magnets on rheumatoid arthritis of the knee. Each constituent magnet had a rating of 190 mT (1900 gauss). Control magnets were similarly constructed, but contained only one true magnet among three blanks. This control magnet had a surface strength of 72 mT (720 gauss). The authors do not stipulate which pole of the one active magnet was against the skin. The authors also stated that they did not use a true placebo magnet[24] (ie, one with no active element, because blinding could not be maintained [presumably, patients and staff would somehow be able to tell that the placebo magnet was not a real magnet]).

Exclusion and inclusion criteria are clearly and extensively detailed. Outcome data obtained before, during, and after treatment included a rheumatologist's global assessment of disease activity, Westergren erythrocyte sedimentation rate (ESR) or C-reactive protein, knee range of motion by goniometry, examination for tenderness, examination for swelling, patient's assessment of physical function, 100 mm VAS score for pain, subject's global assessment of disease activity, the Modified Health Assessment Questionnaire, and the subjects' assessment of treatment outcome.[25]

Following the initial measures, patients were randomly assigned to the MagnaBloc (n=38) and control magnet (n=26) treatment groups. Treatment consisted of placing four blinded devices over specified locations above, below, and on either side of the knee, for 1 week. After completion of the study and breaking the code, it was found that the baseline pain level for the MagnaBloc group was 63/100, and for the control group was 61/100. At the end of 1 week, both groups had reported statistically significant pain reduction (40.4% and 25.9%, respectively, p<0.0001). Although this value was greater for the MagnaBloc group, the difference between the groups was not significant (p<0.23).[25]

Other measures that were not significantly different were serum analysis for acute phase reactants, rheumatologist's assessments of tenderness, swelling, or range of motion. Measures that were significantly different between the groups and in favor of the MagnaBloc treatment were the subjects' assessment of global disease activity and subjects' assessment of treatment outcomes. Two measures showed a trend in favor of the MagnaBloc group, but which did not reach statistical significance were the Modified Health Assessment Questionnaire and the rheumatologist's global assessment of disease activity.

In their conclusion, the authors stated, "Both devices demonstrated statistically significant pain reduction in comparison to baseline, with concordance across multiple indices. However, a significant difference was not observed between the two treatment groups (p<0.23). In future studies, the MagnaBloc treatment should be compared with a nonmagnetic placebo treatment to characterize further its therapeutic potential for treating RA."[24] In other words, maybe there is a beneficial effect, but it is not clearly evident at this time.

Hinman et al[26] enrolled 47 subjects with chronic knee pain into a double-blinded, randomized, placebo-controlled trial (RCT). Data were obtainable on 43 of them (18 in the true-magnet group, and 25 in the placebo group) after a 2-week treatment period. The devices were packaged in pads containing either four true or four placebo magnets that were worn around the knee. The true magnets were unipolar Ne-Fe-Bo disks rated by the manufacturer as being 1.08 T. The authors randomly tested eight of these discs and found that the surface measurements varied from 0.040 to 0.056 T at their centers and 0.14 to 0.18 T at the periphery (this difference between manufacturer ratings and ratings obtained by independent testing will be discussed later). The authors checked on the polarity of the magnets using a compass (as described previously) to verify that the biomagnetic north (negative) pole was properly indicated and applied to the skin.[26]

Outcome measures were the sum of five VAS pain ratings, the sum of 17 functional activity ratings, and a timed 15-meter (50-foot) walk. These measures were performed before being randomly assigned to either treatment group and then at the end of the 2-week period. Treatment logs that recorded the time the pads were worn for each day were also completed by the subjects. After the final data were tabulated for each subject, the magnet manufacturer provided the list of code numbers to distinguish which pads contained the true and placebo magnets.[26]

Analysis of the data showed a statistically significant treatment effect in which subjects wearing the magnets had greater improvements in their pain, physical function, and gait speed than those who wore the placebo magnets.

Harlow et al[27] performed a randomized, placebo controlled trial using 194 men and women, aged 45 to 80 years, with osteoarthritis of the hip or knee, divided into three groups. Although the hips and knees were the source of the pain, the magnets were bracelets worn on the wrist. The three groups received either "a standard strength" bipolar magnetic bracelet (170 to 200 mTesla or 1700 to 2000 gauss), a "weak magnetic bracelet" (21 to 80 mT or 210 to 800 gauss), or a dummy bracelet. The authors state that the choice of the strength for the "weak magnetic bracelet" was because other studies had shown that this strength range "is insufficient to be therapeutic." (Note though that the previous study on chronic pelvic pain used magnets of 500 gauss, yet claimed a benefit.) Subjects were asked to wear their bracelets during all the time they were awake.

Harlow et al[27] also write that an independent physics laboratory tested 5 magnets of each type before the study began as a check on the manufacturer's specifications. All returned magnets were then re-tested at the end of the project. More studies should include this type of before and after verification.

The primary outcome measure was the change in the Western Ontario and McMaster Universities osteoarthritis index (WOMAC A) obtained at baseline and then after 4 and 12 weeks. Secondary outcome measures were a 100 mm visual analogue scale for pain, as well as WOMAC B and C scales for leg stiffness and functioning. In addition, the authors include a power analysis describing how they arrived at the sample size chosen, and they also state that, "Last value carried forward was used to impute missing values for subsequent analysis."

At the end of 12 weeks, analysis of covariance followed by Dunnett's test showed significant changes compared to baseline between the standard and dummy magnet groups, for the WOMAC

A and VAS scores. The p value for differences between the standard and weak magnet groups was 0.07 (thus, not significant).

But just what were these "statistically significant differences" in VAS pain scores? Here is a summary of Table 2 of that paper:

	Standard (n=65)	Weak (n=44)	Dummy (n=64)
Baseline	66.8 (16.2)	64.9 (18.3)	63.75 (9.5)
12 Weeks	54.8 (24.5)	55.7 (22.2)	62.9 (22.2)

It is obvious therefore, that the "average" patient who received the standard magnet was not pain-free at the end of 12 weeks, but still had a moderate amount of pain, although not as severe as before treatment. Similarly, the change in the WOMAC A score for the standard magnet group was a 27% reduction from baseline which, though better than the dummy magnet group, does not translate to "normal" function. My point is that by knowing the real figures, you won't be taken in by a manufacturer or dealer who promotes this paper as "proving" that magnets "relieve" pain. Ask them what they mean by "relieve"? I predict they will not know the details.

Another interesting aspect of this paper is the discussion of how these findings compare with studies using medications. Harlow et al remark that the improvements noted in this study are "similar to that found in trials of frontline osteoarthritis treatments." Therefore, the equivalence of results suggests that magnets, which are less expensive than drugs, and are not accompanied by side effects, might be a better option. Indeed, Harlow et al suggest the need for just such a comparison. I agree, but you can imagine how drug companies would view this concept!

CHRONIC PELVIC PAIN

Brown et al[28] enrolled 33 women (out of 40 screened) with chronic pelvic pain (CPP) in a randomized, double-blind, placebo-controlled trial (see paper for details of inclusion/exclusion criteria and for power analysis that led to this number of subjects). Outcome measures included the McGill Pain Questionnaire (MPG), the Pain Disability Index (PDI), and the Clinical Global Impressions Scale (CGI). Of these, the primary outcome measure was the change from baseline in the Present Pain Intensity (PPI) component of the CGI. Secondary outcome measures were other components of the questionnaires.

An interesting research design was employed. After baseline measurements were obtained, all subjects unknowingly had placebo magnets applied to manually-determined trigger points on two sites on the abdomen for 1 week. Magnets were to be worn continuously. Subjects were told that the strength of the magnets might vary and that "adherence of the device to metal surfaces was not related to their efficacy." At the end of the first week, all 33 subjects repeated their questionnaire ratings, and were then randomly and blindly assigned to either an active-treatment group (n=16) or to continue unknowingly with the sham magnets (n=17). Active devices were 500 gauss, concentric, bipolar magnets, 50 mm in diameter, and 1.5 mm thick, held over the trigger points with adhesive tape. Subjects then completed the questionnaires again after 2 weeks and after 4 weeks of this double-blind period.

Results showed that after the first week, during which all subjects received sham magnets, there were no significant changes in pain measures from baseline, "suggesting no significant placebo effect from the sham magnets."

After 2 weeks of double-blind treatment, no significant differences were noted between the groups, and subjects were given the opportunity to continue for another 2 weeks. At the end of this second 2-week interval, the active magnet group now showed significant improvements compared to the sham-treated group (see paper for details).

However, review of the data shows that only 8 of 16 subjects in the active group completed the entire 4 weeks of treatment compared to 11 of 17 subjects in the sham group. This means that more subjects dropped out of the study than was originally planned for in the power analysis (which we are told required at least 14 subjects to complete the study in each group). Furthermore, the authors did not perform an intention-to-treat (ITT) analysis, which further detracts from the quality of this report.

With respect to the efficacy of the blinding, the authors tell us that "patients receiving active magnets were more likely than those receiving placebo magnets to correctly guess their treatment." At the end of the fourth week of double-blind treatment, all of the subjects in the active magnet group correctly guessed that they had active magnets, while 45.5% of those in the placebo group incorrectly guessed they were wearing active magnets.

The authors conclude that "Static magnetic field therapy significantly improves disability and may reduce pain when active magnets are worn continuously for 4 weeks in patients with CPP, but blinding efficacy is compromised."[28] I, however, wouldn't tout this study as one that has clearly shown such a result.

FIBROMYALGIA

Two papers have been published reporting the effects that sleeping on magnetic mattresses have on certain complaints in patients with fibromyalgia.

Colbert et al[29] enrolled 35 female subjects with fibromyalgia, although only 30 of them met the American College of Rheumatology's diagnostic criteria for fibromyalgia syndrome.[30] Of these 30, five did not complete the study for various reasons. Therefore, the results reported were on 25 patients, 13 in the experimental group and 12 in the sham group. The paper details the demographic characteristics of the patients, as well as their prescribed medications and other therapeutic interventions. The paper specifies that subjects had to agree to start no new pain medications or additional pain management modalities during the 16 weeks of the trial. Patients could continue with whatever medications or modalities they had already been using. Outcome measures were related to pain and sleep. Eight variables were employed (see paper for details).[29]

After completing the baseline measures and physical examination, patients were randomly assigned to receive (at their homes) either an experimental (true magnetic) mattress pad or a sham pad that was identical to the true pad except it was not magnetized. Pads were provided by Magnetherapy Inc (Leicester, United Kingdom), and shipped from the manufacturer to the patients. Only the manufacturer had the code telling which mattresses were experimental and which were sham.[29]

Details of the magnetic pads are provided in the paper. Suffice it to say that each pad contained 270 monopolar domino-shaped ceramic magnets, each with a surface field strength of 1100 gauss. They were arranged in the mattress with the negative poles (as demonstrated by using a compass) facing the body. It was estimated that the field strength delivered to the skin surface at various anatomical sites was between 200 to 600 gauss. The authors also note that this field strength would make it "difficult to detect magnetization with lightweight items such as paperclips." This obviously helped in keeping subjects "blinded" as to whether they were sleeping on a true or sham mattress pad.[29]

Data analysis after completion of the 16 weeks showed how the patients were divided into the experimental and control groups, and also that these groups were not significantly different except for their weight; the sham group was heavier than the experimental. The authors note, however, that this had no effect on outcome "since the magnetic field level would have been within the 200 to 600 gauss range for the sham group had they been treated with the active magnets."[29]

The findings can be summarized as follows[29]:

> *The results demonstrate that subjects with fibromyalgia who slept on mattress pads containing permanent magnets delivering 200 to 600 gauss to the skin surface, for a 16-week period, when compared to sham controls, experienced statistically significant and clinically relevant pain reduction and sleep improvement. This was evidenced by the self-reported improved VAS for pain, sleep, and fatigue; a reduction in the total myalgic score; and the subject's own assessment of her body pain distribution. The diminished pain*

and enhanced sleep also correlated with improvements in the subject's functional abilities for performing tasks of daily living as measured by the modified FIQ [Fibromyalgia Impact Questionnaire].

One statistically significant improvement was noted in the sham group—this was in "tiredness upon awakening." However, this improvement was only noted by week 12 and did not change further after that. Conversely, in the experimental group, this measurement continued improving by week 16. Therefore, some placebo effect was noted with respect to this outcome measure. No adverse effects were reported in either group.[29]

Alfano et al[31] performed a randomized placebo-controlled 6-month trial of the effects of sleeping on one of two magnetic pads (two true treatment groups), or on one of two sham pads of the same materials but with inactive magnets (two sham treatment groups). Functional pad group A (n=37) was exposed to a uniform magnetic field (monopolar arrangement) consisting of a grid of ceramic magnets rated at 3950 gauss (or 395 mT) placed between the subject's mattress and box spring (as recommended by the manufacturer, MagnetiCo Inc, Calgary, Canada). This placed the subject's body approximately 15 to 25 cm above the magnets, which exposed the body to a field strength of 0.3 to 0.6 mT (3 to 6 gauss). Sham pad group A (n=17) slept on a pad made of the same material but with inactive magnets in it. Functional pad group B (n=33) was exposed to a magnetic field that varied spatially and in polarity, rated at 75 mT or 750 gauss. These pads were placed on top of the subject's mattress (as recommended by the manufacturer, Nikken Inc, Irvine, CA). Sham pad group B slept on a pad made of the same material but with inactive magnets.

Outcome measures included changes after 6 months in pain intensity ratings, tender point counts, tender point pain intensity ratings, and functional status (Fibromyalgia Impact Questionnaire). At baseline, the groups did not differ significantly in any of these outcome measures. At the end of 6 months, the findings were[30]:

+ All four groups showed a decline in the number of tender points, but the differences among the groups were not significant (p=0.72).

+ The functional pad groups showed the largest declines in total tender point pain intensity, but overall differences were not significant (p=0.25).

+ Improvement in functional status was greatest in the functional pad groups, but differences among groups were not significant (p=0.23).

+ Functional pad group A showed the greatest decrease in pain intensity rating from baseline to 6 months, which was significant (p=0.03).

This paper also describes measurements of field strengths at different distances above the functional pads (remember inverse square relationship with distance) and found that, indeed, the actual field strength that patients were exposed to was considerably less than the magnets themselves. Not surprisingly, functional pad A had higher field strengths at all the distances measured than did functional pad B, although not nearly as strong as the magnets were rated at their surface.

Wound Healing

Szor and Topp[32] described a 51-year-old female with paraplegia (secondary to surgery to correct a congenital malformation of the spinal cord) with an abdominal wound that had not healed with conventional treatment after a year. Surgery was being considered, but it was first decided to try a short course of magnet therapy. A thin (one-sixteenth of an inch) round (1.5 inch diameter), 650 gauss magnet (not specified whether monopolar or bipolar) was taped over the dressings, which were changed twice daily. Except for the placement of the magnet, no other changes in wound care were initiated. The patient's wound, therefore, was exposed to the magnet essentially 24 hours a day.[31]

On the patient's first return visit 11 days later, "remarkable progress in healing of the wound was observed." By the end of 4 weeks, the wound was closed. A follow-up 9 months later showed continued closure. This case report clearly justifies more appropriately controlled research in this area.[31]

Man et al[33] studied 20 patients randomly assigned to a treatment or sham treatment group (n=10 in each) who underwent suction lipectomy. Immediately after surgery, Tectonic patch magnets of sizes needed to cover the surgical site or sham patches were applied with compression dressings. These magnets are unipolar and were applied with the "negative" pole facing the skin. Magnetic strengths ranged from 150 to 400 gauss, depending upon the size of the patch. The magnets were worn for 14 consecutive days. The surgeon, patients, and a physician "observer" were blinded to whether the patch was a magnet or sham magnet until after the data were obtained (14 days later).[32]

Outcome measures included the pain reported by the patients using a VAS, and two measures determined by an "observer," also using a 0 to 10 analogue scale for ecchymosis within the limits of the area covered by the patches compared to the areas outside the patch, and for edema compared with neighboring regions that had not undergone surgery. The paper describes, for these last two measures, how these determinations were made. These outcome measures were performed on postoperative days 1, 2, 3, 4, 7, and 14. Nonparametric statistical tests were used to compare the discoloration, edema, and pain scores at each time interval.[32]

Findings can be summarized as follows:[33]

1. Discoloration was significantly less (both statistically and clinically) in the treated group on postoperative days 1, 2, and 3. From postoperative days 4 through 14, however, there were no longer any significant differences.

2. Edema was significantly less in the treated group on postoperative days 1 to 4; not significantly different on days 7 or 14.

3. Pain was significantly less in the treated group throughout the first 7 days. By day 14, although pain was still less in the treated group, it was not significantly different from the sham group. The treated group also had less consumption of analgesics than the sham group. No adverse reactions were noted in either group.

This paper presents good evidence that the employed magnets provided a "healing" benefit during the first 7 days postoperatively. Although there were no significant differences between the two groups by the end of 2 weeks, the fact that the treated group progressed faster and required less medication during the first week suggests a clear benefit was obtained.

Other Claims of Efficacy

An oft-repeated claim is that magnets exert their beneficial effects, at least in part, by increasing blood flow to the underlying area. Consider the following two theoretical explanations for how this might occur:

> All of our bodies are full of blood, which contains hemoglobin. The heme in hemoglobin is iron (magnetic) and follows the rule of north-to-south pole orientation of every molecule. Is it any wonder that placed in a powerful magnetic field, our bodies would react accordingly? Assuming that injury or dysfunction causes a misalignment of these molecules, consider the advantages of their realignment in a therapeutic magnetic field.

The reference for this statement is purposely not divulged to avoid embarrassing the writer, although the "article" it appeared in was published in a physical therapy/occupational therapy "newspaper." Before going on to the second example, though, let's examine the above sentences in more detail.

First, the claim implies that because hemoglobin contains iron, it will be influenced by a "powerful magnetic field." Are the magnets we are talking about considered "powerful?" Is there any evidence that a few hundred gauss placed on the surface of the body attracts hemoglobin? The author gives no references for this. Second, and more importantly, the claim requires us to "assume" that injury or dysfunction causes a "misalignment" of these hemoglobin molecules. Just what is a misalignment of a hemoglobin molecule, and what data exists for this misalignment being "corrected" when placed in a magnetic field? Again, no references are given to support these claims. So, are we to believe them?

Consider this second explanation for an effect that appears on a manufacturer's Web site[33]:

> *If we were to take a sample of animal or human blood and spin off the fluid (the plasma) and leave the red blood cells, then place these red blood cells on a slide and insert them into a good microscope, we would see that, when we bring a magnet up under the slide, the red blood cells all spin around and point in one direction. This is **polarisation** or alignment of the iron particles of the red blood cells. When this happens, the blood circulation improves and you have gathered strength, power, and energy. The improved circulation helps reduce body stress because now the body does less work to perform its normal functions.*

Again, a number of questions come to mind. First, since red blood cells are circular, how does one know, when viewing them under a microscope, that under the influence of a magnetic field, they "point in one direction?" How does one determine that a bunch of homogeneous circles are all pointing in one direction? Without more information, this appears patently ridiculous. More importantly, how does one make the giant leap that even if these red blood cells were all pointing the same direction, this necessarily translates into improved circulation, improved strength, power, energy, etc? Talk about making mountains out of molehills! Such unsubstantiated, pseudoscientific statements as these may convince the gullible, but they do nothing to bolster the credibility of the field.

However, even if the above "explanations" are naive at best, perhaps blood flow is indeed increased locally by exposure to the magnets we are talking about. Are there any studies to support this contention?

A Medline search revealed one study in humans, and the results were negative. Reported in the dental literature, Saygili et al[35] employed 10 subjects who wore dental magnets inserted into a retention system on one side, and a similar retention system without magnets on the other. These systems were kept in place continuously, except during sleep, for 45 days. Buccal mucosal blood flow was measured using the 133 Xe clearance technique, before and periodically during the 45 days, comparing each subject's experimental and control sides. No significant differences were found.

In the veterinary medicine literature, Steyn et al[36] reported findings on six healthy adult horses. One metacarpus had a magnetic wrap (270 gauss, bipolar field arrangement) placed around it, while the contralateral metacarpus had a control wrap. Using radio-labeled red blood cells and scintigraphic images, relative perfusion ratios of the two sides were obtained before wrapping, and then 48 hours after continuous application of the field. No significant differences between the before-and-after relative perfusion ratios were found. The authors concluded, "Results suggest that in horses, the static magnetic field associated with application of commercially available magnetic wraps for 48 hours does not increase blood flow to the portion of the metacarpus underneath the wrap."[32] The authors also caution, "Results of the present study do not allow us to conclude that these magnetic wraps do not have any potential advantages, but rather suggest that any effects of these magnetic wraps are not a result of increased local blood flow."[35]

So, at present, we must take the claim that blood flow is increased locally by the static magnets we are talking about with a grain of salt. Perhaps this will be shown in the future, but at present, such evidence is missing.

A Disturbing Report

One aspect concerning the widespread use of static magnets is that these devices can be purchased in drug stores, supermarkets, over the Internet, etc. Manufacturers make all sorts of claims (as already mentioned) and package their products very seductively. When one of these over-the-counter magnets is purchased by a consumer, what guarantee is there that the magnet is of the strength the package claims? Apparently, not much of a guarantee. Blechman et al[37] acquired five "popular magnets" and tested them with two different gaussmeters. For all five magnets, the determined values at multiple sites along the face of the magnets were significantly lower than the claimed values. Of course, when measured 2.5 cm above the surfaces of the magnets, the field strengths were even less. The authors note that this "suggests minimal tissue penetration," and they ask, "How can the public benefit from the results of clinical studies using magnets of a specific strength," if there is no guarantee of the strength of the purchased magnets?[36] Once again, caveat emptor (let the buyer beware).

Some Comparisons

Now that we've reviewed some examples of research papers that have either shown or not shown efficacy of static magnetic fields, let's compare these to some examples taken from popular books on magnets. For example, some chapters in the book by Philpott and Kalita[5] contain "success stories":

> *Richard had a raised and tender area on his buttocks, which rapidly developed into a boil. It was convenient for him to sit on a 4 x 6 x 0.5-inch ceramic magnet for half the day. After the first 2 days of this magnetic exposure, the tender area receded. By the third day, the boil was completely gone. Always use a magnet that is larger than the size of the area affected.*

> *Michael, 20, was diagnosed with an inoperable malignant glioblastoma, a type of brain tumor. He was left unconscious and unresponsive to environmental stimuli. The negative magnetic field from a 4 x 6 x 0.5-inch ceramic magnet was placed on the back of his head where the tumor had started growing and was continued for 24 hours a day.*

> *Three days later, his consciousness returned and he was able to wiggle his fingers and respond to questions. In 3 weeks, he walked out of the hospital with only the assistance of a walker. He continued the treatment on his brain for an extended period of time. After this dramatic turnaround, he has remained well for the past 5 years, and his tumor has not returned.*

What do you think of this as a "report"? What else would you want to know before you start treating malignant glioblastomas with magnets?

Or this from Lawrence and Rosch[7]:

> *Katherine T., a 34-year-old office worker, suffered headaches classified as the muscle contraction or tension type. They occurred on a daily basis. When she wore the magnets as directed in the evening hours, it would alleviate about 50% to 60% of her discomfort. Dr. Lawrence also gave her a Relax Band with a neodymium magnet over the wrist, which helped reduce her tension. She described her job as "high stress," but felt after the headache relief and the Relax Band that she was able to handle it.*

Both the above books, and others like them on the market, offer readers similar examples of people getting relief. Amazing though, little to nothing (mostly nothing) is said about those who did not get better. As mentioned in the beginning of this chapter, it is hard to believe that every patient treated found relief. From the minimum "facts" given, positive outcomes cannot even be attributable only to the magnets.

Such selective reporting is characteristic. Only the positive results are described; the others are forgotten or conveniently ignored. This is the difference between research and anecdote. This is the difference between controlled experimentation and bias. But let's give these individuals the benefit of the doubt and ask how can so many positive results be possible? The answer is fairly simple: Let's assume that in any sample of patients with some painful condition (such as arthritis), 33% of them will be spontaneously getting better during any one time period. If you "treat" 100 such individuals and then report in glowing terms the 33 cases that improved, you have certainly amassed what appears to be an impressive "study." But by ignoring, or forgetting to describe, what happened to the others, that is where "deliberate selectivity," or bias, creeps in. Of course, by not utilizing proper control subjects, etc, the entire "study" becomes more and more suspect. Most people, however, are not sophisticated enough to ask for such details. They are impressed instead by the litany of how many people "got better."

Conclusion

From the above review of published studies, it appears that there is little objective evidence to support the claims of pain relief that can be attributed specifically to using static magnets. The two studies of magnetic mattresses for fibromyalgia are exceptions and clearly suggest more research is warranted for this debilitating condition. The article by Hinman et al[26] is also favorable. For wound healing, there are two positive reports, although only one was randomized and controlled. The other was a case report, which, though promising, needs to be repeated in a more rigorous manner. So the issue is obviously still open to investigation. The "challenge" to those who write the popular books on this topic should be: If you are so convinced from your experiences that these magnets perform the wonders that you describe, do us all a favor and perform the appropriate research. You have the patient populations, so do what has to be done to present scientific evidence of an effect. This means randomized, blinded, controlled studies, along with the proper statistical analyses of results. Collaborate with a research methodologist and/or statistician to make sure that you do the study properly. Do not complain that you cannot get your work into the peer-reviewed literature when the reason is that the "research" does not qualify as being credible. In addition, the field desperately needs comparisons between the bipolar and monopolar configurations to determine if this variable really has an effect. This entire area of static magnets is wide open for exploration, and I encourage serious researchers to get involved. Then, let the chips fall where they may.

References

1. Verschuur GL. *Hidden Attraction: The Mystery and History of Magnetism*. New York, NY: Oxford University Press; 1993.
2. Chiappa KH. *Evoked Potentials in Clinical Medicine*. 2nd ed. New York, NY: Raven Press; 1990.
3. Davis AR, Rawls WC Jr. *Magnetism and Its Effects on the Living System*. Hicksville, NY: Exposition Press, Inc; 1974.
4. Davis AR, Rawls WC Jr. *The Magnetic Blueprint of Life*. Kansas City, MO: Acres USA; 1979.
5. Philpott WH, Kalita DK. *Magnet Therapy*. Available at http://www.alternativemedicine.com. Accessed November 3, 2003.
6. Watkins A. *A Manual of Electrotherapy*. Philadelphia, PA: Lea & Febiger; 1968.
7. Lawrence R, Rosch PJ. *Magnet Therapy: The Pain Cure Alternative*. Rocklin, CA: Prima Publishing; 1998.
8. Edelman A, Teulon J, Puchalska IB. Influence of magnetic fields on frog sciatic nerve. *Biochem Biophys Res Comm*. 1979; 91:118-122.
9. Gaffey CT, Tenforde TS. Bioelectric properties of frog sciatic nerves during exposure to stationary magnetic fields. *Radiat Environ Biophys*. 1983;22:61-73.
10. Liberman EA, Vaintsvaig MN, Tsofina LM. Effects of constant magnetic field on excitation threshold of isolated frog nerve. *Biofizka*. 1959;4:505-506.

11. Schwartz JL. Influence of constant magnetic field on nervous tissues: nerve conduction velocity studies. *IEEE Trans Biomed Eng.* 1978;25:467-473.

12. Cavopol AV, Wamil AW, Holcomb RR, McLean MJ. Measurement and analysis of static magnetic fields which block action potentials in cultured neurons. *Bioelectromagnetics.* 1995;16:197-206.

13. McLean MJ, Holcomb RR, Wamil AW, Pickett JD. Effects of steady magnetic fields on action potentials of sensory neurons in vitro. *Environ Med.* 1991;8:36-44.

14. McLean MJ, Holcomb RR, Wamil AW, Pickett JD, Cavopol AV. Blockade of sensory neuron action potentials by a static magnetic field in the 10 mT range. *Bioelectromagnetics.* 1995;16:20-32.

15. Hong C-Z. Static magnetic field influence on human nerve function. *Arch Phys Med Rehabil.* 1987;68:162-164.

16. Hong C-Z, Lin JC, Bender LF, Schaeffer JN, Meltzer RJ, Causin P. Magnetic necklace: its therapeutic effectiveness on neck and shoulder pain. *Arch Phys Med Rehabil.* 1982;63:462-466.

17. Vallbona C, Hazlewood CF, Jurida G. Response of pain to static magnetic fields in postpolio patients: a double-blind pilot study. *Arch Phys Med Rehabil.* 1997;78:1200-1203.

18. Caselli MA, Clark N, Lazarus S, Velez Z, Venegas L. Evaluation of magnetic foil and PPT insoles in the treatment of heel pain. *J Am Podiatr Med Assoc.* 1997;87:11-16.

19. Borsa PA, Liggett CL. Flexible magnets are not effective in decreasing pain perception and recovery time after muscle microinjury. *J Athletic Training.* 1998;33:150-155.

20. Reeser JC, Smith DT, Fischer V, et al. Static magnetic fields neither prevent nor diminish symptoms and signs of delayed onset muscle soreness. *Arch Phys Med Rehabil.* 2005;86:565-570.

21. Mikesky AE, Hayden MW. Effect of static magnetic therapy on recovery from delayed onset muscle soreness. *Phys Ther Sport* 2005;6:188-194.

22. Weintraub MI. Magnetic biostimulation in painful diabetic peripheral neuropathy: a novel intervention—a randomized, double-placebo crossover study. *AJPM.* 1999;9:8-17.

23. Collacott EA, Zimmerman JT, White DW, Rindone JP. Bipolar permanent magnets for the treatment of chronic low back pain: a pilot study. *JAMA.* 2000;283:1322-1325.

24. Holcomb RR, Worthington AB, McCullough BA, McLean MJ. Static magnetic field therapy for pain in the abdomen and genitals. *Pediatr Neurol.* 2000;23:261-264.

25. Segal NA, Yoshitaka T, Huston J, et al. Two configurations of static magnetic fields for treating rheumatoid arthritis of the knee: a double-blind clinical trial. *Arch Phys Med Rehabil.* 2001;82:1453-1460.

26. Hinman MR, Ford J, Heyl H. Effects of static magnets on chronic knee pain and physical function: a double-blind study. *Alter Ther.* 2002;8:50-55.

27. Harlow T, Greaves C, White A, Brown L, Hart A, Ernst E. Randomized controlled trial of magnetic bracelets for relieving pain in osteoarthritis of the hip and knee. *BMJ.* 2004;329:1450-1454.

28. Brown CS, Ling FW, Wan JY, Pilla AA. Efficacy of static magnetic field therapy in chronic pelvic pain: A double-blind pilot study. *Am J Obstet Gynecol.* 2002;187:1581-1587.

29. Colbert A, Banerji M, Pilla AA. Magnetic mattress pad use in patients with fibromyalgia: a randomized double-blind pilot study. *J Back Musculoskel Rehabil.* 1999;13:19-31.

30. Wolfe F, Smythe HA, Yunus MB. The American College of Rheumatology 1990 criteria for classification of fibromyalgia: report of the Multicenter Criteria Committee. *Arthritis Rheum.* 1990;33:160-172.

31. Alfano AP, Taylor AG, Foresman PA, et al. Static magnetic field for treatment of fibromyalgia: a randomized controlled trial. *J Altern Comp Med.* 2001;7:53-64.

32. Szor JK, Topp R. Use of magnet therapy to heal an abdominal wound: a case study. *Ostomy Wound Manage.* 1998;44:24-29.

33. Man D, Man B, Plosker H. The influence of permanent magnetic field therapy on wound healing in suction lipectomy patients: a double-blind study. *Plast Reconstr Surg.* 1999;104:2261-2266.

34. Just Magnotherapy Plus. The effects of magnetic fields on the living system. http://www.justmagnotherapy.com/magnettherapy2.html. Accessed November 4, 2003.

35. Saygili G, Aydinlik E, Ercan MT, Naldoken S, Ulutuncel N. Investigation of the effect of magnetic retention systems used in prostheses on buccal mucosal blood flow. *Int J Prosthodont.* 1992;5:326-332.

36. Steyn PF, Ramsey DW, Kirschvink J, Uhrig J. Effect of a static magnetic field on blood flow to the metacarpus in horses. *J Am Vet Med Assoc.* 2000;217:874-877.

37. Blechman AM, Mehmet CO, Vijaya N, Ting W. Discrepancy between claimed field flux density of some commercially available magnets and actual gaussmeter measurements. *Altern Ther Health Med.* 2001;7:92-95.

CHAPTER 19

ACUPUNCTURE THEORY AND ACUPUNCTURE-LIKE THERAPEUTICS IN PHYSICAL THERAPY

Patrick J. LaRiccia, MD, MSCE; Mary Lou Galantino, PT, MS, PhD; and Kerri Sowers, DPT

Traditional Chinese Acupuncture Concepts

Acupuncture has been in existence for at least 2000 years. It is a part of traditional Chinese medicine (TCM) which contains concepts of Yin, Yang, Qi (pronounced chee), and meridians among others. TCM has undergone change and evolution.[1,2] The concept of Qi is very important in acupuncture. Qi is considered "vital energy." Qi courses through pathways of the body called meridians (Figure 19-1). Qi moving through the meridians is analogous to blood moving through blood vessels. Disease results if there is a hindrance or obstruction of blood flow (eg, peripheral vascular disease and coronary artery disease). Disease also results if there is a deficiency of blood volume as in anemia. If there is hindrance or obstruction of the flow of Qi through the meridians, disease results. A deficiency of the amount of Qi is signaled in the symptom of fatigue. In acupuncture the goal of therapy is to restore the proper circulation of Qi. Acupuncture points (Figure 19-2) are locations where the Qi coursing through the meridians is transported to the surface of the body.[3] There are 361 "regular points" which fall on the 14 most frequently utilized meridians. In addition, there are 40 extrameridian points (EM points) that are not on the 14 meridians. There are also Ashi Points which are tender spots. "Tender spots can be used as acupoints, and this was the primary method for point selection in early acupuncture and moxibustion treatments. Without specific names and definite locations, Ashi Points are considered to represent the earliest stage of acupoint evolution. Clinically, they are mostly used for pain syndromes."[3] There are 14 frequently used meridians. These meridians travel essentially longitudinally along the body (see Figure 19-1), however, there are interconnections with each other. Also, most of the meridians have a connection to a specific visceral organ (eg, heart, gallbladder, liver, etc).

The acupuncturist must make a decision as to which acupuncture points to stimulate. Then decisions must be made regarding the stimulation technique itself (ie, needle, needle plus moxibustion, moxibustion alone, and needles with electrical stimulation through the needles). Moxibustion involves burning the herb artemisia vulgaris near acupuncture points in one of a number of specific

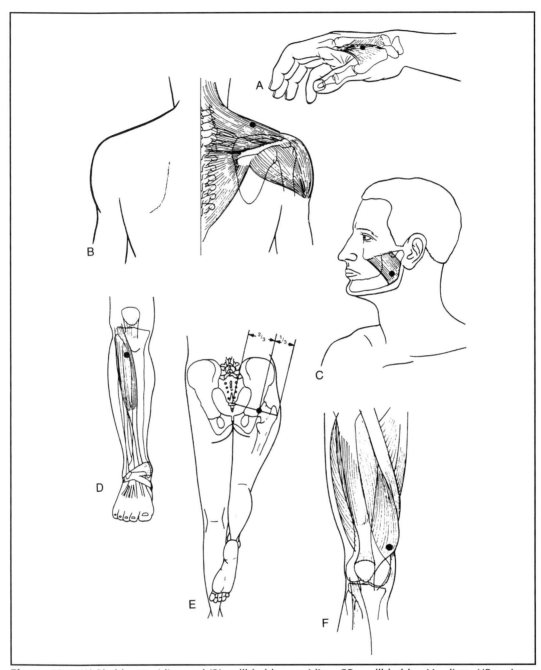

Figure 19-1. (A) Bladder meridian and (B) gallbladder meridian. GB=gallbladder; Liv=liver; UB=urinary bladder. (Reprinted from Orthopaedic *Physical Therapy Clinics of North America*, 9(3), LaRiccia PJ, Acupuncture and physical therapy, 430, ©2000 with permission from Elsevier.)

manners. Decisions must also be made on depth of insertion, direction of insertion, type of needle manipulation, duration needles are left in place, frequency of treatments, and number of treatments. One can see that there is an enormous number of ways a treatment can be performed. Different schools of thought will address the various dimensions of acupuncture treatment (ie, point selection, depth of insertion, needle manipulation, etc) in different ways. In mainland China where the TCM

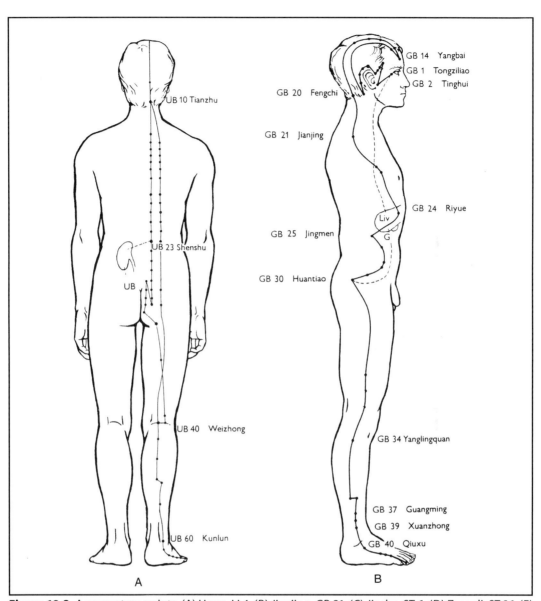

Figure 19-2. Acupuncture points. (A) Hegu, LI 4. (B) Jianjing, GB 21. (C) Jiache, ST 6. (D) Zusanli, ST 36. (E) Huantiao, GB 30. (F) Xuehai, SP 10. (Reprinted from *Orthopaedic Physical Therapy Clinics of North America*, 9(3), LaRiccia PJ, Acupuncture and physical therapy, 432, ©2000 with permission from Elsevier.)

style is dominant, the depth of insertion and needle manipulation will result in a feeling of "de qi" (a temporary feeling of numbness, fullness, or heaviness), while certain Japanese acupuncture styles cause no discomfort at all. Some of the various schools of thought include TCM, Japanese, Korean, French Energetics, Worsley Five Elements, and modern neuroanatomical methods.

An important point selection method for musculoskeletal pain will be described. This point selection method is a method used for what TCM practitioners call Bi syndromes. Bi syndromes are manifested by soreness, pain, numbness and heavy sensation of the limbs and joints, and limitation of movement. Acupuncture points located in the area of pain (local points) along with points distal to the involved area but on meridians running through the involved area are chosen. In addition Ashi Points are also used.[4]

Randomized controlled clinical trials comparing different acupuncture styles are needed to refine acupuncture treatment by guiding point selection, stimulation method, etc.

Modern Physiological Findings

In this section we will look at 1) a spinal cord and brain model of acupuncture analgesia described by Pomeranz,[5] 2) support for the endorphin explanation of acupuncture analgesia, 3) the sympatholytic effect of acupuncture, 4) the relationship of acupuncture to hypnosis, 5) sham acupuncture, 6) characteristics of acupuncture points, and 7) neuroimaging of acupuncture effects.

Among the most notable researchers in the modern physiology of acupuncture are Han[6] of Beijing and Pomeranz[5,7] of Toronto. Both have completed enormous amounts of basic laboratory work along with publishing numerous empirical research reports and reviews. Also, an extensive review of the physiological aspects of acupuncture and human acupuncture research issues has been written by Liao, Lee, and Ng.[2]

SPINAL CORD AND BRAIN MODEL

The following is a simplified version of the model proposed by Pomeranz[5] (Figure 19-3). Type II, III, and IV afferents from muscle transmit the acupuncture stimulus to the spinal cord, while A delta afferents transmit the acupuncture stimulus from the skin. In the spinal cord, ascending pain transmission is blocked in a segmental fashion via enkephalin and dynorphin. When the acupuncture stimulus reaches the midbrain, enkephalin activates a descending pain inhibition system which utilizes serotonin and norepinephrine. After the acupuncture stimulus reaches the hypothalamus the arcuate nucleus releases ß-endorphin into the midbrain resulting in further activation of the descending pain inhibition pathway. Hypothalamic activity also induces the pituitary to release ß-endorphin. ß-endorphin reaches the brain via a retrograde passage in the pituitary-portal system. This ß-endorphin also reinforces activation of the descending pain inhibition system. The pituitary co-releases ß-endorphin and adrenocorticotropic hormone (ACTH) into the systemic circulation. This helps explain anti-inflammatory effects of acupuncture. In addition to the core description above, studies suggest the involvement of the limbic system in acupuncture analgesia, including the amygdala, hippocampus, cingulate, and cerebellar vermis, which may relate to the emotional component of pain.[8,9]

SUPPORT FOR THE ENDORPHIN EXPLANATION OF ACUPUNCTURE ANALGESIA

Converging lines of evidence are powerful arguments in science for validating theories. The endorphin hypothesis as a major mechanism for the analgesic effect of acupuncture has at least 17 lines of converging evidence. We will look at nine of these lines.

1. Naloxone, naltrexone, cyclazocine, and diprenorphine are all opioid antagonists that can block acupuncture analgesia.[5,10]

2. Blockage of acupuncture analgesia by naloxone is stereospecific for the L-isomer. This implicates a receptor mechanism rather than a side effect such as membrane fluidization.[5,10]

3. Macroinjections of naloxone via the systemic circulation can block acupuncture analgesia. However, microinjections are only successful if injection is into areas of the nervous system where there is endorphin activity. Microinjections of antibodies to ß-endorphin, enkephalin, and dynorphin must also be site specific to block acupuncture analgesia. Thus, microinjection of antisera to dynorphin is effective if given intrathecally, but not effective if given in the midbrain.[5,11]

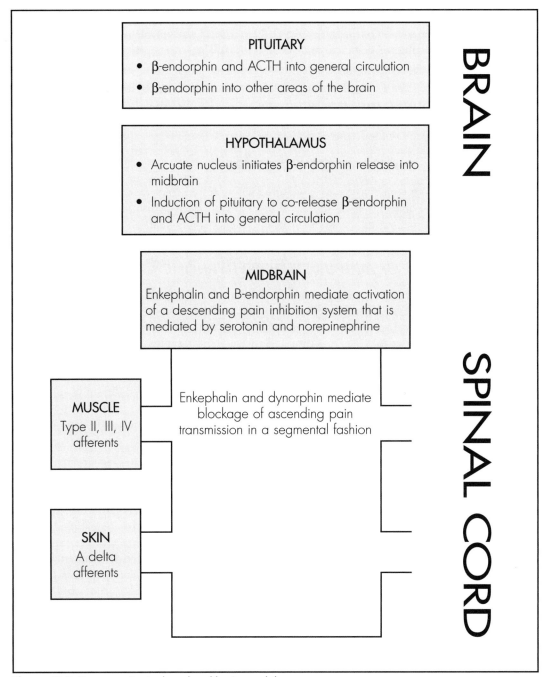

Figure 19-3. Pomeranz' spinal cord and brain model.

4. Mice with endorphin receptor deficiency do less well with acupuncture.[5,12]

5. Endorphin deficient rats respond less well to acupuncture.[5,13]

6. There is an increase in cerebrospinal fluid (CSF) endorphins along with a decrease in brain endorphins after acupuncture.[5,14]

7. Enzyme blockers which retard the breakdown of the endorphins enhance acupuncture analgesia.[5,15]

8. Experiments have been done in which the circulation of one animal subject is crossed into another animal subject of the same species. Only one of the animals received acupuncture, however, both animals demonstrated acupuncture analgesia reversed by naloxone.[5,16]

9. Pituitary ablation and suppression techniques reduce acupuncture analgesia.[5,17]

Pomeranz[5,18] has also addressed the issue of stress analgesia in detail. In one of the studies performed by his group,[19] one of the control groups of mice was handled exactly the same throughout the experiment which included the application of painful stimuli. This group did not exhibit an analgesic effect while the acupuncture group did.

SYMPATHOLYTIC EFFECT OF ACUPUNCTURE

Face, hands, and foot temperature were measured with infrared color thermographs before and after acupuncture.[20] Temperature was increased in all areas. These diffuse nonsegmental sympatholytic effects were long lasting. Sakai et al found evidence for sympatholytic activity resulting from acupuncture,[21] while Knardahl et al did not using a different methodology.[22]

THE RELATIONSHIP OF ACUPUNCTURE TO HYPNOSIS

Studies have evaluated the correlation between hypnotizability and results of acupuncture. Liao and Wen,[23] Peng et al,[24] and Ulett[25] reported no correlation between hypnotizability and acupuncture results. There are studies reporting the failure of naloxone to modify hypnotic analgesia.[26-28] Successful veterinary acupuncture and the fact that acupuncture analgesia has been produced across different species of animals[5] argue against hypnosis as an explanation for the effects of acupuncture. In a study by Lu et al, hypnosis was compared to acupuncture in a quasi-experimental design of subjects with head and neck pain.[29] The outcome of the study suggested that patients with psychogenic pain of nonorganic origin benefit most from hypnosis, those with acute pain have greater pain relief from acupuncture, and those with chronic pain have variable results.

SHAM ACUPUNCTURE

Sham acupuncture is defined in the laboratory as needling at nonacupuncture points. Sham acupuncture fails in acute laboratory pain studies. Placebo pills bring about analgesia in only 3% of cases[5,30,31] in acute laboratory pain. Sham acupuncture in the context of chronic pain in humans is problematic. In clinical human studies placebo analgesia works in 30% to 35% of patients, sham acupuncture works in 33% to 50% of patients, while true points are effective in about 55% to 85% of patients. Therefore, to show statistical significance in studies that incorporate sham acupuncture control groups, a minimum of 122 subjects must be in the study. This criterion is seldom obtained.[5,32]

A major concern about sham needling is the possibility that piercing the skin may activate alternative pain modulation systems, there may also be local effects on healing, a release of vasoactive substances, or trigger point effects.[33] Lund et al investigated whether minimal, superficial, or sham acupuncture could be considered an inert placebo.[34] The authors outlined how light touch on the skin stimulates mechanoreceptors linked to unmyelinated C afferents which may lead to both emotional and hormonal reactions. This may be how sham interventions seem to be as effective as true acupuncture in some conditions, especially those with an increased sensory component. A study by Kong et al investigated brain activity through functional magnetic resonance imaging associated with placebo analgesia via sham acupuncture treatment. The authors concluded that the right anterior insula, bilateral rostral anterior cingulated cortex, dorsal lateral prefrontal cortex, and the parietal cortex play an important role in placebo modulation of pain perception.[35] In light of Lund et al's study,[34] did Kong's study brain map a placebo response or did it brain map the response associated with a treatment that uses light touch instead of needle piercing?

CHARACTERISTICS OF ACUPUNCTURE POINTS

Anatomically, the most notable characteristics of acupuncture points from a physical therapy perspective are: 1) frequent coincidence with trigger points,[5,36] 2) frequency of acupuncture points near motor points of neuromuscular attachments, and 3) frequency of acupuncture points near blood vessels in the vicinity of neuromuscular attachments.[5,37]

Physiologically acupuncture points sometimes have decreased electrical resistance as compared to the surrounding skin.[5] Shang investigated the neurobiology of acupuncture points which suggests that acupuncture points and meridians have higher electrical conductance associated with a higher density of gap junctions. Additionally, acupuncture points have been found to have higher temperatures, higher metabolic rates, and increased carbon dioxide release.[38] A study by Li et al using a rat model showed that acupuncture points may be excitable muscle/skin-nerve complexes with an increased density of peripheral nerve endings and receptive fields.[39] Alternatively, a study by Wick et al performed immunohistochemistry on biopsies of fresh cadaver skin and showed that human acupuncture points are associated with a significantly decreased number and density of subcutaneous nerve structures compared to nonacupuncture points.[40] This study contradicts several animal studies which suggest that acupuncture points have a higher density of nerve endings. This pilot study does point out the need for more research.

Another study looked at the force required to remove the needle from selected acupuncture points where the de qi sensation was present as compared to non-acupuncture locations. It was found that the force necessary to remove the needle from an acupuncture point was significantly greater compared to the non-acupuncture point, suggesting that there may be biomechanical differences at those locations.[41]

Kwang-Sup Soh in Korea has successfully visualized the Bonghan duct which may be the anatomical basis of the acupuncture meridian system which in biophysical terms is a system of optical channels of biophotons.[42]

NEUROIMAGING OF ACUPUNCTURE EFFECTS

Various brain imaging techniques have been used to study the effects of acupuncture. The imagining techniques include electroencephalography (EEG), functional magnetic resonance imaging (fMRI), magnetoencephalography (MEG), positron emission tomography (PET), somatosensory evoked potential (SEP), and single photon emission computed tomography (SPECT).[43] Newberg et al reported a series of SPECT studies in subjects with chronic pain who were treated with acupuncture. The report suggested that there is asymmetrical blood flow to the right and left thalami in patients with chronic pain and that acupuncture improved the blood flow symmetry.[44]

Dhond et al have summarized the findings of imagining studies and report that acupuncture: 1) modulates corticolimbic and brainstem networks supporting endogenous antinociception, 2) alters somatomotor cortex processing and cortical somatotopy in patients with chronic pain and stroke, 3) may modulate autonomic nervous system (ANS) function, and 4) may modulate activity within brain networks supporting attention and higher cognition.[43]

Safety of Acupuncture

The 1997 NIH Consensus Panel[45] on acupuncture and the FDA consider acupuncture safe when done by qualified practitioners using sterile needles. Acupuncture is safer than many of our standard therapies. One study[46] calculated that an acupuncturist might cause less than one serious event per 100 years of full-time practice. Another study conducted in 2000 in the United Kingdom surveyed 34,407 treatments and found no report of serious adverse events which would lead to hospital admission, permanent disability, or death. Additionally, only 43 minor adverse events (1.3 per 1000 treatments) were reported. These included severe nausea or fainting. Other reported events include mild bruising, site pain, and bleeding.[47] In a systematic review of acupuncture safety, the authors concluded that minor complications may be more common than previously thought; the chance of a serious event continues to be rare. Minor complications in this review included bleeding, aggravation of pain (often followed by increased relief after additional sessions), bruising, nausea, vomiting, burns, or failure to have needles removed following treatment.[48]

Clinical Studies

Many clinical studies have been done in acupuncture. Over 2000 acupuncture studies were reviewed for the 1997 NIH Consensus Panel on acupuncture. Previous studies have ranged from single case studies to a randomized controlled double-blind pilot study utilizing laser acupuncture.[49] In addition to the usual design and statistical considerations, there are four issues that are very important in evaluating acupuncture research.

1. Respect for the paradigm. Simply stated, if method A is reported effective in daily practice did the researchers evaluate method A or a different method?
2. Generalizability of research study results across different acupuncture methods.
3. Sham acupuncture controls.
4. The application of acupuncture research results to everyday practice.

RESPECT FOR THE PARADIGM

Hammerslag[50] notes that a considerable proportion of acupuncture trials used acupuncture methods that did not respect the paradigm. Many of these used fixed acupuncture points and did not individualize sessions. An example of evaluating method B instead of method A follows. In 1997 a negative controlled trial of acupuncture was reported.[51] The study was prompted by a retrospective analysis of 27 patients with psoriasis who had an excellent response to classical Chinese acupuncture, complemented with topical needling of the psoriatic lesions, ear acupuncture, and a Chinese herbal remedy. However, for standardization purposes needling of the psoriatic lesions was left out during the conduct of the study, thus changing the method of acupuncture that was observed to be effective.

To allow the reader of a research article to determine if the paradigm has been respected, studies must clearly describe their treatment method and reference their treatment method. The references can be to standard acupuncture texts, acupuncture research literature, and acupuncture experts. The background of the acupuncture expert should be stated. There should be a clear statement as to the opinion of the expert regarding whether or not the study method accurately represents the acupuncture technique being tested. At a minimum the study should follow the standards for reporting interventions in controlled trials of acupuncture (STRICTA).[52]

GENERALIZABILITY OF RESEARCH STUDY RESULTS ACROSS DIFFERENT ACUPUNCTURE METHODS

The 1997 NIH Consensus Panel on acupuncture paper[45] touches on this issue. This is a difficult issue because there are so many different acupuncture methods. This issue applies to both negative and positive results. Shlay et al[53] reported that a standardized acupuncture regimen (SAR) was no better than sham acupuncture for the pain of HIV peripheral neuropathy. This article also reported that 75 mg of amitriptyline was no better than placebo capsules. In both the acupuncture arm and the amitriptyline arm one cannot generalize to another acupuncture method or to a higher dosage of amitriptyline. Berman et al[54] in 1999 reported positive results for the adjunctive use of acupuncture in the treatment of osteoarthritis of the knee. He used a specific method derived from TCM theory regarding Bi syndromes. However, one cannot readily generalize from this that other acupuncture methods derived from Japanese, Korean, or French Energetics will also be effective. Since acupuncture is a group of methods we are not able to test all methods in a single study.

SHAM ACUPUNCTURE CONTROLS

First of all, studies that use sham controls must have enough statistical power to detect a significant difference between real acupuncture and sham acupuncture. This requires a study population of at least 122 subjects.[5] In some recent systematic reviews and meta-analyses looking at neck pain[55] and back pain,[56,57] none of the studies using sham controls had a large enough study population.

Sham controls appear less problematic in areas of study that do not look at pain. A study of acupuncture for stroke recovery[58] using sham controls was positive for acupuncture as was a study of chemotherapy-associated nausea and vomiting.[59] Multiple acupuncture points can turn on the endorphin mechanism. Clinical observation indicates that the effective area of an acupuncture point is increased during chronic processes. Sham points should be nonacupuncture points far removed from real acupuncture points and not situated on an acupuncture meridian. Studies that utilize sham points should describe in detail their locations.

As mentioned earlier there is concern that sham treatments are not truly inert treatments. A systematic review by Dincer and Linde analyzed 47 randomized controlled trials that compared true acupuncture to various types of sham acupuncture including trials that used blunt tipped placebo needles which do not penetrate the skin. The authors concluded that there is no single adequate sham intervention for acupuncture trials.[60]

THE APPLICATION OF ACUPUNCTURE RESEARCH RESULTS TO EVERYDAY PRACTICE

The NIH Consensus Panel[45] paper on acupuncture stated the evidence for acupuncture in the treatment of fibromyalgia, myofascial pain, and tennis elbow was as good as the evidence for our standard treatments of nonsteroid anti-inflammatory drugs (NSAIDs) and steroid injections. Certainly, acupuncture has a better safety record. In 1997, deaths from NSAID toxicity in the United States was almost equal to the number of deaths from AIDS that year.[61] In 1998, the *Journal of the American Medical Association* published an article[62] indicating that deaths from adverse prescription drug reactions ranked between the fourth and sixth leading cause of death in US hospitals. A number of randomized controlled trials have indicated that acupuncture and acupuncture-like treatments are effective adjunctive treatments to standard treatment regimens (eg, osteoarthritis of the knee[51] and stroke rehabilitation[63,64]). Acupuncture has also appeared as effective as standard treatments for temporomandibular joint disorders in some randomized controlled studies.[65] In light of this information, it is not unreasonable to consider acupuncture or acupuncture-like modalities more often in our physical therapy treatment plans.

Application of Acupuncture Concepts and Acupuncture-Like Modalities in Orthopedic Physical Therapy

ACCESSING THE ACUPUNCTURE POINT AND MERIDIAN SYSTEM

In order to access the acupuncture point and meridian system one must have a knowledge of the location of the acupuncture points and their meridians (see Figures 19-1 and 19-2). A detailed exposition of traditional Chinese anatomy is beyond the scope of this chapter. Liao,[2] Stux,[66] and

Xinnong[67] are excellent texts with which to begin. Once the anatomy is known, there are multiple ways to access the system. Access is not restricted to acupuncture needles but can be obtained additionally through manual pressure, surface electrical stimulation, piezo-electric devices, moxibustion, infrared lamps, low energy (cold) lasers, and other direct methods. The system can also be accessed by T'ai Chi movements and Qi gong posture, breathing, and mental practices.

Before proceeding, one must note that some confusion has arisen in the literature regarding the term electrical acupuncture. One must differentiate between electrical stimulation applied to acupuncture needles and electrical stimulation applied to surface electrodes resting on acupuncture points. Originally, electrical acupuncture referred only to electrical stimulation applied to acupuncture needles. This original definition should be maintained. When one stimulates acupuncture points via surface electrodes, one should consider using the acronym SEAPS, which stands for *surface-electrode-acupuncture-point-stimulation*.

There are a number of studies in which the acupuncture system was accessed without needles. Ballegaard et al[68] incorporated Shiatsu (which involves manual pressure to acupuncture points) in a treatment package which also included acupuncture and lifestyle adjustment. A series of 69 patients were treated with this package for angina pectoris. The results were positive.

Dundee and McMillan[69] report successfully using a portable-operated square wave stimulator fixed at 10Hz with a large EKG surface electrode on acupuncture point Pericardium 6 (P6) to control nausea and vomiting. Milne et al[70] did a systematic review of five randomized controlled trials of transcutaneous electrical nerve stimulation (TENS) for chronic low back pain. Active TENS treatment included both conventional and acupuncture-like modes. The variability of the outcome measures across studies and the small number of studies reviewed pointed to a clear need for more and better designed studies. Osiri et al,[71] in a systematic review of TENS, which included acupuncture-like TENS for knee osteoarthritis, reported positive support. However, here again was a need for better designed studies in this area. Chao et al used TENS over acupuncture points for pain relief during the first stage of labor.[72] Their results showed that TENS over acupuncture points provided significantly increased pain relief compared to placebo TENS (very low stimulation; sensory setting). Fargas-Babjak et al[73] used a surface electrical stimulation device designed by Bruce Pomeranz called the codetron (EHM Rehabilitation Technology, Ontario, Canada) to stimulate acupuncture points in patients with chronic pain. This randomized controlled, double-blind study showed benefit to patients. Galantino et al[74] demonstrated in a pilot study that surface electrical stimulation of acupuncture points ST36, LIV3, K1, and BL60 decreased pain in HIV patients with peripheral neuropathy. The source of electrical stimulation was an H-wave machine from Electronic Waveform Lab Inc (Cardiff, CA). Ng et al conducted a randomized controlled trial with knee osteoarthritis participants using electro-acupuncture (2 Hz) or TENS (2 Hz, pulse width of 200) compared to a education-based control group.[75] This study showed both electro-acupuncture and TENS (at acupuncture points) to be effective in significantly reducing osteoarthritis-based knee pain after eight treatment sessions. Wong[64] showed enhanced stroke rehabilitation using electrical stimulation of acupuncture points through surface electrodes. She used the HANS device of Wearnes Technology, Singapore.

Naeser et al[49] showed improvement in carpal tunnel syndrome patients by using a combination of cold laser acupuncture point stimulation and microamps TENS. This was done in a randomized controlled double-blind fashion. The laser device was Dynatronics model 1620 (Salt Lake City, UT) while the microamps TENS device was Microstim model 100 (Microstim Inc, Tamarac, FL). Pontinen[76] has written an entire book on low energy laser therapy. He discusses the stimulation of acupuncture points and trigger points for musculoskeletal disorders. In addition, he discusses cold laser therapy for other medical disorders.

In a literature review, Gur discusses the potential mechanisms of pain relief through laser therapy.[77] These include collagen proliferation, anti-inflammatory effects, circulation enhancement, peripheral nerve stimulation, and analgesic effects. In a study by Allais et al, acupuncture, TENS, and infrared laser therapy at acupuncture points was used for the treatment of transformed migraines.[78] The results showed that all three treatment groups showed a significant decrease in migraine frequency, but the acupuncture group demonstrated the longest-lasting beneficial effects. All three treatment groups utilized the same six acupuncture point locations (with additional points selected on an individual basis). The above studies point to the need for more randomized clinical trials to further determine optimal parameters for use in physical therapy clinical practice.

If one keeps in mind the above examples and remembers the long established practices of acupressure or shiatsu (manual pressure to the acupuncture points) one can easily imagine potential application to physical therapy.

RESEARCH POSSIBILITIES

In addition to randomized controlled trials with double blinding as some of the acupuncture system modalities might allow, individual physical therapists and small group physical therapy facilities might consider well-documented case studies and case series to improve their practices. These smaller studies would contribute to the field by stimulating new ideas and setting the stage for larger studies at university centers. Ottenbacher[79] has written a useful book for doing such research.

Also, some of the acupuncture system modalities can be utilized at home by patients. After initial training by a physical therapist, the physical therapist would act as a coach for setting goals and monitoring adherence to the home program. Research into methods of promoting home therapy adherence for acupuncture system modalities will be very important for our aging population.

DELIVERY OF CARE ISSUES

To do needle acupuncture requires a program of study followed by licensure or registration. To access the acupuncture system without needles may or may not require licensure or registration depending on the modality and individual state laws. However, further training in traditional Chinese anatomy and physiology is a requisite. The use of cold lasers and electrical stimulation of the acupuncture system requires training and/or supervision or collaboration with a physician acupuncturist or a licensed acupuncturist who is knowledgeable regarding the use of cold lasers and electrical stimulation in the acupuncture system. One must be aware of any applicable FDA regulations. For further information on training in TCM for nonphysicians, the reader can contact the following organizations:

✦ ACAOM—Accreditation Commission for Acupuncture and Oriental Medicine
  1010 Wayne Avenue, Suite 1270
  Silver Spring, MD 20910
  Phone: (301) 608-9680

✦ AOBTA—American Oriental Bodywork Therapy Association
  47 Jamaica Street
  Jamaica Plain, MA 02130
  Phone: (617) 522-0257

Medical doctors and doctors of osteopathy can contact:

✦ American Academy of Medical Acupuncture
  4929 Wilshire Boulevard, Suite 428
  Los Angeles, CA 90010
  Phone: (323) 937-5514

✦ American College of Acupuncture
  1021 Park Avenue
  New York, NY 10028
  Phone: (212) 876-9781

Conclusion

Acupuncture and its system of acupuncture points and meridians holds exciting promise for more effective physical therapy and presents opportunities for physical therapy research aimed at greater availability of care utilizing this Asian system of medicine. To move the profession of physical therapy forward, collaboration across borders is essential. The International Accupuncture Association of Physical Therapists (IAAPT) is an network of physical therapy associations and individuals interested in the practice of acupuncture. It was founded in 1991 and became a subgroup of the World Confederation of Physical Therapists in 1999. It was formed by a core group of physiotherapists from five countries, where physiotherapists had been practicing acupuncture from the early 1980s (eg, Australia, South Africa, New Zealand, Sweden, and United Kingdom). Standards of practice for basic safety have been established and accepted by member countries (http://www.iaapt.org). Although in the United States physical therapists are unable to insert needles for treatment, a number of acupuncture points are incorporated into clinical practice through electrical stimulation interventions. Therefore, greater knowledge of specific points relevant to optimizing treatment for various orthopedic conditions may be on the horizon for standardizing SEAPS and cold laser stimulation in clinical practice. Future clinical research is needed to determine dose-effect relationships, optimal timing to integrate acupuncture and/or physical therapy, and when would be ideal time for each therapy to intervene in the progression of treatment whether the condition is acute or chronic. Continued research is needed to develop more refined applications of this knowledge.

References

1. Kaptchuk T. *The Web That Has No Weaver: Understanding Chinese Medicine*. New York, NY: Congdon & Weed; 1993.
2. Liao SJ, Lee MHM, Ng LK. *Principles and Practice of Contemporary Acupuncture*. New York, NY: Marcel Dekker; 1994.
3. Xinnong C. *Chinese Acupuncture and Moxibustion*. Beijing: Foreign Languages Press; 1987:108-109.
4. Xinnong C. *Chinese Acupuncture and Moxibustion*. Beijing: Foreign Languages Press; 1987:439-441.
5. Pomeranz B. Scientific basis of acupuncture. In: Stux G, Pomeranz B, eds. *Acupuncture: Textbook and Atlas*. Berlin: Springer-Verlag; 1987:1-34.
6. Han J. Central neurotransmitters and acupuncture analgesia. In: Stux G, Pomeranz B, eds. *Scientific Basis of Acupuncture*. Berlin: Springer-Verlag; 1989:7-34.
7. Pomeranz B. Acupuncture research related to pain, drug addiction and nerve regeneration. In: Stux G, Pomeranz B, eds. *Scientific Basis of Acupuncture*. Berlin: Springer-Verlag; 1989:35-52.
8. Napadow V, Webb JM, Pearson N, Hammerschlag R. Neurobiological correlates of acupuncture: November 17-18, 2005 conference report. *J Altern Complement Med*. 2006;12(9):931-935.
9. Wu M-T, Hsieh J-C, Xiong J, et al. Central nervous pathway for acupuncture stimulation: localization of processing with functional MR imaging of the brain—preliminary experience. *Neuroradiology*. 1999;212:133-141.
10. Cheng RS, Pomeranz BH. Electroacupuncture analgesia is mediated by stereospecific opiate receptors and is reversed by antagonists of type I receptors. *Life Sci*. 1979;26:631-639.
11. Han JS, Xic GX. Dynorphin: important mediator for electroacupuncture analgesia in the spinal cord of the rabbit. *Pain*. 1984;18:367-377.
12. Peets J, Pomeranz B. CXBX mice deficient in opiate receptors show poor electroacupuncture analgesia. *Nature*. 1978; 273:675-676.
13. Murai M, Takeshige C, et al. Correlation between individual variations in effectiveness of acupuncture analgesia and that in contents of brain endogenous morphine-like factors. In: Takeshige C, ed. *Studies on the Mechanism of Acupuncture Analgesia Based on Animal Experiments*. Tokyo: Showa University Press; 1986:542.
14. Pert A, Dionne R, Ng L, Bragin E, Moody TW, Pert CB. Alterations in rat central nervous system endorphins following transauricular electroacupuncture. *Brain Res*. 1981;224:83-98.
15. Ehrenpreis S. Analgesic properties of enkephalinase inhibitors: animal and human studies. *Prog Clin Biol Res*. 1985; 192:363-370.
16. Lee Peng CH, Yang MMP, et al. Endorphin release: a possible mechanism of AA. *Comp Med East West*. 1978;6:57-60.
17. Cheng R, Pomeranz B, Yu G. Dexamethasone partially reduces and 2% saline treatment abolishes electroacupuncture analgesia: these findings implicate pituitary endorphins. *Life Sci*. 1979;24:1481-1486.

18. Pomeranz B. Relation of stress-induced analgesia to acupuncture analgesia. *Annals of the New York Academy of Sciences.* 1986;467(1):444-447.

19. Pomeranz B, Chiu D. Naloxone blocks acupuncture analgesia and causes hyperalgesia: endorphin is implicated. *Life Sci.* 1976;19:1757-1762.

20. Lee MHM, Ernst M., Clinical and research observations on acupuncture analgesia and thermography. In: Stux G, Pomeranz B, eds. *Scientific Basis of Acupuncture.* Berlin: Springer-Verlag; 1989:157-176.

21. Sakai S, Hori E, Umeno K, et al. Specific acupuncture sensation correlates with EEGs and autonomic changes in human subjects. *Autonomic Neuroscience.* 2007;133:158-169.

22. Knardahl S, Elam M, Bengt O, Wallin G. Sympathetic nerve activity after acupuncture in humans. *Pain.* 1998; 75:19-25.

23. Liao SJ, Wen K. Patient's hypnotizability and their responses to acupuncture treatments for pain relief. A preliminary statistical study. *Am J Acupuncture.* 1976;4:263-268.

24. Peng ATC, Behar S, Yu SJ. Long term therapeutic effects of electroacupuncture for chronic neck and shoulder pain—a double blind study. *Acupunct Electrother Res.* 1987;12:37-44.

25. Ulett G. Studies supporting the concept of physiological acupuncture. In: Stux G, Pomeranz B, eds. *Scientific Basis of Acupuncture.* Berlin: Springer-Verlag; 1989:177-196.

26. Barber J, Mayer DJ. Evaluation of the efficacy and neural mechanism of a hypnotic analgesia procedure in experimental and clinical dental pain. *Pain.* 1977;4:41-48.

27. Goldstein A, Hilgard ER. Failure of opiate antagonist naloxone to modify hypnotic analgesia. *Proc Nat Acad Sci.* 1975;72:2041-2043.

28. Nasrallah HA, Holley TY, Janowsky DS. Opiate antagonism fails to reverse hypnotic-induced analgesia. *Lancet.* 1979;1(8130):1355.

29. Lu DP, Lu GP, Kleinman L. Acupuncture and clinical hypnosis for facial and neck pain: a single crossover comparison. *Am J Clin Hypn.* 2001;44(2):141-148.

30. Chapman CR, Chen AC, Bonica JJ. Effects of intrasegmental electrical acupuncture on dental pain: evaluation by threshold estimation and sensory decision theory. *Pain.* 1977;3:213-227.

31. Stacher G, Wancura I, et al. Effect of acupuncture on pain threshold and pain tolerance determined by electrical stimulation of the skin: a controlled study. *Am J Chin Med.* 1975;3:143-146.

32. Vincent CA, Richardson PH. The evaluation of therapeutic acupuncture: concepts and methods. *Pain.* 1986;24: 1-13.

33. Kleinhenz J, Streitberger K, Windeler J, et al. Randomised clinical trial comparing the effects of acupuncture and a newly designed placebo needle in rotator cuff tendinitis. *Pain.* 1999;83:235-241

34. Lund I, Lundeberg T. Are minimal, superficial or sham acupuncture procedures acceptable as inert placebo controls? *Acupunct Med.* 2006;24(1):13-15.

35. Kong J, Gollub R, Rosman IS, et al. Brain activity associated with expectancy-enhanced placebo analgesia as measured by functional magnetic resonance imaging. *J Neurosci.* 2006;26(2):381-388.

36. Melzack R, Stillwell DM, Fox EJ. Trigger points and acupuncture points for pain: correlations and implications. *Pain.* 1987;3:3-23.

37. Dung H. Anatomical features contributing to the formation of acupuncture points. *Am J Acupunct.* 1984;12:139-143.

38. Shang C. The past, present and future of meridian system research. *Clinical Acupuncture and Oriental Medicine.* 2000; 1:115-124.

39. Li AH, Zhang JM, Xie YK. Human acupuncture points mapped in rats are associated with excitable muscle/skin-nerve complexes with enriched nerve endings. *Brain Res.* 2004;1012:154-159.

40. Wick F, Wick N, Wick MC. Morphological analysis of human acupuncture points through immunohistochemistry. *Am J Phys Med Rehab.* 2007;86(1):7-11.

41. Langevin HM, Churchill DL, Fox JR, et al. Biomechanical response to acupuncture needling in humans. *J Applied Physiol.* 2001;91:2471-2478.

42. Soh K-S. Bonghan duct and acupuncture meridian as optical channel of biophoton. *J Kor Phys Soc.* 2004;45:1196-1198.

43. Dhond RP, Kettner N, Napadow V. Neuroimagining acupuncture effects in the brain. *J Altern Complement Med.* 2007; 13:603-616.

44. Newberg AB, LaRiccia PJ, Lee BY, et al. Cerebral blood flow effects of pain and acupuncture: a preliminary single-photon emission computed tomography imagining study. *J Neuroimagining.* 2005;15:43-49.

45. NIH Consensus Development Panel on Acupuncture. *JAMA.* 1998;280:1518-1524.

46. Norheim AJ, Fønnebø V. Acupuncture adverse effects are more than occasional case reports: results from questionnaires among 1,135 randomly selected doctors and 197 acupuncturists. *Compl Therap Med.* 1996;4:8-13.

47. MacPherson H, Thomas K, Walters S, Fitter M. The York acupuncture safety study: prospective survey of 34,000 treatments by traditional acupuncturists. *BMJ.* 2001;323:486-487.

48. Ernst E, White A. Prospective studies of the safety of acupuncture: a systematic review. *Am J Med.* 2001;110:481-485.

49. Naeser MA, Hahn K, Lieberman B. Real vs. sham laser acupuncture and microamp TENS to treat carpal tunnel syndrome and work-site wrist pain: pilot study. *Lasers Surg Med.* 1996;8(suppl):7.

50. Hammerslag R. Methodological and ethical issues in acupuncture research. NIH Consensus Development Conference on Acupuncture. November, 1997:45-49.

51. Jerner B, Skogh M, Vahlquist A. A controlled trial of acupuncture in psoriasis: no convincing effect. *Acta Dermato-Venereologica.* 1997;77:154-156.

52. MacPherson H, White A, Cummings M, et al. Standards for reporting interventions in controlled trials of acupuncture: the STRICTA recommendations. *J Altern Complement Med.* 2002;8:85-89.

53. Shlay JC, Chaloner K, Max MB, et al. Acupuncture and amitriptyline for pain due to HIV-related peripheral neuropathy: a randomized controlled trial. *JAMA.* 1998;280:1590-1595.

54. Berman BM, Singh B, Lao L, et al. A randomized trial of acupuncture as an adjunctive therapy in osteoarthritis of the knee. *Rheumatology.* 1999;38:346-354.

55. White AR, Eernst E. A systematic review of randomized controlled trials of acupuncture for neck pain. *Rheumatology.* 1999;38:143-147.

56. van Tulder MW, Cherkin DC, Berman B, Lao L, Koes BW. The effectiveness of acupuncture in the management of acute and chronic low back pain: a systematic review within the framework of the Cochrane Collaboration back review group. *Spine.* 1999;24:1113-1123.

57. Ernst E, White A. Acupuncture for back pain: a meta-analysis of randomized controlled trials. *Arch Intern Med.* 1998;158:2235-2241.

58. Naeser MA, Alexander MP, Stiassny-Eder DGV, Hobbs J, Buchman D. Real vs. sham acupuncture in the treatment of paralysis in acute stroke patients—a CT scan lesion site study. *J Neurol Rehab.* 1992;6:163-173.

59. Shen J. Adjunct antiemesis electroacupuncture in stem cell transplantation. *Proc Amer Soc Clin Oncol.* 1997;148:2a.

60. Dincer F, Linde K. Sham interventions in randomized clinical trials of acupuncture—a review. *Compl Therap Med.* 2003;11: 235-242.

61. Wolfe MM, Lichtenstein DR, Singh G. Gastrointestinal toxicity of nonsteroidal antiinflammatory drugs. *N Engl J Med.* 1999;340:1888-1899.

62. Lazarou J, Pomeranz B, Corey PN. Incidence of adverse drug reactions in hospitalized patients: a meta-analysis of prospective studies. *JAMA.* 1998;279:1200-1205.

63. Johansson K, Lindgren I, Widner H, Wiklung I, Johansson BB. Can sensory stimulation improve the functional outcome in stroke patients? *Neurology.* 1993;43:2189-2192.

64. Wong AM, Su TY, Tang FT, Cheng PT, Liaw MY. Clinical trial of electrical acupuncture on hemiplegic stroke patients. *Am J Phys Med Rehab.* 1999;78:117-122.

65. Ernst E, White A. Acupuncture as a treatment for temporomandibular joint dysfunction: a systematic review of randomized trials. *Arch Otolaryngol Head Neck Surg.* 1999;125:269-272.

66. Stux G, Pomeranz BE. *Acupuncture: Textbook and Atlas.* Berlin: Springer-Verlag; 1987.

67. Xinnong C. *Chinese Acupuncture and Moxibustion.* Beijing: Foreign Languages Press; 1987.

68. Ballegaard S, Norrelund S, Smith DF. Cost-benefit use of acupuncture, Shiatsu and lifestyle adjustment for treatment of patients with severe angina pectoris. *Acupunct Electrother Res Int J.* 1966;21:187-97.

69. Dundee JW, McMillan C. Clinical uses of P6 acupuncture antiemesis. *Acupunct Electrother Res Int J.* 1990;15:211-215.

70. Milne S, Welch V, Brosseau L, et al. Transcutaneous electrical nerve stimulation (TENS) for chronic low back pain (Cochrane Review). *Cochrane Database Syst Rev.* 2001;2:CD003008.

71. Osiri M, Welch V, Brosseuau L, et al. Transcutaneous electrical nerve stimulation for knee osteoarthritis (Cochrane Review). *Cochrane Database Syst Rev.* 2000;4:CD002328.

72. Chao, AS, Chao, A, Wang, TH, et al. Pain relief by applying transcutaneous electrical nerve stimulation (TENS) on acupuncture points during the first stage of labor: a randomized double-blind placebo-controlled trial. *Pain.* 2007;127:214.

73. Fargas-Babjak AM, Pomeranz B, Rooney PJ. Acupuncture like stimulation with codetron for rehabilitation of patients with chronic pain syndrome and osteoarthritis. *Acupunct Electrother Res Int J.* 1992;17:95-105.

74. Galantino MLA, Eke-Oro S, Findley TW, Condalucci D. Use of noninvasive electroacupuncture for the treatment of HIV-related peripheral neuropathy: a pilot study. *J Altern Complementary Med.* 1999;3:135-142.

75. Ng MM, Leung MC, Poon DM. The effects of electro-acupuncture and transcutaneous electrical nerve stimulation on patients with painful osteoarthritic knees: a randomized controlled trial with follow-up evaluation. *J Altern Complement Med.* 2003;9(5):641-649.

76. Pontinen P. *Low Level Laser Therapy as a Medical Treatment Modality.* Jarmpere, Findland: Art Urpo Ltd; 1992.

77. Gur A. Physical therapy modalities in management of fibromyalgia. *Curr Pharm Des.* 2006;12(1):29-35.

78. Allais G, De Lorenzo C, Quirico PE, et al. Non-pharmacological approaches to chronic headaches: transcutaneous eletrical nerve stimulation, lasertherapy and acupuncture in transformed migriane treatment. *Neurol Sci.* 2003;24: S138-S142.

79. Ottenbacher K. *Evaluating Clinical Change: Strategies for Occupational and Physical Therapists.* Baltimore, MD: Williams and Wilkins; 1986.

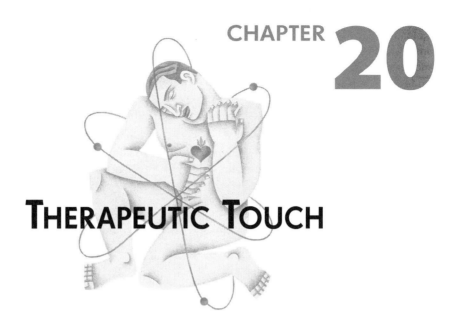

CHAPTER 20

THERAPEUTIC TOUCH

Ellen Zambo Anderson, PT, MA, GCS

Introduction

Therapeutic Touch (TT) is a complementary therapy used to promote health and healing. A modern interpretation of the "laying of hands" but without a religious context, TT is offered as an intervention for reducing pain and anxiety, accelerating the healing process and promoting a sense of well-being.[1] TT was developed in the 1970s by Delores Krieger, RN, PhD and Dora Kunz, and follows a protocol of assessment and intervention that is different from similar sounding approaches such as *Healing Touch, Touch for Health,* or *Therapeutic Massage.* The name TT is nevertheless, misleading because the practitioner does not always need to touch the client or patient to provide a therapeutic intervention. TT is considered by many to be a nursing intervention and is taught in many nursing school curricula across the country. Krieger, herself a nurse, and Kunz, however, believe that any person who wants to facilitate health and healing can become a TT practitioner.[2] Specific medical or psychological training is not required to become a TT practitioner.

History

The work of Krieger and Kunz began in the 1960s when Krieger was studying at New York University's School of Nursing. Krieger, who has since been named professor emeritus at NYU, and Kunz, a psychic healer, set out to investigate the phenomenon and characteristics of people known as "healers." Their observations of healers and research into ancient medical systems led them to the conclusion that healers are not "chosen" by a higher entity. Rather, healers merely possess a heightened sensitivity to their patient's state of health and being and are able to effect change through intention and energy. Krieger's belief that others are capable of developing this heightened sensitivity motivated her to develop a process in which a patient's status could be assessed and enhanced through intention and modulation of energy. Krieger points out, however, that TT does not "cure" diseases or other medical conditions. Rather, TT facilitates an improvement in energy flow, thereby creating an environment in which the body's own healing powers can be maximized.

Therapeutic Touch and Energy Fields

The concept of internal and external subtle energies and their relationship to health has been promoted in many ancient medical systems such as Ayurveda and traditional Chinese medicine.[3,4] Contemporary scientists and philosophers have also suggested theoretical frameworks pertaining to the existence and interaction of biological, environmental, and spiritual energy. Weber[5,6] has integrated ideas from ancient Eastern philosophies of energy with concepts of quantum physics and the work of theoretical physicist David Bohm.[7,8] He suggests that the universe is a unitary flow of energy and that all matter and life are inextricably linked. Similarly, Rogers[9,10] has proposed that humans are multidimensional energy fields indivisible with energy fields of the environment and all matter. Furthermore, Rogers suggests that energy fields are distinguishable by their patterns and that energy fields are infinite, open, and in continuous motion. Defined according to Rogers' framework, TT is a plausible intervention in which the practitioner is able to detect the energy fields and patterns of a client and modulate, if necessary, the energy fields with the intention of promoting health and wellness.

Therapeutic Touch and Chakras

Krieger's writings[1,2,11] reflect a close alignment with the assumptions and teachings of *Ayurveda*, a medical system that has been practiced in India for more that 5000 years.[3] Ayurveda assumes that all life is based on vital life energy known as prana and that that mind, body, spirit, and environment are inextricably linked. Disease is the end result of energetic imbalance among these domains and disharmony with the environment. Ayurveda holds that vital energy is centered in seven major and several lesser chakras located throughout the body. The seven major *chakras*, which means "wheels" in Sanskrit, are described as "whirling vortices of energy."[12] They are located within the body's core and are aligned vertically from the base of the coccyx to the crown. Each chakra is associated with a major endocrine gland and nerve plexus and is responsible for receiving, transforming, and releasing vital life energy. Lesser chakras are located, in addition to other areas, in the palms and feet. Krieger proposes that TT practitioners utilize the hand chakras to perceive and modulate the energy of their clients.

Foundational Premises of Therapeutic Touch

Krieger offers four premises that underpin TT's process and approach to healing. The first assumption is that the body is an open energy system that allows for the transfer of energy between people and the environment. The second assumption is that the body is bilaterally symmetrical, inferring that there is a pattern to the underlying human energy field. The third and fourth are that illness is the result of energy imbalance and the body can often initiate self-healing.[2]

The Practice of Therapeutic Touch

A typical TT session runs about 20 to 30 minutes, but reports from practitioners indicate that some sessions may run as little as 5 minutes or as long as 1 hour. Although TT is not contraindicated for any specific conditions, practitioners are encouraged to limit the time of their intervention for persons who are elderly, young, or very weak. TT is usually performed with the client fully dressed and sitting in a chair or standing. A TT practitioner begins the process by centering his or her consciousness.[1] Centering is considered to be a journey toward one's inner being. In this personal space, the practitioner appreciates a sense of being quiet, fully integrated, and focused.[2] From this state of centeredness, the practitioner is able to initiate an assessment of the client's subtle energy fields. In the "assessment" phase of TT, the practitioner places his or her palms 2 to 3 inches from the client's head, using the spine as a reference for bilateral symmetry. The practitioner then moves his or her hands down the client's body, carefully noting characteristics of the client's energy field and acknowledging the energy flow that is perceived. During this assessment phase, the TT practitioner will make note of how the client's energy feels and begin to determine which centers or areas can benefit from intervention. A practitioner, for example, may describe a client's energy as feeling tingly, vibratory, or cold, or the practitioner may perceive a client's energy flow to be sluggish or blocked in a certain area and will make a mental note to return to that area with the intention of improving that energy flow.

Krieger describes the next step in the TT process to be "unruffling the field," which she explains to be a sweeping away of bound up or congested energy.[2] This activity can also be used to re-establish rhythm in the client's energy field and set the stage for the practitioner to begin directing and modulating the transfer and flow of human energy. During this step, the practitioner can direct his or her own energy to the client and/or direct the client's own energy. Directing and modulating is performed with the intention of balancing the flow and amount of energy so that the client's energy field is perceived to be symmetrical. Lastly, TT practitioners assess the client's energy field to determine that the intervention is complete. Krieger suggests that improving energy flow and balance is critical in creating an environment in which healing can occur.

Training in Therapeutic Touch

Nurse Healers Professional-North America is an organization that was established to promote the work and teaching of TT (http://www.therapeutic-touch.org). Krieger reported teaching TT to more than 48,000 people worldwide and estimated that more than 85,000 people have learned TT.[13] Education and training in TT is usually conducted in full weekend seminars. After two weekends of training and practice, most students feel confident offering TT to their family members, clients, and patients as a healing modality. Although there are no standard requirements or certification to be a TT practitioner, Krieger and Patricia Winstead-Fry, PhD, RN developed the Self-Evaluation of Therapeutic Touch Scale (SETTS).[1] This measurement tool can assist clients and researchers in determining experienced and proficient practitioners from those who are less experienced.

Evidence of Efficacy

Unlike many other energy-based complementary therapies, TT has received much attention in the scientific literature. As with most emerging approaches in health and medicine, descriptive articles and anecdotal reports dominated the early literature. Since the 1980s, however, numerous researchers have investigated TT, and several review articles have been written since 1997 on the state of research on TT.[14-23] Perhaps the most well-known controversial research with TT was published in the April 1, 1998 issue of the *Journal of the American Medical Association*[24] wherein a sixth grade student conducted an experiment in which TT practitioners were asked to detect whether the experimenter's hand was closer to the practitioner's left or right hand. Of the 280 trials conducted, the practitioners identified the correct hand 44% of the time. The results were written in part by the young student's mother, a member of the Questionable Nurse Practices Task Force, National Council Against Health Fraud Inc, and the cofounder of Quackwatch Inc, a Web site dedicated to identifying health fraud and quackery. The authors concluded that failure to accurately detect human energy fields is "...unrefuted evidence that the claims of TT are groundless and that further professional use is unjustified."[20] Critics of the study were quick to identify serious flaws in the study's design.[25-27] and improper statistical analysis.[27] In addition, Leskowitz[26] suggested that the only logical conclusion of this study is that given the described set of experimental conditions, a human energy field could not be reliably detected. The leap to refuting TT is unsubstantiated because the intervention of TT as described by Krieger[2] was never administered.

Reduction of Anxiety

Most research in TT has focused on its effectiveness for the reduction of pain and anxiety, and enhancement of healing processes Although several researchers have investigated the effectiveness of TT in reducing anxiety, Robinson, Biley and Dolk[23] were unable to identify any studies that included subjects with an anxiety disorder as defined by the *Diagnostic and Statistical Manual of Mental Disorders* (DSM-IV), the *International Classification of Diseases* (ICD-10), or any other validated diagnostic instruments. Instead, anxiety has been associated with stress and mood and has not been identified, as a specific diagnosis for subjects in TT research. In fact, comparing the results of the studies that have included anxiety as an outcome measure is often difficult due to subject variability and/or differences in how anxiety is measured. Ireland,[28] for example, demonstrated that children ages 6 to 12 who were HIV positive and received TT experienced a significant reduction in anxiety compared to control subjects who received sham or mock TT. Anxiety was measured using a subscale of the Spielberger State-Trait Anxiety Inventory (STAI) for Children. Kramer[29] also investigated the use of TT with children, but her subjects were 2 weeks to 2 years of age and were not HIV positive. The subjects in Kramer's study were hospitalized for either an acute illness, injury, or surgery; stress or anxiety reduction was determined by measuring heart rate, skin temperature, and galvanic skin response.

Hospitalized patients have been subjects in at least six studies investigating TT and reduction in anxiety. Quinn[30] and Heidt[31] studied patients admitted to a hospital with cardiovascular diagnoses. Both researchers found subjects who received TT reported significant reductions in anxiety on the STAI compared to control groups who received mock or placebo TT. Turner and colleagues[32] measured anxiety using the visual analogue scale (VAS) for anxiety and found that TT was associated with a reduction in anxiety of patients hospitalized for severe burns. Gangne and Toye[33] compared TT with relaxation therapy and sham TT for inpatients with psychiatric diagnoses and found TT was more effective than sham TT in reducing anxiety, but that relaxation therapy was just as effective as TT. In a study of hospitalized pregnant women known to have chemical dependency, daily TT sessions were found to help reduce anxiety and withdrawal symptoms when compared to women who received either standard ward care or a shared activity period with a registered nurse.[34] Simington and Laing[35] investigated the use of TT to reduce anxiety in patients in a long-term care facility rather than patients admitted to an acute care hospital. They found that TT significantly reduced state anxiety in institutionalized elderly. Samarel and colleagues[36] studied the use of dialogue and TT with patients who had to undergo surgery for breast cancer. Treatment was administered in subject's home within 7 days of surgery and 24 hours after hospital discharge. The experimental group received 10 minutes of TT and 20 minutes of dialogue. The control group received 10 minutes of sitting quietly and 20 minutes of dialogue. The experimental group had significantly lower preoperative anxiety scores than the control group, but no difference was found in postoperative measures. Similar results were reported by Frank and colleagues.[37] In this experiment, 82 women received either TT (n=42) or sham TT (n=40) as they underwent a stereotactic core biopsy (SCB) of a breast lesion. Using a VAS, all subjects were found to have less fear and feelings of restlessness and nervousness post-SCB as compared to pre-SCB scores, but no differences were seen between the TT and sham TT groups.

Lin and Taylor[38] investigated the efficacy of TT in reducing anxiety in an elderly population. Unlike other studies that utilized either inpatient or outpatient subjects, these researchers recruited and obtained subjects from long-term care facilities as well as community senior centers and adult day care programs. Anxiety was measured with Form Y-1 of the STAI and was found to be significantly reduced in subjects who received TT as compared to subjects who received mock TT.

Applying TT with healthy subjects has also been investigated. Olson and Sneed[39] administered TT to professional caregiver/health care students who were grouped as either having high anxiety or low-moderate anxiety according to the results of three self-report measures of anxiety: Profile of Mood States, STAI, and VAS. Both groups were then split, with half of the subjects receiving TT and the other half sitting quietly for 15 minutes. No statistically significant reduction of anxiety was found between groups, but reduction of anxiety for the high-anxiety group was greater with TT compared to the high-anxiety group who sat quietly. The authors suggested that a larger sample size would be necessary to determine statistically significant differences. Small sample size is also concern in a study by Engle and Graney[40] in which 11 healthy subjects received one session of either TT or sham TT. Pulse rate and amplitude, blood pressure, skin temperature, anxiety, perceived health status, and time perception were measured pre- and post-intervention. No differences were noted except for significant decreases in total pulse amplitude and perceived duration of time. A reduction of total pulse amplitude may indicate vasoconstriction and a potential adverse effect of TT whereas the clinical importance of a decreased perceived duration of time is unclear. Lafreniere and colleagues[41] investigated TT in healthy subjects and reported that participants who were randomly assigned to receive TT showed a significantly greater reduction in mood disturbance and anxiety compared to subjects who did not receive TT. Although the design of this study included random assignment, the control group did not receive sham TT and thus subjects were aware if they received or did not receive TT. This design flaw seriously limits the conclusions that can be made from this experiment.

A review of the literature suggests that TT's usefulness in reducing anxiety in unclear. Although a number of researchers have reported benefits of TT, others have found no effects when compared to control groups that received sham TT. In particular, it appears that TT is not particularly effective for reducing anxiety in young, healthy subjects. One must consider, however, that researchers of TT have used different definitions of anxiety and measurement tools, making it a challenge to compare results. In addition, research designs have been inconsistent and frequently poor. Variability in assignment methods; blinding, frequency, and duration of the intervention; and lack of an appropriate control group make it difficult to support or refute the application of TT for anxiety. Certainly, facilitating a reduction in anxiety can be beneficial for the therapist-patient/client relationship and rehabilitation process. Perhaps of equal concern for health care providers are interventions that are effective for reducing pain.

Evidence of Efficacy in the Reduction of Pain

Several researchers have investigated the potential of TT to reduce pain in a variety of patient populations. In two previously cited studies measuring anxiety, Samarel et al[36] and Turner et al[32] also included pain measures in their assessment of TT. Samarel and colleagues found a reduction of pain in patients with breast cancer who received TT, but the amount of pain relief did not reach statistical significance. Turner, on the other hand, reported a significant reduction in pain on the McGill Pain Questionnaire with patients who were admitted to the hospital with serious burns. Researchers have also found that TT appears to be helpful in reducing pain in other patient populations.

Leskowitz[42] presented a case report in which a 62-year-old man with a 4-year history of phantom limb pain was successfully treated with TT. Prior to the application of TT, the subject's pain ranged from an 8 to 10 on a self-reported VAS with 10 being the maximum intensity. Previous interventions, such as medication, stress management, hypnosis, transcutaneous nervous stimulation (TENS), and ultrasound, reduced his pain to between 6 and 8, but long-term pain management with all of these techniques were inadequate. In contrast, the subject reported 0 pain on the VAS with the first TT session; and with self-administered TT, the subject has been able to maintain his pain at a 0 to 1 on a VAS.

Two studies were conducted to assess the potential for TT to decrease pain in patients with osteoarthritis.[43,44] In the study by Eckes Peck,[43] a two-group longitudinal design was used in which subjects served as their own controls and repeated VASs were used to measure pain and distress. Subjects in one group received TT, whereas subjects in the other group received progressive muscular relaxation (PMR). A statistically significant decrease in pain was recorded in the TT group from baseline to the first TT session, with further decreases noted in subsequent treatments. Similarly, the mean score for pain decreased progressively with each session of PMR. However, when TT and PMR were compared using multivariate analysis of variance, PMR was found to be more effective for decreasing pain than TT.

In a single-blind, randomized, control experiment, Gordon, Merenstein, D'Amico, and Hudgens[44] also investigated the effect TT might have for reducing pain in patients with OA. Subjects were proportionately randomized based on OA severity into one of three subject groups. Pain was measured using a VAS and the West Haven-Yale Multidimensional Pain Inventory (MPI). The treatment group received TT, the placebo group received mock TT (MTT), and the control group received no intervention. In comparing pain reduction across the groups, the group who received TT had significantly decreased pain when compared to both the placebo and control groups.

Lin and Taylor[38] conducted a single-blind randomized experiment to assess whether TT was helpful in reducing chronic pain in older adults. Subjects either received TT, MTT, or standard care. Similar to Gordon's findings,[44] subjects who received TT were found to have significantly less pain when compared to both the placebo and control groups although the investigators measured pain using an 11-point numeric rating scale rather than a VAS or the MPI. Gregory and Verdouw[45] have also reported that older adults living in a care facility have benefited from TT, including a 40% reduction of pain. The researchers, however, "...sought to be as inclusive as possible in the context of a range of behavioral and physiological conditions," did not seek to control for any confounding variables, and did not include a control group in their design. Giasson and Bouchard[46] did have a control group when they investigated the effect of TT on the well-being of 20 persons with terminal cancer and found that after each of three TT sessions subjects reported improvement in their appetite and sense of inner peace and a reduction of pain. TT was also investigated with subjects who had chronic pain associated with fibromyalgia syndrome.[47] Subjects either received TT (n=10) or listened to tapes about complementary therapies (n=5) once a week for 6 weeks. No statistically significant improvement was noted on the Short From McGill Pain Questionnaire (SF-MPQ), VAS, or Fibromyalgia Health Assessment Questionnaire (FHAQ). In a single-blinded cross-over study by Blankfield and colleagues,[48] persons with chronic pain associated with carpal tunnel syndrome received either six sessions of TT or six sessions of sham TT. Although there were no significant differences between the two groups in terms of changes in median motor nerve distal latencies, pain scores, and relaxation scores, both groups demonstrated significant immediate changes from baseline for all three dependent variables. The researchers have identified several limitations of the study including small sample size and potential bias of the TT practitioners who also collected the electroneurometer data. They have also offered several interpretations of their findings. One interpretation that seems to warrant further investigation is the possibility that both TT and sham TT facilitated a relaxation response that may have influenced physiologic processes and contributed to the observed improvements in median nerve conduction velocities.

The effect of TT on acute pain rather than chronic pain has also been explored. Keller and Bzdek[49] demonstrated that subjects who received TT had their tension headaches reduced by an average of 70% on the McGill-Melzack Pain Questionnaire (MMPQ). This reduction was significant when compared to subjects who received MTT and reported an average 35% decline in their headaches. Meehan[50] assessed pain reduction in subjects who had postoperative pain from abdominal or pelvic surgery. Using a single-blind, randomized, single trial design, Meehan randomly assigned subjects to one of three groups: TT group, MTT group, and standard intervention (narcotic analgesic group). Subjects who received TT reported a reduction in pain of 13%, whereas subjects who received MTT did not report any pain control. Subjects who received standard intervention, however, experienced a 42% reduction in pain, indicating that analgesics were the intervention of choice for pain management in this patient population. Several researchers have investigated the use of TT for pain reduction in subjects across a wide range of diagnoses and conditions. The literature provides some preliminary evidence to support the use of TT with older adults and persons with osteoarthritis. Other research suggests that TT may be helpful in managing phantom limb pain, headaches, and pain associated with burns, although many studies have been of limited quality with issues related to the studies' design and methods. Inclusion of a control group, use of sham or MTT, duration and frequency and TT, and type of outcome measures are fairly inconsistent across the studies, limiting the ability to draw firm conclusions about the efficacy of TT for reducing pain. Most investigators have also identified small sample size as a factor that challenges the measurement of TT's effect and the studies' external validity.

Evidence of Efficacy in Wound Healing

Although most of the experimental studies in TT have assessed TT's efficacy for reduction of pain and anxiety, a few studies have been conducted to assess TT's capacity to facilitate wound healing. In 1992, Wirth[51] published the results of a study he conducted in which subjects received incised, full-thickness dermal wounds in their lateral deltoid muscle. Half the subjects received TT; the other half received no intervention. The subjects in the TT group healed significantly faster than the control group, with complete healing noted in 57% of treated subjects compared to 0% of the 23 controls. Wirth attempted to advance his research by replicating experiments and conducting double-blind, randomized studies,[52-54] but he cited many problematic variables and inconsistent results.

Therapeutic Touch and Immune System Function

Researchers have begun to consider the interdisciplinary field of psychoneuroimmunology as a potential way of explaining the mechanism by which TT may act on the body and whether measurable physiologic changes are associated with the commonly used self-report outcome measures such as the VAS and STAI. Quinn and Strelkauskas[30] investigated the effects of TT on both bereaved subjects and the TT practitioners providing the intervention. Psychological measures included the STAI and Affect Balance Scale (ABS). A profile of immune functioning was established for practitioners and recipients by measuring lymphocyte subset composition, mixed lymphocyte reactivity (MLC), cell-mediated toxicity (CML), lymphocyte stimulation (mitogen responsiveness), and natural killer cells. In general, changes identified in each participant's immunological profile were extremely varied from person to person except in percentage of T8 cells. T8 or suppressor T-cells were identified in terms of lymphocyte subset composition using cytoflurographic analysis. The percentage of suppressor T-cells was found to be dramatically reduced in subjects following TT and at very low levels for the practitioners at all times. The authors concluded that TT appears to have an impact on lymphocyte subset composition through a diminution of T8 cells. From this conclusion, the researchers hypothesized that TT might enhance immune function by reducing immune suppression.

Olson, Sneed, LaVia, Virella, Bonadonna, and Michel[55] also sought to determine whether TT would have an effect on the immunological profile of highly stressed subjects. Subjects were randomly assigned to either the experimental group, who received three sessions of TT, or to the control group, who did not receive any intervention. In addition to measuring stress, anxiety, and mood, the researchers obtained blood from each subject to measure three immunoglobulin classes (IgG, IgA, IgM), the IgG subclasses, and lymphocyte subpopulations. Serum immunoglobulin levels and quantification of lymphocyte subpopulations are frequently used as indicators for immune system functioning. The results of the study did not support the hypothesis of the authors. Subjects who received TT did not have significantly different levels of IgA, IgM, IgG, or lymphocyte levels when compared to the control subjects. The authors noted that the direction of change in the immunoglobulin and lymphocyte levels was supportive of their hypothesis, but that statistical significance had not been reached. A subsequent power calculation suggests that the sample size for this experiment should be 90 subjects per group. The pilot study by Olson and her colleagues was conducted with 22 subjects.[55]

Therapeutic Touch and Muscle and Autonomic Nervous System Activity

Wirth and Cram[56] also sought a physiologic explanation for the therapeutic effects of TT, but did not use immune function measures in their study. Instead, they measured physiologic variables, including surface electromagnetic (EMG) activity at four different muscle groups, heart rate, hand temperature, head temperature, and end tidal CO_2 levels. Wirth and Cram's study also differed from others in that they utilized subjects who were daily meditators and, for the most part, had no acute or chronic health or psychological abnormalities. Several issues regarding the experimental design, subject selection, and independent variables raise concern for the reliability of the results, but subjects who received TT had a significant reduction in EMG activity at the C4, T6, and L3 paraspinals. The autonomic indicators showed a general trend toward lower arousal, but the decline was not significant.

The effect that TT may or may not have on bodily systems requires much more research. Links between stress, anxiety, and pain reduction with psychoneuroimmunological changes seem logical, but determining the appropriate dependent variables requires additional study. Researchers may need to consider a multitude of physiologic responses that together facilitate improvement in one's sense of well-being. At the same time, scientists may need to expand the work of Quinn and Strelkauskas[30] to understand what, if any, physiological changes occur in TT practitioners as they provide TT to their clients.

Limitations in Research Design in Many Studies

Several authors have written reviews of the TT literature and concluded that further despite preliminary research that supports the use of TT for pain, much more study and better research is required before clear recommendations about TT can be made.[14-21]

One methodological issue often discussed is the duration of the TT intervention. TT, as described by Krieger, may be offered in sessions from 5 minutes to over 30 minutes, depending on the needs of the client. It is up to the practitioner to assess the client's energy field, intervene appropriately, and reassess. Some research studies, however, have required TT practitioners to administer TT for a designated period of time regardless of what the practitioner determines to be the needs of the client. Supporters argue that this method allows for greater control of the independent variables. Opponents of this practice argue that limiting the duration of the TT intervention interferes with the potential for physiological and psychological changes to occur.

Another methodological concern is that all the studies reviewed in this chapter and all studies included in Peters' meta-analysis[21] were conducted with samples of convenience. Although several had two or more groups and reported random assignment to the groups, the assignment methods were not well described and drop-out rates were not adequately addressed. A few reviewers also raised issues related to potential bias of subjects and researchers.[16,21]

Therapeutic Touch and Placebo Effect

Meehan[18] raises the issue that controlled efficacy studies need to differentiate between the effects of TT and placebo effect. Several researchers[28,44,49,50] have attempted to use "mock" or "mimic" TT in their studies as a way to control for placebo effect. Mock or mimic TT has the appearance of TT, but is performed by a health care provider without TT training who engages in some form of mental activity to avoid a positive intention to help or heal. Debate and discussion continue as to whether mock TT is adequate for ensuring a single-blind control. One needs to consider also that double-blind control experiments will probably not be possible in TT research because the intent of the practitioner will always be subject to scrutiny.

Winstead-Fry and Kijek[16] acknowledge that the scientific literature in TT has evolved over the past 20 years from anecdotal reports to single-blind, randomized studies. Nevertheless, the need to increase the scientific rigor in the study of TT continues to exist. Suggestions include improving the descriptions of the study sample, increasing the sample sizes, and utilizing physiologic outcome measures in combination with the more commonly used self-report measures.

Conclusion

Therapists inclined to consider including complementary therapies into their plans of care will find support for TT as an intervention to reduce pain and to a lesser extent, anxiety. As a noninvasive, nonpharmaceutical intervention, TT seems to have little potential for causing negative interactions with medications or other physiological conditions. Research that assesses the mechanism by which TT may alleviate pain will further advance the acceptance of TT into the medical and rehabilitation communities. In addition, assessment of the physiologic changes that occur with TT may further suggest patient diagnoses and conditions that might benefit the most from incorporating TT into a rehabilitation program. As experts in impairment, dysfunction, and pain management, physical and occupational therapists are well suited to collaborate with other scientists to conduct research in complementary therapies such as TT.

References

1. Krieger D. *Accepting Your Power to Heal: The Personal Practice of Therapeutic Touch.* Santa Fe, NM: Bear and Company; 1993.
2. Krieger D. *The Therapeutic Touch. How to Use Your Hands to Help or Heal.* New York, NY: Simon and Schuster; 1979.
3. Mishra L, Singh BB, Dagenais S. Ayurveda: a historical perspective and principles of the traditional. *Altern Ther Health Med.* 2001;7(2):36-42.
4. Veith I (trans). *The Yellow Emperor's Classic of Internal Medicine.* Berkeley, CA: University of California Press; 1970.
5. Weber R. Philosophical foundations and frameworks for healing. In: Borelli MD, Heidt P, eds. *Therapeutic Touch: A Book of Readings.* New York, NY: Springer; 1981.
6. Weber R. A philosophical perspective on touch. In: Barnard KE, Bazelton TB, eds. *Touch: The Foundation of Experience.* Madison, WI: International Universities Press; 1990.
7. Bohm D. *Wholeness and the Implicate Order.* Boston, MA: Routledge & Kegan Paul; 1980.
8. Bohm D. The implicate order and the super-implicate order. In: Weber E, ed. *Dialogues with Scientists and Sages: The Search for Unity.* New York, NY: Routledge & Kegan Paul; 1986.

9. Rogers ME. *Introduction to the Theoretical Basis of Nursing*. Philadelphia: FA Davis; 1970.

10. Rogers ME. Science of unitary, irreducible human being: update 1990. In: Barrett E, ed. *Visions of Rogers' Science Based Nursing*. New York, NY: National League for Nursing; 1990.

11. Krieger D. *Therapeutic Touch Inner Workbook: Ventures in Transpersonal Healing*. Santa Fe, NM: Bear and Company, Inc; 1997.

12. Gerber R. *Vibrational Medicine: New Choices for Healing Ourselves*. Rev ed. Santa Fe, NM: Bear and Company; 1988.

13. Freeman L. Therapeutic touch: healing with energy. In: Freeman LW, Lawlis GF, eds. *Complementary & Alternative Medicine: A Research-Based Approach*. St. Louis, MO: Mosby; 2001.

14. Ireland M, Olson O. Massage therapy and therapeutic touch in children: state of the science. *Altern Ther Health Med*. 2000;6(5):54-63.

15. Ramnarine-Singh S. The surgical significance of therapeutic touch. *Association of Operating Room Nurses*. 1999; 69(2):358-369.

16. Winstead-Fry P, Kijek J. An integrative review and meta-analysis of therapeutic touch research. *Altern Ther Health Med*. 1999;5(6):58-67.

17. Easter A. The state of research on the effects of therapeutic touch. *J Holistic Nurs*. 1997;15(2):158-175.

18. Meehan TC. Therapeutic touch as a nursing intervention. *J Adv Nurs*. 1998;28(1):117-125.

19. Spence JE, Olsen MA. Quantitative research of therapeutic touch. An integrative review of the literature 1985-1995. *Scand J Caring Sci*. 1997;11(3):183-190.

20. Daley B. Therapeutic touch, nursing practive and contemporary cutaneous wound healing research. *J Adv Nurs*. 1997;25(6):1123-1132.

21. Peters RM. The effectiveness of therapeutic touch: a meta-analytic review. *Nurs Sci Q*. 1999;12(1):52-61.

22. O'Mathuna DP, Ashford RL. Therapeutic touch for healing acute wounds. *Cochrane Database of Sytematic Reviews*. 2003;4: CD002766. DOI: 10.1002/14651858.CD002766.

23. Robinson J, Biley FC, Dolk H. Therapeutic touch for anxiety disorders. *Cochrane Database of Systematic Reviews* 2007;3: CD006240. DOI: 10.1002/14651858.CD006240.pub2.

24. Rosa L, Rosa R, Sarner L, Barrett S. A close look at therapeutic touch. *JAMA*. 1998;279:1005-1010.

25. Achterberg J. Clearing the air in the therapeutic touch controversy. *Altern Ther Health Med*. 1998;4(4):100.

26. Leskowitz ED. Undebunking therapeutic touch. *Altern Ther Health Med*. 1998;4(4):101-102.

27. Cox T. A nurse-statistician reanalyzes data from the Rosa therapeutic touch study. *Altern Ther Health Med*. 2003; 9(1):58-64.

28. Ireland M. Therapeutic touch with HIV-infected children: a pilot study. *J Assoc Nursing AIDS Care*. 1998;9(4):68.

29. Kramer NA. Comparison of therapeutic touch and casual touch in stress reduction of hospitalized children. *Pediatr Nurs*. 1990;16(5):483-485.

30. Quinn JF, Strelkauskas AJ. Psychoimmunologic effects of therapeutic touch on practitioners and recently bereaved recipients: a pilot study. *Adv Nurs Sci*. 1993;15(4):13-26.

31. Heidt P. Effect of therapeutic touch on the anxiety level of hospitalized patients. *Nurs Res*. 1981;30(1):32-37.

32. Turner JG, Clark AJ, Gauthier DK, Williams M. The effect of therapeutic touch on pain and anxiety in burn patients. *J Adv Nurs*. 1998;28(1):10-28.

33. Gagne D, Toye RC. The effects of therapeutic touch and relaxation therapy in reducing anxiety. *Arch Psychiatr Nurs*. 1984;8(3):184-187.

34. Larden C, Palmer M, Lynne M, Janssen P. Efficacy of therapeutic touch in treating pregnant inpatients who have a chemical dependency. *J Holistic Nurs*. 2004;22(4):320-322.

35. Simington JA, Laing GP. Effects of therapeutic touch on anxiety in the institutionalized elderly. *Clin Nurs Res*. 1993; 2(4):438-450.

36. Samarel N, Fawcett J, Davis MM, Ryan FM. Effects of dialogue and therapeutic touch on preoperative and postoperative experiences of breast cancer surgery: an exploratory study. *Oncol Nurs Forum*. 1998;25(8):1369-1376.

37. Frank LS, Frank JL, March D, Makari-Judson G, Barham RB, Mertens WC. Does therapeutic touch ease the discomfort or distress of patients undergoing stereotactic core breast biopsy? A randomized clinical trial. *Pain Med*. 2007; 8(5):419-424.

38. Lin Y, Taylor AG. Effects of therapeutic touch in reducing pain and anxiety in an elderly population. *Integrative Medicine*. 1998;1(4):155-162.

39. Olson M, Sneed N. Anxiety and therapeutic touch. *Issues Ment Health Nurs*. 1995;16:97-108.

40. Engle VF, Graney MJ. Biobehavioral effects of therapeutic touch. *J Nurs Scholarsh*. 2003;32(3):287-293.

41. Lafreniere KD, Mutus B, Cameron S, et al. Effect of therapeutic touch on biochemical and mood indicators in women. *J Altern Complement Med*. 1999;5(4):367-370.

42. Leskowitz ED. Phantom limb pain treated with therapeutic touch: a case report. *Arch Phys Med Rehab*. 2000;81:552-524.

43. Eckes Peck, SD. The effectiveness of therapeutic touch for decreasing pain in elders with degenerative arthritis. *J Holistic Nurs*. 1997;15(2):176-198.

44. Gordon A, Merenstein JH, D'Amico F, Hudgens D. The effects of therapeutic touch on patients with osteoarthritis of the knee. *J Fam Pract*. 1998;47(4):271-276.

45. Gregory S, Verdouw. Therapeutic touch: its application for residents in aged care. *Aust Nurs J*. 2005;12(7):

46. Giasson M, Bouchard L. Effect of therapeutic touch on the well-being of persons with terminal cancer. *J Holistic Nurs.* 1998;16(3):383-398.

47. Denison B. Touch the pain away. New research on therapeutic touch and persons with fibromyalgia syndrome. *Holistic Nurs Pract.* 2004;12(3):142-151.

48. Blankfield RP, Sulzmann C, Fradle LG, Tapolyai AA, Zyzanski SJ. Therapeutic touch in the treatment of carpal tunnel syndrome. *J Am Board Fam Pract.* 2001;14(5):335-342.

49. Keller E, Bzdek VM. Effects of therapeutic touch on tension headache pain. *Nurs Res.* 1986;35(2):102-106.

50. Meehan TC. Therapeutic touch and postoperative pain: a Rogerian research study. *Nurs Sci Q.* 1993;6(2):69-78.

51. Wirth DP. The effect of non-contact therapeutic touch on the healing rate of full thickness dermal wounds. *Subtle Energies.* 1992;1(1):1.

52. Wirth DP, Richardson JT, Eidleman WS, O'Malley AC. Full thickness dermal wounds treated with non-contact therapeutic touch: a replication and extension. *Complement Ther Med.* 1993;1(3):127-132.

53. Wirth DP, Barrett MJ, Eidleman WS. Non-contact therapeutic touch and wound re-epithelializational: an extension of previous research. *Complement Ther Med.* 1994;2(4):187-192.

54. Wirth DP, Richardson JT, Martinez RD, Eidelman WS, Lopez ME. Non-contact therapeutic touch intervention and full-thickness cutaneous wounds: a replication. *Complement Ther Med.* 1996;4(4):237-240.

55. Olson M, Sneed N, LaVia M, Virella G, Bonadonna R, Michel Y. Stress-induced immunosuppression and therapeutic touch. *Altern Ther Health Med.* 1997;3(2):68-74.

56. Wirth DP, Cram JR. Multi-site electromyographic analysis of non-contact therapeutic touch. *International Journal of Psychosomatics.* 1993;40(1-4):47-55.

Bibliography

Becker RO, Selden G. *The Body Electric.* New York, NY: William Morrow and Company; 1985.

Nurse Healers-Professional Associates International. The official organization of Therapeutic Touch. http://www.therapeutic-touch.org. Accessed November 6, 2003.

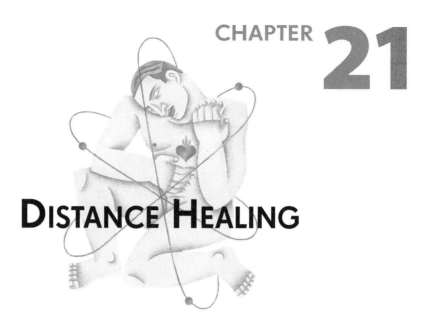

CHAPTER 21

DISTANCE HEALING

Susan Morrill Ramsey, PT, MA

> *Modern medicine has become one of the most spiritually malnourished professions in our society. Because we have so thoroughly disowned the spiritual component to healing, most healers throughout our history would view our profession today as inherently perverse. They would be aghast at how we have squeezed the life juices out of our calling. Physicians have spiritual needs like anyone else, and we have paid a painful price for ignoring them. It simply does not feel good to practice medicine as if the only thing that matters is the physical; something feels left out and incomplete.*

> —Larry Dossey, MD

Introduction

Many may wonder why there is a chapter on distance healing in a book about evidence-based complementary therapies. The truth is that, in the future, distance healing may be considered a complementary therapy. This is a topic that is very complex and emotionally charged, and could have a profound influence on the way we practice medicine in the future.

In a survey study of 2055 Americans in 1997, Eisenberg et al[1] found that more than 25% of the people surveyed had seen a practitioner of distance healing (including energetic and spiritual healing) within the previous 12 months. King and Bushwick's study[2] showed that 50% of hospitalized patients wanted their physicians to pray, not only *for* them, but also *with* them. A national survey conducted in the United States in 1996 found that 82% of Americans believed in the healing power of prayer.[3] In the United Kingdom, there are more distance healers (about 14,000) than there are therapists from other branches of complementary and alternative medicine.[4]

In a recent systematic review of randomized trials testing the efficacy of distance healing, Astin, Harkness, and Ernst[4] found that in the 23 trials they chose to investigate in regard to distance healing, 57% of the trials showed a positive result.[4] In the face of this type of evidence, it is imperative that we explore the healing potential in distance healing methods.

Distance Healing

Distance healing has been defined as "a conscious, dedicated act of mentation attempting to benefit another person's physical and emotional well-being at a distance."[5] Distance healing is a broad category that includes prayer, spiritual healing, and energetic healing. The common thread in all distance healing techniques is that a person or group of persons sends a positive intention of healing to another.

There are many categories in the area of distant healing. For the purposes of this chapter, we will describe prayer, spiritual healing, and energetic healing. Each of these categories describes a particular theoretical, cultural, and pragmatic approach to attempts to mediate a healing or biological change through mental intention.[6]

PRAYER

Prayer makes up the largest category in distance healing. Prayer is a highly personal event that defies exact definition. A general definition of prayer is that it is the simple act of turning our mind to the sacred.[7] A belief in God is not a necessary prerequisite for prayer. Prayer can be performed in a religious or spiritual context.

According to Krieder, prayer may be individual or communal, private, or public. Prayer may be offered in words, signs, gestures, or silence.[8] According to Dr. Larry Dossey, "prayer may be a conscious activity, of course, but it may flow also from the depths of the unconscious."[9]

Dr. Jeffrey Levin, an epidemiologist, has found more than 250 empirical studies published in the epidemiological and medical literature that show that spiritual and religious practices have been statistically associated with particular health outcomes. Levin is an expert on the local effects of prayer. These local effects include a positive effect on morbidity and mortality for cardiovascular disease, stroke, and all types of cancers, hypertension, and colitis.[10] There are more than two dozen studies that demonstrate the health promoting effects of simply attending a church or synagogue.[10]

In this chapter, we will look at the effects of prayer at a distance. In the research on distance healing, the most frequent type of prayer used is intercessory prayer. Intercessory prayer is an active form of prayer that seeks an outcome for another person. It is through intercessory prayer that we ask for healing for ourselves or for our patients. The formal definition of intercessory prayer is any form of prayer requesting God to bring about a desired result (God's own will or an outcome specified to the person praying). Intercessory prayer can be either directed or non-directed:

+ *Directed prayer*: Intercessory prayer in which the person praying specifies a particular outcome he or she desires.

+ *Nondirected prayer*: Intercessory prayer in which the person praying wishes only that God's will be done in the life of the subject.

SPIRITUAL HEALING

Dr. David Benor defines spiritual healing as "the intentional influence of one or more people upon another living system without utilizing known physical means of intervention."[11] Spiritual healing includes techniques such as visualization, meditation, and imagery, which can be performed at a distance.

Spiritual healing can include broad requests to the universal energies. For example, a person may ask for the universal energies of love to assist a person or for the life force of the universe to assist a person. During this process, the healer adopts a dispassionate, loving, and compassionate attitude toward the person in need.[9] Spiritual healing can be practiced in a nonreligious or religious context.

ENERGETIC HEALING

Some authors, such as Astin and Harkness, consider energetic healing as a type of distance healing method.

Energetic healing includes complementary therapy practices such as Therapeutic Touch (TT) and Reiki, where the practitioner does not have to actually touch the patient for a transfer of energy to occur. Both methods incorporate the concept of intentionality, whereby the practitioner clearly intends for the person to receive the energy he or she needs to assist in the healing process.

Nonlocal Mind or Consciousness

In order to understand the research in the area of distance healing, a key concept must be introduced. This concept is called nonlocal mind or consciousness, and it is one possible theory that explains the phenomenon of distance healing. Dr. Larrey Dossey coined the term *nonlocal mind* in 1989.

Dossey defines all known mind-body events as either local or nonlocal. Local events are those that are mediated by the senses (speech, hearing, touch, smell, taste, and sight).[9] These local events are explainable through the known laws of physics and human physiology. These events exist in the present moment and occur within an individual or between two or more people. Nonlocal mind-body events are initiated between individuals who are too far apart to communicate by the senses.[9] All types of distance healing are classified as nonlocal mind-body events.

The main premise of nonlocal mind is that a person's consciousness is not limited to distance or time, thus, we can influence our world at a distance. If, according to Dossey, the mind is nonlocal, in principle the mind cannot be walled off and be separate from other minds, thus at some level all minds are unitary.[9]

BELL'S THEOREM

One landmark physics theorem, called Bell's theorem, is often used to elucidate this concept.[9] In 1964, Bell, an Irish physicist, paired two electrons in a vacuum tube. The electrons were then separated by a great distance. Bell discovered that if one electron turned, the other did also, regardless of the distance between them. In essence, once paired, the electrons would respond to each other, even if there was a universe between them. Some physicists believe that this concept of nonlocality does not just apply to subatomic particles, but to the mind as well.

Physicists such as Nick Herbert[12] explain distance healing using the term *nonlocal* world. In this theory, neither information nor energy travels from one mind to another because the two minds involved are not separate, discrete entities; rather they are interconnected, omniscient, and instances of a holographic reality.

Sean O'Laire states that "it may be that consciousness is a field in the same sense as gravity and electromagnetism (hence an infinite, unbounded, unmanifest reality). Taken holistically, it is possible that intelligence (consciousness/mind) is the wave-like aspect of a unitary phenomenon of which matter (in this case the brain) is the particle-like aspect. As particles, we might experience ourselves as 5 billion separate, discrete entities; as waves we might experience a nonlocal connectivity that inextricably weaves our fate together."[13]

So how could this theoretical model assist in explaining the effects of distance healing?

HUMAN INTENTIONALITY

There is a large body of research that is not well-known in the medical community studying the effects of human intentionality on biological systems. The US National Institutes of Health

(NIH) has a category of studies that evaluate the research done in this area. Since this area has been highly controversial in the medical community, these studies have not been well-publicized. Dr. David Benor[14] has cited 131 controlled research trials in this area and reviews each study in his book Healing Research.

The main premise underlying all of these studies is that a human being can intentionally cause a change in a biological system. Bernard Grad,[15-20] a psychologist at McGill University, performed a series of experiments in the 1960s suggesting that the mental intention of a healer could bring about changes nonlocally in distant biological systems. In his carefully controlled studies, he showed how nonlocal healing could significantly increase the healing rate of surgical wounds in mice, retard the rate of tumor growth in animals, and affect the growth rate of seedlings.[15-21]

Grad worked with the healer Oscar Estebany in these studies. Estebany never actually touched any of the plants or animals used in the studies. For example, Estebany sent a mental intention of growth into a vial of saline that would be used to water the experimental seed group. Grad found that the seeds that received the saline water that Estebany had held sprouted and grew far more successfully than the control seed group. His work was highly significant in that he demonstrated that the results of his experiments were not due to the effects of suggestion, expectation, positive thinking, or any other placebo-related idea because they were done on plant and animal subjects.

Grad's revolutionary worked spawned much continued research in the area of distance healing on biological organisms. Since Grad, researchers have developed techniques for measuring possible distance intentionality effects on living systems and for assessing probabilities so that chance expectation can be determined and criteria can be established for rejecting the null hypothesis.[9,22-24] An example of how these studies are performed follows.

In a small study, 10 subjects tried to inhibit the growth of fungus cultures in a lab using conscious intent by concentrating on inhibiting the growth of the fungus for 15 minutes. The subjects were 1.5 yards away from the cultures. The cultures were then incubated for several hours. Researchers found that 151 out of 194 cultures showed significant retarded growth.[25]

In a replication of this study, one group of subjects demonstrated the same effect in 16 out of 17 trials, while standing from 1 to 15 miles away from the fungus culture.[26] Why would the ability for a human being to intentionally inhibit fungus growth be meaningful to us? There are many times in medicine that it would be beneficial to inhibit the growth of a pathogen. Learning to inhibit or increase the growth of biological organisms could be a valuable health resource.

Other important studies in this area include biologist Carroll Nash's work, which showed that the growth rate of bacteria could be influenced by conscious intention in controlled, double-blind studies.[27] Braud's studies demonstrated the mental ability of individuals nonlocally to affect the rate of hemolysis of human red blood cells in hypotonic saline solution.[28] Muehsam found that mental intentions could nonlocally affect specific biochemical reactions in test tubes.[29]

Well-controlled laboratory experiments involving nonhuman systems have found replicable results of direct mental influence on fungi,[30,31] yeast,[32] bacteria cells,[27,33] and cancer cells[34,35] under blinded conditions. Other researchers have also reported significant evidence of distance healing in animal disease models, including studies done by Snel and Hol on distance healing with hamsters with amyloidosis,[36] and Snel and Van der Sijde's studies on decreased tumor weight in mice using distance healing.[35] All of the above experiments provide a strong suggestion of the existence of the nonlocal mind.

Distance Healing Research With Human Subjects

It might be surprising to learn that the medical community has been performing research in the area of distance healing for decades. Benor[37] has identified 130 controlled investigations in the area of spiritual healing, and Rosa et al[38] has identified 74 qualitative studies of TT.

For the purposes of this chapter, we will take a closer look at two well-known research projects: Dr. Randolph Byrd's pivotal research[39] in the use of intercessory prayer in a coronary care unit population, and Sicher, Targ, Moore, and Smith's[5] research in the effectiveness of distance healing in a population with advanced AIDS. We will also look at the results of Astin, Harkness, and Ernst's[4] recent research to systematically review the randomized trials that have been done in the area of distant healing.

BYRD'S STUDY

Dr. Randolph Byrd, a cardiologist, performed a study in 1982 and 1983 that attempted to assess the therapeutic effectiveness of intercessory prayer in a coronary care unit population.

Byrd's study was designed to answer the following questions[39]: does intercessory prayer to the Judeo-Christian God have any effect on the patient's medical condition and recovery while in the hospital, and how are these effects characterized, if present? This was a large study in which 393 patients were entered into a prospective, double-blind, randomized protocol to assess the therapeutic effects of intercessory prayer. Patients were randomly assigned via a computer-generated list either to receive or not receive intercessory prayer. The patients gave informed consent prior to participating in the study. The patients, staff, and doctors remained blind throughout the study. The people performing the intercessory prayer were primarily categorized as "born again" Christians, with an active Christian life based on their commitment to daily devotional prayer and active involvement with a local church. Other people involved in the intercessory prayer for the study were members of the local Protestant and Roman Catholic churches.

Following the randomization process, each patient was assigned to several people who would pray for him or her. The intercessors (people praying for the patients) were given the patients' first names, diagnoses, and general condition. They were also given updates on the patients' condition while in the hospital. Under the supervision of a coordinator, each intercessor was asked to pray daily for a rapid recovery, prevention of complications and death, and, in addition, the intercessor could pray for any additional things that he or she thought would benefit the patient.[39]

Byrd collected data on each patients' status upon entry to the hospital (Table 21-1). There were no statistical differences between the two groups at entry. After entry into the hospital, patients had follow-up for the remainder of their hospitalization. New problems, new diagnoses, and new therapeutic interventions that occurred after hospitalization were recorded and summarized (Table 21-2).[39]

Byrd's results showed that of the many variables that were measured, the data showed that congestive heart failure, heart attack, pneumonia, diuretics, antibiotics, and intubation/ventilation were seen less frequently in the prayer group. Multivariant analysis of the data showed that there was a significant difference between the two groups, and that fewer patients in the prayer group required ventilatory support, antibiotics, or diuretics. Based on his findings, Byrd concluded that there was a positive therapeutic effect from intercessory prayer in a coronary care unit.[39]

Byrd's study has become a landmark in the areas of both medicine and religion. It certainly was one of the largest studies ever done on the effects of intercessory prayer on hospitalized patients and gives us much information to consider.

There are, of course, obvious limitations to this study. Byrd could not control other people who may be praying for the patients in both groups. For example, friends and family of the person in the hospital may have prayed for the person, regardless of which group he or she was in. We could assume that some patients in the control group were receiving prayer as well. In this sense, the control group may not be "pure." However, this does not invalidate the fact that there was a differential effect seen between the two groups.

Another limitation to the study relates to the instructions that each intercessor was given. The intercessors were given specific instructions in what they should pray for, and then they were given the opportunity to pray in other areas that they thought were beneficial to the patient. We could surmise that the prayers were not standardized for each patient. Byrd also selected a specific

Table 21-1

PATIENTS' STATUS ON ENTRY

ENTRY VARIABLES	INTERCESSORY PRAYER GROUP (192)	CONTROL GROUP (201)	P
Age (mean ± SD)	58.2±14.8	60.1±15.0	NS
Sex: Female	65	63	NS
Male	127	138	NS
Time (days, mean ± SD)	0.9±1.2	0.9±1.1	NS
PRIMARY CARDIAC DIAGNOSIS	**% (NO.)**	**% (NO.)**	**P**
Congestive heart failure	33 (66)	33 (66)	NS
Cardiomegaly	32 (62)	32 (64)	NS
Prior myocardial infarction	30 (57)	26 (50)	NS
Acute myocardial infarction	27 (51)	29 (58)	NS
Unstable angina	25 (48)	30 (61)	NS
Chest pain, cause unknown	19 (36)	15 (31)	NS
Acute pulmonary edema	13 (25)	13 (27)	NS
Syncope	11 (21)	6 (12)	NS
Cardimyopathy	8 (16)	9 (17)	NS
Supraventricular tachyarrhythmia	8 (15)	12 (24)	NS
VT/VF	8 (14)	9 (17)	NS
Intubation/ventilation	6 (11)	10 (19)	NS
Valvular heart disease	5 (8)	8 (15)	NS
Hypotension (systolic <90 torr)	4 (8)	5 (10)	NS
Cardiopulmonary arrest	4 (8)	6 (12)	NS
Third-degree heart block	2 (3)	1 (1)	NS
PRIMARY NONCARDIAC DIAGNOSIS	**% (NO.)**	**% (NO.)**	**P**
Diabetes mellitus	8 (16)	9 (18)	NS
COPD	8 (15)	10 (19)	NS
Gastrointestinal bleeding	5 (10)	2 (3)	NS
Severe hypertension	5 (10)	7 (13)	NS
Pneumonia	5 (9)	4 (7)	NS
Chronic renal failure	4 (8)	4 (8)	NS
Trauma	4 (7)	3 (6)	NS
Cerebrovascular accident	4 (7)	2 (4)	NS
Drug overdose	3 (5)	3 (5)	NS
Sepsis	2 (3)	2 (4)	NS
Cirrhosis of the liver	2 (3)	1 (2)	NS
Pulmonary emboli	1 (2)	1 (1)	NS
Systemic emboli	1 (2)	0 (0)	NS
Hepatitis	0 (0)	1 (2)	NS

Time from admission to the coronary care unit to randomization.

Key: *=192 people; †=201 people; NS = P>0.05. VT/VF=ventricular tachycardia/ventrical fibrilation; COPD=chronic obstructive pulmonary disease.

Reprinted with permission from Byrd R. Positive therapeutic effects of intercessory prayer in a coronary care unit population. *South Med J.* 1988;81(7):826.

Table 21-2

RESULTS OF INTERCESSORY PRAYER

STUDY VARIABLE	INTERCESSORY PRAYER GROUP	CONTROL GROUP	P
Days in coronary care unit after entry	2.0±2.5	2.4±4.1	NS
Days in hospital after entry	7.6±8.9	7.6±8.7	NS
Number of discharge medications	3.7±2.2	4.0±2.4	NS
NEW PROBLEMS, DIAGNOSES, & THERAPEUTIC EVENTS AFTER ENTRY	**% (NO.)**	**% (NO.)**	**P**
Antianginal agents	11(21)	10 (19)	NS
Unstable angina	10 (20)	9 (18)	NS
Antiarrhythmics	9 (17)	13 (27)	NS
Coronary angiography	9 (17)	11 (21)	NS
VT/VF	7 (14)	9 (17)	NS
Readmissions coronary care unit	7 (14)	7 (14)	NS
Mortality	7 (13)	9 (17)	NS
Congestive heart failure	4 (8)	10 (20)	<0.03
Inotropic agents	4 (8)	8 (16)	NS
Vasodialators	4 (8)	6 (12)	NS
Supraventricular tachyarrhythmia	4 (8)	8 (15)	NS
Arterial pressure monitoring	4 (7)	8 (15)	NS
Central pressure monitoring	3 (6)	7 (15)	NS
Diuretcis	3 (5)	8 (15)	<0.05
Major surgery before discharge	3 (5)	7 (14)	NS
Temporary pacemaker	2 (4)	1 (1)	NS
Sepsis	2 (4)	4 (7)	NS
Cardiopulmonary arrest	2 (3)	7 (14)	<0.02
Third-degree heart block	2 (3)	1 (2)	NS
Pneumonia	2 (3)	7 (13)	<0.03
Hypotension (systolic <90 torr)	2 (3)	4 (7)	NS
Extension of infarction	2 (3)	3 (6)	NS
Antibiotics	2 (3)	9 (17)	<0.005
Permanent pacemaker	2 (3)	1 (1)	NS
Gastrointestinal bleeding	1 (1)	2 (3)	NS
Intubation/ventilation	0 (0)	6 (12)	<0.002

NS=$P>0.05$; VT/VF=ventricular tachycardia or ventricular fibrillation.

Reprinted with permission from Byrd R. Positive therapeutic effects of intercessory prayer in a coronary care unit population. *South Med J.* 1988;81(7):826.

and perhaps narrow group of intercessors with very similar beliefs. What would have happened if he had chosen a broad-based group of intercessors, with varying beliefs about religion and spirituality?

Another problem with the study is that it focused on the patients only while they were hospitalized. Medical follow-up did not continue after discharge, and this data would have been interesting to analyze. Finally, one of the major limitations of this study and of all studies in distance healing, as stated by Targ,[40] is "the need to separate distant effects from subjective factors such as hope, expectation, or simply the act of participating in a healing project."

Byrd's study helped other researchers assert that distance healing is a valid object of investigation. Despite its design flaws, this study represents an important first step in demonstrating that distance healing, in this case intercessory prayer, may have a positive effect on patients. Byrd's study also pushes us to investigate the possibility of the reality of the nonlocal mind. In this case, that a person's consciousness (the intercessor) is not limited to space or time and can, thus, influence a person (the patient) at a distance. We are just beginning to look at the effects of distant intentionality on the health of patients, and this study gives us a chance to look at both the possible benefits and difficulties of researching this question.

SICHER, TARG, MOORE, AND SMITH'S RESEARCH

A study done almost 10 years later by Fred Sicher et al[5] looked at the effects of distance healing in a population with advanced AIDS. This small study was done following a double-blind pilot study of 10 treated and 10 control subjects conducted between 1995 and 1996. The pilot study suggested that there were both medical and psychological benefits from distance healing; this study was then performed.

Based on the results from their pilot study, Sicher and Targ hypothesized that the distance healing treatments could be associated with improved disease progression (ie, fewer and less severe AIDS-defining diseases and improved CD4+ levels, decreased medical utilization, and improved psychological well-being).[5] This study was designed as a pro of of principle trial (ie, to determine if there is an effect on healing over a distance. The study was not designed to investigate the mechanism of the possibility of a distance healing effect).[5]

Forty subjects were recruited from a variety of sociodemographic populations. Each subject had to meet the criteria of the Centers for Disease Control AIDS category. Each subject signed an informed consent, was photographed, and then randomly assigned on a double-blind basis to either a control group or the distance healing group. Each subject came to the lab or was visited at home to obtain the initial baseline measurements. Measurements were then taken at the end of the 10-week treatment intervention and at a follow-up 12 to 14 weeks later. The measurements used included the CD4+ count, psychological distress measured by the Profile of Mood States, and physical symptoms measured by the Medical Outcomes Survey for HIV. The subjects also reported doctor visits, hospitalizations, illness recovery, and any new onset of illness.[5]

To control for the variation in severity and prognosis of different AIDS-related illnesses, Sicher and Targ scored all illnesses according to the Boston Health Study Opportunistic Disease Score, which includes both AIDS-defining and secondary AIDS-related diseases.[5]

Forty distance healing practitioners were recruited via professional healing associations and schools of healing. Each distance healer had to have at least 5 years of experience in an ongoing healing practice. This group of distance healers had an average of 17 years of experience. The healers were from the Christian, Jewish, Buddhist, and Native American and shamanistic traditions. The healers also included graduates of secular schools of bioenergetic and meditative healing.[5]

A rotating healing schedule was created that randomized healers to subjects on a weekly basis to minimize the possible differences in healer effectiveness. Each subject in the distance healing group was treated by a total of 10 distance healers. Each healer received a packet including the subject's photograph, first name, CD4+ count, and current symptoms. Healers were asked to work on the assigned subject for approximately 1 hour per day for 6 consecutive days, with the instruction to direct an intention for health and well-being to each subject. The healers kept written logs for each healing session indicating the time spent in the distant healing session, the technique used, and any impressions they had from the session.[5] Please refer to Figure 21-1 for the study flow chart.

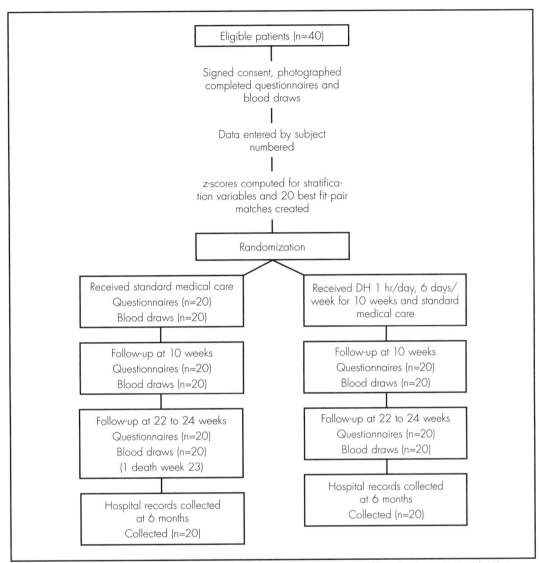

Figure 21-1. Study flow chart. (Reprinted with permission from Sicher F, Targ E, Moore D, Smith HS. A randomized double blind study of the effect of distant healing in a population with advanced AIDS. Report of a small scale study. *West J Med*. 1998;169:358,361-362.)

The results of this study showed that over a 6-month period of time, the distance healing group experienced significantly fewer outpatient doctor visits, fewer hospitalizations, fewer new AIDS-related diseases, and a significantly lower illness severity level as defined by the Boston Health Study Opportunistic Disease Score. Subjects in the distance healing group also showed significant improvement in mood compared with the control group.[5] Please refer to Tables 21-3 and 21-4 to view the detailed results of this study.

The authors concluded that their results showed a positive therapeutic effect from distance healing in advanced AIDS patients. This study was impeccably done using the highest level of research design. The researchers carefully improved on Byrd's method and design in his study by utilizing experienced healers who performed distance healing for 1 hour each day, for a 10-week period of time.[5]

Table 21-3

BASELINE AND AIDS MANAGEMENT-RELATED VARIABLES

	TREATED (20)	CONTROL (20)	TWO-SIDED P[1]
Age (years)	42.9±7.2	43.2±6.4	0.80
Sex (% female subjects)	10	5	1.00
Ethnic minority (% subjects)	0	20	0.12
Education[2]	4.1±0.6	3.9±1.0	0.38
Baseline AIDS-related factors			
Years HIV positive	9.0±3.5	7.3±3.1	0.11
CD4 cell number/mL	90.3±66.0	83.8±70.9	0.55
No. existing ADDs	1.4±1.3	1.3±1.4	0.65
No. prior ADDs	1.9±1.3	2.1±1.4	0.58
ADD severity[3]	5.4±3.0	5.0±3.3	0.49
Interventions during study			
Triple drug therapy[4]			
Throughout study	70	80	0.72
At least 2 months	20	15	1.00
Protease inhibitors	90	95	1.00
Pneumonia carinii prophylaxis	100	100	1.00
No. alternative therapies[5]	4.2±2.6	2.7±2.0	0.10
Support[6]	85	95	0.61
Baseline subjective measures			
WPSI score	1.64±0.72	1.69±0.80	0.86
POMS score	62.3±46.7	42.8±39.9	0.16
MOS score[7]	−0.01±0.8	−0.01±0.8	1.00
Baseline personal habits			
Smokers	0	25	0.06
Recreational drug use[8]	20	20	1.00
Alcohol use[9]	0.4±0.6	0.8±1.1	0.27
Exercise[10]	1.4±1.3	1.9±1.4	0.34
Meditation practice	60	75	0.50
Religious/spiritual practice	90	80	0.66
Belief in DH	2.8±0.6	2.9±0.4	0.33

Data are means ±SD or %.

[1]Paired t test for continuous variables with outliers, McNemar's test for binary variables; all tests are of matched paired differences. "Matched" refers to variables used for pair matching. [2]Some high school=1; high school graduate=2; some college=3; college graduate=4; graduate degree=5. [3]Boston Health Study opportunistic disease score. [4]Simultaneous use of a protease inhibitor and at least two antiretroviral drugs. [5]Acupuncture, psychic healing or prayer, Chinese herbs, yoga, biofeedback, guided imagery, Qi gong, nutrional supplements or vitamins, special diet, group therapy, or other. [6]Number of subjects reporting study participation support from family or community members. [7]Normalized mean score for 10 factors. [8]Four subjects in each group used crack cocaine or oral amphetamines; one treatment subject also used IV amphetamines. [9]No alcohol=0; once or twice a week=1; several times a week=2, heavily on weekends=3; daily=4. [10]No exercise=0; once a week=1, two or three times a week=2; four or five times a week=3; daily=4. [11]"I doubt it"=0; "Maybe"=1; "Probably"=2; "Yes, definitely"=3.

Reprinted with permission from Sicher F, Targ E, Moore D, Smith HS. A randomized double blind study of the effect of distant healing in a population with advanced AIDS. Report of a small scale study. *West J Med.* 1998; 169:358,361-362.

Table 21-4

MEDICAL COURSE OVER 6-MONTH STUDY

MEDICAL OUTCOME	TREATED (20)	CONTROL (20)	TWO-TAILED P[1]
Outpatient visits	185 (9.2±5.9)	260 (13.0±7.0)	0.01
Hospitalizations	3 (0.15±0.5)	12 (0.6±1.0)	0.04
Days of hospitalization	10 (0.5±1.7)	68 (3.4±6.2)	0.04
Illness severity[2]	16 (0.80±1.15)	43 (2.65±2.41)	0.03
ADDs acquired	2 (0.1±0.3)	12 (0.6±0.9)	0.04
ADD recoveries	6 (0.3±0.6)	2 (0.1±0.3)	0.23
CD4 change (/ul)[3]	31.1±54.9	55.5±102.0	0.55
Deaths	0	1	1.00
Change in POMS score (distress)	−25.7±46.0	14.2±49.0	0.02
Change in MOS	0.2±0.8	−0.2±0.8	0.15
Change in WPSI	−0.2±0.6	0.1±0.9	0.31

Data are *n* (means ±SD) or means ±SD.

[1]Wilcoxon signed-rank test for the first seven outcomes; paired *t* tests for the last three outcomes; McNemar's test for number of deaths. Due to clumpiness of the data for variables near P=0.05, the randomization test was also performed with the following results: hospitalizations, P=0.06; days of hospitalization. P=0.04; ADD severity score, P=0.03; ADDs acquired, P=0.06.

[2]Boston Health Survey opportunistic disease severity score, includes ADD and AIDS-related illness.

[3]n=19 in the control group (one subject died).

Reprinted with permission from Sicher F, Targ E, Moore D, Smith HS. A randomized double blind study of the effect of distant healing in a population with advanced AIDS. Report of a small scale study. *West J Med.* 1998; 169:358,361-362.

The authors also looked at different possibilities for their results other than distance healing, which include the placebo effect, and baseline medical or treatment differences. After analyzing both theories, the authors stated that they could not show that either influence was responsible for the clear and significant outcomes they found in the study. One obvious limitation of this study was its size. However, the researchers started out with a small pilot study, then expanded it to 40 patients. It will be interesting to see if the study can be replicated with a larger number of patients.

The authors also concluded that "existing medical understanding offers no mechanism to account for a finding of healing at a distance, however science does not require a known mechanism to prove the existence of a phenomenon. As pointed out by Dossey, for years, no one knew how colchicines, morphine, aspirin, or quinine worked, yet they were known to be effective."[5]

This study is exciting because it begins to look at the long-term effect of distance healing in the course of a progressive illness. It also showed that distance healing may have economic benefits as well. That is, the subjects in the distance healing group had less medical utilization; therefore they had fewer medical costs versus the control group. The thought of using distance healing for both prevention of disease-related complications and in medical cost reduction is a fascinating concept.

ASTIN, HARKNESS, AND ERNST'S SYSTEMATIC REVIEW OF RANDOMIZED TRIALS RELATING TO DISTANCE HEALING

One of the most recent and thorough reviews of distance healing research was done by Astin, Harkness, and Ernst. Their work was published in the *Archives of Internal Medicine* in 2001.[4]

The authors did a comprehensive literature search to identify studies of distance healing that included spiritual healing, mental healing, faith healing, prayer, TT, Reiki, psychic healing, and external Qi gong.[4] The search included all research done through the end of 1999.

They created specific criteria for literature inclusion in their review. The authors only included studies that met the following criteria:

1. Random assignment of study participants
2. Adequate control interventions (including placebo or sham controls)
3. Publication of the study in a peer-reviewed journal
4. Clinical research-based studies
5. Medical conditions were present in the subjects

The authors also utilized a Jadad score (ie, specific criteria that assesses the methodological quality of a study).[41] They also examined whether a study had successful randomization, controlled baseline differences, and patients that were lost in the follow-up portion of the study. The criteria also included sample size, type of intervention, type of control, and the results.[4]

The authors found more than 100 clinical trials of distance healing. Of those trials, 23 met their inclusion criteria. Tables 21-5 through and 21-7 show the methodological details and results of these trials. The studies were categorized into three types: prayer, TT, and other types of distance healing. These 23 trials included 2774 patients, and 1295 of the patients received the experimental interventions being studied.[4]

Five studies met their inclusion of prayer as a distance healing intervention. In each study, the intercessors did not have any physical or direct contact with the persons for whom they were praying. Two of the five trials showed significant effects on at least one outcome in patients being prayed for, and three studies showed no effect (see Table 21-5).

Eleven studies met their inclusion of noncontact TT. A specific inclusion criteria for these studies was that the TT treatment be compared to an adequate placebo such as a sham or mock TT treatment. Of the 11 trials, seven showed a positive treatment effect on at least one outcome. Three studies showed no effect and one study showed a negative treatment effect (ie, the control group healed faster) (see Table 21-6).

Seven studies met the inclusion criteria for other forms of distance healing. These included interventions such as remote mental healing and distance healing. Four of the clinical trials showed a positive effect, and three showed no effect from the healing intervention (see Table 21-7).

The authors found through their systematic review of these 23 randomized controlled trials that in all forms of distance healing research, 13 studies, or 57%, showed a positive treatment effect. Nine studies showed no effect, and one showed a negative effect.[4]

The authors were very candid about the limitations of their work. They cited the heterogeneity of the trials as the major limitation of this systematic analysis. They also agree that it is difficult to obtain "pure" control groups in distance healing research, as researchers cannot control the prayers and positive intention that a control subject may receive from his or her friends and family. Sample size was also noted as an overall limitation in this study. The authors note that well-designed and randomized controlled trials of prayer and distance healing with larger sample sizes (more than 1000 patients) are in progress.[42,43]

Another consideration in these studies has to do with the possibility of the experimenter effect[44] (ie, that previous skeptical beliefs of trial volunteers or investigators might contribute to unsuccessful outcomes). The authors suggest that one way to empirically test this is to have investigators who are skeptical of and investigators who are believers of spiritual healing conduct

Table 21-5

RANDOMIZED, PLACEBO-CONTROLLED TRIALS OF PRAYER

AUTHOR, YEAR	DESIGN	SAMPLE SIZE	EXPERIMENTAL INTERVENTION	CONTROL INTERVENTION*	RESULT	COMMENTS	JADAD SCORE
Joyce and Welldon, 1965	Double-blind; 2 parallel groups	48 patients with psychological or rheumatic disease	Prayer in Christian or Quaker tradition; patients received 15 hours of daily prayer for 6 months	Usual care	No signifcant differences in clinical or attitude state	Inclusion and exclusion criteria not stated; heterogeneous patient groups; results of only 16 pairs available	5
Collipp, 1969	Triple-blind; 2 parallel groups	18 children with leukemia	Daily prayer for 15 months	Usual care	Higher death rate in a control group, but difference was not significant (P=0.1)	Heterogeneity of groups makes findings inconclusive; inclusion criteria not stated	4
Byrd, 1988	Double-blind; 2 parallel groups	393 coronary care patients	Prayer in Christian tradition; 3 to 7 intercessors per patient until patient was released from hospital	Usual care	Treatment group required less ventilatory support and treatment with antibiotics or diuretics	Outcomes combined into "severity score" to handle multiple comparisons, score was lower in treatment group	5
Walker et al, 1997	Double-blind; 2 parallel groups	40 patients receieving alcohol abuse treatment	Prayer for 6 months	Usual care	No treatment effect on alcohol consumption	Insufficiently powered	4
Harris et al, 1999	Double-blind; 2 parallel groups	990 coronary care patients	Remote intercessory prayer in Christian tradition for 28 days	Usual care	Significant treatment effects for summed and weighted coronary care unit score; no differences in length of hospital stay	No differences were observed when the summed scoring system developed in Byrd's study 23 was used; unclear whether baseline differences were adequately controlled	5

*A placebo was unnecessary because patients were unaware of whether prayers were made on their behalf.

Reprinted with permission from Astin J, Harkness E, Ernst E. The efficacy of "distant healing": a systematic review of randomized trials. *Ann Intern Med.* 2000;132:11:907.

Table 21-6

RANDOMIZED, PLACEBO-CONTROLLED TRIALS OF THERAPEUTIC TOUCH

AUTHOR, YEAR	DESIGN	SAMPLE SIZE	EXPERIMENTAL INTERVENTION	CONTROL INTERVENTION	RESULT	COMMENTS	JADAD SCORE
Quinn, 1984	Double-blind	60 patients in cardiovascular unit	Noncontact Therapeutic Touch for 5 minutes	Simulated or mock Therapeutic Touch in treatment group	17% decrease in post-test anxiety scores		2
Keller and Bzdek, 1986	Single-blind; 2 parallel groups	60 patients with tension headache	Noncontact Therapeutic Touch for 5 minutes	Mock Therapeutic Touch	Treated group showed pain reduction after trial	Treatment effects were no longer present at 4 hours of follow-up; however, when participants who used intervening therapy were removed from analysis, 4-hour changes became significant	3
Quinn, 1988	Single-blind; 3 parallel groups	153 patients awaiting open-heart surgery	Noncontact Therapeutic Touch for 5 minutes	Mock Therapeutic Touch; no treatment	No significant treatment effects	Negative findings suggest importance of eye and face contact	2
Meehan, 1992	Single-blind; 3 parallel groups	108 postoperative patients	Noncontact Therapeutic Touch for 5 minutes	Mock Therapeutic Touch; usual care (analgesic drugs)	Nonsignificant reductions in postoperative pain ($P < 0.06$) treatment group showed reduced need for analgesic medication	Used conservative "intention-to-treat" analyses	3
Simington and Laing, 1993	Double-blind; 3 parallel groups	105 institutionalized elderly patients	Noncontact Therapeutic Touch with back rub for 3 minutes	Mock Therapeutic Touch with back rub; back rub alone	Lower levels of post-test anxiety observed in treatment group compared with back rub only	No differences between Therapeutic Touch and mock therapy; no pretest given	2
Wirth et al, 1993	Double-blind	24 participants with experimentally induced puncture wounds	Noncontact Therapeutic Touch (healer behind 1-way mirror) 5 min/d for 10 days	No treatment (placebo not necessary)	More rapid healing in treatment group		4

continued

Table 21-6 continued

Randomized, Placebo-Controlled Trials of Therapeutic Touch

AUTHOR, YEAR	EXPERIMENTAL DESIGN	CONTROL SAMPLE SIZE	INTERVENTION	INTERVENTION	RESULT	COMMENTS	JADAD SCORE
Wirth et al, 1996	Double-blind; 2 parallel groups	38 participants with experimentally induced puncture	Noncontact Therapeutic Touch (healer behind 1-way mirror), 5 min/d for 10 days	No treatment (placebo not necessary)	No treatment effect in terms of healing of dermal wounds	Control group healed significantly faster than treatment group	3
Gordon et al, 1998	Single-blind	31 patients with osteoarthritis of knee	Noncontact Therapeutic Touch, 1 session/wk for 6 weeks	Mock Therapeutic Touch; usual care	Treatment group showed improvements in pain, health status, and function	No change in functional disability	3
Turner et al, 1998	Single-blind; 2 parallel groups	99 burn patients	Noncontact Therapeutic Touch for 5 days; time varied from 5 to 20 mins	Mock Therapeutic Touch	Treatment group showed reductions in pain and anxiety and had lower CD8 counts		3
Wirth et al, 1994	Double-blind crossover study	25 participants with experimentally induced puncture	Noncontact Therapeutic Touch with visualization and wounds	Visualization and relaxation without Therapeutic Touch relaxation	No treatment effect	Authors note that the number of healed wounds was insufficient to compare for analyses	4
Wirth, 1990	Double-blind	44 men with experimentally induced puncture wounds	Noncontact Therapeutic Touch (healer not visible to participants), 5 min/d for 10 days	Mock Therapeutic Touch	Treatment group showed accelerated wound healing at days 8 and 16		4

Reprinted with permission from Astin J, Harkness E, Ernst E. The efficacy of "distant healing": a systematic review of randomized trials. *Ann Intern Med.* 2000;132: 11:907.

Table 21-7

RANDOMIZED, PLACEBO-CONTROLLED TRIALS OF OTHER DISTANT HEALING METHODS

AUTHOR, YEAR	DESIGN	SAMPLE SIZE	EXPERIMENTAL INTERVENTION	CONTROL INTERVENTION*	RESULT	COMMENTS	JADAD SCORE
Braud and Schlitz, 1983	Single-blind within and between participants	32 participants with high levels of autonomic arousal	Distant mental influence (intension to decrease arousal with 10 30-second sessions)	No-influence control conditions	10% reduction in galvanic skin response between control and influence sessions	No effect in participants with initially low galvanic skin response levels	3
Beutler et al, 1998	Double-blind; 3 parallel groups	120 patients with hypertension	Laying on of hands by 12 healers, 20 min/week for 15 weeks	Healing at a distance; usual care	No treatment effect	Unclear hat precisely the healers did; acute increase in diastolic blood pressure after laying on of hands	4
Wirth et al, 1993	Double-blind crossover study	21 patients with bi-lateral asymptomatic-impacted third molar who were undergoing surgery	Distance healing (Reiki, LeShan) for 15 to 20 minutes, 3 hours after surgery	No treatment (placebo not necessary)	Treatment group showed decrease in pain intensity and and greater pain relief after surgery		4
Greyson, 1996	Double-blind	40 patients with depression	Distance healing (LeShan Technique)	Usual care	No treatment effect	May have been under-powered	5
Sicher et al, 1998	Double-blind; 2 parallel groups	40 patients with AIDS	Distance healing (40 healers from different spiritual traditions; each patient treated by 10 healers)	Usual care (no placebo necessary)	Healing group had fewer new AIDS-defining illnesses, less illness severity, fewer physician visits and hospitalizations, and improved mood.	Mood changes may have been due to base-line differences; no apparent statistical adjustment for multiple comparisons	5
Miller, 1982	Double-blind; 2 parallel groups	96 patients with hypertension	"Remote mental heal-ing" in Church of Rel-ious Science tradition	No treatment (no placebo necessary)	Decrease in systolic blood pressure in treatment group	Unclear how many partic-ipants were lost to follow-up; results given for only 4 of 8 healers; use of medication not controlled	1
Harkness, et al	Double-blind	84 patients with warts	6 weeks of distant healing ("channeling of energy") by 10 healers	No treatment (no placebo necessary)	No significant treat-ment effect on size or number of warts	Seems that baseline values were not con-trolled for in analysis	5

Reprinted with permission from Astin J, Harkness E, Ernst E. The efficacy of "distant healing": a systematic review of randomized trials. *Ann Intern Med.* 2000;132: 11-907.

the same trials and assess whether in fact such beliefs influence outcomes. Such an experiment was done by Wiseman and Schlitz,[44] and their experiment suggests that the intentionality of the experimenter may be an important variable in the outcome of the distance intentionality studies.

Astin, Harkness, and Ernst's systematic review further supports that the clinical research that has been done to date supports the view that distance healing warrants further and more serious study in the scientific community.

Views For and Against Distance Healing Research

Distance healing research is, by its very nature, controversial. Before we look at how the results of these studies could be applied in a rehabilitation setting, let us first look at the pros and cons of researching distance healing. One of the main objections that faces researchers in this area is that the research is blasphemous, and that the research is trying to prove or disprove the existence of God or organized religion. Targ refutes this type of thinking by stating that "research in distant healing is neither a test of faith nor a test of religious teachings. It is an exploration of the relationship of human consciousness to the universal." She continues to say that[45]:

> No experiment can prove or disprove the existence of God, but if in fact (mental) intentions can be shown to facilitate healing at a distance, this would clearly imply that human beings are more connected to each other and more responsible to each other than previously believed. That connection could be actuated through the agency of God, consciousness, love electrons, or a combination. The answers to such questions await further research.

Thompson contends that establishing a control group for whom there is no prayer is impossible. He contends that people all over the world pray for "all the sick," which would include any control group. He also says that it is impossible to measure a dose or treatment of prayer. He feels that the research is "hideously blasphemous and arrogant at best."[45]

Benor suggests numerous reasons why scientists and skeptics reject scientific evidence for distance healing[46]:

1. Western materialistic beliefs exclude the possibility of prayer-based healing. In our modern scientific worldview, there is no room for the possibility of healing at a distance, so scientists ignore the evidence presented. It is unthinkable for many scientists to believe that nonmaterial types of healing may exist.

2. It is human nature to resist change. When we are faced with evidence that contradicts our belief systems, we resist it.

3. Cognitive dissonance can occur when people feel there is a conflict between their beliefs and their perceptions. Cognitive dissonance describes the discomfort a person is feeling when he or she faces this conflict. One way in which scientists deal with this feeling of discomfort is to reject the evidence without studying it closely.

4. Spiritual healing is often associated with mysticism, and intellectually oriented people tend to dismiss anything associated with mysticism.

5. Prayer-type healing may occur outside of conscious control. This is very threatening to people who feel the need to be in control most of the time.

6. The thought that the power of others may be feared is a concern for some. This is the thought that if someone can use prayer for benefit, he or she could also use it for harm. It is easier to reject the evidence than consider this possibility.

7. One's own healing power may be feared. It can be easier to reject that healing powers may exist rather than consider the possibility that this healing power actually resides within each of us.

8. Healing power is believed to be possessed only by people who are strange or different. Scientists and skeptics may associate healing abilities with weird people or fanatics. They may deny that average people have healing abilities and dismiss scientific evidence based on this fact.

9. The lack of consistent replicability of the research is often used to dismiss the research on distance healing. However, it is important to note that many of the studies on distance healing have been replicated and will continued to be replicated.

10. Healing has laws that appear to differ from those of other sciences. Scientists insist that all phenomena obey the same laws. As Benor states,[46]

   It is ludicrous that scientists from other fields suggest that their rules for evidence should be applied in healing. It would certainly be nicer, neater, and less complicated if this worked...

   [Healing] appears to be influenced by multiple factors (so many in fact that is virtually impossible to establish a repeatable experiment in which all would occur in the same combination more than once). As it is difficult to control any one of these, much less all of them in concert, it is of little wonder that only approximately equivalent results have been obtained in experiments over a number of trials. We will have to be content with our human limitations and settle for approximate results, measured in probabilities over large numbers of trials. No apologies are needed. These are the limitations of healing.

11. Healing is often allied with specific religions that emphasize faith and belief. For many scientists, mixing concepts of religion and medicine is a step backward for science, and they then can easily dismiss the evidence for distance healing.

12. Careers and financial investment are at stake. The majority of all research grants, funding, professorships, etc, are associated with the physically based view of reality. Scientists are fearful of research that calls these assumptions into question.

Given these fears, it is understandable that some scientists and skeptics would refute all scientific evidence that supports distance healing.

However, researchers in the area of distance healing feel differently. Targ states, "The scientific method does not require mechanistic explanations. It has the power to study paradigms that we neither understand nor believe in. Experiments to test the distant healing hypothesis are in fact surprisingly easy to design."[45] She also is very clear about the design challenges and the need to replicate studies and do further exploratory studies in this field.

Targ points out that in many of the studies with positive results, volunteers not trained in distance healing were used, and they apparently successfully sent a healing intention.[47-49] She believes that perhaps distance healing largely functions in the unconscious, subtly a part of each medical procedure, each healing goal, and each intention as set by the medical practitioner.[48] This idea sets up a larger research paradigm to explore in the area of distance healing.

Dossey predicts that the experimental evidence supporting the concept of the nonlocal mind will continue to accumulate.[9] This includes distance healing and specifically the effects of prayer. He also predicts that the use of prayer will become part of mainstream medicine.

Koopman and Blasband[40] cite the burgeoning quantity of serious scientific research that indicates distance healing is becoming a valid object of investigation. They add that their hope is that modern technology, combined with shifting paradigms and the use of nonlinear logic, may assist in defining the answers to the mechanistic questions.

Targ also points out that many distance healers charge for their work, and many patients commit their time and money to this type of healing. She surmises that if mental intention itself does not support healing, patients should be directed away from relying on it, but if mental intentions can support healing, "it is both an ethical obligation and a great opportunity to study it and make it as available and effective as possible."[45]

Finally, researchers in the field of distance healing point to the fact that of 131 formal laboratory and clinical studies that were done before 1992, 77 found statistically significant effects.[7]

Combined with Astin, Harkness, and Ernst's review,[4] which showed that out of 23 clinical trials in the area of distant healing, 57% of the studies showed a positive treatment effect, we have information that cannot be ignored and must be pursued through more research.

Application of Distance Healing in the Rehabilitative Setting

As Dossey points out,[9] one of the implications of distance healing may be that other people can participate in creating our health reality, and that we may participate in creating theirs. He further states that the evidence (of distance healing) cannot be avoided, and it causes havoc with the belief that the conscious "I" is the sole creator of my medical reality.

Many other medical systems, including Chinese, Ayurvedic, and Native American medicine, have always believed in the universality of healing, and that healing includes the totality of existence—those things that we can see—and others we cannot. These medical systems acknowledge the holistic nature of the universe and through thousands of years of observation, created healing methods that include the premise that others can participate in our healing reality, and we can participate in theirs.

How can this information be applied in the rehabilitation setting? One of the primary similarities in all of the evidence presented in the distance healing studies is the concept of intentionality. The intercessors and healers all prayed for, or used other distance healing methods to transmit or send a healing intention to, the patients in the studies. Indeed, just the process of intending health for someone could be a powerful force in the healing process. Many rehabilitation professionals do this on a regular basis through prayer, spiritual practice, or through using energetic therapies such as TT or Reiki. However, the topic of intentionality is rarely discussed or explored candidly among rehabilitation providers.

The exception to this is the nursing field, which through its Holistic Nursing Association discusses the concept of intention in great detail. According to Lynne Rew, "Holistic nursing is about intentions: commitment to the well-being of another, responsibility for self and others, an integration of caring and communication."[50] McKivergin writes about the nurse as an instrument of healing and defines intention as "the conscious alignment with creative essence and divine purpose that allows the highest good to flow through a healing intervention or through life itself."[51]

Intentionality is a primary concept in the practice of TT. Delores Krieger states that there are at least three main conditions that have to be met for a person to become a really helpful healer. Those conditions are intentionality, motivation in the interests of the patient, and the ability and willingness to confront oneself.[52] She continues to say that intentionality is essential in that the intentional act has a goal in view, and that the healer knows what he or she is going to do. This implies that the intervention will be done from a knowledgeable and intelligent base.

Janet Macrae emphasizes that intentionality is not an emotional or personal desire but the much deeper force by which we mobilize and focus ourselves (mind and body) to carry out a specific purpose.[53] Macrae states that in the case of TT, the purpose is to become an instrument of healing and to help living organisms restore their wholeness.

Intentionality can be taught to rehabilitation professionals using techniques such as meditation, centering, prayer, and spiritual and energetic therapies. Therapists who already use distance healing methods in their lives could begin to teach other professionals how to practice intentionality exercises. In addition, those therapists who use distance healing techniques would be the perfect people to pilot research projects to further investigate the benefits of using intentionality to assist their patients in their healing process.

The Philadelphia Panel[54] found that many of the modalities that physical therapists use for pain management actually do not show evidence of efficacy in controlled trials, yet our patients get better. Is it the therapist's intention that contributes to the patient's health? The patient's expectation that the therapy will be beneficial? Or a combination of both? Carol Davis advocates expanding our narrow view of clinical studies to include research paradigms that look into outcomes that are not so easy to measure, such as "motivation, mood, hope, belief in self, belief in the health care professional, prayer, optimism, and locus of control."[55] She also believes that it is time to expand our ways of collecting data and to stop denigrating research efforts other than randomized controlled trials. By broadening our scope of research efforts, we could truly begin to investigate the many facets of distance healing effects.

Distance healing research generates a multitude of questions to explore in the rehabilitation setting. Questions such as:

✦ How reliable is distance healing?

✦ Is distance healing potent enough to work as a single modality, or should it be combined with other modalities?

✦ Can the ability to be an effective distance healer be acquired? If so, how can we effectively teach these skills to health care providers?

✦ Are there certain conditions that enhance the use of distance healing in the clinical setting?

✦ What conditions inhibit them?

It will be exciting to see the answers to these questions emerge as more research is developed and performed in the area of distance healing.

Conclusion

The increasing body of research investigating distance healing as a valuable therapeutic intervention is compelling. This research may challenge our view of what constitutes a complementary therapy. There will be a continuing debate over the relevance of funding research in this arena, however this type of research is essential in understanding how human beings can help each other to heal. Perhaps distance healing will become central to a new type of health care delivery, as described by Davis[56]:

> What is being asked for, indeed, demanded by many, is health care based on the principles of holism that emphasize healing over curing, and that is safe, supported by systematic research whenever possible, and that is less costly and toxic. This new health care will bring to the world the safest, most cost-effective and most flexible system possible both for prevention and healing. And then what it means to help someone, really help a person, will become clear to many of us for the first time.

References

1. Targ E. Prayer and distant healing: Sicher et al. *Advances in Mind-Body Medicine*. 1998;17:2-59.
2. King E, Bushwick B. Beliefs and attitudes of hospital inpatients about faith healing and prayer. *J Fam Pract*. 1994; 39:210-213.
3. Wallis C. Faith and healing: can prayer, faith and spirituality really improve your physical health? A growing and surprising body of scientific evidence says they can. *Time*. 1996;147:58.
4. Astin J, Harkness E, Ernst E. The efficacy of "distant healing": a systematic review of randomized trials. *Ann Intern Med*. 2000;132:903-910.
5. Sicher F, Targ E, Moore D, Smith HS. A randomized double blind study of the effect of distant healing in a population with advanced AIDS. Report of a small-scale study. *West J Med*. 1998;169:356-363.
6. Targ E. Research methodology for studies of prayer and distant healing. *Complementary Therapies in Nursing and Midwifery*. 2002;8:29-41.
7. Ameling A. Prayer and ancient healing practice becomes new again. *Holist Nurs Pract*. 2000;14(3):40-48.

8. Krieder E. Learning and teaching prayer. In: Sponheim P, ed. *A Primer on Prayer*. Philadelphia, PA: Fortress Press; 1988.

9. Dossey L. *Healing Words: The Power of Prayer and the Practice of Medicine*. New York, NY: Harper Books; 1993.

10. Levin J, Vandrpool H. Is frequent religious attendance really conducive to better health? *Soc Sci Med*. 1987;589-600.

11. Benor D. Survey of spiritual healing research. *Complementary Medical Research*. 1990;4:9-33.

12. Herbert N. *Quantum Reality*. New York, NY: Anchor Books; 1987.

13. O'Laire S. An experimental study of the effects of distant intercessory prayer on self-esteem, anxiety and depression. *Altern Ther Health Med*. 1997;3:6-40.

14. Benor D. *Healing Research*. Munich: Heliz Verlag; 1993.

15. Grad BR. A telekinetic effect on plant growth I. *International Journal of Parapsychology*. 1963;5(2):117-134.

16. Grad BR. A telekinetic effect on plant growth II. Experiments involving treatment of saline in stoppered bottles. *International Journal of Parapsychology*. 1964;6:473-498.

17. Grad BR. A telekinetic effect on plant growth III. Stimulating and inhibiting effects. Research Brief presented to the Seventh Annual Convention of the Parapsychological Association, Oxford University, Oxford England; 1964.

18. Grad BR. Some biological effects of laying-on of hands. A review of experiments with animals and plants. *J Am Soc Psychical Res*. 1965;59:95-127.

19. Grad BR. Effects of fermentation of yeast. *Proceedings of the Parapsychological Association*. 1965;2:15-16.

20. Grad BR. The laying-on of hands: implications for psychotherapy, gentling and the placebo effect. *J Am Soc Psychical Res*. 1967;61(4):286-305.

21. Dossey L. Non-local mind: the seminal experiments of Bernard Grad. *Advances in Mind-Body Medicine*. 2001;17:8-10.

22. Benor DJ. *Healing Research: Holistic Medicine and Spiritual Healing*. Munich: Helix Verlag; 1993.

23. Solvin J. Mental healing. In: Krippner S, ed. *Advances in Parapsychological Research*. Vol 4. Jefferson, NC: McFarland and Company; 1984:31-63.

24. May E, Vilenskaya L. Some aspects of parapsychological research in the former Soviet Union. *Subtle Energies*. 1994;3:1-24.

25. Barry J. General and comparative study of the psychokinetic effect on a fungus culture. *J Parapsych*. 1968;32:237-243.

26. Tedder W, Monty M. Exploration of long distance PK: conceptual replication of the influence on a biological system. *Research in Parapsychology*. 1980;1981:90-93.

27. Nash CB. Psychokinetic control of bacterial growth. *J Am Soc Psychical Res*. 1982;51:217-221.

28. Braud W. Distant mental influence of rate of hemolysis of human red blood cells. *J Am Soc Psychical Res*. 1990;84(1):1-24.

29. Muehsam DJ, et al. Effects of Qi gong on cell free myosin phosphorylation: preliminary experiments. *Subtle Energies*. 1994;5(1):93-108.

30. Barry J. Generalized and comparative study of the psychokinetic effect on a fungus culture. *J Parapsych*. 1968;32:237-243.

31. Tedder WH, Monty ML. Exploration of long-distance PK: a conceptual replication of the influence on a biological system. In: Roll WG, Beloff J, eds. *Research in Parapsychology*. Metuchen, NJ: Scarecrow; 1980:90-93.

32. Haraldsson E, Thorsteinson T. Psychokinetic effects on yeast: an exploratory experiment. In: Roll WG, Beloff J, eds. *Research in Parapsychology*. Metuchen, NJ: Scarecrow; 1980:20-21.

33. Rauscher EA, Rubik BA. Effects on motility behavior and growth of salmonella typhimurium in the presence of a psychic subject. In: Roll WG, Beloff J, eds. *Research in Parapsychology*. Metuchen, NJ: Scarecrow; 1980.

34. Rein G. *Quantum Biology: Healing with Subtle Energy*. Paolo Alto, CA: Quantum Biology Research Labs; 1992.

35. Snel FWJ. PK influences on malignant cell growth research. *Lett Univ Utrecht*. 1980;10:19-27.

36. Snel FWJ, Hol PR. Psychokinesis experiments in casein induced amyloidosis of the hamster. *J Parapsychol*. 1983;5(1):51-76.

37. Benor DJ. *Healing Research*. Vol F. Deddington, UK: Helix Editions Ltd; 1992.

38. Rosa L, Rosa E, Sarner L, Barret S. A close look at therapeutic touch. *JAMA*. 1998;279:1005-10.

39. Byrd R. Positive effects of intercessory prayer in a coronary care unit population. *South Med J*. 1988;81(7):826.

40. Koopman B, Blasband R. Distant healing revisited: time for a new epistemology. *Altern Ther Med*. 2002;8(1):101.

41. Jadad AR, Moore RA, Carroll D, et al. Assessing the quality of reports of randomized clinical trials: is blinding necessary? *Control Clin Trials*. 1996;17:1-12.

42. Roberts L, Ahmed I, Hall S, Sargent C. Intercessory prayer for the alleviation of ill health. *The Cochrane Database of Systematic Reviews*. 1992:2.

43. Krucoff MW, Crater SW, Green CL, et al. Randomized integrative therapies in interventional patients with unstable angina. The monitoring and activation of noetic training (mantra) feasibility pilot [abstract]. *Circulation*. 1998; A1458.

44. Wiseman R, Schlitz M. Experimenter effects and the remote detection of staring. *J Parapsychol*. 1997;61:197-201.

45. Targ E, Thomson K. Can prayer and intentionality be researched? Should they be? *Altern Ther Health Med*. 1997; 3(6):92-97.

46. Benor D. A psychiatrist examines fears of healing. In: Dossey L, ed. *Healing Words: The Power of Prayer and the Practice of Medicine*. New York, NY: Harper Books; 1993:278-284.

47. Snel FWJ, Van der Sijde PC. The effect of paranormal healing on tumor growth. *J Sci Exploration*. 1995;9:2:209-221.

48. Targ E. Evaluating healing a research review. *Altern Therapies*. 1997;3(6):74-77.

49. Braud WG, Schlitz M. Consciousness interaction with remote biological systems: anomalous intentionality effects. *Subtle Energies*. 1992;2(1):1-46.

50. Rew L. Intentionality in holistic nursing. *J Holistic Nurs*. 2000;18(2):91-93.

51. McKivergin M. The nurse as an instrument of healing. In: Dossey B, Keegan L, Guzzetta C, eds. *Holistic Nursing: A Handbook for Practice*. Gaithersburg, MD: Aspen Press; 2000.

52. Krieger D. *The Therapeutic Touch: How to Use Your Hands to Help and Heal*. New York, NY: Prentice Hall; 1986.

53. Macrae J. *Therapeutic Touch: A Practical Guide*. New York, NY: Alfred Knopf; 1995.

54. The Philadelphia Panel. Evidence-based clinical practice guidelines on selected rehabilitation interventions. *Journal of the American Physical Therapy Association*. 2001;81(10):1622-1730.

55. Davis C. Unpublished editorial. 2001.

56. Davis C, ed. *Complementary Therapies in Rehabilitation: Holistic Approaches for Prevention and Wellness*. Thorofare, NJ: SLACK Incorporated; 1997.

CHAPTER 22

Biomedical Applications of Low-Energy Lasers

G. Kesava Reddy, PhD

Introduction

L ASER is an acronym for *light amplification by the stimulated emission of radiation*. Laser therapy is a form of photobiostimulation that has been used in Europe for more than 30 years. Researchers in other parts of the world such as the Soviet Republic and Japan, for example, used low-intensity lasers to irradiate areas of skin and claim the low-intensity laser therapy accelerated wound healing. During the past decade, the clinical application of low-intensity laser therapy has also gained widespread acceptance in Canada and Australia.

History of the Evolution of Laser

In medicine, the use of light to treat various medical problems is not entirely new. Reports indicate that Galen (A.D. 131-201) routinely prescribed sunbaths for his patients. In the 13th century, Henri de Mondeville (A.D. 1260-1320) used light to treat smallpox, a method he had learned from the Arabians, who in turn had acquired the technique from the Chinese.[1,2] Albert Einstein (1879-1955) was first to postulate the theory that paved the way for the development of lasers. In 1917, he discovered that the existence of equilibrium between electromagnetic radiation and its interactions with matter required a previously undiscovered radiation process called stimulated emission. However, his theoretical work remained largely unexplored until 1954, when Townes and coworkers[3] developed the maser, a microwave amplifier based on the stimulated emission of radiation. Schawlow and Townes[4] then adapted the principle of masers to light. In 1960, Maiman[5] succeeded in building the first laser device, the ruby laser, which emitted monochromatic red light at a wavelength of 694.3 nanometers (nm). Within months, Javan and associates[6] developed the first gas laser, the helium-neon laser, which emitted radiation in both the infrared and visible spectral regions. Since then, laser has come to the forefront of modern technology, has been the subject of numerous investigations, and has become an integral scientific tool. Further advancements in laser research have led to the conclusions that different forms of light and other photonic radiation have a potential to modulate a variety of biological processes and can be used as powerful therapeutic tools for the treatment of various disorders. Although controversy still exists with regard to the mechanisms of the action of low-power lasers, recent progress in laser research warrants special attention to the role of low-power lasers in biology and medicine.

Low-Level Laser Therapy

Low-level laser therapy, also known as *photostimulation* or *photobiostimulation*, is thought to work through a photochemical response to the laser that induces biochemical alterations in cells, leading to physiological changes. The interaction of cells with light at different wavelengths produces physiological changes leading to alterations in cellular metabolism. Certain chromophores, like rhodopsin, bilirubin, and porphyrins, absorb light energy and cause chemical reactions in the cell, resulting in changes in the metabolic activities of the cell. These photochemical reactions between the cells and light thus form the basis for the fundamental mechanism of action of the modern therapeutic low-intensity laser photostimulation.

There have been many claims for the therapeutic effects of low-power laser therapy on a broad range of disorders. A short list of laser applications promoted by some users and manufacturers of laser devices include promotion of tissue repair, acceleration of wound healing, stimulation of bone repair, pain attenuation, restoration of normal neural function following injury, and modulation of the immune system.

Conversion of Light Energy into Laser

Basic atomic theory is used to explain the principles of laser generation. The atom is divisible into fundamental particles called neutrons, protons, and electrons. When an atom absorbs energy from light, an orbiting electron is excited to a higher orbit. When it returns to its original orbit, the electron releases energy in the form of a photon. According to Einstein's principle, the photon that is released from the exited atom would stimulate another similarly exited atom to release an identical photon, and in doing so, returns to its original orbit. The triggering photon would continue on its way unchanged, and subsequent photons generated would be identical in phase, direction, and frequency. To contain them and to generate a large number of photons, mirrors are placed at both ends of a chamber, one of which is totally reflective and the other is partially reflective. The photons are then reflected within the chamber, and light amplification occurs and stimulates the emission of other photons from excited atoms. When a specific level of energy is attained, photons of a particular wavelength are ejected through the partially reflective mirror, resulting in amplified light through stimulated emissions known as laser.

Characteristics of the Laser

Light, including laser, is a source of electromagnetic radiation. Laser light is emitted in an organized manner rather than in the random pattern of nonlaser radiation, such as in an incandescent light bulb. Besides sharing the common characteristics of electromagnetic radiation, laser radiation has three distinguishing features: monochromaticity, coherence, and unidirectionality or collimation.

+ *Monochromaticity.* Of a single wavelength and hence one color, is the characteristic emission produced by a laser. Because of this property, when the laser beam is passed through a prism, only one color will appear at the opposite side of the prism.

✦ *Coherence.* The waves are generated in phase with each other, that is, the troughs and crests of the waves are "locked" together. Coherence is one of the most specific and critical properties of laser radiation and is intimately related to the stimulated emission mechanism or source of the laser radiation. There are two types of coherences: spatial coherence and temporal coherence. In spatial coherence, a laser beam originating from two different points of the same laser interferes when superposed in the same point, producing interference fringes. Temporal coherence occurs when laser radiation emitted from a given point of the laser source at a given moment interferes with the laser radiation emitted from the same point at a later time providing that both beams are incident in the same point. The time interval within which the interference may be obtained is called coherence time, and the laser is defined as a temporally coherent source of electromagnetic radiation.

✦ *Unidirectionality or Collimation.* The lack of divergence of the laser beam. The laser beam is well collimated and travels uniformly in the same direction without diverging in the manner that nonlaser radiation does. Ordinary light spreads rapidly in any direction; laser light usually is emitted in one direction and, in the best of situations, along a straight line. This means that the photons move in a parallel fashion and thus concentrate in a narrow beam of light, focusing the power of the light into narrow space.

Basic Components of Laser

There are four primary components of a laser regardless of style, size, or application.

✦ *Active medium.* The active medium may be solid crystals, liquid dyes, gases such as carbon dioxide or helium/neon, or semiconductors. These active media contain atoms whose electrons may be excited to a metastable energy level by an energy source.

✦ *Excitation mechanism.* Excitation mechanisms pump energy into the active medium by one or more of three basic methods: optical, electrical, or chemical.

✦ *Totally reflective mirror.* A mirror that reflects essentially 100% of the laser light.

✦ *Partially reflective mirror.* A mirror that reflects less than 100% of the laser light and transmits the remainder. In other words, some of the light is reflected and some of the light passes through this mirror.

Lasing Action: A Summary

Photons are produced following the application of energy to an atom, raising an electron to a higher orbit (unstable energy level). This excited electron will then randomly return to its stable state and release a photon of light or of a nonvisible radiation in the process. Light produced in this manner is called incoherent light and has many different directions and phases with a number of wavelengths. When energy is applied to a laser active medium, electrons are raised to an unstable energy level from which they spontaneously decay to a lower, relatively long-lived metastable state. Electrons in this state will not spontaneously return to their ground energy level; therefore, it is possible to pump large amounts of energy into the material and obtain a population inversion in which most of the atoms exist in a metastable state. After this population inversion has been achieved, lasing action is then initiated by an electron that spontaneously returns to its ground state, producing a photon. If the photon released is of exactly the right wavelength, it will stimulate an atom in a metastable state to emit a photon of the same wavelength (stimulated emission). Many of these stimulated photons will be lost when they hit the side of the lasing medium. However, those photons that travel parallel to the long axis of the optical cavity continue to stimulate emissions of photons having the same wavelengths, which travel coherently until they reach the mirrored ends of the optical cavity. When the beam strikes the totally reflecting mirror in the optical cavity, the beam is reversed while maintaining its coherence and continues to stimulate emissions of photons. The radiation increases in intensity until the beam reaches the partially reflecting surface of the optical cavity. A small portion of the coherent light is released while the rest is reflected back through the lasing medium to continue the process of stimulating photon emission. Laser radiation will continue to be produced as long as energy is applied to the lasing medium.

Continuous Wave Form

If energy is continuously pumped into the active medium, equilibrium may be achieved between the number of atoms raised to a metastable state and the number of photons emitted, which produces a continuous laser output. Output for continuous wave lasers is expressed as a power (W=watts). The concentration of a laser beam on a given area is described as the power density, that is, power/unit area (watts/cm^2). The output is also recorded as energy density (Joules [J]/cm^2), where 1 J is 1 watt per second.

Pulsed Laser and Q-Switched Laser Waves

Just as with pulsed electricity, pulsed laser emissions are produced when the excitation medium is modulated, producing a pulse of laser radiation lasting usually less than 0.25 seconds. Pulsed output may also be produced by blocking the beam with a rotating mirror or prism. "Q-switching or Q-spoiling" is a technique employed to produce a very high output pulse. Q-switching is accomplished by using a device that prevents the reflection of photons back and forth in the active medium. This produces a higher population of electrons in the metastable state. At a predetermined instant, the Q-switch is turned off, allowing the lasing action to continue producing very intense short pulses of laser radiation. Q-switched lasers produce pulses of 10 to 250 nanoseconds (ns). Output for pulsed lasers is expressed as radiant exposure (H), which is the concentration of laser energy (power x time in seconds) on a given area energy/unit area (J/cm^2)—energy density.

Types of Lasers

Depending on the lasing medium placed between two reflecting surfaces, different types of laser beams will be produced. Each of these laser beams is very specific in its wavelength and has unique characteristics. The media used to create lasers include gas and excimer, crystal and glass (solid-state) semiconductor, liquid dye, and chemical.

GAS LASERS

Gas lasers were developed in early 1960s shortly after the first ruby laser. There are several types of gas lasers available, including helium-neon, carbon dioxide, and argon lasers.

Helium-Neon Laser

The most common and inexpensive gas laser, the helium-neon laser, is usually constructed to operate in the red at 632.8 nm. It can also be constructed to produce laser action in the green at 543.5 nm and in the infrared at 1523 nm. One of the excited levels of helium at 20.61 electron volts (eV) is very close to a level in neon at 20.66 eV, so close in fact that upon collision of a helium and a neon atom, the energy can be transferred from the helium to the neon atom. Helium-neon laser is the most studied device among other lasers for its therapeutic applications in medicine and biology, particularly for wound healing, tissue repair, and pain attenuation.

Carbon Dioxide Laser

The carbon dioxide gas laser is capable of continuous output powers above 10 kilowatts (kW). It is also capable of extremely high-powered pulsed operation. It exhibits laser action at several infrared frequencies but none in the visible range. Operating in a manner similar to the helium-neon laser, it employs an electric discharge for pumping, using a percentage of nitrogen gas as a pumping gas. The carbon dioxide laser is the most efficient laser, capable of operating at more than 30% efficiency, much more efficient than an incandescent light bulb, which has an efficiency of only about 10%. As a therapeutic modality, these lasers have been successfully used to treat wrinkles and scars as well as benign skin growths such as warts, linear epidermal nevi (birthmarks), rhinophyma (enlarged oil glands on the nose), and other skin conditions.

Argon Laser

The argon ion laser can be operated as a continuous gas laser at about 25 different wavelengths in the visible spectrum between 408.9 and 686.1 nm, but is best known for its most efficient transmissions in the green spectrum at 488 nm and 514.5 nm. Operating at much higher powers than the helium-neon gas laser, it is not uncommon to achieve 30 to 100 watts of continuous power. This output is produced in hot plasma and takes extremely high power, typically 9 to 12 kW, so argon lasers are large and expensive devices. They are commonly employed in dentistry for teeth whitening and to cure the resin materials used for tooth fillings.

SEMICONDUCTOR (DIODE) LASERS

After the expansion of gas lasers, semiconductor or diode lasers were developed. The gallium-arsenide (Ga-As) was the first diode laser developed and is used as a therapeutic modality for wound healing and tissue repair. Diode lasers are also used for hair removal and dermatological surgeries.

CRYSTAL LASERS

Several types of crystal lasers have been developed using synthetic materials. These include neodymium-yttrium-aluminum-garnet (Nd: YAG) and synthetic ruby lasers. These lasers are commonly used for the removal of tattoos and are also used in certain dental procedures.

LIQUID LASERS

In the production of liquid lasers, an organic dye is used as the lasing medium. Another name of liquid lasers is dye lasers. Some of the medical applications of these lasers include the treatment of port-wine stains and other vascular lesions.

CHEMICAL LASERS

Chemical lasers are extremely high-power lasers and mostly used in the military as weapons.

High-Power vs Low-Power Lasers

Depending on the intensity of energy emitted, lasers are categorized into high or low power. Since high-power lasers generate high thermal energy, they are know also as hot lasers and are primarily used for surgical cutting and coagulation, dermatology, ophthalmology, oncology, vascular surgery, and other surgical specialties.

Low-power lasers are intended to work at lower intensities and generate minimal thermal energy. These lasers produce a maximal output of less than 500 mW. A majority of low-power lasers are used for therapeutic purposes, including tissue repair, wound healing and pain attenuation. Unlike high-power lasers, low-power lasers cause a photochemical reaction rather than thermal effects. Clinically, no significant tissue warming occurs while using low-power lasers. These include the helium-neon (He-Ne) laser, the argon laser, the gallium-arsenide (Ga-As) laser, the gallium-aluminum-arsenide laser, the carbon dioxide laser, and the nitrogen laser.

Although the medical applications of low-power lasers remain controversial in the United States, the clinical use of these devices for a variety of conditions, including promotion of tissue repair processes, acceleration of wound healing, stimulation of bone repair, pain attenuation, restoration of normal neural function following injury, and modulation of the immune system, is steadily increasing. There are numerous biological and physiological effects of low-power lasers reported in the literature (Table 22-1), which may help to support the various applications of these devices in biology and medicine. Together with other reports, these findings offer ample explanation of photochemical, photobiological, and photomedical effects of low-power lasers on living cells and tissues.

Biological Effects of Low-Power Lasers

The biological effects of low-power lasers can be explained on the basis of photobiological interactions between electromagnetic radiation light and atoms. From a light source, when an atom absorbs a photon, an electron of that atom is raised to a higher energy state. This excited atom then loses its extra energy either by re-emitting a photon, by giving off heat, or by undergoing photochemical changes. The biological effects of low-power lasers are a response to the photochemical reactions between light and atoms. Both visible and infrared low-power lasers produce similar clinical and biological responses. For instance, Abergel et al[7] and Lam et al[8] found that the irradiation of fibroblasts in culture either at 633 nm (visible red) or at 904 nm (infrared) stimulated the synthesis of collagen. Karu[9] offers an explanation. When visible red light is absorbed, a chain of events is triggered following the absorption of light by photoreceptors in the mitochondria, which leads to signal transduction and amplification that modulates nucleic acid synthesis and finally induction of cell proliferation. Infrared radiation initiates the response at the membrane level and, in that way, promotes the cell proliferation (Figure 22-1).

The biological effects of low-power lasers have been established using both in vivo and in vitro systems. Studies using an in vitro system of cell culture showed that low-power laser irradiation stimulates the proliferation of fibroblasts through the modulation of the production of fibroblast growth factor.[10] Other investigators showed the release of soluble factors, which promotes fibroblast proliferation following laser treatment using macrophage cell lines.[11] A nonlinear dose and intensity dependence of mitosis rate of human fibroblasts following light irradiation had been reported earlier.[12] Similar results were reported using diode laser to irradiate human fibroblasts.[13] Their results suggest a relationship between fibroblast proliferation and succinic dehydrogenase, a mitochondrial enzyme. An increased synthesis of DNA has been observed in fibroblast cultures following laser irradiation.[14] A further effect of low-power laser irradiation showed a direct and massive transformation of cultured fibroblasts into myofibroblasts.[15] A dose-dependent enhancement of cell proliferation resulting from laser irradiation of fibroblasts has been reported previously.[16] Increases in fibroblast proliferation and collagen production have been observed in vitro by several investigators.[17,18]

While low-power lasers have been shown to increase both the phagocytic and chemotactic activity of human leukocytes in vitro, there have also been claims that laser irradiation can act directly and selectively on the immune system.[22] Low-power laser irradiation of human peripheral blood mononuclear cells has been shown to increase the production of cytokines including inter-

Table 22-1

AN EXTENSIVE REVIEW OF LITERATURE FOCUSING ON THE BIOLOGICAL EFFECTS OF LOW-POWER LASER THERAPY

BIOLOGICAL EFFECTS	STUDY DESCRIPTION	REFERENCES
Increased cell proliferation, cell activation, cell division, cell maturation, transformation into myofibroblasts, release of interleukins, secretion of growth factors, collagen synthesis, DNA synthesis, and ATP production	**Cell culture system**: Using fibroblasts, macrophages mitochondria, keratinocytes, epithelial cells, endothelial cells, lymphocytes, and osteoblasts	Atabey et al[16] Almeida-Lopes et al[19] Yu et al[20] Haas et al[21] Tadakuma et al[22] Passarella et al[23] Rajaratnam et al[11] Bolton et al[13] Pereira et al[17] Funk et al[24] Ghali et al[25] Coombe et al[26] Yamada et al[27]
Improved wound healing, increased vascularity, increased collagen production, enhanced wound strength, elevated mRNA levels, proliferation of myofibroblasts and fibroblasts, increased rate of wound closure, enhanced granulation tissue formation, earlier epithelialization, acceleration of wound healing, and improved biomechanical properties of healing tissue	**Wound healing**: Using rat, mice, rabbit, and studies in humans	Mester et al[28] Braverman et al[29] Bisht et al[30] Lyons et al[31] Saperia et al[32] Surinchak et al[33] Strassl et al[34] Al-Watban et al[35] Reddy et al[36] Reddy et al[37]
Improved wound epithelialization, enhanced granulation tissue formation, increased collagen deposition, increased cellular contents, enhanced collagen production, decreased collagen solubility, increased wound tensile properties, improved skin circulation, and shortened healing phase	**Impaired wound healing**: Using diabetic rat, mice, and studies in human diabetic patients' healing phase	Yu et al[38] Schindl et al[39] Stadler et al[40] Reddy et al[41] Reddy et al[42] Reddy et al[43] Reddy et al[44] Kuliev et al[45] Chentsova et al[46] Sugrue et al[47]

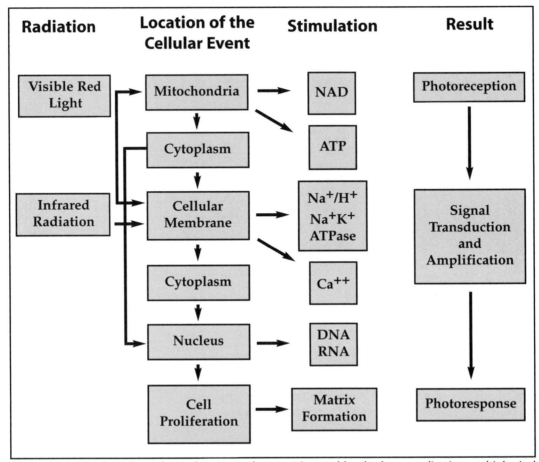

Figure 22-1. The flow chart shows the events that are triggered by the laser application on biological system. In addition, the possible mechanism of the action of the laser photostimulation at visible-red and infrared radiations was outlined at cellular level.

leukin-1 alpha (IL-1 alpha), interleukin-2, tumor necrosis factor-alpha, and interferon-gamma.[24] Ghali and Dyson[25] reported alterations in the proliferation rate of human umbilical vein endothelial cells after irradiation with low-power lasers. Studies on bone cells reveal that laser irradiation exerts pronounced effects on proliferation, differentiation, and calcification of cultured osteoblast cells.[27]

In summary, these in vitro studies demonstrated low-level laser therapy can stimulate cell proliferation, enhance the ATP synthesis, augment the cell division, induce the secretion of growth factors such as interleukin-1 and interleukin-8 from macrophages, increase DNA synthesis, and augment collagen production, which are all required for wound healing and tissue repair.

Clinical Applications of Low-Power Lasers

WOUND HEALING

Wound healing is a complex process with an orchestrated sequence of biochemical changes involving the interactions of many different cell types, matrix components, proteases, and cytokines. Normal wound healing proceeds in three distinct but overlapping phases: inflammation, proliferation, and remodeling. Wound healing involves a dynamic series of events including clotting, inflammation, granulation tissue formation, epithelialization, matrix synthesis, and tissue remodeling.[48] Many of the regimens and therapeutic interventions designed to facilitate the wound healing process influence the various phases wound healing.

Most early studies of low-power laser applications on wound healing were performed in Europe using animal models. Many of these studies have utilized rats, mice, rabbits, dogs, and pigs to investigate the effects of laser on wound healing. These studies have evaluated the efficacy of low-intensity laser irradiation using healthy animals. A study by Mester et al[49] in Hungary revealed that a ruby laser treatment accelerated the healing of mechanical wounds and burns in mice. Kana et al[50] showed that treatment with He-Ne laser at low intensities increases the rate of wound closure in rats. Similarly, Dyson and Young[51] reported the acceleration of wound healing in mice following treatment with a combined low-intensity He-Ne and diode laser.

Al-Watban and his group examined the influence of variety of irradiation protocols and other factors related to wound healing in rats.[35,52-54] These investigators reported that He-Ne laser was most effective in the enhancement of wound healing. More evidence for efficacy of He-Ne lasers in wound healing comes from a study by Strassl et al,[34] who investigated healing times, fibroblast numbers, collagen content, and strength of surgical wounds in dogs after He-Ne laser and placebo treatment. The results revealed an increased numbers of fibroblasts, greater content of collagen, and faster healing in the laser-treated wounds compared with the contralateral sham-treated wounds. Other investigators reported increased granulation tissue, earlier epithelialization, increased fibroblast proliferation, and matrix synthesis in healing wounds following laser therapy.[30]

Other reports found that the low-intensity He-Ne laser treatment improved wound tensile strength in rats[33] and mice.[31] However, in rabbits, no significant differences were detected in healing between laser treated and control wounds.[33] Saperia et al[32] proposed a mechanism for enhanced wound healing by demonstrating the increased mRNA levels for collagen of cutaneous wounds of pigs treated with He-Ne laser. Braverman et al[29] showed that laser irradiation increases wound tensile strength in rabbits. Recently, it has been shown that laser therapy modified inflammation and induced collagen deposition along with the higher proliferation of myofibroblasts in experimental cutaneous wounds.[55]

Only a few studies examined the efficacy of low-intensity lasers using severely impaired wound healing models. It is well known that diabetes interferes with normal wound healing and, as a consequence, diabetic patients have significant morbidity. Therefore, impaired wound healing in diabetics poses a serious challenge in clinical medicine. Although the exact nature of the pathogenesis of the poor wound healing in diabetics is not well understood, evidence from studies involving both human and animal models of diabetes reveal several abnormalities in the various phases of the wound healing process. Diabetes-induced impairment of wound healing is characterized by an inhibition of the inflammatory response, angiogenesis, fibroplasia, defects in collagen deposition, and differentiation of the extracellular matrix.[56-59] The impaired wound healing in diabetes may thus provide a sensitive and suitable model for evaluating the efficacy and mechanism of low-power laser therapy.

In an effort to determine the specific effects and mechanism of low-energy laser therapy, Yu et al[38] studied the wound healing processes by evaluating the percentage of wound closure and histologic score using genetically diabetic mice. They compared the effect of laser irradiation (Argon dye laser at 630 nm wavelength), basic fibroblast growth factor (bFGF), and combination of laser and growth factor on healing resistant wounds of diabetic mice. Their results indicated that all three treatment regimens significantly improved the wound epithelialization, cellular content, granulation tissue formation, and collagen deposition with laser treatment alone, or in combination with a topical application of growth factor.

Recent studies from the author's laboratory involve the evaluation of the efficacy of low-power laser therapy on healing resistant wounds in experimental diabetic rats.[41-44] In these studies, experimental diabetes was induced in rats by the administration of streptozotocin. Following establishment of uncontrolled diabetes in rats, two circular wounds were created on the either side of the spine, and the left side of the wound of each diabetic rat was treated with laser photostimulation. The potential beneficial effects of laser irradiation on healing wounds were evaluated by measuring and comparing biomechanical and biochemical indices of wounded tissue with and without laser treatments. The results of these studies revealed that a significant improvement in biomechanical indices (maximum load, stress, strain, energy absorption, and toughness) as well as biochemical indices (collagen production and collagen extractability) in laser-treated wounds compared to control wounds. Other investigators showed that laser irradiation increased wound tensile strength using a diabetic murine model.[40]

In a clinical study of wound healing involving 152 diabetic patients with purulent injuries of the skin and underlying soft tissues, low-level laser therapy resulted in a shortened healing phase.[45] In another study involving 512 patients with corneal wounds, burns, or ulcers, it was reported that laser therapy accelerated the rate of healing.[46] Similarly, other investigators reported positive effects of laser therapy for patients with chronic venous leg ulcers that had not responded to other conventional treatments.[47] An improvement in skin circulation was observed in patients with diabetic microangiopathy following laser irradiation.[39]

Case reports are used to support claims that low-level laser therapy can shrink keloid scars, accelerate wound healing, and modulate the healing of diabetic foot ulcers.[60,61] Successful treatment was achieved for a persistent radiation ulcer using low power laser therapy.[62]

In summary, these in vivo studies collectively demonstrate that laser photostimulation accelerates wound healing where healing has been delayed.

TISSUE REPAIR PROCESSES

Compared to studies on cutaneous wound healing, research concerning the effects of laser photostimulation on other types of tissue repair is still in its infancy. The effect of low-level laser therapy on soft tissue repair has been studied using rabbit Achilles' tendon as the model. In this experimental model, the Achilles' tendons were severed, sutured, and used to examine the effects of laser irradiation at various intensities during tendon repair. A dose of 1 to 5 mJ/cm^2 He-Ne laser augments the force per unit area (tensile stress) acquired by the tendons after 21 days of healing, albeit without significantly increasing the ultimate tensile strength or energy absorption capacity of the tissue.[63] No dose-dependent effects were observed within this dose range. Similarly, 1 to 5 mJ/cm^2 He-Ne laser modulates collagen synthesis, as evidenced by altered collagen fibril morphometry, and promotes the formation of membrane-bound intracytoplasmic collagen fibrils in tendon fibroblasts and myofibroblasts.[64,65]

In contrast to the biomechanical effects of the lower dose range described above (ie, 1 to 5 mJ/cm^2) He-Ne laser of 0.5 or 1.0 J/cm^2 induces a significant (30% to 40%) increase in the ultimate tensile strength, and tensile stress of the tendons after just 14 days of healing. These beneficial effects are slightly better with the 1.0 J/cm^2 dose than with other doses.[66] Similarly, Ga-As laser of 0.5, 1.0, or 1.5 J/cm^2 significantly increases the ultimate tensile strength and tensile stress of tendons by as much as 40% after 14 days of healing. As with the He-Ne laser study, these beneficial effects are slightly better with the 1.0 J/cm^2 dose than other dose levels.[67] With both He-Ne and Ga-As lasers, photostimulation in the continuous mode produced a slightly better effect than stimulation in the pulsed model.[66,67] Photostimulation of repaired tendons during the first 7 days of healing yielded a better result than irradiation during the next 7 days of healing. This may relate to the modulating effects of He-Ne lasers on specific events during the first two phases of tendon repair (ie, the inflammation phase and the collagen synthesis phase). Collectively, these findings indicate that the period of intervention may be as critical with Ga-As laser as it is with He-Ne laser. Subsequent studies from the author's laboratory have shown that laser photostimulation of surgically tenotomized rabbit Achilles' tendons produced significantly more collagen, marginally improved tensile strength, and other biomechanical indices than controls.[36,37]

Few studies have been reported in the literature regarding the effects of low-level laser therapy on bone repair. Trelles and Mayayo[68] reported a faster formation of callus and vascularization in induced fractures in mice by laser irradiation. Barushka et al[69] found that laser irradiation on drill-hole injuries in the tibia of the rat affected the population of osteoblasts and osteoclasts, altered alkaline phosphatase activities, and promoted bone repair. Glinkowsky and Rowinsky[70] reported that laser irradiation promoted the healing of tibial fractures in mice. Similarly, enhanced bone fracture healing was observed following low-level laser therapy in rats.[71] Other investigators reported positive effects of laser irradiation on bone healing using microscopic measurements.[72] Thus, these studies collectively indicate that laser photostimulation can modulate tissue repair and fracture healing.

PAIN ATTENUATION

Clinically, low-power laser therapy has been used successfully in the treatment of chronic pain, but many have questioned the scientific basis for its use. There have been many reports on the applications of low-reactive-level laser therapy for pain attenuation or pain removal. Evidence indicates that low-level laser therapy is effective in reducing pain from several musculoskeletal conditions, including shoulder injuries,[73] tendonitis,[74] myofasciitis,[75] muscle spasm,[76] calcaneal spur,[77] osteoarthritis,[78,79] and rheumatoid arthritis.[79] In studying the effect of laser therapy on painful conditions, Baxter et al[80] reported that lasers achieved the premier overall ranking for pain relief compared with the other electrophysical modalities. Moreover, other investigators found a rapid relief from neck pain[81] and back pain[82,83] with laser therapy. Beneficial effects of laser irradiation were also observed against vascular headaches.[73] The mechanisms for the neuropharmacological analgesic action of laser irradiation have been explained in several ways. When the laser is applied to key points on the surface of the skin, muscle tension can be released and circulation of blood can be increased. Stimulating these key points triggers the release of endorphins, which are the neurochemicals that relieve pain.[84] With the release of this chemical comes relief from the pain and reduced inflammation, together with increases in blood flow and oxygen supply to the affected area. In addition, low-level laser therapy appears to modulate the release of neurotransmitters such as serotonin and acetylcholine, which are known to play important roles in pain attenuation. Reports also indicate that laser therapy is effective in attenuating pain from experimentally induced inflammation. Honmura et al[85,86] have shown the potential beneficial effects of laser irradiation with experimentally induced inflammation in rats. Collectively, these studies suggest that laser therapy is an effective modality for pain attenuation.

OTHER MEDICAL APPLICATIONS

A list of other medical applications of laser photostimulation can be found in a recent book on laser therapy by Tuner and Hode.[87] Some of the medical conditions that the authors suggest can be treated with laser therapy include carpal tunnel syndrome, fibromyalgia, herpes simplex, modulation of the immune system, muscle regeneration, nerve condition and regeneration, edema, ophthalmic problems, spinal cord injuries, sports injuries, tinnitus, and some urological problems.

Controversies About Low-Level Laser as a Therapeutic Modality

In this chapter, thus far, only studies that reported positive effects of low-level laser therapy in biology and medicine have been considered. However, there have been many studies that reported either no effects or negative effects of laser irradiation. The most striking arguments against the therapeutic effects of laser stimulation come from a variety of studies conducted both in vitro and in vivo settings. These studies reported no detectable effects of laser therapy in general. It appears that the lack of detectable effects of laser therapy observed in many of these studies could be due to major experimental design flaws, inappropriate selection of clinical conditions, the absence of biological responses in the selected setting, and inappropriate dosimetry of laser application.[88] Experiments using either too low[89,90] or too high[91,92] dosages of laser therapy are unlikely to yield positive effects since low-level laser irradiation-inducible biological responses were found to occur at energy densities between 1.0 J/cm^2 and 10 J/cm^2. The power density is also of biological and clinical significance. Moreover, incorrectly calculated radiation parameters and inappropriate specification of dosimetric terms predispose serious consequences on the outcomes of a study.[93] In addition, methodological differences preclude valid comparison of these studies with that of studies with positive findings. The units of measurement that should be specified when low-level laser therapy is used are listed below.

Units of Measurement

The following parameters are important for clinicians to record so that they and others can repeat their work:
+ Wavelength (in nanometers)
+ Treatment duration (in minutes)
+ Power output (in mW)
+ Power density (in mW/centimeter squared)
+ Energy density (in Joules/centimeter squared)

The power density can be calculated by dividing the power output by the irradiating area (or spot size) of the laser. The spot of a semiconductor diode is typically 0.1 to 0.125 cm^2. Similarly, the energy density can be calculated by multiplying the power density by the irradiation time in seconds. In addition, when low-intensity laser photostimulation is used in pulsed mode, the pulse repetition rate in Hertz (ie, number of pulses per second) should also be documented.

Conclusion

The use of lasers in biology and medicine is increasing tremendously. Laser is a form of light or infrared radiation, both of which are electromagnetic radiations. In contrast to nonlaser radiation, which is made up of divergent and generally multiple wavelengths, laser beam is monochromatic, coherent, and collimated. Because of these properties, laser became an important tool in the scientific community. The number of studies on the medical applications of low-level laser therapy is steadily growing. The clinical use of laser for a variety of medical conditions is rising. Several recent studies have confirmed their potential beneficial effects for wound healing and other types of tissue repair using both in vivo and in vitro settings. The medical use of lasers warrants further research.

The granting of US Food and Drug Administration marketing approval to some low-level laser therapy devices during the past year is expected to increase awareness of laser therapy to the benefit of both patients and clinicians.

References

1. Garrison FH. *An Introduction to the History of Medicine.* Philadelphia: WB Saunders; 1929.
2. Kleinkort JA, Foley RA. Laser acupuncture: its use in physical therapy. *Am J Acupuncture.* 1984;12:51-56.

3. Gordon JP, Zeiger HJ, Townes CH. Molecular microwave oscillator and new hyperfine structure in the microwave spectrum of NH3. *Phys Rev Lett.* 1954;95:282-284.

4. Schawlow AL, Townes CH. Infrared and optical masers. *Phys Rev Lett.* 1958;112:1940-1949.

5. Maiman TH. Stimulated optical radiation in ruby. *Nature.* 1960;187:493-494.

6. Javan A, Bennett WR, Harriott DR. Population inversion and continuous maser oscillation in a gas discharge containing He-Ne mixtures. *Phys Rev Lett.* 1961;6:106-110.

7. Abergel RP, Meeker CA, Lam TS, Dwyer RM, Lesavoy MA, Uitto J. Control of connective tissue metabolism by lasers: recent developments and future prospects. *J Am Acad Dermatol.* 1984;11:1142-1150.

8. Lam TS, Abergel RP, Castel JC, Dwyer RM, Lesavoy MA, Uitto J. Laser stimulation of collagen synthesis in human skin fibroblast cultures. *Lasers Life Sci.* 1986;1:61-77.

9. Karu T. Molecular mechanism of the therapeutic effect of low intensity laser radiation. *Lasers Life Sci.* 1988;2:53-74.

10. Yu W, Naim JO, Lanzafame RJ. The effect of laser irradiation on the release of bFGF from 3T3 fibroblasts. *Photochem Photobiol.* 1994;59:167-170.

11. Rajaratnam S, Bolton P, Dyson M. Macrophage responsiveness to laser therapy with varying pulsing frequencies. *Laser Therapy.* 1994;6:107-112.

12. Lubart R, Friedmann H, Peled I, Grossmann N. Light effect on fibroblast proliferation. *Laser Therapy.* 1993;5:55-57.

13. Bolton P, Young S, Dyson M. The direct effect of 860 nm light on cell proliferation and on succinic dehydrogenase activity of human fibroblasts in vitro. *Laser Therapy.* 1995;7:55-60.

14. Loevschall H, Arenholt-Bindslev D. Effect of low level diode laser irradiation of human oral mucosa fibroblasts in vitro. *Lasers Surg Med.* 1994;14:347-354.

15. Pourreau-Schneider N, Ahmed A, Soudry M, et al. Helium-neon laser treatment transforms fibroblasts into myofibroblasts. *Am J Pathol.* 1990;137:171-178.

16. Atabey A, Karademir S, Atabey N, Barutcu A. The effects of the helium neon laser on wound healing in rabbits and on human skin fibroblasts. *Eur J Plast Surg.* 1995;18:99-102.

17. Pereira AN, Eduardo Cde P, Matson E, Marques MM. Effect of low-power laser irradiation on cell growth and procollagen synthesis of cultured fibroblasts. *Lasers Surg Med.* 2002;31:263-267.

18. Labbe RF, Skogerboe KJ, Davis HA, Rettmer RL. Laser photobioactivation mechanisms: in vitro studies using ascorbic acid uptake and hydroxyproline formation as biochemical markers of irradiation response. *Lasers Surg Med.* 1990;10:201-7.

19. Almeida-Lopes L, Rigau J, Zangaro RA, Guidugli-Neto J, Jaeger MM. Comparison of the low level laser therapy effects on cultured human gingival fibroblasts proliferation using different irradiance and same fluence. *Lasers Surg Med.* 2001;29:179-184.

20. Yu HS, Chang KL, Yu CL, Chen JW, Chen GS. Low-energy helium-neon laser irradiation stimulates interleukin-1 alpha and interleukin-8 release from cultured human keratinocytes. *J Invest Dermatol.* 1996;107:593-596.

21. Haas AF, Isseroff RR, Wheeland RG, Rood PA, Graves PJ. Low-energy helium-neon laser irradiation increases the motility of cultured human keratinocytes. *J Invest Dermatol.* 1990;94:822-826.

22. Tadakuma T. Possible application of the laser in immunobiology. *Keio J Med.* 1993;42:180-182.

23. Passarella S, Casamassima E, Molinari S, et al. Increase of proton electrochemical potential and ATP synthesis in rat liver mitochondria irradiated in vitro by helium-neon laser. *FEBS Lett.* 1984;175:95-99.

24. Funk JO, Kruse A, Kirchner H. Cytokine production after helium-neon laser irradiation in cultures of human peripheral blood mononuclear cells. *J Photochem Photobiol B.* 1992;16:347-355.

25. Ghali L, Dyson M. The direct effect of light therapy on endothelial cell proliferation in vitro. In: Steiner R, Weisz P, Langer R, eds. *Principles: Science-Technology-Medicine.* Basel, Switzerland: Birkhauser Verlag; 1992:411-414.

26. Coombe AR, Ho CT, Darendeliler MA, et al. The effects of low level laser irradiation on osteoblastic cells. *Clin Orthod Res.* 2001;4:3-14.

27. Yamada K. Biological effects of low power laser irradiation on clonal osteoblastic cells (MC3T3-E1). *Nippon Seikeigeka Gakkai Zasshi.* 1991;65:787-799.

28. Mester E, Jaszsagi-Nagy E. The effect of laser radiation on wound healing and collagen synthesis. *Studia Biophysica.* 1973;35:227-230.

29. Braverman B, McCarthy RJ, Ivankovich AD, Forde DE, Overfield M, Bapna MS. Effect of helium-neon and infrared laser irradiation on wound healing in rabbits. *Lasers Surg Med.* 1989;9:50-58.

30. Bisht D, Gupta SC, Misra V, Mital VP, Sharma P. Effect of low intensity laser radiation on healing of open skin wounds in rats. *Indian J Med Res.* 1994;100:43-46.

31. Lyons RF, Abergel RP, White RA, Dwyer RM, Castel JC, Uitto J. Biostimulation of wound healing in vivo by a helium-neon laser. *Ann Plast Surg.* 1987;18:47-50.

32. Saperia D, Glassberg E, Lyons RF, et al. Demonstration of elevated type I and type III procollagen mRNA levels in cutaneous wounds treated with helium-neon laser. Proposed mechanism for enhanced wound healing. *Biochem Biophys Res Commun.* 1986;138:1123-1128.

33. Surinchak JS, Alago ML, Bellamy RF, Stuck BE, Belkin M. Effects of low-level energy lasers on the healing of full-thickness skin defects. *Lasers Surg Med.* 1983;2:267-74.

34. Strassl H, Porteder H, Zenter K. The influence of laser beam treatment on wound healing in dogs. *Acta Chir Austriaca.* 1983;2:33-40.
35. Al-Watban FH, Zhang XY. Comparison of the effects of laser therapy on wound healing using different laser wavelengths. *Laser Therapy.* 1996;8:127-135.
36. Reddy GK, Stehno-Bittel L, Enwemeka CS. Laser photostimulation of collagen production in healing rabbit Achilles' tendons. *Lasers Surg Med.* 1998;22:281-287.
37. Reddy GK, Gum S, Stehno-Bittel L, Enwemeka CS. Biochemistry and biomechanics of healing tendon: part II. Effects of combined laser therapy and electrical stimulation. *Med Sci Sports Exerc.* 1998;30:794-800.
38. Yu W, Naim JO, Lanzafame RJ. Effects of photostimulation on wound healing in diabetic mice. *Lasers Surg Med.* 1997; 20:56-63.
39. Schindl A, Schindl M, Schon H, Knobler R, Havelec L, Schindl L. Low-intensity laser irradiation improves skin circulation in patients with diabetic microangiopathy. *Diabetes Care.* 1998;21:580-584.
40. Stadler I, Lanzafame RJ, Evans R, et al. 830-nm irradiation increases the wound tensile strength in a diabetic murine model. *Lasers Surg Med.* 2001;28:220-226.
41. Reddy GK, Childs E, Ogle A, Enwemeka CS, Stehno-Bittel L. In: *World Association for Laser Therapy, Second World Congress.* Kansas City, MO; 1998:124-125.
42. Reddy GK, Stehno-Bittel L, Enwemeka CS. In: *World Association for Laser Therapy, Third World Congress.* Athens, Greece; 2000:58.
43. Reddy GK, Stehno-Bittel L, Enwemeka CS. Laser photostimulation accelerates wound healing in diabetic rats. *Wound Repair Regen.* 2001;9:248-255.
44. Reddy GK, Stehno-Bittel L, Enwemeka CS. *World Association for Laser Therapy. Fourth World Congress.* Tokyo, Japan; 2002:110.
45. Kuliev RA, Babaev RF. Therapeutic action of laser irradiation and immunomodulators in purulent injuries of the soft tissues in diabetic patients. *Probl Endokrinol Mosk.* 1991;37:31-32.
46. Chentsova OB, GL P, Mozherenkov VP, Kharchenko LN, Balarev AI, Sergushev SG. Low intensity helium-neon laser irradiation in multimodel treatment of corneal injuries. *Vestn Oftalmol.* 1991;107:23-26.
47. Sugrue ME, Carolan J, Leen EJ, Feeley TM, Moore DJ, Shanik GD. The use of infrared laser therapy in the treatment of venous ulceration. *Ann Vasc Surg.* 1990;4:179-81.
48. Singer AJ, Clark RA. Cutaneous wound healing. *N Engl J Med.* 1999;341:738-46.
49. Mester E, Spiry T, Szende B, Tota JG. Effect of laser rays on wound healing. *Am J Surg.* 1971;122:532-535.
50. Kana JS, Hutschenreiter G, Haina D, Waidelich W. Effect of low-power density laser radiation on healing of open skin wounds in rats. *Arch Surg.* 1981;116:293-296.
51. Dyson M, Young S. Effect of laser therapy on wound contraction and cellularity in mice. *Lasers Med Sci.* 1986;1:126-130.
52. Al-Watban FA, Zhang XY. Comparison of wound healing process using Argon and Krypton lasers. *J Clin Laser Med Surg.* 1997;15:209-215.
53. Al-Watban FH, Zhang XY. Dosimetry related wound healing response in the rat model following helium neon laser LLLT. *Laser Therapy.* 1994;6:119-124.
54. Zhang XY, Al-Watban FH. The effect of low power He-Ne and He-Cd laser therapy on wound healing in rats. *J Clin Laser Med Surg.* 1994;12:327-329.
55. Medrado AR, Pugliese LS, Reis SR, Andrade ZA. Influence of low level laser therapy on wound healing and its biological action upon myofibroblasts. *Laser Surg Med.* 2003;32:239-244.
56. Prakash A, Pandit PN, Sharman LK. Studies in wound healing in experimental diabetes. *Int Surg.* 1974;59:25-28.
57. Goodson WHd, Hung TK. Studies of wound healing in experimental diabetes mellitus. *J Surg Res.* 1977;22:221-227.
58. Goodson WHD, Hunt TK. Wound healing and the diabetic patient. *Surg Gynecol Obstet.* 1979;149:600-8.
59. Fahey TJ, Sadaty A, Jones WG, Barber A, Smoller B, Shires GT. Diabetes impairs the late inflammatory response to wound healing. *J Surg Res.* 1991;50:308-13.
60. Kleinkort JA, Foley RA. Laser: a preliminary report on its use in physical therapy. *Clin Manage Phys Ther.* 1982;2:30-32.
61. Schindl A, Schindl M, Pernerstorfer-Schon H, Kerschan K, Knobler R, Schindl L. Diabetic neuropathic foot ulcer: successful treatment by low-intensity laser therapy. *Dermatology.* 1999;198:314-6.
62. Schindl A, Schindl M, Schindl L. Successful treatment of a persistent radiation ulcer by low power laser therapy. *J Am Acad Dermatol.* 1997;37:646-8.
63. Enwemeka CS. Connective tissue plasticity: ultrastructural, biomechanical, and morphometric effects of physical factors on intact and regenerating tendons. *J Orthop Sports Phys Ther.* 1991;14:198-212.
64. Enwemeka CS, Rodriguez O, Gall NG, Walsh NE. Morphometric of collagen fibril population in He:Ne laser photostimulated tendons. *J Clin Laser Med Surg.* 1990;8:47-51.
65. Enwemeka CS. Ultrastructural morphometry of membrane-bound intracytoplasmic collagen fibrils in tendon fibroblasts exposed to He:Ne laser beam. *Tissue Cell.* 1992;24:511-523.
66. Enwemeka CS. Frontiers of laser photostimulation of wounds, ulcers and bedsores. *Med Biol Eng Computing.* 1991;(Suppl)29:723.

67. Enwemeka CS, Cohen-Kornberg E, Duswalt EP, Weber DM, Rodriguez IM. Biomechanical effects of three different periods of gas laser photostimulation on tenotomized tendons. *Laser Therapy*. 1994;6:181-188.

68. Trelles MA, Mayayo E. Bone fracture consolidates faster with low-power laser. *Lasers Surg Med*. 1987;7:36-45.

69. Barushka O, Yaakobi T, Oron U. Effect of low-energy laser (He-Ne) irradiation on the process of bone repair in the rat tibia. *Bone*. 1995;16:47-55.

70. Glinkowsky W, Rowinsky J. Effect of low incident levels of infrared laser energy on the healing of experimental bone fractures. *Laser Therapy*. 1995;7:67-70.

71. Luger EJ, Rochkind S, Wollman Y, Kogan G, Dekel S. Effect of low-power laser irradiation on the mechanical properties of bone fracture healing in rats. *Lasers Surg Med*. 1998;22:97-102.

72. Tang XM, Chai BP. Effect of CO2 laser irradiation on experimental fracture healing: a transmission electron microscopic study. *Lasers Surg Med*. 1986;6:346-52.

73. Calderhead G, Ohshiro T, Itoh E, Okada T, Kato Y. The Nd-YAG and Ga-Al-As lasers: a comparative analysis in pain therapy. *Laser Acupuncture*. 1982;21:1-4.

74. England S, Farrell AJ, Coppock JS, Struthers G, Bacon PA. Low power laser therapy of shoulder tendonitis. *Scand J Rheumatol*. 1989;18:427-431.

75. Ceccherelli F, Altafini L, Lo Castro G, Avila A, Ambrosio F, Giron GP. Diode laser in cervical myofascial pain: a double-blind study versus placebo. *Clin J Pain*. 1989;5: 301-304.

76. Gur A, Karakoc M, Nas K, Cevik R, Sarac J, Demir E. Efficacy of low power laser therapy in fibromyalgia: a single-blind, placebo-controlled trial. *Lasers Med Sci*. 2002;17:57-61.

77. McKibbin LS, Downie R. A statistical study on the use of the infrared 904-nm low energy laser on calcaneal spurs. *J Clin Laser Med Surg*. 1991;9:71-77.

78. Ozdemir F, Birtane M, Kokino S. The clinical efficacy of low-power laser therapy on pain and function in cervical osteoarthritis. *Clin Rheumatol*. 2001;20:181-184.

79. Brosseau L, Welch V, Wells G, et al. Low level laser therapy for osteoarthritis and rheumatoid arthritis: a metanalysis. *J Rheumatol*. 2000;27:1961-1969.

80. Baxter GD, Bell AJ, Allen JM, Ravey J. Low level laser therapy: current clinical practice in Northern Ireland. *Physiotherapy*. 1991;77:171-178.

81. Airaksinen O, Airaksinen K, Rantanen P. Effects of He-Ne laser irradiation on the trigger points of patients with chronic tension in the neck. *Scand J App Electrother*. 1991;4:63-65.

82. Gur A, Karakoc M, Cevik R, Nas K, Sarac AJ. Efficacy of low power laser therapy and exercise on pain and functions in chronic low back pain. *Lasers Surg Med*. 2003;32:233-238.

83. Basford JR, Sheffield CG, Harmsen WS. Laser therapy: a randomized, controlled trial of the effects of low-intensity Nd:YAG laser irradiation on musculoskeletal back pain. *Arch Phys Med Rehabil*. 1999;80:647-652.

84. Laakso E, Cramond T, Richardson C. Plasma ACTH and B-endorphin levels in response to low level laser therapy for myofascial trigger points. *Laser Therapy*. 1994;7:133-142.

85. Honmura A, Ishii A, Yanase M, Obata J, Haruki E. Analgesic effect of Ga-Al-As diode laser irradiation on hyperalgesia in carrageenin-induced inflammation. *Lasers Surg Med*. 1993;13:463-469.

86. Honmura A, Yanase M, Obata J, Haruki E. Therapeutic effect of Ga-Al-As diode laser irradiation on experimentally induced inflammation in rats. *Lasers Surg Med*. 1992;12:441-449.

87. Tuner J, Hode L. *Laser Therapy: Clinical Practice and Scientific Background*. Grangesberg, Sweden: UP Print; 2002.

88. Tuner J, Hode L. Are all the negative studies really negative? *Laser Therapy*. 1998;10:165-174.

89. Colver GB, Priestley GC. Failure of a helium-neon laser to affect components of wound healing in vitro. *Br J Dermatol*. 1989;121:179-186.

90. Hallman HO, Basford JR, O'Brien JF, Cummins LA. Does low-energy helium-neon laser irradiation alter "in vitro" replication of human fibroblasts? *Lasers Surg Med*. 1988;8:125-129.

91. Hardie EM, Carlson CS, Richardson DC. Effect of Nd:YAG laser energy on articular cartilage healing in the dog. *Lasers Surg Med*. 1989;9:595-601.

92. Cambier DC, Vanderstraaten GG, Mussen MJ. Low level laser therapy and bacterial infections: a comparative in vitro assay. *Eur J Phys Med Rehabil*. 1995;5:189-192.

93. Pogrel MA, Chen JW, Zhang K. Effects of low-energy gallium-aluminum-arsenide laser irradiation on cultured fibroblasts and keratinocytes. *Laser Surg Med*. 1999;20:426-32.

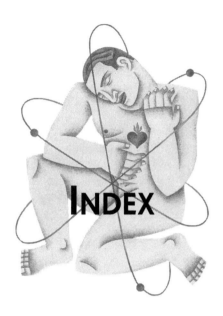

INDEX